IMPORTANT

Here is your registration code to access *Connect Core Co...*
11e (Brief Edition). This registration code is valid if you ha...
book.

You need this code to gain access to
Connect Core Concepts in Health, Brief Edition.

To gain access to *Connect Core Concepts in Health*:

1. Your instructor will provide you with a web address (URL) to *Connect Core Concepts in Health*. Click on that link.

2. At the Connect registration site, click the "Register Now" button.

3. When prompted, enter your email address, and then click the "Submit" button.

4. Enter the personal access code that is found on this card.

5. Follow the instructions to setup your personal UserID and Password

6. Write your UserID and Password down for future reference. Keep it in a safe place.

If you forget your password and would like to reset it, please visit the Support website at www.mhhe.com/support for help. Support hours and telephone numbers can be found at this site.

Thank you. Welcome to *Connect Core Concepts in Health*!

D0817887

WNJN-UJW7-69GJ-YAPX-MU3T

REGISTRATION CODE

ISBN 978-0-07-734042-1
MHID 0-07-734042-6

EAN
9 780077 340421

90000

www.mhhe.com

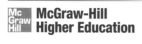

The McGraw-Hill Companies

McGraw-Hill
Higher Education

CORE CONCEPTS IN HEALTH

connect
|PERSONAL HEALTH

The McGraw-Hill Companies

McGraw-Hill
Higher Education

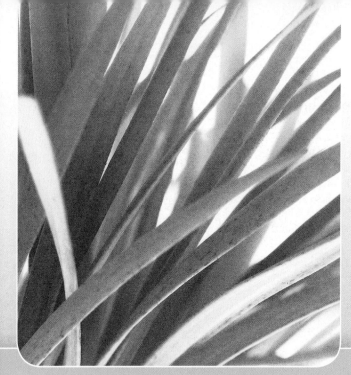

connect™
CORE CONCEPTS
IN HEALTH

BRIEF
ELEVENTH EDITION

Paul M. Insel
Stanford University

Walton T. Roth
Stanford University

Boston   Burr Ridge, IL   Dubuque, IA   Madison, WI   New York
San Francisco   St. Louis   Bangkok   Bogotá   Caracas   Kuala Lumpur
Lisbon   London   Madrid   Mexico City   Milan   Montreal   New Delhi
Santiago   Seoul   Singapore   Sydney   Taipei   Toronto

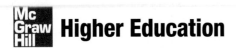

Higher Education

Published by McGraw-Hill, an imprint of The McGraw-Hill Companies, Inc., 1221 Avenue of the Americas, New York, NY 10020. Copyright © 2010. All rights reserved. No part of this publication may be reproduced or distributed in any form or by any means, or stored in a database or retrieval system, without the prior written consent of The McGraw-Hill Companies, Inc., including, but not limited to, in any network or other electronic storage or transmission, or broadcast for distance learning.

2 3 4 5 6 7 8 9 0 DOW/DOW 0 9

ISBN: 978-0-07-338078-0
MHID: 0-07-338078-4

Editor in Chief: *Michael Ryan*
Editorial Director: *William R. Glass*
Executive Editor: *Christopher Johnson*
Marketing Manager: *William Minick*
Director of Development: *Kathleen Engelberg*
Developmental Editor: *Tim Huddleston*
Developmental Editor for Technology: *Julia D. Akpan*
Editorial Coordinator: *Lydia Kim*
Production Editor: *Carey Eisner*
Design Manager and Cover Designer: *Andrei Pasternak*
Text Designer: *Glenda King*
Manager, Photo Research: *Brian J. Pecko*
Illustrators: *John and Judy Waller*
Senior Production Supervisor: *Richard DeVitto*
Composition: *10.5/12 Berkeley Oldstyle Book by Thompson Type*
Printing: *45# New Era Thin Plus Recycle, R. R. Donnelley & Sons*

Front and Back Cover: © *Keate/Masterfile www.masterfile.com*

Credits: The credits appear at the end of the book and are considered an extension of the copyright page.

Library of Congress Cataloging-in-Publication Data

Connect core concepts in health / [compiled by] Paul M. Insel, Walton T. Roth. — Brief 11th ed.
    p. cm.
  Rev. ed. of: Core concepts in health. Brief 10th ed. update. c2008.
  Includes bibliographical references and index.
  ISBN-13: 978-0-07-338078-0 (pbk. : alk. paper)
  ISBN-10: 0-07-338078-4 (pbk. : alk. paper)
  1. Health—Handbooks, manuals, etc. I. Insel, Paul M. II. Roth, Walton T. III. Core concepts in health.

  RA776.C83 2010b
  613—dc22   2009007902

The Internet addresses listed in the text were accurate at the time of publication. The inclusion of a Web site does not indicate an endorsement by the authors or McGraw-Hill, and McGraw-Hill does not guarantee the accuracy of the information presented at these sites.

www.mhhe.com

BRIEF CONTENTS

CHAPTER 1   TAKING CHARGE OF YOUR HEALTH   1

CHAPTER 2   STRESS: THE CONSTANT CHALLENGE   24

CHAPTER 3   PSYCHOLOGICAL HEALTH   47

CHAPTER 4   INTIMATE RELATIONSHIPS AND COMMUNICATION   69

CHAPTER 5   SEXUALITY, PREGNANCY, AND CHILDBIRTH   90

CHAPTER 6   CONTRACEPTION AND ABORTION   122

CHAPTER 7   THE USE AND ABUSE OF PSYCHOACTIVE DRUGS   149

CHAPTER 8   ALCOHOL AND TOBACCO   175

CHAPTER 9   NUTRITION BASICS   205

CHAPTER 10   EXERCISE FOR HEALTH AND FITNESS   240

CHAPTER 11   WEIGHT MANAGEMENT   262

CHAPTER 12   CARDIOVASCULAR DISEASE AND CANCER   283

CHAPTER 13   IMMUNITY AND INFECTION   318

CHAPTER 14   ENVIRONMENTAL HEALTH   346

CHAPTER 15   CONVENTIONAL AND COMPLEMENTARY MEDICINE   362

CHAPTER 16   PERSONAL SAFETY   383

CHAPTER 17   THE CHALLENGE OF AGING   406

APPENDIX   NUTRITIONAL CONTENT OF POPULAR ITEMS FROM FAST-FOOD
             RESTAURANTS   A-1

CREDITS   C-1

INDEX   I-1

CONTENTS

1 TAKING CHARGE OF YOUR HEALTH 1

WELLNESS: THE NEW HEALTH GOAL 1
The Dimensions of Wellness 1
New Opportunities, New Responsibilities 3
The Healthy People Initiative 5
Health Issues for Diverse Populations 6

CHOOSING WELLNESS 11
Factors That Influence Wellness 11

REACHING WELLNESS THROUGH LIFESTYLE
MANAGEMENT 14
Getting Serious About Your Health 14
Building Motivation to Change 15
Enhancing Your Readiness to Change 17
Dealing with Relapse 18
Developing Skills for Change: Creating a Personalized
Plan 18
Putting Your Plan into Action 20

BEING HEALTHY FOR LIFE 21

Tips for Today and the Future 21
Summary 21
For More Information 22
Selected Bibliography 23

2 STRESS: THE CONSTANT CHALLENGE 24

WHAT IS STRESS? 24
Physical Responses to Stressors 24
Emotional and Behavioral Responses to Stressors 27

STRESS AND HEALTH 28
The General Adaptation Syndrome 28
Allostatic Load 29
Psychoneuroimmunology 30
Links Between Stress and Specific Conditions 30

COMMON SOURCES OF STRESS 31
Major Life Changes 31
Daily Hassles 32
College Stressors 32
Job-Related Stressors 33
Social Stressors 33
Other Stressors 34

MANAGING STRESS 34
Social Support 34
Communication 35

Exercise 35
Nutrition 36
Sleep 36
Time Management 37
Striving for Spiritual Wellness 38
Confiding in Yourself Through Writing 38
Cognitive Techniques 38
Relaxation Techniques 39
Counterproductive Coping Strategies 42

CREATING A PERSONAL PLAN FOR MANAGING
STRESS 42
Identifying Stressors 42
Designing Your Plan 43
Getting Help 43

Tips for Today and the Future 43
Behavior Change Strategy 44
Summary 44
For More Information 45
Selected Bibliography 45

3 PSYCHOLOGICAL HEALTH 47

DEFINING PSYCHOLOGICAL HEALTH 47
Self-Actualization 47
What Psychological Health Is Not 49

MEETING LIFE'S CHALLENGES 49
Growing Up Psychologically 49
Achieving Healthy Self-Esteem 50
Being Less Defensive 51
Being Optimistic 52
Maintaining Honest Communication 53
Dealing with Loneliness 53
Dealing with Anger 54

PSYCHOLOGICAL DISORDERS 54
Anxiety Disorders 55
Mood Disorders 58
Schizophrenia 62

GETTING HELP 64
Self-Help 64
Peer Counseling and Support Groups 64
Professional Help 64

Tips for Today and the Future 65
Summary 66
Behavior Change Strategy 67
For More Information 67
Selected Bibliography 68

4 INTIMATE RELATIONSHIPS AND COMMUNICATION 69

DEVELOPING INTIMATE RELATIONSHIPS 69
Self-Concept and Self-Esteem 69
Friendship 70
Love, Sex, and Intimacy 71
Challenges in Relationships 72
Unhealthy Relationships 74
Ending a Relationship 74

COMMUNICATION 75
Nonverbal Communication 75
Communication Skills 75
Gender and Communication 75
Conflict and Conflict Resolution 75

PAIRING AND SINGLEHOOD 78
Choosing a Partner 78
Dating 78
Living Together 78
Same-Sex Partnerships 81
Singlehood 81

MARRIAGE 83
Benefits of Marriage 83
Issues in Marriage 83
The Role of Commitment 83
Separation and Divorce 84

FAMILY LIFE 84
Becoming a Parent 84
Parenting 85
Single Parents 86
Stepfamilies 87
Successful Families 87

Tips for Today and the Future 88
Summary 88
For More Information 89
Selected Bibliography 89

5 SEXUALITY, PREGNANCY, AND CHILDBIRTH 90

SEXUAL ANATOMY 90
Female Sex Organs 90
Male Sex Organs 91

HORMONES AND THE REPRODUCTIVE LIFE CYCLE 93
Differentiation of the Embryo 93
Female Sexual Maturation 94
Male Sexual Maturation 95
Aging and Human Sexuality 96

SEXUAL FUNCTIONING 96
Sexual Stimulation 97
The Sexual Response Cycle 97
Sexual Problems 98

SEXUAL BEHAVIOR 100
Sexual Orientation 100
Varieties of Human Sexual Behavior 100
Atypical and Problematic Sexual Behaviors 102
Commercial Sex 103
Responsible Sexual Behavior 104

UNDERSTANDING FERTILITY 104
Conception 105
Infertility 106

PREGNANCY 107
Pregnancy Tests 107
Changes in the Woman's Body 107
Fetal Development 108
The Importance of Prenatal Care 113
Complications of Pregnancy and Pregnancy Loss 114

CHILDBIRTH 116
Choices in Childbirth 116
Labor and Delivery 116
The Postpartum Period 118

Tips for Today and the Future 119
Summary 120
For More Information 120
Selected Bibliography 121

6 CONTRACEPTION AND ABORTION 122

PRINCIPLES OF CONTRACEPTION 122

REVERSIBLE CONTRACEPTION 123
Oral Contraceptives: The Pill 123
Contraceptive Skin Patch 125
Vaginal Contraceptive Ring 125
Contraceptive Implants 126
Injectable Contraceptives 126
Emergency Contraception 127
The Intrauterine Device (IUD) 127
Male Condoms 129
Female Condoms 131
The Diaphragm with Spermicide 131
Lea's Shield 132
FemCap 133
The Contraceptive Sponge 133
Vaginal Spermicides 133
Abstinence, Fertility Awareness, and Withdrawal 134
Combining Methods 135

PERMANENT CONTRACEPTION:
STERILIZATION   136
    Male Sterilization: Vasectomy   136
    Female Sterilization   137

WHICH CONTRACEPTIVE METHOD IS RIGHT FOR
YOU?   139

THE ABORTION ISSUE   140
    The History of Abortion in the United States   141
    Current Legal Status   141
    Public Opinion   141
    Personal Considerations   141
    Abortion Statistics   143
    Methods of Abortion   144
    Complications of Abortion   146

Tips for Today and the Future   146
Summary   147
For More Information   147
Selected Bibliography   148

7   THE USE AND ABUSE OF PSYCHOACTIVE
    DRUGS   149

ADDICTIVE BEHAVIOR   149
    What Is Addiction?   149
    Characteristics of Addictive Behavior   150
    The Development of Addiction   150
    Characteristics of People with Addictions   151
    Examples of Addictive Behaviors   151

DRUG USE, ABUSE, AND DEPENDENCE   152
    Drug Abuse and Dependence   153
    Who Uses Drugs?   153
    Why Do People Use Drugs?   155
    Risk Factors for Dependence   155
    Other Risks of Drug Use   156

HOW DRUGS AFFECT THE BODY   157
    Changes in Brain Chemistry   157
    Drug Factors   157
    User Factors   158
    Social Factors   158

REPRESENTATIVE PSYCHOACTIVE DRUGS   158
    Opioids   160
    Central Nervous System Depressants   160
    Central Nervous System Stimulants   162
    Marijuana and Other Cannabis Products   164
    Hallucinogens   165
    Inhalants   166

DRUG USE: THE DECADES AHEAD   167
    Drugs, Society, and Families   167
    Legalizing Drugs   167
    Drug Testing   167
    Treatment for Drug Dependence   169

    Preventing Drug Abuse   170
    The Role of Drugs in Your Life   171

Tips for Today and the Future   171
Summary   171
Behavior Change Strategy   172
For More Information   173
Selected Bibliography   173

8   ALCOHOL AND TABACCO   175

THE NATURE OF ALCOHOL   175
    Alcoholic Beverages   176
    Absorption   176
    Metabolism and Excretion   176
    Alcohol Intake and Blood Alcohol
        Concentration   176

ALCOHOL AND HEALTH   178
    The Immediate Effects of Alcohol   178
    Drinking and Driving   180
    The Effects of Chronic Use   180
    The Effects of Alcohol Use During Pregnancy   182
    Possible Health Benefits of Alcohol   182

ALCOHOL ABUSE AND DEPENDENCE   183
    Abuse versus Dependence   183
    Binge Drinking   183
    Alcoholism   184
    Gender and Ethnic Differences   186
    Helping Someone with an Alcohol Problem   188

WHO USES TOBACCO?   188

WHY PEOPLE USE TOBACCO   189
    Nicotine Addiction   189
    Social and Psychological Factors   189
    Why Start in the First Place?   189

HEALTH HAZARDS   191
    Tobacco Smoke: A Toxic Mix   191
    The Immediate Effects of Smoking   192
    The Long-Term Effects of Smoking   192
    Other Forms of Tobacco Use   194

THE EFFECTS OF SMOKING ON THE
NONSMOKER   196
    Environmental Tobacco Smoke   196
    Smoking and Pregnancy   196
    The Cost of Tobacco Use to Society   197

WHAT CAN BE DONE?   197
    Action at Many Levels   197
    Individual Action   198

HOW A TOBACCO USER CAN QUIT   198
    The Benefits of Quitting   198
    Options for Quitting   198
Tips for Today and the Future   199

Summary 200
For More Information 201
Behavior Change Strategy 202
Selected Bibliography 204

9 NUTRITION BASICS 205

NUTRITIONAL REQUIREMENTS: COMPONENTS OF A HEALTHY DIET 205
Proteins—The Basis of Body Structure 206
Fats—Essential in Small Amounts 207
Carbohydrates—An Ideal Source of Energy 209
Fiber—A Closer Look 212
Vitamins—Organic Micronutrients 213
Minerals—Inorganic Micronutrients 213
Water—Vital but Often Ignored 216
Other Substances in Food 216

NUTRITIONAL GUIDELINES: PLANNING YOUR DIET 217
Dietary Reference Intakes 217
Dietary Guidelines for Americans 218
USDA's MyPyramid 221
The Vegetarian Alternative 225
Dietary Challenges for Special Population Groups 226

A PERSONAL PLAN: MAKING INFORMED CHOICES ABOUT FOOD 228
Reading Food Labels 228
Reading Dietary Supplement Labels 228
Protecting Yourself Against Foodborne Illness 228
Organic Foods 231
Additives in Food 232
Food Irradiation 232
Genetically Modified Foods 232
Food Allergies and Food Intolerances 233

Tips for Today and the Future 233
Summary 233
Behavior Change Strategy 234
For More Information 235
Selected Bibliography 235

10 EXERCISE FOR HEALTH AND FITNESS 240

WHAT IS PHYSICAL FITNESS? 240
Cardiorespiratory Endurance 240
Muscular Strength 241
Muscular Endurance 241
Flexibility 242
Body Composition 242
Skill-Related Components of Fitness 242

PHYSICAL ACTIVITY AND EXERCISE FOR HEALTH AND FITNESS 242

THE BENEFITS OF EXERCISE 243
Improved Cardiorespiratory Functioning 243
More Efficient Metabolism 244
Improved Body Composition 244
Disease Prevention and Management 245
Improved Psychological and Emotional Wellness 247
Improved Immune Function 247
Prevention of Injuries and Low-Back Pain 247
Improved Wellness for Life 247

DESIGNING YOUR EXERCISE PROGRAM 247
First Steps 248
Cardiorespiratory Endurance Exercises 250
Developing Muscular Strength and Endurance 250
Flexibility Exercises 252
Training in Specific Skills 254
Putting It All Together 254

GETTING STARTED AND STAYING ON TRACK 254
Selecting Instructors, Equipment, and Facilities 254
Eating and Drinking for Exercise 255
Managing Your Fitness Program 256

Tips for Today and the Future 258
Summary 258
Behavior Change Strategy 259
For More Information 260
Selected Bibliography 260

11 WEIGHT MANAGEMENT 262

BASIC CONCEPTS OF WEIGHT MANAGEMENT 262
Body Composition 262
Energy Balance 263
Evaluating Body Weight and Body Composition 264
Excess Body Fat and Wellness 265
What Is the Right Weight for You? 268

FACTORS CONTRIBUTING TO EXCESS BODY FAT 268
Genetic Factors 268
Physiological Factors 269
Lifestyle Factors 269
Psychosocial Factors 270

ADOPTING A HEALTHY LIFESTYLE FOR SUCCESSFUL WEIGHT MANAGEMENT 270
Diet and Eating Habits 270
Physical Activity and Exercise 271
Thinking and Emotions 271
Coping Strategies 272

APPROACHES TO OVERCOMING A WEIGHT PROBLEM 272
Doing It Yourself 272
Dietary Supplements and Diet Aids 272

Weight-Loss Programs 274
Prescription Drugs 275
Surgery 275

BODY IMAGE 276
Severe Body Image Problems 276
Acceptance and Change 276

EATING DISORDERS 276
Anorexia Nervosa 276
Bulimia Nervosa 278
Binge-Eating Disorder 278
Borderline Disordered Eating 278
Treating Eating Disorders 279

Tips for Today and the Future 279
Summary 279
Behavior Change Strategy 280
For More Information 281
Selected Bibliography 281

12 CARDIOVASCULAR DISEASE AND CANCER 283

THE CARDIOVASCULAR SYSTEM 283

RISK FACTORS FOR CARDIOVASCULAR DISEASE 285
Major Risk Factors That Can Be Changed 285
Contributing Risk Factors That Can Be Changed 288
Major Risk Factors That Can't Be Changed 290
Possible Risk Factors Currently Being Studied 291

MAJOR FORMS OF CARDIOVASCULAR DISEASE 292
Atherosclerosis 293
Heart Disease and Heart Attack 293
Stroke 295
Congestive Heart Failure 297
Other Forms of Heart Disease 297

PROTECTING YOURSELF AGAINST CARDIOVASCULAR DISEASE 298
Eat Heart-Healthy 298
Exercise Regularly 299
Avoid Tobacco 299
Know and Manage Your Blood Pressure 299
Know and Manage Your Cholesterol Levels 299
Develop Effective Ways to Handle Stress and Anger 299

WHAT IS CANCER? 299
Tumors 299
Metastasis 300
Types of Cancer 300
The Incidence of Cancer 301

COMMON CANCERS 301
Lung Cancer 301

Colon and Rectal Cancer 302
Breast Cancer 302
Prostate Cancer 303
Cancers of the Female Reproductive Tract 305
Skin Cancer 306
Oral Cancer 307
Testicular Cancer 309

THE CAUSES OF CANCER 309
The Role of DNA 309
Tobacco Use 309
Dietary Factors 310
Inactivity and Obesity 310
Carcinogens in the Environment 310

DETECTING, DIAGNOSING, AND TREATING CANCER 312
Detecting Cancer 312
Diagnosing and Treating Cancer 312

PREVENTING CANCER 314

Tips for Today and the Future 314
Summary 314
Behavior Change Strategy 315
For More Information 316
Selected Bibliography 317

13 IMMUNITY AND INFECTION 318

THE CHAIN OF INFECTION 318

THE BODY'S DEFENSE SYSTEM 319
Physical and Chemical Barriers 319
The Immune System 320
Immunization 322
Allergy: The Body's Defense System Gone Haywire 322

PATHOGENS AND DISEASE 323
Bacteria 323
Viruses 326
Fungi 328
Protozoa 328
Parasitic Worms 328
Prions 328
Emerging Infectious Diseases 328
Other Immune Disorders: Cancer and Autoimmune Diseases 330

SUPPORTING YOUR IMMUNE SYSTEM 330

THE MAJOR STDS 330
HIV Infection and AIDS 330
Chlamydia 337
Gonorrhea 338
Pelvic Inflammatory Disease 339
Human Papillomavirus Infection 339
Genital Herpes 340

Hepatitis B   341
Syphilis   341
Other STDs   342

WHAT YOU CAN DO   342
Education   342
Diagnosis and Treatment   342
Prevention   342

Tips for Today and the Future   343
Summary   344
For More Information   344
Selected Bibliography   345

14 ENVIRONMENTAL HEALTH   346

ENVIRONMENTAL HEALTH DEFINED   346

POPULATION GROWTH AND CONTROL   347

AIR QUALITY AND POLLUTION   348
Air Quality and Smog   348
The Greenhouse Effect and Global Warming   348
Thinning of the Ozone Layer   350
Energy Use and Air Pollution   350
Indoor Air Pollution   352
Preventing Air Pollution and Conserving Energy   352

WATER QUALITY AND POLLUTION   352
Water Contamination and Treatment   352
Water Shortages   352
Sewage   353
Protecting the Water Supply   353

SOLID WASTE POLLUTION   353
Solid Waste   353
Reducing Solid Waste   354

CHEMICAL POLLUTION AND HAZARDOUS WASTE   355
Asbestos   355
Lead   355
Pesticides   356
Mercury   356
Other Chemical Pollutants   356
Preventing Chemical Pollution   357

RADIATION   357
Medical Uses of Radiation   358
Radiation in the Home and Workplace   358
Avoiding Radiation   358

NOISE POLLUTION   358

YOU AND THE ENVIRONMENT   359

Tips for Today and the Future   359
Summary   359
For More Information   360
Selected Bibliography   361

15 CONVENTIONAL AND COMPLEMENTARY MEDICINE   362

SELF-CARE   362
Self-Assessment   362
Knowing When to See a Physician   363
Self-Treatment   363

PROFESSIONAL CARE   364

CONVENTIONAL MEDICINE   366
Premises and Assumptions of Conventional Medicine   366
The Providers of Conventional Medicine   367
Choosing a Primary Care Physician   368
Getting the Most Out of Your Medical Care   369

COMPLEMENTARY AND ALTERNATIVE MEDICINE   370
Alternative Medical Systems   372
Mind-Body Interventions   374
Biological-Based Therapies   375
Manipulative and Body-Based Methods   375
Energy Therapies   375
Evaluating Complementary and Alternative Therapies   377

PAYING FOR HEALTH CARE   378
Health Insurance   378
Choosing a Policy   380

Tips for Today and the Future   380
Summary   380
For More Information   381
Selected Bibliography   381

16 PERSONAL SAFETY   383

DIFFERENTIATING INJURIES   383

UNINTENTIONAL INJURIES   384
What Causes an Injury?   384
Motor Vehicle Injuries   384
Home Injuries   388
Leisure Injuries   390
Work Injuries   390

VIOLENCE AND INTENTIONAL INJURIES   391
Factors Contributing to Violence   391
Assault   393
Homicide   394
Gang-Related Violence   394
Hate Crimes   394
School Violence   394
Workplace Violence   394
Terrorism   395
Family and Intimate Violence   396
Sexual Violence   398
What You Can Do About Violence   401

PROVIDING EMERGENCY CARE 402

Tips for Today and the Future 402
Behavior Change Strategy 403
Summary 403
For More Information 404
Selected Bibliography 404

17 THE CHALLENGE OF AGING 406

GENERATING VITALITY AS YOU AGE 406
What Happens as You Age? 406
Life-Enhancing Measures: Age-Proofing 407

DEALING WITH THE CHANGES OF AGING 409
Planning for Social Changes 409
Adapting to Physical Changes 410
Handling Psychological and Mental Changes 411

AGING AND LIFE EXPECTANCY 413
America's Aging Minority 413
Family and Community Resources for Older
    Adults 414
Government Aid and Policies 414

WHAT IS DEATH? 415
Defining Death 415
Learning About Death 416
Denying Versus Welcoming Death 416

PLANNING FOR DEATH 416
Making a Will 416
Considering Options for End-of-Life Care 417
Deciding to Prolong Life or Hasten Death 418
Completing an Advance Directive 419
Becoming an Organ Donor 420
Planning a Funeral or Memorial Service 420

COPING WITH DYING 420
The Tasks of Coping 421
Supporting a Dying Person 421

COPING WITH LOSS 421
Experiencing Grief 421
Supporting a Grieving Person 423

COMING TO TERMS WITH DEATH 425

Tips for Today and the Future 425
Summary 425
For More Information 426
Selected Bibliography 426

APPENDIX

NUTRITIONAL CONTENT OF POPULAR ITEMS FROM FAST-FOOD RESTAURANTS A-1

CREDITS C-1
INDEX I-1

BOXES

IN THE NEWS

A "Planet in Peril": Healing the Environment 13
Coping After Violence on the Campus 35
Antidepressant Use in Young People 63
Same-Sex Marriage and Civil Unions 82
Sexsomnia: Sleep Disorders and Sex 103
Access to Emergency Contraception 128
Key Abortion Decisions and Legislation 142
The Meth Epidemic 163
College Binge Drinking 185
Going Trans Fat–Free 220
Drugs and Supplements for Improved Athletic
    Performance 253
Are Diet Sodas Bad for You? 270
Cancer Myths and Misperceptions 311
MRSA: The Superbug? 325
Global Warming, Local Action 351
Medical Errors, Adverse Events, and Their Prevention 371
Emergency Preparedness 396
Profound Trauma and Loss 424

MIND/BODY/SPIRIT

Occupational Wellness 3
Stress and Your Brain 31
Are Intimate Relationships Good for Your Health? 84
Sexual Decision Making 101
Spirituality and Drug Abuse 156
Tobacco Use and Religion: Global Views 190
Exercise and Total Wellness 243
Exercise, Body Image, and Self-Esteem 272
Anger, Hostility, and Heart Disease 289
Stress and Genital Herpes 341
Expressive Writing and Chronic Conditions 364
The Power of Belief: The Placebo Effect 374
In Search of a Good Death 422

TAKE CHARGE

Meditation and the Relaxation Response 40
Breathing for Relaxation 41
Realistic Self-Talk 52
Being a Good Friend 71
Strategies for Enhancing Support in Relationships 74
Guidelines for Effective Communication 76
Communicating About Sexuality 105
Talking with a Partner About Contraception 139

If Someone You Know Has a Drug Problem . . .   170
Dealing with an Alcohol Emergency   179
Drinking Behavior and Responsibility   187
Setting Intake Goals for Protein, Fat, and Carbohydrate   210
Choosing More Whole-Grain Foods   211
Eating for Healthy Bones   216
Judging Portion Sizes   224
Eating Strategies for College Students   227
Safe Food Handling   231
Making Time for Physical Activity   245
Determining Your Target Heart Rate Range   251
Lifestyle Strategies for Successful Weight Management   273
What to Do in Case of a Heart Attack, Stroke, or Cardiac
   Arrest   295
How to Perform a Breast Self-Exam   304
Testicle Self-Examination   309
Preventing HIV Infection and Other STDs   337
Making Your Letters Count   360
Preventing Date Rape   399
Staying Safe on Campus   401

CRITICAL CONSUMER

Evaluating Sources of Health Information   16
Alternative Remedies for Depression   62
Sex Enhancement Products   99
Buying and Using Over-the-Counter Contraceptives   130
Smoking Cessation Products   200
Using Food Labels   229
Using Dietary Supplement Labels   230
Choosing Exercise Footwear   255
Is Any Diet Best for Weight Loss?   274
Choosing and Using Sunscreens and Sun-Protective
   Clothing   308
Avoiding Cancer Quackery   313
Getting an HIV Test   335
How to Be a Green Consumer   355
Evaluating Health News   368
Avoiding Health Fraud and Quackery   372
Choosing a Bicycle Helmet   388

DIMENSIONS OF DIVERSITY

Health Disparities Among Ethnic Minorities   9
Diverse Populations, Discrimination, and Stress   34
Ethnicity, Culture, and Psychological Disorders   56
Interfaith and Intrafaith Partnerships   79
Ethnicity and Genetic Diseases   112
Contraceptive Use Among American Women   138
Drug Use and Ethnicity: Risk Factors and Protective
   Factors   168
Metabolizing Alcohol: Our Bodies Work Differently   177
Exercise for People with Special Health Concerns   246
Ethnicity and CVD   291
HIV/AIDS Around the World   332
Poverty and Environmental Health   356
Who Are the Uninsured?   379

Violence and Health: A Global View   395
El Día de los Muertos: The Day of the Dead   417

GENDER MATTERS

Women's Health/Men's Health   8
Women, Men, and Stress   29
Depression, Anxiety, and Gender   60
Gender and Communication   77
Pregnancy Tasks for Fathers   109
Men's Involvement in Contraception   140
Gender Differences in Drug Use and Abuse   155
Gender and Tobacco Use   195
How Different Are the Nutritional Needs of Women and
   Men?   226
Gender Differences in Muscular Strength   252
Gender, Ethnicity, and Body Image   277
Women and CVD   290
Women Are Hit Hard by STDs   338
Gender and Environmental Health   357
Injuries Among Young Men   385
Why Do Women Live Longer?   413

IN FOCUS

Wellness Matters for College Students   12
Headaches: A Common Symptom of Stress 32
Shyness   57
Online Relationships   80
Sexual Activity Among College Students   102
The Adoption Option   144
Drug Use Among College Students   154
Club Drugs   161
Diabetes   267
The Next Influenza Pandemic—When, Not If?   327
Herbal Remedies: Are They Safe?   377
Cell Phones and Distracted Driving   386
Carpal Tunnel Syndrome   392
Stem Cells   407
Alzheimer's Disease   412

TOPICS OF SPECIAL CONCERN TO WOMEN

Aging among women, 409–410, 411, 413
Alcohol metabolism in women, 177
Alcohol use, special risks for women, 177, 181, 182
Alcoholism, patterns among women, 184, 186
Amenorrhea, 269
Anxiety disorders, 55–58, 60
Arthritis, 246, 320, 330, 376, 410, 411, 413
Body composition, 242, 262–263, 264–265
Body image, negative, 268
Breast cancer, 302–303, 312
Breast self-examinations, 303, 304
Cancer and women, 301, 302, 303, 305–306

Cardiovascular disease, risk among women, 287, 290, 292
Caregiving for older adults, 417–418
Carpal tunnel syndrome, 390, 391, 392
Causes of death among women, 125, 290, 292, 301, 302, 306
Cervical cancer, 305–306
Communication styles among women, 77
Contraception, female methods, 123–129, 130, 131–135, 137–139
Depression, risk among women, 9
Dietary recommendations for women, 213, 216, 226–227
Drug use, rates and special risks for women, 155, 158, 163
Eating disorders, 276–279
Ectopic pregnancy, 114
Environmental health risks, 196, 356, 357
Family violence, 396–398
Female athlete triad, 268, 269
Financial planning for retirement, 409
Folic acid, 292, 298
Gender roles, 28, 29, 70, 385
Health concerns and status, general, 6–8
Heart attack risk among women, 9, 290
HIV infection rates and transmission, 331–333
Hormone replacement therapy, 303, 410
Hormones, female, 93–96
Infertility, female, 106–107
Life expectancy of women, 8, 9, 413
Marital status, 78, 79, 80–81, 84, 85
Menopause, 96, 410–411
Menstrual cycle, 94, 95
Migraine, 42
Muscular strength, development of, 250–252
Osteoporosis, 411
Ovarian cancer, 306
Pap tests and pelvic exams, 107, 124, 134, 305, 337, 343
Parenting, single, by women, 86–87
Pelvic inflammatory disease, 124, 128–129, 136, 157, 338, 339
Post-traumatic stress disorder, 58, 59
Poverty rates among older women, 356
Pregnancy and childbirth, 107–120
Premenstrual syndrome and premenstrual dysphoric disorder, 95
Psychological disorders among women, 60
Rape, 162, 163, 398–401
Sexual anatomy, female, 90–91
Sexual functioning, female, 96–98
Sexual harassment, 400–401
Sexual health problems and dysfunctions, female, 98–99
Sexually transmitted diseases and pregnancy, 114, 342
Sexually transmitted diseases, symptoms and special risks among women, 338, 342
Stalking and cyberstalking, 396, 397
Sterilization, female, 137
Stressors and responses to stress among women, 29
Tobacco use, rates and special risks among women, 9, 188, 194, 195, 196–197
Uterine cancer, 306, 312
Violence against women, 398–401

TOPICS OF SPECIAL CONCERN TO MEN

Aging among men, 413
Alcohol abuse and dependence, patterns among men, 187
Alcohol metabolism in men, 177–178
Body composition, 242, 262–263, 264–265
Body image, negative, 268
Cancer and men, 84, 301, 307
Cardiovascular disease risk among men, 289
Causes of death among men, 395
Cigars and pipes, 195
Circumcision, 93, 305, 332
Cluster headaches, 32
Communication styles among men, 75, 77
Contraception, male methods, 129–131, 136–137
Dietary recommendations for men, 213, 226
Drug use, rates of, 150, 155
Environmental health risks, 196, 357
Family violence, 396–398
Firearm-related injuries, 389–390
Gambling, 151–152
Gender roles, 28, 29, 70, 385
Health concerns and status, general, 6–8
Heart attack risk among men, 9, 290
HIV infection rates and transmission, 331–333
Homicide, rates among men, 394, 395
Hormones, male, 93
Infertility, male, 106
Injuries, rates of, 385
Life expectancy of men, 265, 413
Marital status, 81, 85
Motor vehicle injuries, 384–387
Motorcycle and moped injuries, 387
Muscular strength, development of, 250–252
Oral cancer, 307, 309
Parenting, single, by men, 87
Poverty rates among older men, 409–410, 414
Pregnancy, men's roles, 109
Prostate cancer, 303–304, 312
Psychological disorders among men, 60, 62
Rape, 398–400
Schizophrenia, 62–64
Sexual anatomy, male, 91–92
Sexual functioning, male, 96–98
Sexual harassment, 400–401
Sexual health problems and dysfunctions, male, 98–100
Sexually transmitted diseases, symptoms and special risks among men, 9, 332–333, 337, 338, 339–340, 341
Spit tobacco, 194–195
Stalking and cyberstalking, 396, 397
Sterilization, male, 136–137
Stressors and responses to stress among men, 29
Suicide, 7, 59–60
Testicular cancer, 309
Testicular self-examination, 309
Tobacco use, rates and special risks among men, 188, 194, 195
Violent behavior among men, 392–393
Violent deaths of men, 394–395

Note: The health issues and conditions listed here include those that disproportionately influence or affect women or men. For more information, see the Index under gender, women, men, and any of the special topics listed here.

DIVERSITY TOPICS RELATED TO ETHNICITY

Alcohol metabolism, 177
Alcohol use and abuse patterns, 177, 184, 186, 187–188
Asthma, 7, 10
Body image, 277
Cancer, rates and risk, 7, 10, 306
Cardiovascular disease patterns and risks, 286, 291, 292
Contraceptive use, patterns of, 138
Cystic fibrosis, 7
Death, attitudes toward, 11, 420
Diabetes, 112, 267
Dietary patterns and considerations, 270
Discrimination and health, 9, 34
Drug use, risk and protective factors, 168
Environmental health, 355–356
Genetic disorders, 112
Glaucoma, 409
Hate crimes, 394
Health disparities, general, 7, 9, 10
Health insurance status, 379
Health status and concerns, general, 6–11
Heart disease, 12, 292
Hemochromatosis, 112
HIV/AIDS rates, 11, 332–333
Homicide rates, 394
Hypertension, 286
Lactose intolerance, 112
Lead poisoning, 355–356
Marketing, targeted
Metabolic syndrome, 291–292
Osteoporosis, 112
Overweight/obesity, rates and trends, 6
Poverty rates among older adults, 409, 413, 414
Prostate cancer, 303–305
Psychological disorders, symptoms and rates, 9, 56
Sickle cell disease, 8, 112
Single-parent families, 86–87
Smoking rates, 188
Stress and discrimination, 9, 34
Suicide rates, 59
Tay-Sachs disease, 8, 112
Thallasemia, 112
Tobacco use, 188–199
Violence, rates of, 391, 393, 394, 395, 397–398

Note: The health issues and conditions listed here include those that disproportionately influence or affect specific U.S. ethnic groups or for which patterns may appear along ethnic lines. For more information, see the Index under ethnicity, culture, names of specific population groups, and any of the topics listed here.

PREFACE

Core Concepts in Health has maintained its leadership in the field of personal health education for more than 30 years. Since we pioneered the concept of self-responsibility for personal health in 1976, millions of students have used our book to become active, informed participants in their own health care. Our commitment to these principles is reflected in both the larger edition of the text and in this Brief Edition, which we have prepared to accommodate instructors whose courses afford too little time for the complete range of topics and level of detail included in the larger version.

In keeping with twenty-first-century technology, we are adding an exciting digital dimension to the eleventh edition, reflected in the title *Connect Core Concepts in Health*. McGraw-Hill *Connect Personal Health* is an online platform that allows instructors to connect with their students and students to connect with their instructors and coursework. *Connect* adds a level of enhanced online teaching and learning potential to *Core Concepts in Health* that benefits both instructors and students. More information about *Connect* is included later in the preface.

OUR GOALS

Every edition of *Core Concepts in Health* has brought improvements and refinements, but our goals and principles have remained the same:

- To present scientifically based, accurate, up-to-date information in an accessible format
- To involve students in taking responsibility for their health and well-being
- To instill a sense of competence and personal power in students

The first of these goals means making expert knowledge about health and health care available to the individual. *Core Concepts* brings scientifically based, accurate, up-to-date information to students about topics and issues that concern them—exercise, stress, nutrition, weight management, contraception, intimate relationships, HIV infection, drugs, alcohol, and a multitude of others. Current, complete, and straightforward coverage is balanced with user-friendly features designed to make the text appealing. Written in an engaging, easy-to-read style and presented in a colorful, open format, *Core Concepts* invites the student to read, learn, and remember. Boxes, tables, artwork, photographs, and many other features highlight areas of special interest throughout the book.

Our second goal is to involve students in taking responsibility for their health. *Core Concepts* uses innovative pedagogy and unique interactive features to get students thinking about how the material they're reading relates to their lives. We invite them to examine their emotions about the issues under discussion, to consider their personal values and beliefs, to develop their critical thinking skills, and to analyze their health-related behaviors. Beyond this, for students who want to change behaviors that detract from a healthy lifestyle, we offer guidelines and tools, ranging from samples of health journals and personal contracts to detailed assessments and behavior change strategies.

Perhaps our third goal is the most important: to instill a sense of competence and personal power in the students who read the book. Everyone has the ability to monitor, understand, and affect his or her health. Although medical and health professionals possess impressive skills and have access to a huge body of knowledge that benefits everyone in our society, people can help to minimize the amount of professional care they actually require in their lifetime by taking care of themselves—taking charge of their health—from an early age. Our hope is that *Core Concepts* will continue to help young people make this exciting discovery—that they have the power to shape their futures.

ORGANIZATION AND CONTENT OF THE ELEVENTH EDITION

The Brief Edition of *Connect Core Concepts in Health* focuses on the health issues and concerns of greatest importance to students. Topics include behavior change, stress, psychological health, intimate relationships and communication, sexuality, substance use and abuse, nutrition, exercise, weight management, cardiovascular health, cancer, infectious diseases, environmental health, consumer health, personal safety, and aging. Taken together, the chapters of the book provide students with a complete guide to promoting and protecting their health, now and through their entire lives.

For the eleventh edition, all chapters were carefully reviewed, revised, and updated. The latest information from scientific and health-related research is incorporated in the text, and newly emerging topics and issues are discussed. The following list gives a sample of some of the topics and concerns addressed in this edition:

- Global warming and climate change; human causes and human health effects; and strategies for reducing one's environmental footprint

- The latest recommendations on physical activity and exercise from the American College of Sports Medicine, the American Cancer Society, and other organizations, as well as new information on the impact of exercise on multiple dimensions of wellness and guidelines for distinguishing light, moderate, and vigorous exercise

- Stress in America and the impact of stress on wellness, including current statistics from the American Psychological Association

- The continuing overweight and obesity epidemic, with the latest from the CDC and the National Center for Health Statistics

- The growing prevalence of diabetes, prediabetes, insulin resistance, and metabolic syndrome; their causes, warning signs, and health effects; and strategies for prevention

- Fat cells and the role of abdominal fat in chronic conditions, along with a distinction between visceral fat and subcutaneous fat and clarification of the impact of both types of fat on health

- Foodborne illness and the safety of the U.S. food supply

- Violence on school and college campuses; current statistics on personal safety, injuries, and violence from the FBI, the National Safety Council, and other organizations; and strategies for coping with violence

- Disparities in access to emergency contraception among American women

- Updated statistics on HIV/AIDS in the United States, showing that rates are higher than previously believed

- The "Healthy Campus 2010" initiative

- Diet sodas and their health implications

- New hands-only CPR guidelines from the American Heart Association

- The possible role of vitamin D in heart disease and other chronic conditions and the growing use of aspirin therapy for CVD

- Exercise guidelines for older adults from the American College of Sports Medicine

- The importance of sleep in health and wellness; sleep disorders; and sleep aids and their side effects

- The importance of friendships and social connectedness in overall wellness

- Emerging infections and antibiotic resistance; MRSA and *Clostridium difficile*; and strategies for prevention

(A complete, chapter-by-chapter list of changes to this edition is included on the Instructor Resource Site at www.mhhe.com/insel11e.)

For the eleventh edition, the chapter on environmental health has been moved up to highlight the importance of environmental issues in our time, and an environmental theme runs through the text, expressed in **Thinking About the Environment** boxes in each chapter. The text emphasizes that students are not just individuals but also participants in communities and citizens of a "planet in peril"—one that needs care and protection if it is to continue providing us with the means to healthy lives. The chapters on Conventional and Complementary Medicine and on Personal Safety have also been moved forward to highlight growing interest in these two important areas of personal health.

A new feature in the eleventh edition is **Quick Stats**—a marginal notation highlighting a particularly striking statistic related to the chapter topic. Quick Stats appear several times in each chapter, calling students' attention to key data. Also new to the eleventh edition are **Questions for Critical Thinking and Reflection**, which appear at the ends of major sections within chapters. These questions prompt students to think critically about chapter topics, relate them to their own lives, and probe more deeply into their own attitudes, values, and beliefs. Instructors may want to use these questions to stimulate classroom discussion.

The eleventh edition also features a new, more visually appealing design. New and updated graphics have been added, along with more readable tables and figures and many colorful points of interest throughout each chapter.

FEATURES OF THE ELEVENTH EDITION

This Brief edition of *Core Concepts in Health* builds on the features that attracted and held our readers' interest in the previous editions. One of the most popular features has always been the **boxes**, which allow us to explore a wide range of current topics in greater detail than is possible in the text itself. Each type of box is a different color and marked with a distinctive icon and label. Refer to the table of contents for a complete list of all the boxes in each category.

Boxes with the *Connect* icon feature a student activity in *Connect*, typically a short multiple-choice quiz and a question for personal reflection. Instructors can assign the *Connect* activities to ensure that their students are getting the most from the boxes.

In the News boxes focus on current health issues that have recently been highlighted in the media. Topics include environmental issues, such as global warming and climate change; access to emergency contraception; sleep aids and sexsomnia; same-sex marriage; health issues related to trans fats and diet sodas; and aspirin and medical errors.

 Mind/Body/Spirit boxes focus on spiritual wellness and the close connections between people's feelings and states of mind and their physical health. Included in Mind/Body/Spirit boxes are topics such as occupational and financial wellness, sexual decision making and personal values, how exercise fosters total wellness, and the placebo effect.

 Take Charge boxes distill from each chapter the practical advice students need in order to apply information to their own lives. By referring to these boxes, students can find ways to foster friendships; to become more physically active; to perform deep-breathing exercises for stress reduction; or to help a friend who has a problem with drugs.

Critical Consumer boxes help students develop and apply the critical thinking skills they need to make sound health-related choices. Critical Consumer boxes provide specific guidelines for evaluating health news and advertising, using food and dietary supplement labels to make smart choices, choosing a bicycle helmet, avoiding quackery, selecting exercise footwear, getting an HIV test, and making environmentally friendly shopping choices, among others.

Dimensions of Diversity boxes reflect and respond to the diversity of the student population. These boxes give students the opportunity to identify any specific health risks that affect them as individuals or as members of a group. Topics covered in these boxes include factors contributing to health disparities among ethnic minorities, diverse populations and stress, ethnic and cultural influences on psychological disorders, rates of drug use among ethnic populations, exercise for people with special health concerns, links between poverty and environmental health, and the global pattern of HIV infection.

 Gender Matters boxes highlight key gender differences related to wellness as well as areas of particular concern to men or women. An over-

view of key gender-related wellness concerns is provided in Chapter 1. Topics covered in later chapters include gender differences in rates of anxiety, depression, drug use, and tobacco use; in responses to stress; and in rates of unintentional injuries.

 In Focus boxes highlight current wellness topics of particular interest. Topics include diabetes, headaches, carpal tunnel syndrome, herbal remedies, and Alzheimer's disease.

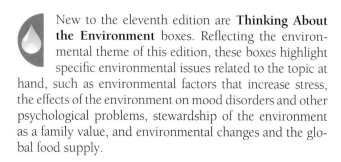 New to the eleventh edition are **Thinking About the Environment** boxes. Reflecting the environmental theme of this edition, these boxes highlight specific environmental issues related to the topic at hand, such as environmental factors that increase stress, the effects of the environment on mood disorders and other psychological problems, stewardship of the environment as a family value, and environmental changes and the global food supply.

In addition to the boxes, many carefully refined features and learning aids are included in the eleventh edition. **Vital Statistics** tables and figures highlight important facts and figures in a memorable format that often reveals surprising contrasts and connections. For students who grasp a subject best when it is displayed graphically, numerically, or in a table, the Vital Statistics feature provides alternative ways of approaching and understanding the text. As noted earlier, the new feature **Quick Stats** highlights striking statistics related to chapter topics, and **Questions for Critical Thinking and Reflection** prompt students to relate chapter material to their own lives.

Like previous editions, the eleventh edition features a wealth of attractive and helpful **illustrations.** The anatomical art, which has been prepared by medical illustrators, is both visually appealing and informative. These illustrations help students understand such important information as how blood flows through the heart, how diabetes affects the body, and how to use a condom. These illustrations will particularly benefit those students who learn best from visual images.

Chapter-ending **Tips for Today and the Future** sections provide brief distillations of the major message of each chapter, followed by suggestions for a few simple things that students can try right away and in the weeks and months ahead. Tips for Today and the Future are designed to encourage students and to build their confidence by giving them easy steps they can take immediately to start changing their behaviors.

The **Behavior Change Strategies** that conclude many chapters offer specific behavior management/modification plans relating to the chapter's topic. Based on the principles of behavior management that are carefully explained in Chapter 1, these strategies will help students change unhealthy or counterproductive behaviors. Included are strategies for dealing with test anxiety, quitting smoking, developing responsible drinking habits, planning a personal exercise program, phasing in a healthier diet, and many other practical plans for change.

The **Appendix**, "Nutritional Content of Popular Items from Fast-Food Restaurants," provides information on commonly ordered menu items.

The latest emergency care guidelines for choking and cardiac arrest (the Heimlich maneuver and CPR) appear inside the back cover of the text, providing information that can save lives.

In addition, several specific learning aids have been incorporated into the text. Learning objectives labeled **Looking Ahead** appear on the opening page of each chapter, identifying major concepts and helping guide students in their reading and review of the text. Important terms appear in boldface type in the text and are defined in a **running glossary**, helping students handle a large and complex new vocabulary.

Chapter summaries offer a concise review and a way to make sure students have grasped the most important concepts in the chapter. **For More Information** sections contain annotated lists of books, newsletters, hotlines, organizations, and Web sites that students can use to extend and broaden their knowledge or pursue subjects of interest to them. Also found at the end of every chapter are **Selected Bibliographies**. A complete **Index** at the end of the book includes references to glossary terms in boldface type.

TEACHING AND LEARNING TOOLS

Available with the eleventh edition is a comprehensive package of supplementary materials designed to enhance teaching and learning.

Connect Core Concepts in Health

McGraw-Hill *Connect Personal Health* is a Web-based assignment and assessment platform that makes it easy for instructors to connect with their students and students to connect with their instructors and coursework. With *Connect*, you can choose interactive activities organized by chapter learning objectives, or you can create activities that align with your coursework. Available with *Connect Core Concepts in Health* are interactive Wellness Worksheets, video activities, Internet activities, the Fitness and Nutrition Log, the Behavior Change Workbook, and more.

Also available are activities aligned with boxes from the text. For example, in Chapter 1, there are activities associated with the Mind/Body/Spirit box on occupational wellness and the Dimensions of Diversity box on factors contributing to health disparities among ethnic minorities. You can deliver all these assignments, assessments, quizzes, and tests online and have the results automatically reported to your grade book. *Connect* is available to accompany the eleventh edition via an access code that can be packaged with each copy of the text.

With easy, 24/7 access to *Connect*, your students can practice important skills at their own pace and on their own schedule. *Connect* provides students with immediate feedback on assignments so they can see how they performed on each question. Students can conveniently complete and submit assignments for online grading, creating a paperless classroom. Every chapter-opening page in the text has the *Connect* icon and Web site address to remind students to log on to study, review, and complete their assignments.

Also available is *Connect Plus*, which includes all the features of *Connect* plus an interactive, media-rich eBook—an online version of the eleventh edition text. With *Connect Plus*, students have access to a wide range of additional online resources and learning aids embedded in the eBook, including videos, key terms and definitions, chapter quizzes, student handouts, behavior change tools, links to health-related Web sites and national organizations, and the fast food appendix. *Connect Plus* provides students with everything they need online to successfully complete their work wherever and whenever they choose.

Instructor's Resource Site

The **Instructor's Resource Site** (www.mhhe.com/insel11e) presents key teaching resources in an easy-to-use format. It includes the following teaching tools:

• The **Course Integrator Guide** includes learning objectives, extended chapter outlines, suggested activities, and lists of additional resources. It also describes all the print and electronic supplements available with the text and shows how to integrate them into lectures and assignments for each chapter. For the eleventh edition, the guide was prepared by Cathy Kennedy, Colorado State University.

• The **test bank** includes more than 1500 true-false, multiple-choice, and short essay questions; it also includes two 100-question multiple-choice tests that cover the content of the entire text. The answer key lists the page number in the text where each answer is found. Contributors to the test bank for the eleventh edition are Majella Smith, Los Medanos Community College; Patricia Rhea, Community College of Baltimore County, Catonsville; Leonard Williams, Tougaloo College; Cynthia Bunwell, Norfolk State University; and Karen Vail-Smith, East Carolina University.

The test bank is also available with the EZ Test **computerized testing software.** EZ Test provides a powerful, easy-to-use test maker to create printed quizzes and exams. EZ Test runs on both Windows and Macintosh systems. For secure online testing, exams created in EZ Test can be exported to WebCT, Blackboard, PageOut, and EZ Test Online. EZ Test is packaged with a Quick Start Guide; once the program is installed, users have access to the complete User's Manual, including multiple Flash tutorials. Additional help is available at www.mhhe.com/eztest.

• The **PowerPoint slides** provide a lecture tool that you can alter or expand to meet the needs of your course. The slides include key lecture points and images from the text and other sources. For the eleventh edition, the PowerPoint presentations were created by Andrew Shim, Indiana University of Pennsylvania, and updated by Rob Hess, Community College of Baltimore County, Catonsville. As an aid for instructors who wish to create their own presentations, a complete **image bank,** including all the illustrations from the text, is also included on the Instructor's Resource Site.

• **Transparency masters and student handouts**— more than 150 in all—are provided as additional lecture resources. The transparency masters feature tables showing key statistics and data, illustrations from the text and other sources, and key points from the text. Illustrations of many body systems are also provided. The student handouts provide additional information and can be used to extend student knowledge on topics such as pre-diabetes, glycemic index, yoga for relaxation, and dealing with alcohol emergencies.

Tegrity Campus

Tegrity Campus is a service that makes class time available all the time by automatically capturing every lecture in a searchable format for students to review when they study and complete assignments. With a simple one-click start and stop process, you capture all computer screens and corresponding audio. Students replay any part of any class with easy-to-use browser-based viewing on a PC or Mac.

Educators know that the more students can see, hear, and experience class resources, the better they learn. With Tegrity Campus, students quickly recall key moments by using Tegrity Campus's unique search feature. This search helps students efficiently find what they need, when they need it, across an entire semester of class recordings. Help turn all your students' study time into learning moments immediately supported by your lecture. Contact your local sales representative for more information about Tegrity Campus.

Classroom Performance System

Classroom Performance System (CPS) brings interactivity into the classroom or lecture hall. CPS is a wireless response system that gives instructors and students immediate feedback from the entire class. Each student uses a wireless response pad similar to a television remote to respond instantly to polling or quiz questions. Contact your local sales representative for more information about CPS.

Student Resources Available with *Connect Core Concepts in Health*

Contact your local representative to find out about packaging any of the following student resources with the text.

• More than 100 **Wellness Worksheets** (ISBN 0-07-727321-4) are available to help students become more involved in their wellness and better prepared to implement successful behavior change. The worksheets include assessment tools, Internet activities, and knowledge-based reviews of key concepts. They are available shrink-wrapped with the text in an easy-to-use pad.

• **NutritionCalc Plus** (ISBN 0-07-321925-8) is a dietary analysis program with an easy-to-use interface that allows users to track their nutrient and food group intakes, energy expenditures, and weight control goals. It generates a variety of reports and graphs for analysis, including comparisons with the latest Dietary Reference Intakes (DRIs). The ESHA database includes thousands of ethnic foods, supplements, fast foods, and convenience foods, and users can add their own foods to the food list. NutritionCalc Plus is available on CD-ROM (Windows only) or in an online version.

• **The Daily Fitness and Nutrition Journal** (ISBN 0-07-302988-2) is a handy booklet that guides students in planning and tracking a fitness program. It also helps students assess their current diet and make appropriate changes.

• The **Health and Fitness Pedometer** (ISBN 0-07-320933-3) can be packaged with copies of the text. It allows students to count their daily steps and track their level of physical activity.

• The interactive **HealthQuest CD-ROM** (ISBN 0-07-295117-6) helps students explore and change their wellness behavior. It includes tutorials, assessments, and behavior change guidelines in such key areas as stress, fitness, nutrition, cardiovascular disease, cancer, tobacco, and alcohol.

A NOTE OF THANKS

The efforts of innumerable people have gone into producing the eleventh edition of this text. The book has benefited immensely from their thoughtful commentaries, expert knowledge and opinions, and many helpful suggestions. We are deeply grateful for their participation in the project.

Academic Contributors

Thomas D. Fahey, Ed.D., California State University, Chico
Exercise for Health and Fitness

James V. Freeman, M.D., M.P.H., Stanford University
Cardiovascular Disease and Cancer

Michael R. Hoadley, Ph.D., Assistant Vice-President for Academic Affairs, Center for Academic Technology Support, Eastern Illinois University
Personal Safety

Paul M. Insel, Ph.D., Stanford University
Taking Charge of Your Health

Mary Iten, Ph.D., University of Nebraska at Kearney
The Challenge of Aging

Robert Jarski, Ph.D., Professor, School of Health Sciences, Director, Complementary Medicine and Wellness Program, Oakland University
Conventional and Complementary Medicine

Nancy Kemp, M.D.
Sexuality, Pregnancy, and Childbirth; Immunity and Infection

John Kowalczyk, Ph.D., University of Minnesota, Duluth
Environmental Health

Inna Landres, M.D., Stanford Hospital and Clinics
Contraception and Abortion

Howard Lee, M.D., M.P.H., Hematology and Oncology, San Mateo County General Hospital
Cardiovascular Disease and Cancer

Javier Lopez-Zetina, Associate Professor, Health Science Department, California State University, Long Beach
The Use and Abuse of Psychoactive Drugs

Jacob W. Roth, M.D., Chief of Adult Psychiatry, Kaiser Permanente San Jose Medical Center, Adjunct Clinical Faculty, Stanford University
The Challenge of Aging

Walton T. Roth, M.D., Stanford University
Stress: The Constant Challenge; Psychological Health

Judith Sharlin, Ph.D., R.D., Department of Nutrition, Simmons College
Weight Management

Rachel Stern, M.S., R.D., Nutrition Consultant
Alcohol and Tobacco

Phillip Takakjian, Ph.D.
Intimate Relationships and Communication

Mae Tinklenberg, R.N., N.P., M.S.
Contraception and Abortion

R. Elaine Turner, Ph.D., R.D., University of Florida
Nutrition Basics

Sarah Waller, M.D., Stanford University
Sexuality, Pregnancy, and Childbirth

Patrick Zickler, Senior Health and Science Writer, Circle Solutions, Inc.
Alcohol and Tobacco

Martha C. Zúñiga, Ph.D., University of California, Santa Cruz
Immunity and Infection

Academic Advisers and Reviewers of the Eleventh Edition

Rachel Abbott, University of West Georgia
Jimmy Anderson, Macon State College
Tami Ashford-Carroll, Benedict College
Debra Atkinson, Iowa State University
Faye Avard, Mississippi Valley State University
Brian Barthel, Utah Valley State College
Autumn Benner, Minnesota State University
Stephanie Bennett, University of Southern Indiana
Sheri Bollinger, Northampton Community College
Liz Brown, Rose State College
Mary Chalupsky, Eastern Connecticut State University
Michael Cleary, Slippery Rock University
Holly Clemens, Cuyahoga Community College
Nicholas DiCicco, Camden County College
Paul Finnicum, Arkansas State University
Daniel Gerber, University of Massachusetts, Amherst
Brian Goslin, Oakland University
Mary Iten, University of Nebraska at Kearney
Linda Jenuwine, Macomb Community College
Cathy Kennedy, Colorado State University
Brian Kipp, Grand Valley State University
Deneen Long, Howard University
Mary Miller, Morehead State University
Irene O'Boyle, Central Michigan University
Pam Rost, Buffalo State College

Andrea Salis, Queensborough Community College, City
University of New York

Patrick Sierer, Coastal Carolina Community College

Barbara Spatz, Cuyahoga Community College

William Swanson, South Texas College

Paul Villas, University of Texas-Pan American

Debbi Ware, Gardner-Webb University

Finally, we would like to thank the members of the *Core Concepts* book team at McGraw-Hill Higher Education. We are indebted to Kirstan Price, whose dedication and extraordinary creative energies have contributed so much to the success of this book; we are also indebted to Tim Huddleston for so ably taking on the role of developmental editor for this edition. Thanks also go to Chris Johnson, executive editor; Bill Minick, marketing manager; Kate Engelberg, director of development; Julia D. Akpan, developmental editor for technology; Lydia Kim, editorial coordinator; Ron Nelms, Jr., media project manager; Carey Eisner, production editor; Randy Hurst and Rich DeVitto, production supervisors; Andrei Pasternak, design manager; Brian Pecko, photo research manager; and Marty Moga, permissions editor. To all we express our deep appreciation.

Paul M. Insel
Walton T. Roth

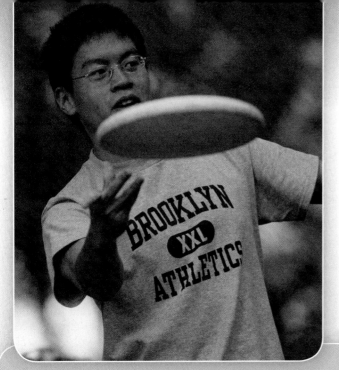

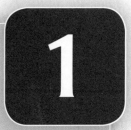

TAKING CHARGE OF YOUR HEALTH

A college sophomore sets the following goals for herself:

- To join in new social circles and make new friends whenever possible
- To exercise every day
- To clean up trash and plant trees in blighted neighborhoods in her community

These goals may differ, but they have one thing in common. Each contributes, in its own way, to this student's health and well-being. Not satisfied merely to be free of illness, she wants more. She has decided to live actively and fully—not just to be healthy, but to pursue a state of overall wellness.

WELLNESS: THE NEW HEALTH GOAL

Generations of people have viewed health simply as the absence of disease. That view largely prevails today; the word **health** typically refers to the overall condition of a person's body or mind and to the presence or absence of illness or injury. **Wellness** is a relatively new concept that expands our idea of health. Beyond the simple presence or absence of disease, wellness refers to optimal health and vitality—to living life to its fullest.

Wellness involves making conscious decisions to enhance your health and to control **risk factors** that contribute to illness or injury. Some risk factors, such as genetic predisposition to a particular disease or condition, are beyond the control of the individual. Other risk factors, such as the kinds of food you eat, are well within individual control. People of every age can reduce their health risks and pursue wellness by choosing healthy behaviors, such as exercising, not smoking, and managing stress.

The Dimensions of Wellness

Experts have defined six dimensions of wellness, which are listed in Table 1.1. These dimensions are interrelated; each has an effect on the others. Further, the process of

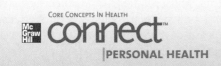

Table 1.1	Examples of Qualities and Behaviors Associated with the Dimensions of Wellness				
Physical	**Emotional**	**Intellectual**	**Interpersonal**	**Spiritual**	**Environmental**
• Eating well • Exercising • Avoiding harmful habits • Practicing safer sex • Recognizing symptoms of disease • Getting regular checkups • Avoiding injuries	• Optimism • Trust • Self-esteem • Self-acceptance • Self-confidence • Ability to understand and accept one's feelings • Ability to share feelings with others	• Openness to new ideas • Capacity to question • Ability to think critically • Motivation to master new skills • Sense of humor • Creativity • Curiosity • Lifelong learning	• Communication skills • Capacity for intimacy • Ability to establish and maintain satisfying relationships • Ability to cultivate support system of friends and family	• Capacity for love • Compassion • Forgiveness • Altruism • Joy • Fulfillment • Caring for others • Sense of meaning and purpose • Sense of belonging to something greater than oneself	• Having abundant, clean natural resources • Maintaining sustainable development • Recycling whenever possible • Reducing pollution and waste

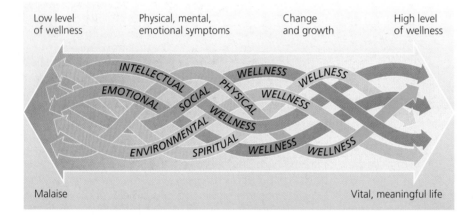

FIGURE 1.1 The wellness continuum. The concept of wellness includes vitality in six interrelated dimensions, all of which contribute to overall wellness.

achieving wellness is constant and dynamic (Figure 1.1), involving change and growth. Wellness is not static; ignoring any dimension of wellness can have harmful effects on your life.

Physical Wellness Your physical wellness includes not just your body's overall condition and the absence of disease but your fitness level and your ability to care for yourself. The higher your fitness level, the higher your level of physical wellness will be. Similarly, as you develop the ability to take care of your own physical needs, you ensure a greater level of physical wellness. To achieve optimum physical wellness, you need to make choices that will help you avoid illnesses and injuries.

Emotional Wellness Your emotional wellness reflects your ability to understand and deal with your feelings. Emotional wellness involves attending to your own thoughts and feelings, monitoring your reactions, and identifying obstacles to emotional stability. Achieving this type of wellness means finding solutions to emotional problems, with professional help if necessary.

Intellectual Wellness Those who enjoy intellectual (or mental) wellness constantly challenge their minds. An active mind is essential to wellness because it detects problems, finds solutions, and directs behavior. People who enjoy intellectual wellness never stop learning; they try to learn new things throughout their lifetime. They seek out new experiences and challenges.

TERMS

health The overall condition of body or mind and the presence or absence of illness or injury.

wellness Optimal health and vitality, encompassing all the dimensions of well-being.

risk factor A condition that increases one's chances of disease or injury.

Occupational Wellness

Many experts contend that occupational (or career) wellness is a seventh dimension of wellness, in addition to the six dimensions described in this chapter. Whether or not occupational wellness appears on every list of wellness dimensions, a growing body of evidence suggests that our daily work has a considerable effect on our overall wellness.

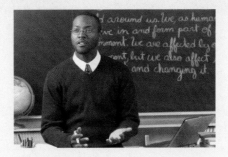

Defining Occupational Wellness

The term *occupational wellness* refers to the level of happiness and fulfillment you gain through your work. Although high salaries and prestigious titles are nice, they alone generally do not bring about occupational wellness. An occupationally well person truly likes his or her work, feels a connection to others in the workplace, and has opportunities to learn and be challenged.

Key aspects of occupational wellness include the following:

- Enjoyable work
- Job satisfaction
- Recognition and acknowledgment from managers and colleagues
- Feelings of achievement
- Opportunities to learn and grow

An ideal job draws on your passions and interests, as well as your vocational skills, and allows you to feel that you are contributing to society in your everyday work.

Financial Wellness

Another important facet of occupational wellness is financial wellness. A person's economic situation is a key factor in his or her overall well-being. People with low socioeconomic status have higher rates of death, injury, and disease; are less likely to have access to preventive health services; and are more likely to engage in unhealthy habits.

Although money and possessions in themselves won't necessarily make you happy, financial security can contribute to your peace of mind. If you are financially secure, you can worry less about daily expenses and focus on personal interests and your future. On the other hand, money problems are a source of stress for individuals and families and are a contributing factor in many divorces and suicides.

You don't need to be rich to achieve financial wellness. Instead, you need to be comfortable with your financial situation. Financially well people understand the limits of their income and live within their means by keeping expenses in check. They know how to balance a checkbook and interpret their bank statements. The financially well person may not strive to be wealthy but at least tries to save money for the future.

Achieving Occupational Wellness

How do you achieve such wellness? Career experts suggest setting career goals that reflect your personal values. For example, a career in sales may be a good way to earn a high income but may not be a good career choice for someone whose highest values involve service to others. Such a person might find more personal satisfaction in teaching or nursing.

Aside from career choices, education is a critical factor in occupational and financial wellness. For starters, learn to manage money *before* you start making it. Classes on personal money management are available through many sources and can help you on your way to financial security, whether you dream of being wealthy or not.

Interpersonal Wellness Your interpersonal (or social) wellness is defined by your ability to develop and maintain satisfying and supportive relationships. Such relationships are essential to physical and emotional health. Social wellness requires participating in and contributing to your community and to society.

Spiritual Wellness To enjoy spiritual wellness is to possess a set of guiding beliefs, principles, or values that give meaning and purpose to your life, especially in difficult times. The spiritually well person focuses on the positive aspects of life and finds spirituality to be an antidote for negative feelings such as cynicism, anger, and pessimism. Organized religions help many people develop spiritual health. Religion, however, is not the only source or form of spiritual wellness. Many people find meaning and purpose in their lives on their own—through nature, art, meditation, or good works—or with loved ones.

Environmental Wellness Your environmental wellness is defined by the livability of your surroundings. Personal health depends on the health of the planet—from the safety of the food supply to the degree of violence in society. Your physical environment either supports your wellness or diminishes it. To improve your environmental wellness, you can learn about and protect yourself against hazards in your surroundings and work to make your world a cleaner and safer place.

In addition, see the box "Occupational Wellness" to learn about another important aspect of wellness.

New Opportunities, New Responsibilities

Wellness is a fairly new concept. A century ago, Americans considered themselves lucky just to survive to adulthood.

Table 1.2 Leading Causes of Death in the United States, 2006

Rank	Cause of Death	Number of Deaths	Percent of Total Deaths*	Death Rate†	Lifestyle Factors
	All causes	2,425,901	100.0	776.4	
1	Heart disease	629,191	25.9	199.4	D I S A
2	Cancer	560,102	23.1	180.8	D I S A
3	Stroke	137,265	5.7	43.6	D I S A
4	Chronic lower respiratory diseases	124,614	5.1	40.4	S
5	Unintentional injuries (accidents)	117,748	4.9	38.5	I S A
6	Alzheimer's disease	72,914	3.0	22.7	
7	Diabetes mellitus	72,507	3.0	23.3	D I S
8	Influenza and pneumonia	56,247	2.3	17.7	S
9	Kidney disease	44,791	1.8	14.3	D I S A
10	Septicemia (systemic blood infection)	34,031	1.4	10.9	A
11	Intentional self-harm (suicide)	32,185	1.3	10.6	A
12	Chronic liver disease and cirrhosis	27,299	1.1	8.7	A
13	Hypertension (high blood pressure)	23,985	1.0	7.6	D I S A
14	Parkinson's disease	19,660	0.8	6.3	
15	Assault (homicide)	18,029	0.7	6.0	A
	All other causes	455,333	18.8		

Key
D Diet plays a part S Smoking plays a part
I Inactive lifestyle plays a part A Excessive alcohol use plays a part

NOTE: Although not among the overall top 15 causes of death, HIV/AIDS (approximately 12,000 deaths in 2006) is a major killer. In 2006, HIV/AIDS was the 8th leading cause of death for Americans age 15–24 years and the 6th leading cause of death for those age 25–44 years.

*Percentages may not total 100% due to rounding.

†Age-adjusted death rate per 100,000 persons.

SOURCE: National Center for Health Statistics. 2008. Deaths: Preliminary data for 2006. *National Vital Statistics Report* 56(16).

QUICK STATS

75% of teens killed in car accidents are not wearing seat belts.

—National Center for Health Statistics, 2007

TERMS

infectious disease A disease that can spread from person to person; caused by microorganisms such as bacteria and viruses.

chronic disease A disease that develops and continues over a long period of time, such as heart disease or cancer.

lifestyle choice A conscious behavior that can increase or decrease a person's risk of disease or injury; such behaviors include smoking, exercising, eating a healthy diet, and others.

A child born in 1900, for example, could expect to live only about 47 years. Many people died from common **infectious diseases** (such as pneumonia, tuberculosis, or diarrhea) and poor environmental conditions (such as water pollution and poor sanitation).

Since 1900, however, life expectancy has nearly doubled, due largely to the development of vaccines and antibiotics to fight infections and to public health measures to improve living conditions. Today, a different set of diseases has emerged as our major health threat, and heart disease, cancer, and stroke are now the three leading causes of death for Americans (Table 1.2). Treating such **chronic diseases** is costly and difficult.

The good news is that people have some control over whether they develop chronic diseases. People make choices every day that increase or decrease their risks for such diseases. These **lifestyle choices** include behaviors such as smoking, diet, exercise, and alcohol use. As Table 1.3 (p. 5) makes clear, lifestyle factors contribute to many deaths in the United States, and people can influence their own health risks.

The need to make good choices is especially true for teens and young adults. For Americans age 15–24, for example, the top three causes of death are unintentional injuries (accidents), homicide, and suicide (Table 1.4, p. 5).

VITAL STATISTICS

Table 1.3	Key Contributors to Death Among Americans	
	Number of Deaths per Year	Percentage of Total Deaths per Year
Tobacco	440,000	18.1
Obesity*	112,000	4.6
Alcohol consumption	85,000	3.5
Microbial agents	75,000	3.1
Toxic agents	55,000	2.3
Motor vehicles	43,000	1.8
Firearms	29,000	1.2
Sexual behavior	20,000	0.8
Illicit drug use	17,000	0.7

NOTE: The factors listed here are defined as lifestyle and environmental factors that contribute to the leading killers of Americans. Microbial agents include bacterial and viral infections like influenza and pneumonia; toxic agents include environmental pollutants and chemical agents such as asbestos.

*The number of deaths due to obesity is an area of ongoing controversy and research. Recent estimates have ranged from 112,000 to 365,000.

SOURCES: Centers for Disease Control and Prevention. 2005. *Frequently Asked Questions About Calculating Obesity-Related Risk* (http://www.cdc.gov/PDF/Frequently_Asked_Questions_About_Calculating_Obesity-Related_Risk.pdf; retrieved December 6, 2007); Mokdad, A. H., et al. 2005. Correction: Actual causes of death in the United States, 2000. *Journal of the American Medical Association* 293(3): 293–294; Mokdad, A. H., et al. 2004. Actual causes of death in the United States, 2000. *Journal of the American Medical Association* 291(10): 1238–1245.

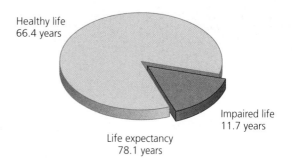

VITAL STATISTICS

FIGURE 1.2 Quantity of life versus quality of life. Years of healthy life as a proportion of life expectancy in the U.S. population.

SOURCES: National Center for Health Statistics. 2008. Deaths: Preliminary data for 2006. *National Vital Statistics Reports* 56(16); National Center for Health Statistics. *Healthy People 2010.* Midcourse Review. Hyattsville, Md.: Public Health Service.

The Healthy People Initiative

Wellness is a personal concern, but the U.S. government has financial and humanitarian interests in it, too. A healthy population is the nation's source of vitality, creativity, and wealth. Poor health drains the nation's resources and raises health care costs for all.

The national Healthy People initiative aims to prevent disease and improve Americans' quality of life. Healthy People reports, published each decade since 1980, set national health goals based on 10-year agendas.

The latest report, *Healthy People 2010*, proposes two broad national goals:

• ***Increase quality and years of healthy life.*** One way to measure quality of life is to count the number of "sick days" people endure–days they can't function due to illness. About 18% of Americans take 14 or more sick days each year, a number that continually rises. Along those same lines, Americans increasingly describe their health as fair or poor rather than excellent or very good. Further, although the life expectancy of Americans has increased significantly in the past century, people can expect poor health to limit their activities and cause distress during the last 15% of their lives (Figure 1.2).

• ***Eliminate health disparities among Americans.*** Many health problems today disproportionately affect certain American populations (issues of special concern

VITAL STATISTICS

Table 1.4	Leading Causes of Death Among Americans Age 15–24		
Rank	Cause of Death	Number of Deaths	Percent of Total Deaths
1	Accidents:	15,859	45.8
	Motor vehicle	10,845	31.3
	All other accidents	5,014	14.5
2	Homicide	5,596	16.2
3	Suicide	4,097	11.8
4	Cancer	1,643	4.7
5	Heart disease	1,021	2.9
	All causes	34,632	

SOURCE: National Center for Health Statistics. 2008. Deaths: Preliminary data for 2006. *National Vital Statistics Report* 56(16).

Table 1.5	Selected *Healthy People 2010* Objectives		
Objective		Estimate of Current Status (%)	Goal (%)
Increase the proportion of people age 18 and older who engage regularly in moderate physical activity.		31	50
Increase the proportion of people age 2 and older who consume at least 3 daily servings of vegetables, with at least one-third being dark-green or orange vegetables.		4	50
Increase the prevalence of healthy weight among people age 20 and older.		32	60
Reduce the proportion of adults 18 and older who use cigarettes.		21	12
Reduce the proportion of college students reporting binge drinking during the past 2 weeks.		40	20
Increase the proportion of adults who take protective measures to reduce the risk of skin cancer (sunscreens, sun-protective clothing, and so on).		71	85
Increase the use of safety belts by motor vehicle occupants.		82	92
Increase the number of residences with a functioning smoke alarm on every floor.		90	100
Increase the proportion of persons with health insurance.		83	100

SOURCE: National Center for Health Statistics. 2008. *DATA 2010: The Healthy People 2010 Database, May 2008 Edition* (http://wonder.cdc.gov/data2010/obj.htm; retrieved December 27, 2008).

to specific groups are discussed later in this chapter). *Healthy People 2010* calls for eliminating disparities in health status, health risks, and use of preventive services among all population groups within the next decade.

Examples of individual health promotion objectives from *Healthy People 2010,* as well as estimates of how we are tracking toward the goals, appear in Table 1.5.

Healthy Campus 2010 Based on the guidelines of *Healthy People 2010* but designed specifically for college students, the *Healthy Campus 2010* program assists colleges in developing plans to improve student health. The American College Health Association's manual for the program, titled *Healthy Campus: Making It Happen,* is a companion to *Healthy People 2010.* The Healthy Campus program was developed through a broad consultation process built on scientific consensus.

Healthy Campus 2010 provides planning guidelines and more than 200 health-related objectives. Using baselines and targets for meeting these objectives, schools can customize their health programs. For example, a school might choose goals such as increasing the proportion of students who exercise at least 3 days a week, or increasing the proportion of students who follow responsible sexual practices.

Health Issues for Diverse Populations

Americans are a diverse people. Our ancestry is European, African, Asian, Pacific Islander, Latin American, and Native American. We live in cities, suburbs, and rural areas and work at every imaginable occupation.

When it comes to health, most differences among people are insignificant; most health issues concern us all equally. We all need to eat well, exercise, manage stress, and cultivate satisfying personal relationships. We need to know how to protect ourselves from heart disease, cancer, sexually transmitted diseases, and injuries. We need to know how to use the health care system.

But some of our differences, as individuals and as members of groups, have important implications for health. Some of us, for example, have a genetic predisposition for developing certain health problems, such as high cholesterol. Some of us have grown up eating foods that raise our risk of heart disease or obesity. Some of us live in an environment that increases the chance that we will smoke cigarettes or abuse alcohol. These health-related differences among individuals and groups can be biological—determined genetically—or cultural—acquired as patterns of behavior through daily interactions with our families, communities, and society. Many health conditions are a function of biology and culture combined. A person can have a genetic predisposition for a disease, for example, but won't actually develop the disease itself unless certain lifestyle factors are present, such as stress or a poor diet.

Health-related differences among groups can be identified and described in the context of several different dimensions. Those highlighted in *Healthy People 2010* are gender, ethnicity, income and education, disability, geographic location, and sexual orientation.

71% of American men are overweight.

—Centers for Disease Control and Prevention, 2007

Sex and Gender Sex and gender profoundly influence wellness. The World Health Organization (WHO) defines **sex** as the biological and physiological characteristics that define men and women; these characteristics are related to chromosomes and their effects on reproductive organs and the functioning of the body. Menstruation in women and the presence of testicles in men are examples of sex-related characteristics. **Gender** is defined as roles, behaviors, activities, and attributes that a given society considers appropriate for men and women. A person's gender is rooted in biology and physiology, but it is shaped by experience and environment—how society responds to individuals based on their sex. Examples of gender-related characteristics that affect wellness include higher rates of smoking and drinking among men and lower earnings among women (compared with men doing similar work).

Both sex and gender have important effects on wellness, but they can be difficult to separate (see the box "Women's Health/Men's Health" on p. 8). For example, more women began smoking with changes in culturally defined ideas about women's behavior (a gender issue). Because women are more vulnerable to the toxins in tobacco smoke (a sex issue), cancer rates also increased.

Ethnicity Achieving the *Healthy People 2010* goal of eliminating all health disparities will require a national effort to identify and address the underlying causes of ethnic health disparities. Compared with the U.S. population as a whole, American ethnic minorities have higher rates of death and disability from many causes. These disparities result from a complex mix of genetic variations, environmental factors, and health behaviors.

Some diseases are concentrated in certain gene pools, the result of each ethnic group's relatively distinct history. Sickle-cell disease is most common among people of African ancestry. Tay-Sachs disease afflicts people of Eastern European Jewish heritage and French Canadian heritage. Cystic fibrosis is more common among Northern Europeans. In addition to biological differences, many cultural differences occur along ethnic lines. Ethnic groups may vary in their traditional diets; their family and interpersonal relationships; their attitudes toward tobacco, alcohol, and other drugs; and their health beliefs and practices. All of these factors have implications for wellness. (See the box "Health Disparities Among Ethnic Minorities" on p. 9 for more information.)

The federal government collects population and health information on five broad ethnic minority groups in American society. (Figure 1.3 shows the current ethnic distribution of the United States.) Each group has some specific health concerns:

• *Latinos* are a diverse group, with roots in Mexico, Puerto Rico, Cuba, and South and Central America. Many Latinos are of mixed Spanish and American Indian descent or of mixed Spanish, Indian, and African American descent. Latinos on average have lower rates of heart disease, cancer, and suicide than the general population, but

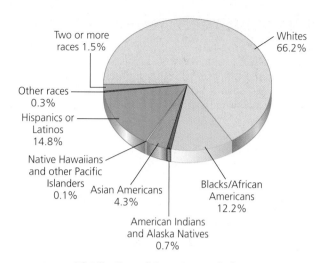

FIGURE 1.3   Distribution of the U.S. population.
SOURCE: U.S. Census Bureau. 2006. *2006 American community survey: Hispanic or Latino origin by race—Universe: Total population.* Washington, D.C.: U.S. Census Bureau.

higher rates of infant mortality and a higher overall birth rate; other areas of concern include gallbladder disease and obesity. At current rates, about one in two Latinas will develop diabetes in her lifetime.

• *African Americans* have the same leading causes of death as the general population, but they have a higher infant mortality rate and lower rates of suicide and osteoporosis. Health issues of special concern for African Americans include high blood pressure, stroke, diabetes, asthma, and obesity. African American men are at significantly higher risk of prostate cancer than men in other groups, and early screening is recommended for them.

• *Asian Americans* include people who trace their ancestry to countries in the Far East, Southeast Asia, or the Indian subcontinent, including Japan, China, Vietnam, Laos, Cambodia, Korea, the Philippines, India, and Pakistan. Asian Americans have a lower death rate and a longer life expectancy than the general population. They have lower rates of coronary heart disease and obesity. However, health differences exist among these groups. For example, Southeast Asian men have higher rates of smoking and lung cancer, and Vietnamese American women have higher rates of cervical cancer.

• *American Indians and Alaska Natives* typically embrace a tribal identity, such as Sioux, Navaho, or Hopi. American Indians and Alaska Natives have lower death

sex The biological and physiological characteristics that define men and women.

gender The roles, behaviors, activities, and attributes that a given society considers appropriate for men and women.

Women's Health/Men's Health

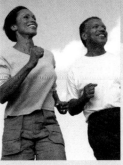

In terms of their health, women and men differ in many ways. They have different life expectancies, for one thing, and suffer from various diseases at different rates. Men and women tend to differ in some health-related behaviors, and they respond in dissimilar ways to some medications and medical treatments. The following table highlights some of the gender differences that can affect wellness.

Health Issues	Women	Men
Life expectancy	On average, live about 5 years longer but have higher rates of disabling health problems such as arthritis, osteoporosis, and Alzheimer's disease	Have a shorter life expectancy but lower rates of disabling health problems
Height and weight	Shorter on average, with a lower proportion of muscle; tend to have a "pear" shape with excess body fat stored in the hips; obesity is more common in women than men	Taller on average, with a higher proportion of muscle; tend to have an "apple" shape with excess body fat stored in the abdomen
Skills and fluencies	Score better on tests of verbal fluency, speech production, fine motor skills, and visual and working memory	Score better on tests of visual-spatial ability (such as the ability to imagine the relationships between shapes and objects when rotated in space)
Heart attacks	Experience heart attacks about 10 years later than men, on average, with a poorer 1-year survival rate; more likely to experience atypical heart attack symptoms (such as fatigue and difficulty breathing) or "silent" heart attacks that occur without chest pain	Experience heart attacks about 10 years earlier than women, on average, with a better 1-year survival rate; more likely to have "classic" heart attack symptoms (such as chest pain)
Stroke	More likely to have a stroke or die from one, but also more likely to recover language ability after a stroke that affects the left side of the brain	Less likely to die from a stroke, but also more likely to suffer permanent loss of language ability after a stroke that affects the left side of the brain
Immune response	Stronger immune systems; less susceptible to infection by certain bacteria and viruses, but more likely to develop autoimmune diseases such as lupus	Weaker immune systems; more susceptible to infection by certain bacteria and viruses, but less likely to develop autoimmune diseases
Smoking	Lower rates of smoking than men, but higher risk of lung cancer at a given level of exposure to smoke	Higher rates of smoking and spit tobacco use
Alcohol	Become more intoxicated at a given level of alcohol intake	Become less intoxicated at a given level of alcohol intake, but are more likely to use or abuse alcohol or to develop alcoholism
Stress	More likely to react to stress with a "tend-and-befriend" response that involves social support; may have a longevity advantage because of a reduced risk of stress-related disorders	More likely to react to stress with aggression or hostility; this pattern may increase the rate of stress-related disorders
Depression	More likely to suffer from depression and to attempt suicide	Lower rates of depression than women and less likely to attempt suicide, but four times more likely to succeed at suicide
Headaches	More commonly suffer migraine and chronic tension headaches	More likely to suffer from cluster headaches
Sexually transmitted diseases (STDs)	More likely to be infected with an STD during a heterosexual encounter; more likely to suffer severe, long-term effects from STDs, such as chronic infection and infertility	Less likely to be infected with an STD during a heterosexual encounter

Health Disparities Among Ethnic Minorities

connect™

In studying the underlying causes of health disparities, it is often difficult to separate the many potential contributing factors.

Income and Education

Poverty and low educational attainment are the most important factors underlying health disparities. People with low incomes and less education have higher rates of death from all causes, especially chronic disease and injury, and they are less likely to have preventive health services such as vaccinations and Pap tests. They are more likely to live in an area with a high rate of violence and many other environmental stressors. They also have higher rates of unhealthy behaviors.

Although ethnic disparities in health are significantly reduced when comparing groups with similar incomes and levels of education, they are not eliminated. For example, people living in poverty report worse health than people with higher incomes; but, within the latter group, African Americans and Latinos rate their health as worse than do whites. Infant mortality rates go down as the education level of mothers goes up; but among mothers who are college graduates, African Americans have significantly higher rates of infant mortality than whites, Latinos, and Asian Americans. These variations point to the complexity of health disparities.

Access to Appropriate Health Care

People with low incomes are less likely to have health insurance and more likely to have problems arranging for transportation to access care. They are also more likely to lack information about services and preventive care. But disparities persist even at higher income levels; for example, among nonpoor Americans, many more Latinos than whites or African Americans report having no insurance, no usual source of health care, and no health care visits within the past year. Ongoing studies continually find that racial minorities have less access to better health care (such as complex surgery at high-volume hospitals) and receive lower quality care than whites.

Factors affecting such disparities may include the following:

• *Local differences in the availability of high-tech health care and specialists.* Minorities, regardless of income, may be more likely to live in medically underserved areas.

• *Problems with communication and trust.* People whose primary language is not English are more likely to be uninsured and to have trouble communicating with health care providers; they may also have problems interpreting health information from public health education campaigns. Language and cultural barriers may be exacerbated by an underrepresentation of minorities in the health professions.

• *Cultural preferences relating to health care.* Groups may vary in their assessment of when it is appropriate to seek medical care and what types of treatments are acceptable.

• *State and federal laws and programs.* Eligibility for Medicaid (a form of government insurance) varies by state and group. For example, Puerto Ricans are U.S. citizens and Cubans are classified as refugees, so people from these groups are immediately eligible for Medicaid; immigrants from other countries may not be able to access public insurance programs until 5 years after they enter the United States.

Culture and Lifestyle

As described in the chapter, ethnic groups may vary in health-related behaviors such as diet, tobacco and alcohol use, coping strategies, and health practices—and these behaviors can have important implications for wellness, both positive and negative. For example, African Americans are more likely to report consuming five or more servings of fruits and vegetables per day than peo-

ple from other ethnic groups. American Indians report high rates of smoking and smoking-related health problems.

Cultural background can be an important protective factor. For example, poverty is strongly associated with increased rates of depression; but some groups, including Americans born in Mexico or Puerto Rico, have lower rates of mental disorders at a given level of income and appear to have coping strategies that provide special resilience.

Discrimination

Racism and discrimination are stressful events that can cause psychological distress and increase the risk of physical and psychological problems. Discrimination can contribute to lower socioeconomic status and its associated risks. Bias in medical care can directly affect treatment and health outcomes.

Conversely, recent research shows that better health care results when doctors ask patients detailed questions about their ethnicity. (Most medical questionnaires ask patients to put themselves in a vague racial or ethnic category, such as Asian or Caucasian). Armed with more information on patients' backgrounds, medical professionals may find it easier to detect some genetic diseases or to overcome language or cultural barriers.

SOURCES: U.S. Department of Health and Human Services, Agency for Healthcare Research and Quality. 2008. *2007 National Healthcare Disparities Report.* Rockville, Md.: U.S. Department of Health and Human Services, Agency for Healthcare Research and Quality, AHRQ Pub. No. 08-0041; National Center for Health Statistics. 2008. *Early Release of Selected Estimates Based on Data from the January–June 2008 National Health Interview Survey* (http://www.cdc.gov/nchs/about/major/ nhis/released200812.htm; retrieved December 27, 2008); National Center for Health Statistics. 2007. *Health, United States, 2007, with Chartbook on Trends in the Health of Americans.* Hyattsville, Md.: National Center for Health Statistics.

Continues on page 10

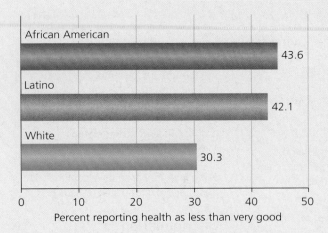

0   10   20   30   40   50
Percent reporting health as less than very good

African American 43.6
Latino 42.1
White 30.3

Self-rated health status. White Americans are significantly more likely than other ethnic groups to rate their health as very good or excellent.

rates from heart disease, stroke, and cancer than the general population, but they have higher rates of early death from causes linked to smoking and alcohol use, including injuries and cirrhosis. Diabetes is a special concern for many groups; for example, the Pimas of Arizona have the highest known prevalence of diabetes of any population in the world.

• *Native Hawaiian and Other Pacific Islander Americans* trace their ancestry to the original peoples of Hawaii, Guam, Samoa, and other Pacific Islands. Pacific Islander Americans have a higher overall death rate than the general population and higher rates of diabetes and asthma. Smoking and obesity are special concerns for this group.

Income and Education   Inequalities in income and education underlie many of the health disparities among Americans. In fact, poverty and low educational attainment are far more important predictors of poor health than any ethnic factor. Income and education are closely related, and groups with the highest poverty rates and least education have the worst health status. These Americans have higher rates of infant mortality, traumatic injury and violent death, and many diseases, including heart disease, diabetes, tuberculosis, HIV infection, and some cancers. They are more likely to eat poorly, be overweight, smoke, drink, and use drugs. They are exposed to more day-to-day stressors (such as the need to hold multiple jobs or deal with unreliable transportation) and have less access to health care services. Many impoverished families are not only uninsured but rely on the local emergency room for their medical needs.

Disability   People with disabilities have activity limitations, need assistance, or perceive themselves as having a disability. About one in five people in the United States has some level of disability, and the rate is rising, especially among younger segments of the population. People with disabilities are more likely to be inactive and overweight. They report more days of depression than people without disabilities. Many also lack access to health care services.

27% of U.S. Latino adults have no usual health care provider.
—Pew Hispanic Center, 2008

QUICK STATS

Geographic Location   About one in four Americans currently lives in a rural area—a place with fewer than 10,000 residents. People living in rural areas are less likely to be physically active, to use safety belts, or to obtain screening tests for preventive health care. They have less access to timely emergency services and much higher rates of some diseases and injury-related death than people living in urban areas (Figure 1.4). They are also more likely to lack health insurance. Children living in dangerous neighborhoods—rural or urban—are four

QUESTIONS FOR CRITICAL THINKING AND REFLECTION
How often do you feel exuberant? Vital? Joyful? What makes you feel that way? Conversely, how often do you feel downhearted, de-energized, or depressed? What makes you feel that way? Have you ever thought about how you might increase experiences of vitality and decrease experiences of discouragement?

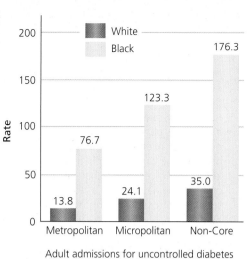

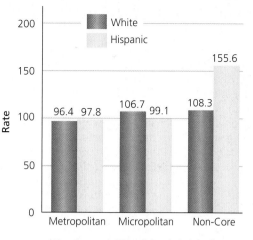

FIGURE 1.4 **Health issues in rural areas.** Ethnic minorities experience a higher proportion of certain diseases than whites, and this problem is compounded for people who live in rural (non-core) areas. **SOURCE**: Agency for Healthcare Research and Quality 2005. *Health Care Disparities in Rural Areas: Selected Findings from the 2004 National Healthcare Disparities Report.* Rockville, Md.: Agency for Healthcare Research and Quality. AHRQ Publication No. 05-P022.

Adult admissions for uncontrolled diabetes per 100,000 population, by race and location

Deaths per 1,000 adult admissions for heart attack, by race and location

Metropolitan ≧ 50,000 inhabitants   Micropolitan = 10,000–50,000 inhabitants
Non-Core (Rural) ≦ 10,000 inhabitants

times more likely to be overweight than children living in safer areas.

Sexual Orientation The 1–5% of Americans who identify themselves as homosexual or bisexual make up a diverse community with varied health concerns. Their emotional wellness and personal safety are affected by factors relating to personal, family, and social acceptance of their sexual orientation. Gay, lesbian, bisexual, and transgender teens are more likely to engage in risky behaviors such as unsafe sex and drug use; they are also more likely to be depressed and to attempt suicide. HIV/AIDS is a major concern for gay men, and gay men and lesbians may have higher rates of substance abuse, depression, and suicide.

CHOOSING WELLNESS

Wellness is something everyone can have. Achieving it requires knowledge, self-awareness, motivation, and effort—but the benefits last a lifetime. Optimal health comes mostly from a healthy lifestyle, patterns of behavior that promote and support your health now and as you get older. In the pages that follow, you'll find current information and suggestions you can use to build a better lifestyle.

Factors That Influence Wellness

Our behavior, family health history, environment, and access to health care are all important influences on wellness. These factors, which vary for both individuals and groups, can interact in ways that produce either health or disease.

Health Habits Scientific research is continuously revealing new connections between our habits and health. For example, heart disease is associated with smoking, stress, hostile and suspicious attitudes, a poor diet, and a sedentary way of life. Unfortunately, poor health habits take hold before many Americans reach adulthood. (See the box "Wellness Matters for College Students" for more information on health habits and wellness concerns of college-age Americans.)

Other habits, however, are beneficial. Regular exercise can help prevent heart disease, high blood pressure, diabetes, osteoporosis, and depression and may reduce the risk of colon cancer, stroke, and back injury. A balanced and varied diet helps prevent many chronic diseases. As we learn more about how our actions affect our bodies and minds, we can make informed choices for a healthier life.

Heredity/Family History Your **genome** consists of the complete set of genetic material in your cells; it contains about 25,000 genes, half from each of your parents. **Genes** control the production of proteins that serve both as the structural material for your body and as the regulators of all your body's chemical reactions and metabolic processes. The human genome varies only slightly from person to person, and many of these

genome   The complete set of genetic material in an individual's cells.

gene   The basic unit of heredity; a section of genetic material containing chemical instructions for making a particular protein.

TERMS

Wellness Matters for College Students

If you are like most college students, you probably feel pretty good about your health right now. Most college students are in their late teens or early twenties, lead active lives, have plenty of friends, and look forward to a future filled with opportunity. With all these things going for you, why shouldn't you feel good?

A Closer Look

Although most college-age people look healthy, appearances can be deceiving. Each year, thousands of students lose productive academic time to physical and emotional health problems—some of which can continue to plague them for life.

The following table shows the top 10 health issues affecting students' academic performance, according to the 2007 National College Health Assessment.

Health Issue	Students Affected (%)
Stress	32.9
Sleep difficulties	25.4
Cold/flu/sore throat	24.8
Concern for a friend or family member	18.1
Relationship problems	15.5
Depression/anxiety	15.5
Internet use/games	15.1
Death of a friend or family member	9.8
Sinus or ear infection/ bronchitis/strep throat	9.4
Attention deficit disorder	7.0

Each of these issues is related to one or more of the six dimensions of wellness, and most can be influenced by choices students make daily. Although

some troubles—such as the death of a friend—cannot be controlled, other physical and emotional concerns can be minimized by choosing healthy behaviors. For example, there are many ways to manage stress, the top health issue affecting students. By reducing unhealthy choices (such as using alcohol to relax) and by increasing healthy choices (such as using time-management techniques), even busy students can reduce the impact of stress on their lives.

The survey also estimated that, based on students' reporting of their height

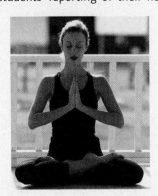

and weight, more than 36% of college students are either overweight or obese. Although heredity plays a role in determining one's weight, lifestyle is also a factor in weight and weight management. In many studies over the past few decades, a large percentage of students have reported behaviors such as these:

- Overeating

- Snacking on junk food

- Frequently eating high-fat foods

- Using alcohol and binge drinking

Clearly, eating behaviors are often a matter of choice. Although students may not see (or feel) the effects of their dietary habits today, the long-term health risks are significant. Overweight and obese persons run a higher-than-normal risk of developing diabetes, heart disease, and cancer later in life. We now know with certainty that improving one's eating habits, even a little, can lead to weight loss and improved overall health.

Other Choices, Other Problems

Students commonly make other unhealthy choices. Here are some examples from the 2007 National College Health Assessment:

- Nearly 50% of students reported that they did not use a condom the last time they had vaginal intercourse.

- About 80% of students had as many as 6 drinks the last time they partied.

- Almost 19% of students had used tobacco at least once during the past month.

What choices do you make in these situations? Remember: It's never too late to change. The sooner you trade an unhealthy behavior for a healthy one, the longer you'll be around to enjoy the benefits.

SOURCE: American College Health Association. 2008. *American College Health Association— National College Health Assessment: Reference Group Executive Summary, Fall 2007.* Baltimore, Md.: American College Health Association.

differences do not affect health. However, some differences have important implications for health, and knowing your family health history can help you determine which conditions may be of special concern for you. Chapter 8 includes more information about creating a family health tree.

Errors in our genes are responsible for about 3500 clearly hereditary conditions, including sickle-cell disease and cystic fibrosis. Altered genes also play a part in heart disease, cancer, stroke, diabetes, and many other common conditions. However, in these more common and complex disorders, genetic alterations serve only to increase an individual's risk, and the disease itself results

from the interaction of many genes with other factors. An example of the power of behavior and environment can be seen in the more than 60% increase in the incidence of diabetes that has occurred among Americans since 1990. This huge increase is not due to any sudden change in our genes; it is the result of increasing rates of obesity caused by poor dietary choices and lack of physical activity.

Environment Your environment includes not only the air you breathe and the water you drink but also substances and conditions in your home, workplace, and community. Are you frequently exposed to environmental tobacco smoke or the radiation in sunlight? Do you live in an area

A "Planet in Peril": Healing the Environment

Our treatment of the environment determines—to a far greater extent than many people want to believe—how the Earth will treat us. This lesson has gradually become clear over several generations, but our troubled environment began attracting intensive worldwide attention only in the last few years. Today, the evidence is irrefutable: Our continuing abuse of the environment has led to a natural backlash that includes the extinction of entire species, shifts in global weather patterns, dying oceans, and the disappearance of polar ice fields.

Climate experts are now sounding the alarm: If we don't immediately begin reducing our impact on the environment, the damage may become irreversible. The compounded effects of humanity's environmental neglect could make our planet a much less hospitable and livable place, possibly within two or three short decades.

The Root of the Problem

Pollution, of course, is not a new problem. People have contaminated the air by burning coal, wood, and oil for millennia. Age-old industries such as forestry and mining have laid waste to vast stretches of land, and processes such as tanning and printing have dumped untold amounts of lethal toxins into the ground and water. People began to take serious notice of pollution even before the dawn of the Industrial Revolution, when a few scientists reported that the smoke from factories and trains was fouling the air, and that industrial runoff was polluting rivers.

Over time, improvements in technology made manufacturing easier and cheaper, while an increasing population and greater prosperity created an insatiable demand for manufactured goods. Industrial growth gave rise to explosive growth of urban areas—population centers that drove the need for transportation and electricity. As a result, industries

and individuals consume ever-larger amounts of fuel and other resources, creating ever more waste and pollution in the process. Combine this with the pollution generated by our use of fossil-fueled transportation, and the result is a recipe for global catastrophe.

Global Warming

Human practices affect the environment on every level. Our food chain is contaminated with pesticides, water must be cleaned of sewage and chemicals before we can drink it, and in some cities the air is so polluted with exhaust that it can actually be dangerous to breathe. But the most ravaging—and frightening—

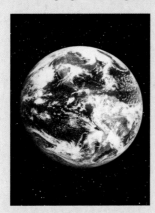

consequence of environmental abuse is the phenomenon known as global warming: the gradual rise in the Earth's temperature that is causing polar ice caps to shrink, creating unfavorable weather patterns, and contributing to rapid devastation of land and oceans.

What causes global warming? As you will learn in Chapter 19, global warming is largely due to human activity. As we burn fossil fuels (such as coal, oil, and fuels derived from them) to power vehicles and factories, the process releases many kinds of waste gases into the skies. Some of these gases, chiefly carbon dioxide (CO_2), rise up into the air and stay there, acting as an invisible insulating blanket.

These gases create a "greenhouse" effect by trapping some of the heat that radiates from the Earth—heat that would normally dissipate through the atmosphere. By defeating the planet's natural temperature controls, CO_2 and other "greenhouse gases" are causing the Earth to get warmer.

As already mentioned, this rise in temperature can wreak havoc on the Earth, especially if temperatures increase unchecked over a long period of time. Experts are trying to determine how high Earth's temperature must climb before we reach the tipping point (when damage from climate change becomes irreversible), and how soon that point may be reached.

Reversing the Warming Trend

Until then, however, one fact is obvious. People, industries, societies, and governments must start taking action now to reduce their "imprint" on the environment. Legislation such as the Clean Water Act have helped, but it is important to understand that pollution and global warming are not problems just for governments to solve. The environment affects every person in an individual way. The more we do as individuals, the more benefits will result from our collective efforts.

This is why *Core Concepts in Health* has been revised with current environmental issues in mind. Not only does Chapter 19 examine the environment in detail, but every chapter briefly addresses the environment's impact on a specific aspect of your well-being—from the way you exercise, to the foods you eat, to your reproductive health. In each chapter, you will see a short feature called "Thinking About the Environment." This feature relates the chapter's main theme to the environment, and poses questions for you to consider or suggests actions you can take to improve the environment—and promote your personal health and wellness, as well.

with poor air quality or high rates of crime and violence? Has alcohol or drug abuse been a problem in your family? These and other environmental factors all have an impact on wellness. (See the box "The Environment" for more information on current environmental issues.)

Access to Health Care Adequate health care helps improve both quality and quantity of life through preventive care and the treatment of disease. For example, vaccinations prevent many dangerous infections, and screening tests help identify key risk factors and diseases in their early, treatable stages. As described earlier in the chapter, inadequate access to health care is tied to factors such as low income and lack of health insurance. Cost is one of many issues surrounding the development of advanced health-related technologies.

Behavior *Can* Make a Difference   In many cases, behavior can tip the balance toward good health, even when heredity or environment is a negative factor. For example, breast cancer can run in families, but it also may be associated with being overweight and inactive. A woman with a family history of breast cancer is less likely to develop and die from the disease if she controls her weight, exercises regularly, and has regular mammograms to help detect the disease in its early, most treatable stage.

Similarly, a young man with a family history of obesity can maintain a normal weight by being careful to balance calorie intake against activities that burn calories. If your life is highly stressful, you can lessen the chances of heart disease and stroke by learning ways to manage and cope with stress. If you live in an area with severe air pollution, you can reduce the risk of lung disease by not smoking. You can also take an active role in improving your environment. Behaviors like these enable you to make a difference in how great an impact heredity and environment will have on your health.

REACHING WELLNESS THROUGH LIFESTYLE MANAGEMENT

As you consider the behaviors that contribute to wellness—being physically active, choosing a healthy diet, and so on—you may be doing a mental comparison with your own behaviors. If you are like most young adults, you probably have some healthy habits and some habits that place your health at risk. For example, you may be physically active and have a healthy diet but indulge in binge drinking on weekends. You may be careful to wear your safety belt in your car but smoke cigarettes or use chewing tobacco. Moving in the direction of wellness means cultivating healthy behaviors and working to

QUESTIONS FOR CRITICAL THINKING AND REFLECTION
We frequently hear news about the ways people harm the environment, but do you ever think about the ways your environment may be harming you? How would you describe the quality of the air you breathe (indoors and outdoors) and the water you drink? Is it easy to make healthy food choices in your neighborhood? Do you find your home or school environment stressful?

overcome unhealthy ones. This approach to lifestyle management is called **behavior change.**

As you may already know from experience, changing an unhealthy habit can be harder than it looks. When you embark on a behavior change plan, it may seem like too much work at first. But as you make progress, you will gain confidence in your ability to take charge of your life. You will also experience the benefits of wellness—more energy, greater vitality, deeper feelings of appreciation and curiosity, and a higher quality of life.

In the rest of this chapter, we outline a general process for changing unhealthy behaviors that is backed by research and that has worked for many people. We also offer many specific strategies and tips for change.

Getting Serious About Your Health

Before you can start changing a wellness-related behavior, you have to know that the behavior is problematic and that you *can* change it. To make good decisions, you need information about relevant topics and issues, including what resources are available to help you change.

Examine Your Current Health Habits   Have you considered how your current lifestyle is affecting your health today and how it will affect your health in the future? Do you know which of your current habits enhance your health and which detract from it? Begin your journey toward wellness with self-assessment: Think about your own

behavior, and talk with friends and family members about what they've noticed about your lifestyle and your health. Challenge any unrealistically optimistic attitudes or ideas you may hold—for example, "To protect my health, I don't need to worry about quitting smoking until I'm 40 years old," or "Being overweight won't put *me* at risk for diabetes." Health risks are very real, and health habits throughout life are important.

Many people start to consider changing a behavior when friends or family members express concern, when a landmark event occurs (such as turning 30), or when new information raises their awareness of risk. If you find yourself reevaluating some of your behaviors as you read this text, take advantage of the opportunity to make a change in a structured way.

Choose a Target Behavior   Changing any behavior can be demanding. This is why it's a good idea to start small, by choosing one behavior you want to change—called a **target behavior**—and working on it until you succeed.

Your chances of success will be greater if your first goal is simple, such as resisting the urge to snack between classes. As you change one behavior, make your next goal a little more significant, and build on your success.

Learn About Your Target Behavior Once you've chosen a target behavior, you need to learn its risks and benefits for you—both now and in the future. Ask these questions:

- How is your target behavior affecting your level of wellness today?
- What diseases or conditions does this behavior place you at risk for?
- What effect would changing your behavior have on your health?

As a starting point, use this text and the resources listed in the For More Information section at the end of each chapter; see the box "Evaluating Sources of Health Information" for additional guidelines.

Find Help Have you identified a particularly challenging target behavior or mood, something like alcohol addiction, binge eating, or depression, that interferes with your ability to function or places you at a serious health risk? Help may be needed to change behaviors or conditions that are too deeply rooted or too serious for self-management. Don't be stopped by the seriousness of the problem; many resources are available to help you solve it. On campus, the student health center or campus counseling center can provide assistance. To locate community resources, consult the yellow pages, your physician, or the Internet.

Building Motivation to Change

Knowledge is necessary for behavior change, but it isn't usually enough to make people act. Millions of people have sedentary lifestyles, for example, even though they know it's bad for their health. This is particularly true of young adults, who may not be motivated to change because they feel healthy in spite of their unhealthy behaviors. To succeed at behavior change, you need strong motivation.

Examine the Pros and Cons of Change Health behaviors have short-term and long-term benefits and costs. Consider the benefits and costs of an inactive lifestyle:

- Short-term, such a lifestyle allows you more time to watch TV and hang out with friends, but it leaves you less physically fit and less able to participate in recreational activities.
- Long-term, it increases the risk of heart disease, cancer, stroke, and premature death.

To successfully change your behavior, you must believe that the benefits of change outweigh the costs.

Carefully examine the pros and cons of continuing your current behavior and of changing to a healthier one. Focus on the effects that are most meaningful to you, including those that are tied to your personal identity and values. For example, if you see yourself as an active person who is a good role model for others, then adopting behaviors such as engaging in regular physical activity and getting

adequate sleep will support your personal identity. If you value independence and control over your life, then quitting smoking will be consistent with your values and goals. To complete your analysis, ask friends and family members about the effects of your behavior on them. For example, a younger sister may tell you that your smoking habit influenced her decision to take up smoking.

The short-term benefits of behavior change can be an important motivating force. Although some people are motivated by long-term goals, such as avoiding a disease that may hit them in 30 years, most are more likely to be moved to action by shorter-term, more personal goals. Feeling better, doing better in school, improving at a sport, reducing stress, and increasing self-esteem are common short-term benefits of health behavior change.

Boost Self-Efficacy When you start thinking about changing a health behavior, a big factor in your eventual success is whether you have confidence in yourself and in your ability to change. **Self-efficacy** refers to your belief in your ability to successfully take action and perform a specific task. Strategies for boosting self-efficacy include developing an internal locus of control, using visualization and self-talk, and getting encouragement from supportive people.

---

behavior change A lifestyle management process that involves cultivating healthy behaviors and working to overcome unhealthy ones.

target behavior An isolated behavior selected as the object for a behavior change program.

self-efficacy The belief in one's ability to take action and perform a specific task.

TERMS

Evaluating Sources of Health Information

Believability of Health Information Sources

A 2007 survey conducted by the American College Health Association indicated that college students are smart about evaluating health information. They trust the health information they receive from health professionals and educators and are skeptical about popular information sources.

Rank	Source	Rank	Source
1	Health educators	8	Resident assistants/ advisers
2	Health center medical staff	9	Religious centers
3	Parents	10	Internet/World Wide Web
4	Faculty/coursework	11	Friends
5	Leaflets, pamphlets, flyers	12	Magazines
6	Campus newspaper articles	13	Television
7	Campus peer educators	14	Other sources

How smart are you about evaluating health information? Here are some tips.

General Strategies

Whenever you encounter health-related information, take the following steps to make sure it is credible:

• *Go to the original source.* Media reports often simplify the results of medical research. Find out for yourself what a study really reported, and determine whether it was based on good science. What type of study was it? Was it published in a recognized medical journal? Was it an animal study or did it involve people? Did the study include a large number of people? What did the authors of the study actually report?

• *Watch for misleading language.* Reports that tout "breakthroughs" or "dramatic proof" are probably hype. A study may state that a behavior "contributes to" or is "associated with" an outcome; this does not prove a cause-and-effect relationship.

• *Distinguish between research reports and public health advice.* Do not change your behavior based on the results of a single report or study. If an agency such as the National Cancer Institute urges a behavior change, however, you should follow its advice. Large, publicly funded organizations issue such advice based on many studies, not a single report.

• *Remember that anecdotes are not facts.* A friend may tell you he lost weight on some new diet, but individual success stories do not mean the plan is truly safe or effective. Check with your doctor before making any serious lifestyle changes.

• *Be skeptical.* If a report seems too good to be true, it probably is. Be wary of information contained in advertisements. An ad's goal is to sell a product, even if there is no need for it.

• *Make choices that are right for you.* Friends and family members can be a great source of ideas and inspiration, but you need to make health-related choices that work best for you.

Internet Resources

Online sources pose special challenges; when reviewing a health-related Web site, ask these questions:

• *What is the source of the information?* Web sites maintained by government agencies, professional associations, or established academic or medical institutions are likely to present trustworthy information. Many other groups and individuals post accurate information, but it is important to look at the qualifications of the people who are behind the site. (Check the home page or click the "About Us" link.)

• *How often is the site updated?* Look for sites that are updated frequently. Check the "last modified" date of any Web page.

• *Is the site promotional?* Be wary of information from sites that sell specific products, use testimonials as evidence, appear to have a social or political agenda, or ask for money.

• *What do other sources say about a topic?* Be cautious of claims or information that appear at only one site or come from a chat room, bulletin board, or blog.

• *Does the site conform to any set of guidelines or criteria for quality and accuracy?* Look for sites that identify themselves as conforming to some code or set of principles, such as those set forth by the Health on the Net Foundation or the American Medical Association. These codes include criteria such as use of information from respected sources and disclosure of the site's sponsors.

LOCUS OF CONTROL Who do you believe is controlling your life? Is it your parents, friends, or school? Is it "fate"? Or is it you? **Locus of control** refers to the figurative "place" a person designates as the source of responsibility for the events in his or her life. People who believe they are in control of their own lives are said to have an *internal locus of control*. Those who believe that factors beyond their control determine the course of their lives are said to have an *external locus of control.*

For lifestyle management, an internal locus of control is an advantage because it reinforces motivation and commitment. An external locus of control can sabotage efforts to change behavior. For example, if you believe that you are destined to die of breast cancer because your mother died from the disease, you may view monthly breast self-exams and regular checkups as a waste of time. In contrast, if you believe that you can take action to reduce your risk of breast cancer in spite of hereditary factors, you will be motivated to follow guidelines for early detection of the disease.

If you find yourself attributing too much influence to outside forces, gather more information about your wellness-related behaviors. List all the ways that making lifestyle changes will improve your health. If you believe you'll succeed, and if you recognize that you are in charge of your life, you're on your way to wellness.

VISUALIZATION AND SELF-TALK One of the best ways to boost your confidence and self-efficacy is to visualize yourself successfully engaging in a new, healthier behavior. Imagine yourself going for an afternoon run 3 days a week or no longer smoking cigarettes. Also visualize yourself enjoying all the short-term and long-term benefits that your lifestyle change will bring. Create a new self-image: What will you and your life be like when you become a regular exerciser or a nonsmoker?

You can also use self-talk, the internal dialogue you carry on with yourself, to increase your confidence in your ability to change. Counter any self-defeating patterns of thought with more positive or realistic thoughts: "I am a strong, capable person, and I can maintain my commitment to change." See Chapter 3 for more on self-talk.

ROLE MODELS AND OTHER SUPPORTIVE INDIVIDUALS Social support can make a big difference in your level of motivation and your chances of success. Perhaps you know people who have reached the goal you are striving for; they could be role models or mentors for you, providing information and support for your efforts. Gain strength from their experiences, and tell yourself, "If they can do it, so can I." In addition, find a buddy who wants to make the same changes you do and who can take an active role in your behavior change program. For example,

an exercise buddy can provide companionship and encouragement when you might be tempted to skip your workout.

IDENTIFY AND OVERCOME BARRIERS TO CHANGE Don't let past failures at behavior change discourage you; they can be a great source of information you can use to boost your chances of future success. Make a list of the problems and challenges you faced in any previous behavior change attempts; to this, add the short-term costs of behavior change that you identified in your analysis of the pros and cons of change. Once you've listed these key barriers to change, develop a practical plan for overcoming each one. For example, if you always smoke when you're with certain friends, decide in advance how you will turn down the next cigarette you are offered.

Enhancing Your Readiness to Change

The transtheoretical, or "stages of change," model has been shown to be an effective approach to lifestyle self-management. According to this model, you move through distinct stages as you work to change your target behavior. It is important to determine what stage you are in now so that you can choose appropriate strategies for progressing through the cycle of change. This approach can help you enhance your readiness and intention to change. Read the following sections to determine what stage you are in for your target behavior.

Precontemplation People at this stage do not think they have a problem and do not intend to change their behavior. They may be unaware of the risks associated with their behavior or may deny them. They may have tried unsuccessfully to change in the past and may now think the situation is hopeless. They may also blame other people or external factors for their problems. People in the precontemplation stage believe that there are more reasons or more important reasons not to change than there are reasons to change.

Contemplation People at this stage know they have a problem and intend to take action within 6 months. They acknowledge the benefits of behavior change but are also aware of the costs of changing—to be successful, people must believe that the benefits of change outweigh the costs. People in the contemplation stage wonder about possible courses of action but don't know how to proceed. There may also be specific barriers to change that appear too difficult to overcome.

Preparation People at this stage plan to take action within a month or may already have begun to make small changes in their behavior. They may be engaging in their new, healthier behavior but not yet regularly or consistently. They may have created a plan for change but may be worried about failing.

THINKING ABOUT THE ENVIRONMENT

As you think about target behaviors you may want to change, consider your behavior toward the environment. By making simple changes to your daily routine or by using more environmentally friendly products, you can make a positive difference to the planet. For example, do you:

- Recycle paper, glass, plastic, and metal products?

- Use energy-efficient compact fluorescent light bulbs instead of standard incandescent bulbs?

- Keep your car well maintained to get the best possible gas mileage and emit the lowest possible amount of pollution?

- Avoid using aerosol products, pesticides, and other chemicals that could pollute the ground, air, or water?

For more information on the environment and environmental health, see Chapter 14.

Action During the action stage, people outwardly modify their behavior and their environment. The action stage requires the greatest commitment of time and energy, and people in this stage are at risk for reverting to old, unhealthy patterns of behavior.

Maintenance People at this stage have maintained their new, healthier lifestyle for at least 6 months. Lapses may have occurred, but people in maintenance have been successful in quickly reestablishing the desired behavior. The maintenance stage can last a few months or many years.

Termination For some behaviors, a person may reach the sixth and final stage of termination. People at this stage have exited the cycle of change and are no longer tempted to lapse back into their old behavior. They have a new self-image and total self-efficacy with regard to their target behavior.

Dealing with Relapse

People seldom progress through the stages of change in a straightforward, linear way; rather, they tend to move to a certain stage and then slip back to a previous stage before resuming their forward progress. Research suggests that most people make several attempts before they successfully change a behavior; four out of five people experience some degree of backsliding. For this reason, the stages of change are best conceptualized as a spiral, in which people cycle back through previous stages but are further along in the process each time they renew their commitment.

QUICK STATS

45.7 million living Americans have stopped smoking.

—Centers for Disease Control and Prevention, 2007

If you experience a lapse—a single slip—or a relapse—a return to old habits—don't give up. Relapse can be demoralizing, but it is not the same as failure; failure means stopping before you reach your goal and never changing your target behavior. During the early stages of the change process, it's a good idea to plan for relapse so you can avoid guilt and self-blame and get back on track quickly.

If relapses keep occurring or if you can't seem to control them, you may need to return to a previous stage of the behavior change process. If this is necessary, reevaluate your goals and your strategy. A different or less stressful approach may help you avoid setbacks when you try again.

Developing Skills for Change: Creating a Personalized Plan

Once you are committed to making a change, it's time to put together a plan of action. Your key to success is a well-thought-out plan that sets goals, anticipates problems, and includes rewards.

1. Monitor Your Behavior and Gather Data Keep a record of your target behavior and the circumstances surrounding it. Record this information for at least a week or two. Keep your notes in a health journal or notebook or on your computer (see the sample journal entries in Figure 1.5). Record each occurrence of your behavior, noting the following:

- What the activity was
- When and where it happened

Date November 5 Day M [TU] W TH F SA SU

Time of day	M/S	Food eaten	Cals.	H	Where did you eat?	What else were you doing?	How did someone else influence you?	What made you want to eat what you did?	Emotions and feelings?	Thoughts and concerns?
7:30	M	1 C Crispix cereal 1/2 C skim milk coffee, black 1 C orange juice	110 40 — 120	3	home	reading newspaper	alone	I always eat cereal in the morning	a little keyed up & worried	thinking about quiz in class today
10:30	S	1 apple	90	1	hall outside classroom	studying	alone	felt tired & wanted to wake up	tired	worried about next class
12:30	M	1 C chili 1 roll 1 pat butter 1 orange 2 oatmeal cookies 1 soda	290 120 35 60 120 150	2	campus food court	talking	eating w/ friends; we decided to eat at the food court	wanted to be part of group	excited and happy	interested in hearing everyone's plans for the weekend

M/S = Meal or snack H = Hunger rating (0–3)

FIGURE 1.5 Sample health journal entries.

- What you were doing
- How you felt at that time

If your goal is to start an exercise program, track your activities to determine how to make time for workouts.

2. Analyze the Data and Identify Patterns

After you have collected data on the behavior, analyze the data to identify patterns. When are you most likely to overeat? What events trigger your appetite? Perhaps you are especially hungry at midmorning or when you put off eating dinner until 9:00. Perhaps you overindulge in food and drink when you go to a particular restaurant or when you're with certain friends. Note the connections between your feelings and such external cues as time of day, location, situation, and the actions of others around you.

3. Be "SMART" About Setting Goals

If your goals are too challenging, you will have trouble making steady progress and will be more likely to give up altogether. If, for example, you are in poor physical condition, it will not make sense to set a goal of being ready to run a marathon within 2 months. If you set goals you can live with, it will be easier to stick with your behavior change plan and be successful.

Experts suggest that your goals meet the "SMART" criteria; that is, your behavior change goals should be:

- *Specific.* Avoid vague goals like "eat more fruits and vegetables." Instead, state your objectives in specific terms, such as "eat 2 cups of fruit and 3 cups of vegetables every day."
- *Measurable.* Recognize that your progress will be easier to track if your goals are quantifiable, so give your goal a number. You might measure your goal in terms of time (such as "walk briskly for 20 minutes a day"), distance ("run 2 miles, 3 days per week"), or some other amount ("drink 8 glasses of water every day").
- *Attainable.* Set goals that are within your physical limits. For example, if you are a poor swimmer, it might not be possible for you to meet a short-term fitness goal by swimming laps. Walking or biking might be better options.
- *Realistic.* Manage your expectations when you set goals. For example, it may not be possible for a long-time smoker to quit cold turkey. A more realistic approach might be to use nicotine-replacement patches or gum for several weeks while getting help from a support group.
- *Time frame–specific.* Give yourself a reasonable amount of time to reach your goal, state the time frame in your behavior change plan, and set your agenda to meet the goal within the given time frame.

Using these criteria, a sedentary person who wanted to improve his health and build fitness might set a goal of being able to run 3 miles in 30 minutes, to be achieved within a time frame of 6 months. To work toward that goal, he might set a number of smaller, intermediate goals that are easier to achieve. For example, his list of goals might look like this:

Week	Frequency (days/week)	Activity	Duration (minutes)
1	3	Walk < 1 mile	10–15
2	3	Walk 1 mile	15–20
3	4	Walk 1–2 miles	20–25
4	4	Walk 2–3 miles	25–30
5–7	3–4	Walk/run 1 mile	15–20
⋮			
21–24	4–5	Run 2–3 miles	25–30

4. Devise a Plan of Action

Develop a strategy that will support your efforts to change. Your plan of action should include the following steps:

- *Get what you need.* Identify resources that can help you. For example, you can join a community walking club or sign up for a smoking cessation program. You may also need to buy some new running shoes or nicotine-replacement patches. Get the items you need right away; waiting can delay your progress.
- *Modify your environment.* If there are cues in your environment that trigger your target behavior, try to control them. For example, if you normally have alcohol at home, getting rid of it can help prevent you from indulging. If you usually study with a group of friends in an environment that allows smoking, try moving to a nonsmoking area. If you always buy a snack at a certain vending machine, change your route so you don't pass by it.
- *Control related habits.* You may have habits that contribute to your target behavior; modifying these habits can help change the behavior. For example, if you usually plop down on the sofa while watching TV, try putting an exercise bike in front of the set so you can burn calories while watching your favorite programs.
- *Reward yourself.* Giving yourself instant, real rewards for good behavior will reinforce your efforts. Plan your rewards; decide in advance what each one will be and how you will earn it. Tie rewards to achieving specific goals or subgoals. For example, you might treat yourself to a movie after a week of avoiding snacks. Make a list of items or events to use as rewards; they should be special to you and preferably unrelated to food or alcohol.
- *Involve the people around you.* Tell family and friends about your plan, and ask them to help. To help them respond appropriately to your needs, create a specific list of dos and don'ts. For example, ask them to support you when you set aside time to exercise or avoid second helpings at dinner.
- *Plan for challenges.* Think about situations and people that might derail your program, and develop ways to cope with them. For example, if you think it will be hard to stick to your usual exercise program during

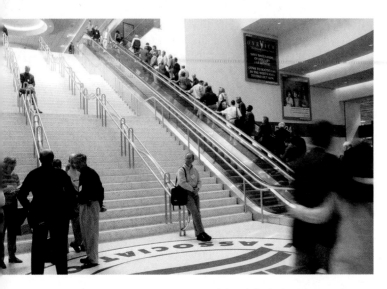

Your environment contains powerful cues for both positive and negative lifestyle choices. Identifying and using the healthier options available to you throughout the day is a key part of a successful behavior change program.

exams, schedule short bouts of physical activity (such as a brisk walk) as stress-reducing study breaks.

5. Make a Personal Contract A serious personal contract—one that commits you to your word—can result in a higher chance of follow-through than a casual, off-hand promise. Your contract can help prevent procrastination by specifying important dates and can also serve as a reminder of your personal commitment to change.

Your contract should include a statement of your goal and your commitment to reaching it. The contract should also include details, such as the following:

- The date you will start
- The steps you will take to measure your progress
- The strategies you plan to use to promote change
- The date you expect to reach your final goal

Have someone—preferably someone who will be actively helping you with your program—sign your contract as a witness.

QUESTIONS FOR CRITICAL THINKING AND REFLECTION
Think about the last time you made an unhealthy choice instead of a healthy one. How could you have changed the situation, the people in the situation, or your own thoughts, feelings, or intentions to avoid making that choice? What can you do in similar situations in the future to produce a different outcome?

Figure 1.6 shows a sample behavior change contract for someone who is committing to eating more fruit every day. You can apply the general behavior change planning framework presented in this chapter to any target behavior. Additional examples of behavior change plans appear in the Behavior Change Strategy sections at the end of many chapters in this text. In these sections, you wil find specific plans for quitting smoking, starting an exercise program, and making other positive lifestyle changes.

Putting Your Plan into Action

The starting date has arrived, and you are ready to put your plan into action. This stage requires commitment, the resolve to stick with the plan no matter what temptations you encounter. Remember all the reasons you have to make the change—and remember that *you* are the boss. Use all your strategies to make your plan work. Make sure your environment is change-friendly, and get as much support and encouragement from others as possible. Keep track of your progress in your health journal, and give yourself regular rewards. And don't forget to give yourself a pat on the back—congratulate yourself, notice how much better you look or feel, and feel good about how far you've come and how you've gained control of your behavior.

Behavior Change Contract

1. I, <u>Tammy Lau</u>, agree to <u>increase my consumption of fruit from 1 cup per week to 2 cups per day.</u>

2. I will begin on <u>10/5</u> and plan to reach my goal of <u>2 cups of fruit per day</u> by <u>12/7</u>

3. To reach my final goal, I have devised the following schedule of mini-goals. For each step in my program, I will give myself the reward listed.

   <u>I will begin to have ½ cup</u>   <u>10/5</u>   <u>see movie</u>
   <u>of fruit with breakfast</u>
   <u>I will begin to have ½ cup</u>   <u>10/26</u>   <u>new cd</u>
   <u>of fruit with lunch</u>
   <u>I will begin to substitute fruit</u>   <u>11/16</u>   <u>concert</u>
   <u>juice for soda 1 time per day</u>

   My overall reward for reaching my goal will be <u>trip to beach</u>

4. I have gathered and analyzed data on my target behavior and have identified the following strategies for changing my behavior: <u>Keep the fridge stocked with easy-to-carry fruit. Pack fruit in my backpack every day. Buy lunch at place that serves fruit.</u>

5. I will use the following tools to monitor my progress toward my final goal:
   <u>Chart on fridge door</u>
   <u>Health journal</u>

   I sign this contract as an indication of my personal commitment to reach my goal: <u>Tammy Lau</u>   <u>9/28</u>
   I have recruited a helper who will witness my contract and <u>also increase his consumption of fruit; eat lunch with me twice a week.</u>
   <u>Eric March</u>   <u>9/28</u>

FIGURE 1.6 A sample behavior change contract.

BEING HEALTHY FOR LIFE

Your first few behavior change projects may never go beyond the planning stage. Those that do may not all succeed. But as you begin to see progress and changes, you'll start to experience new and surprising positive feelings about yourself. You'll probably find that you're less likely to buckle under stress. You may accomplish things you never thought possible—winning a race, climbing a mountain, quitting smoking. Being healthy takes extra effort, but the paybacks in energy and vitality are priceless.

Once you've started, don't stop. Remember that maintaining good health is an ongoing process. Tackle one area at a time, but make a careful inventory of your health strengths and weaknesses and lay out a long-range plan. Take on the easier problems first, and then use what you

QUESTIONS FOR CRITICAL THINKING AND REFLECTION

Have you tried to change a behavior in the past, such as exercising more or quitting smoking? How successful were you? Do you feel the need to try again? If so, what would you do differently to improve your chances of success?

TIPS FOR TODAY AND THE FUTURE

You are in charge of your health. Many of the decisions you make every day have an impact on the quality of your life, both now and in the future. By making positive choices, large and small, you help ensure a lifetime of wellness.

RIGHT NOW YOU CAN

- Go for a 15-minute walk.
- Have a piece of fruit for a snack.
- Call a friend and arrange for a time to catch up with each other.
- Start thinking about whether you have a health behavior you'd like to change. If you do, consider the elements of a behavior change strategy. For example, begin a mental list of the pros and cons of the behavior, or talk to someone who can support you in your attempts to change.

IN THE FUTURE YOU CAN

- Stay current on health- and wellness-related news and issues.
- Participate in health awareness and promotion campaigns in your community—for example, support smoking restrictions in local venues.
- Be a role model for someone else who is working on a health behavior you have successfully changed.

have learned to attack more difficult areas. Keep informed about the latest health news and trends; research is constantly providing new information that directly affects daily choices and habits.

You can't completely control every aspect of your health. At least three other factors—heredity, health care, and environment—play important roles in your well-being. After you quit smoking, for example, you may still be inhaling smoke from other people's cigarettes. Your resolve to eat better foods may suffer a setback when you can't find any healthy choices in vending machines.

But you can make a difference—you can help create an environment around you that supports wellness for everyone. You can help support nonsmoking areas in public places. You can speak up in favor of more nutritious foods and better physical fitness facilities. You can include non-alcoholic drinks at your parties.

You can also work on larger environmental challenges: air and water pollution, traffic congestion, overcrowding and overpopulation, global warming and climate change, toxic and nuclear waste, and many others. These difficult issues need the attention and energy of people who are informed and who care about good health. On every level, from personal to planetary, we can all take an active role in shaping our environment.

SUMMARY

- Wellness is the ability to live life fully, with vitality and meaning. Wellness is dynamic and multidimensional; it incorporates physical, emotional, intellectual, spiritual, interpersonal and social, and environmental dimensions.

- As chronic diseases have become the leading cause of death in the United States, people have recognized that they have greater control over, and greater responsibility for, their health than ever before.

- The Healthy People initiative seeks to achieve a better quality of life for all Americans. The broad goals of the *Healthy People 2010* report are to increase quality and years of healthy life and to eliminate health disparities among Americans.

- Health-related differences among people that have implications for wellness can be described in the context of gender, ethnicity, income and education, disability, geographic location, and sexual orientation.

- Although heredity, environment, and health care all play roles in wellness and disease, behavior can mitigate their effects.

- To make lifestyle changes, you need information about yourself, your health habits, and resources available to help you change.

- You can increase your motivation for behavior change by examining the benefits and costs of change, boosting self-efficacy, and identifying and overcoming key barriers to change.

• The "stages of change" model describes six stages that people move through as they try to change their behavior: precontemplation, contemplation, preparation, action, maintenance, and termination.

• A specific plan for change can be developed by (1) monitoring behavior by keeping a journal; (2) analyzing the recorded data; (3) setting specific goals; (4) devising strategies for modifying the environment, rewarding yourself, and involving others; and (5) making a personal contract.

• To start and maintain a behavior change program you need commitment, a well-developed plan, social support, and a system of rewards.

• Although we cannot control every aspect of our health, we can make a difference in helping create an environment that supports wellness for everyone.

FOR MORE INFORMATION

BOOKS

American Medical Association. 2006. *American Medical Association Concise Medical Encyclopedia.* New York: Random House. *Includes more than 3000 entries on health and wellness topics, symptoms conditions, and treatments.*

Claiborn, J., and C. Pedrick. 2001. *The Habit Change Workbook: How to Break Bad Habits and Form Good Ones.* Oakland, Ca.: New Harbinger Publications. *Provides step-by-step instructions for identifying and overcoming a variety of unhealthy behaviors, such as poor eating habits, reluctance to exercise, and addictive behavior.*

Komaroff, A. L., ed. 2005. *Harvard Medical School Family Health Guide.* New York: Free Press. *Provides consumer-oriented advice for the prevention and treatment of common health concerns.*

Litin, S.C. (ed). 2004. *Mayo Clinic Family Health Book,* 3rd Ed. New York: HarperCollins Publishers. *A complete health reference for every stage of life, covering thousands of conditions, symptoms, and treatments.*

Murat, B., and G. Stewart. 2009. *Do I Need to See the Doctor? The Home-Treatment Encyclopedia—Written by Medical Doctors—That Lets You Decide,* 2nd Ed. New York: John Wiley & Sons. *Fully illustrated, easy-to-read guide to hundreds of common symptoms and ailments, designed to help consumers determine whether they can treat themselves or should seek professional medical attention.*

Prochaska, J. O., J. C. Norcross, and C. C. DiClemente. 1994. *Changing for Good: The Revolutionary Program That Explains the Six Stages of Change and Teaches You How to Free Yourself from Bad Habits.* New York: Morrow. *Outlines the authors' model of behavior change and offers suggestions and advice for each stage of change.*

U.S. Government. 2007. *2007 American Health and Medical Encyclopedia: Authoritative, Practical Guide to Health and Wellness.* FDA, CDC, NIH, Surgeon General Publications (CD-ROM). Washington,

D.C.: Progressive Management. *Contains thousands of documents from various federal agencies on myriad health issues, as well as links to dozens of health- and wellness-related Web sites.*

NEWSLETTERS

Consumer Reports on Health (800-274-7596;
    http://www.consumerreports.org/oh/index.htm)
Harvard Health Publications (877-649-9457;
    http://www.health.harvard.edu)
Harvard Men's Health Watch (877-649-9457)
Harvard Women's Health Watch (877-699-9457)
Mayo Clinic Health Letter (800-291-1128)
University of California, Berkeley, Wellness Letter (800-829-9170;
    http://www.wellnessletter.com)

ORGANIZATIONS, HOTLINES, AND WEB SITES

The Internet addresses (also called uniform resource locators, or URLs) listed here were accurate at the time of publication.
Centers for Disease Control and Prevention. Through phone, fax, and the Internet, the CDC provides a wide variety of health information.
    http://www.cdc.gov
Federal Trade Commission: Consumer Protection — Health. Includes online brochures about a variety of consumer health topics, including fitness equipment, generic drugs, and fraudulent health claims.
    http://www.ftc.gov/bcp/menus/consumer/health.shtm
FirstGov for Consumers: Health. Provides links to online brochures from a variety of government agencies.
    http://www.consumer.gov/health.htm
Healthfinder. A gateway to online publications, Web sites, support and self-help groups, and agencies and organizations that produce reliable health information.
    http://www.healthfinder.gov
Healthy Campus 2010. The American College Health Association's introduction to the Healthy Campus program.
    http://www.acha.org/info_resources/hc2010.cfm
Healthy People 2010. Provides information on Healthy People objectives and priority areas.
    http://www.healthypeople.gov
MedlinePlus. Provides links to news and reliable information about health from government agencies and professional associations; also includes a health encyclopedia and information on prescription and over-the-counter drugs.
    http://www.medlineplus.gov
National Health Information Center (NHIC). Puts consumers in touch with the organizations that are best able to provide answers to health-related questions.
    http://www.health.gov/nhic
National Institutes of Health. Provides information about all NIH activities as well as consumer publications, hotline information, and an A to Z listing of health issues with links to the appropriate NIH institute.
    http://www.nih.gov
National Wellness Institute. Serves professionals and organizations that promote optimal health and wellness.
    http://www.nationalwellness.org
National Women's Health Information Center. Provides information and answers to frequently asked questions.
    http://www.4woman.gov

Office of Minority Health Resource Center. Promotes improved health among racial and ethnic minority populations.

http://www.omhrc.gov

Surgeon General. Includes information on activities of the Surgeon General and the text of many key reports on such topics as tobacco use, physical activity, and mental health.

http://www.surgeongeneral.gov

World Health Organization (WHO). Provides information about health topics and issues affecting people around the world.

http://www.who.int

The following are just a few of the many sites that provide consumer-oriented information on a variety of health issues:

CNN Health: http://www.cnn.com/health
FamilyDoctor.Org: http://www.familydoctor.org
InteliHealth: http://www.intelihealth.com
MayoClinic.com: http://www.mayoclinic.com
MedlinePlus News: http://www.nlm.nih.gov/medlineplus/newsbydate.html
MedPage Today Medical News: http://www.medpagetoday.com
WebMD: http://www.webmd.com
Yahoo Health News: http://news.yahoo.com/i/751

SELECTED BIBLIOGRAPHY

American Cancer Society. 2008. *Cancer Facts and Figures—2008.* Atlanta: American Cancer Society.

American Heart Association. 2008. *Heart Disease and Stroke Statistics—2009 Update.* Dallas: American Heart Association.

Banks, J., et al. 2006. Disease and disadvantage in the United States and in England. *Journal of the American Medical Association* 295(17): 2037–2045.

Barr, D.A. 2008. *Health Disparities in the United States: Social Class, Race, Ethnicity, and Health.* Baltimore: The Johns Hopkins University Press.

Beckman, M. 2007. Help wanted: In the pursuit of a healthy lifestyle, sheer grit only takes you so far. *Stanford Medicine Magazine* 24(3).

Bren, L. 2005. Does sex make a difference? *FDA Consumer,* July–August.

Casciano, D. A. 2005. Paving the way for safer, more effective drugs, food, and medical products. *FDA Consumer,* November–December.

Centers for Disease Control and Prevention. 2008. *Racial and Ethnic Approaches to Community Health (REACH U.S.): Finding Solutions to Health Disparities, 2008* (http://www.cdc.gov/nccdphp/publications/aag/pdf/reach.pdf; retrieved December 27, 2008).

Centers for Disease Control and Prevention. 2008. Racial/Ethnic Disparities in Self-Rated Health Status among Adults with and without Disabilities—United States, 2004–2006. *Morbidity and Mortality Weekly Report* 57(39): 1069–1073.

Finkelstein, E. A., et al. 2008. Do obese persons comprehend their personal health risks? *American Journal of Health Behavior* 32(5): 508–516.

Flegal, K.M., et al. 2005. Excess deaths associated with underweight, overweight, and obesity. Journal of the American Medical Association 293 (15): 1861–1867.

Flegal, K.M., et al. 2007. Cause-specific excess deaths associated with underweight, overweight, and obesity. *Journal of the American Medical Association* 298(17): 2028–2037.

⋮

Gorman, B. K., and J. G. Read.. 2006. Gender disparities in adult health: An examination of three measures of morbidity. *Journal of Health and Social Behavior* 47(2): 95–110.

Herd, P., et al. 2007. Socioeconomic position and health: The differential effects of education versus income on the onset versus progression of health problems. *Journal of Health and Social Behavior* 48(3): 223–238.

Horneffer-Ginter, K. 2008. Stages of change and possible selves: Two tools for promoting college health. *Journal of American College Health* 56(4): 351–358.

How to keep those New Year's resolutions. 2006. *Harvard Health Letter,* January, 31.

Jemal, A., et al. 2008. Cancer statistics, 2008. *CA: A Cancer Journal for Clinicians* 58(2): 71–96.

Martin, G., and J. Pear. 2007. *Behaviour Modification: What It Is and How to Do It,* 8th ed. Upper Saddle River, N.J.: Prentice-Hall.

Mokdad, A. H., et al. 2004. Actual causes of death in the United States, 2000. *Journal of the American Medical Association* 291(10): 1238–1245.

Mokdad, A. H., et al. 2005. Correction: Actual causes of death in the United States, 2000. *Journal of the American Medical Association* 293(3): 293–294.

National Center for Health Statistics. 2006. Health behaviors of adults: United States, 2002–04. *Vital and Health Statistics* 10(230).

National Center for Health Statistics. 2007. *Health, United States, 2007, with Chartbook on Trends in the Health of Americans.* Hyattsville, Md.: National Center for Health Statistics.

National Center for Health Statistics. 2008. Deaths: Preliminary data for 2006. *National Vital Statistics Report* 56(16).

Nothwehr, F., et al. 2008. Age group differences in diet and physical activity-related behaviors among rural men and women. *Journal of Nutrition, Health and Aging* 12(3): 169–174.

Ogden, C. L., et al. 2006. Prevalence of overweight and obesity in the United States, 1999–2004. *Journal of the American Medical Association* 295(13): 1549–1555.

O'Loughlin, J., et al. 2007. Lifestyle risk factors for chronic disease across family origin among adults in multiethnic, low-income, urban neighborhoods. *Ethnicity and Disease* 17(4): 657–663.

Song, J., et al. 2006. Gender differences across race/ethnicity in use of health care among Medicare-aged Americans. *Journal of Women's Health* 15(10): 1205–1213.

U.C. Berkeley. 2007. Do men get their fair share? University of California, *Berkeley, Wellness Letter,* April, 1–2.

U.C. Berkeley. 2008. *Evaluating Web Pages: Techniques to Apply and Questions to Ask* (http://www.lib.berkeley.edu/TeachingLib/Guides/Internet/Evaluate.html; retrieved December 27, 2008).

Walker, B., and C. P. Mouton. 2008. Environmental influences on cardiovascular health. *Journal of the National Medical Association* 100(1): 98–102.

U.S. Census Bureau. 2005. *We the People: Women and Men in the United States.* Washington, D.C.: U.S. Census Bureau.

Walsh, T., et al. 2006. Spectrum of mutations in BRCA1, BRCA2, CHEK2, and TP53 in families at high risk of breast cancer. *Journal of the American Medical Association* 295: 1379–1388.

World Health Organization. 2008. Gender Inequalities and HIV/AIDS (http://www.who.int/gender/hiv_aids/en; retrieved December 27, 2008).

World Health Organization. 2008. *Why Gender and Health?* (http://www.who.int/gender/genderandhealth/en; retrieved December 27, 2008).

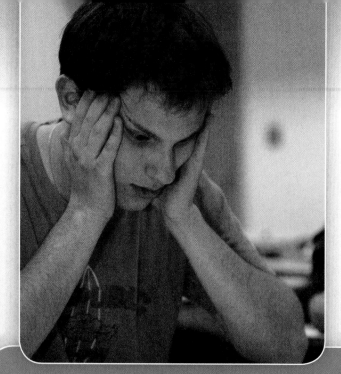

LOOKING AHEAD>>>>>

AFTER READING THIS CHAPTER, YOU SHOULD BE ABLE TO:

- Explain what stress is and how people react to it—physically, emotionally, and behaviorally

- Describe the relationship between stress and disease

- List common sources of stress

- Describe techniques for preventing and managing stress

- Put together a plan for successfully managing the stress in your life

STRESS: THE CONSTANT CHALLENGE

2

Like the term *wellness, stress* is a word many people use without really understanding its precise meaning. Stress is popularly viewed as an uncomfortable response to a negative event, which probably describes *nervous tension* more than the cluster of physical and psychological responses that actually constitute stress. In fact, stress is not limited to negative situations; it is also a response to pleasurable physical challenges and the achievement of personal goals. Whether stress is experienced as pleasant or unpleasant depends largely on the situation and the individual. Because learning effective responses to stress can enhance psychological health and help prevent a number of serious diseases, stress management can be an important part of daily life.

As a college student, you may be in one of the most stressful times of your life. This chapter explains the physiological and psychological reactions that make up the stress response and describes how these reactions can be risks to good health. The chapter also presents methods of managing stress.

WHAT IS STRESS?

In common usage, the term *stress* refers to two different things: situations that trigger physical and emotional reactions, *and* the reactions themselves. This text uses the more precise term **stressor** for a situation that triggers physical and emotional reactions and the term **stress response** for those reactions. A first date and a final exam are examples of stressors; sweaty palms and a pounding heart are symptoms of the stress response. We'll use the term **stress** to describe the general physical and emotional state that accompanies the stress response. So, a person taking a final exam experiences stress.

Physical Responses to Stressors

Imagine a near miss: As you step off the curb, a car careens toward you. With just a fraction of a second to spare, you leap safely out of harm's way. In that split sec-

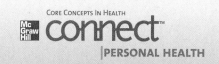

CORE CONCEPTS IN HEALTH

connect

|PERSONAL HEALTH

http://www.mcgrawhillconnect.com/personalhealth

ond of danger and in the moments following it, you experience a predictable series of physical reactions. Your body goes from a relaxed state to one prepared for physical action to cope with a threat to your life.

Two systems in your body are responsible for your physical response to stressors: the nervous system and the endocrine system. Through rapid chemical reactions affecting almost every part of your body, you are primed to act quickly and appropriately in time of danger.

Actions of the Nervous System   The nervous system consists of the brain, spinal cord, and nerves. Part of the nervous system is under voluntary control, as when you tell your arm to reach for a chocolate. The part that is not under conscious supervision—for example, the part that controls the digestion of the chocolate—is the **autonomic nervous system**. In addition to digestion, it controls your heart rate, breathing, blood pressure, and hundreds of other involuntary functions.

The autonomic nervous system consists of two divisions:

- The **parasympathetic division** is in control when you are relaxed; it aids in digesting food, storing energy, and promoting growth.
- The **sympathetic division** is activated during times of arousal, including exercise, and when there is an emergency, such as severe pain, anger, or fear.

Sympathetic nerves use the neurotransmitter **norepinephrine** to exert their actions on nearly every organ, sweat gland, blood vessel, and muscle to enable your body to handle an emergency. In general, the sympathetic division commands your body to stop storing energy and to use it in response to a crisis.

Actions of the Endocrine System   During stress, the sympathetic nervous system triggers the **endocrine system**. This system of glands, tissues, and cells helps control body functions by releasing **hormones** and other chemical messengers into the bloodstream to influence metabolism and other body processes. These chemicals act on a variety of targets throughout the body. Along with the nervous system, the endocrine system prepares the body to respond to a stressor.

The Two Systems Together   How do both systems work together in an emergency? Let's go back to your near collision with a car. Both reflexes and higher cognitive areas in your brain quickly make the decision that you are facing a threat—and your body prepares to meet the danger. Chemical messages and actions of sympathetic nerves cause the release of key hormones, including **cortisol** and **epinephrine**. These hormones trigger the physiological changes shown in Figure 2.1 (p. 26), including these:

- Heart and respiration rates accelerate to speed oxygen through the body.
- Hearing and vision become more acute.

- The liver releases extra sugar into the bloodstream to boost energy.
- Perspiration increases to cool the skin.
- The brain releases **endorphins**—chemicals that can inhibit or block sensations of pain—in case you are injured.

Taken together, these almost-instantaneous physical changes are called the **fight-or-flight reaction.** They give you the heightened reflexes and strength you need to dodge the car or deal with other stressors. Although these physical changes may vary in intensity, the same basic set of physical reactions occurs in response to any type of stressor—positive or negative, physical or psychological.

The Return to Homeostasis   Once a stressful situation ends, the parasympathetic division of your autonomic

stressor   Any physical or psychological event or condition that produces stress.

stress response   The physical and emotional changes associated with stress.

stress   The general physiological and emotional state that accompanies the stress response.

autonomic nervous system   The branch of the nervous system that controls basic body processes; consists of the sympathetic and parasympathetic divisions.

parasympathetic division   A division of the autonomic nervous system that moderates the excitatory effect of the sympathetic division, slowing metabolism and restoring energy supplies.

sympathetic division   A division of the autonomic nervous system that reacts to danger or other challenges by almost instantly accelerating body processes.

norepinephrine   A neurotransmitter released by the sympathetic nervous system onto specific tissues to increase their function in the face of increased activity; when released by the brain, causes arousal (increased attention, awareness, and alertness); also called *noradrenaline*.

endocrine system   The system of glands, tissues, and cells that secrete hormones into the bloodstream to influence metabolism and other body processes.

hormone   A chemical messenger produced in the body and transported in the bloodstream to target cells or organs for specific regulation of their activities.

cortisol   A steroid hormone secreted by the cortex (outer layer) of the adrenal gland; also called *hydrocortisone*.

epinephrine   A hormone secreted by the medulla (inner core) of the adrenal gland that affects the functioning of organs involved in responding to a stressor; also called *adrenaline*.

endorphins   Brain secretions that have pain-inhibiting effects.

fight-or-flight reaction   A defense reaction that prepares an individual for conflict or escape by triggering hormonal, cardiovascular, metabolic, and other changes.

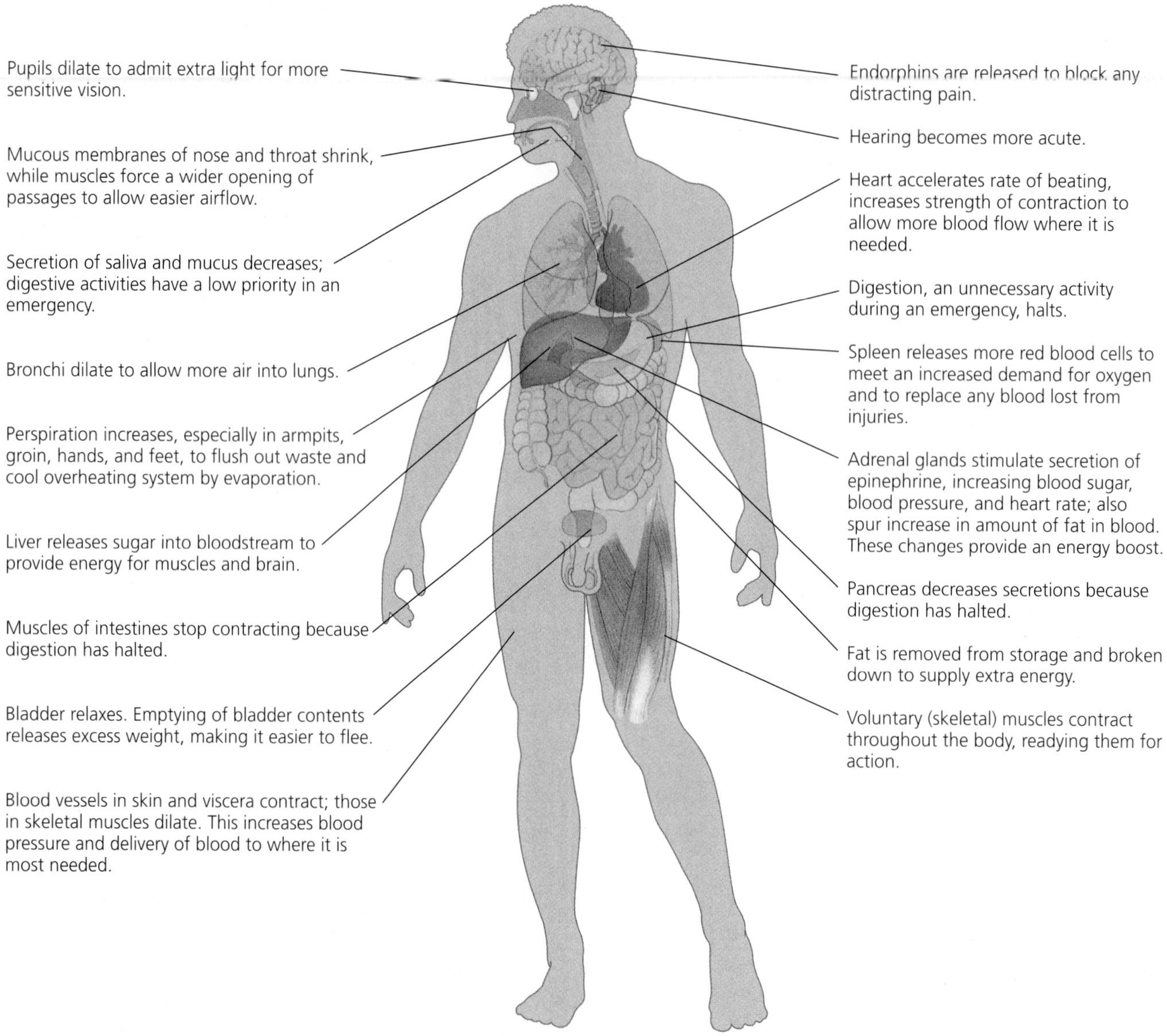
Pupils dilate to admit extra light for more sensitive vision.
Mucous membranes of nose and throat shrink, while muscles force a wider opening of passages to allow easier airflow.
Secretion of saliva and mucus decreases; digestive activities have a low priority in an emergency.
Bronchi dilate to allow more air into lungs.
Perspiration increases, especially in armpits, groin, hands, and feet, to flush out waste and cool overheating system by evaporation.
Liver releases sugar into bloodstream to provide energy for muscles and brain.
Muscles of intestines stop contracting because digestion has halted.
Bladder relaxes. Emptying of bladder contents releases excess weight, making it easier to flee.
Blood vessels in skin and viscera contract; those in skeletal muscles dilate. This increases blood pressure and delivery of blood to where it is most needed.
Endorphins are released to block any distracting pain.
Hearing becomes more acute.
Heart accelerates rate of beating, increases strength of contraction to allow more blood flow where it is needed.
Digestion, an unnecessary activity during an emergency, halts.
Spleen releases more red blood cells to meet an increased demand for oxygen and to replace any blood lost from injuries.
Adrenal glands stimulate secretion of epinephrine, increasing blood sugar, blood pressure, and heart rate; also spur increase in amount of fat in blood. These changes provide an energy boost.
Pancreas decreases secretions because digestion has halted.
Fat is removed from storage and broken down to supply extra energy.
Voluntary (skeletal) muscles contract throughout the body, readying them for action.

FIGURE 2.1 The fight-or-flight reaction. In response to a stressor, the autonomic nervous system and the endocrine system prepare the body to deal with an emergency.

nervous system takes command and halts the stress response. It restores **homeostasis,** a state in which blood pressure, heart rate, hormone levels, and other vital functions are maintained within a narrow range of normal. Your parasympathetic nervous system calms your body down, slowing a rapid heartbeat, drying sweaty palms, and returning breathing to normal. Gradually, your body resumes its normal "housekeeping" functions, such as digestion and temperature regulation. Damage that may have been sustained during the fight-or-flight reaction is repaired. The day after you narrowly dodge the car, you feel fine. In this way, your body can grow, repair itself, and acquire reserves of energy. When the next crisis comes, you'll be ready to respond—instantly—again.

TERMS

homeostasis A state of stability and consistency in an individual's physiological functioning.

somatic nervous system The branch of the peripheral nervous system that governs motor functions and sensory information, largely under conscious control.

personality The sum of behavioral, cognitive, and emotional tendencies.

The Fight-or-Flight Reaction in Modern Life The fight-or-flight reaction is a part of our biological heritage, and it's a survival mechanism that has served humans well. In modern life, however, it is often absurdly inappropriate. Many stressors we face in everyday life do not require a physical response—for example, an exam, a mess left by a roommate, or a stop light. The fight-or-flight reaction prepares the body for physical action regardless of whether such action is a necessary or appropriate response to a particular stressor.

Emotional and Behavioral Responses to Stressors

We all experience a similar set of physical responses to stressors, which make up the fight-or-flight reaction. These responses, however, vary from person to person and from one situation to another. People's perceptions of potential stressors—and of their reactions to such stressors—also vary greatly. Remember, however, that not all stressors are negative. A certain amount of stress, if coped with appropriately, can help promote optimal performance (Figure 2.2).

Effective and Ineffective Responses Common emotional responses to stressors include anxiety, depression, and fear. Although emotional responses are determined in part by inborn personality or temperament, we often can moderate or learn to control them. Coping techniques are discussed later in the chapter.

Behavioral responses to stressors—controlled by the **somatic nervous system,** which manages our conscious actions—are entirely under our control. Effective behavioral responses such as talking, laughing, exercising, meditating, learning time-management skills, and becoming more assertive can promote wellness and enable us to function at our best. Ineffective behavioral responses to stressors include overeating, expressing hostility, and using tobacco, alcohol, or other drugs.

Personality and Stress Some people seem to be nervous, irritable, and easily upset by minor annoyances; others are calm and composed even in difficult situations. Scientists remain unsure just why this is or how the brain's complex emotional mechanisms work. But **personality,** the sum of cognitive, behavioral, and emotional tendencies, clearly affects how people perceive and react to stressors. To investigate the links among personality, stress, and overall wellness, researchers have looked at different constellations of characteristics, or "personality types."

- *Type A.* People with Type A personality are described as ultracompetitive, controlling, impatient, aggressive, and even hostile. Type A people have a higher perceived stress level and more problems coping with stress. They react explosively to stressors and are upset by events that others would consider only annoyances. Studies indicate that certain characteristics of the Type A pattern—anger, cynicism, and hostility—increase the risk of heart disease.
- *Type B.* The Type B personality is relaxed and contemplative. Type B people are less frustrated by daily events and more tolerant of the behavior of others.
- *Type C.* The Type C personality is characterized by anger suppression, difficulty expressing emotions, feel-

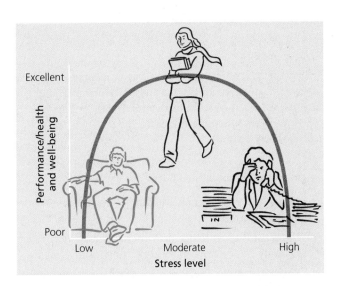

FIGURE 2.2 Stress level, performance, and well-being. A moderate level of stress challenges individuals in a way that promotes optimal performance and well-being. Too little stress, and people are not challenged enough to improve; too much stress, and the challenges become stressors that can impair physical and emotional health.

ings of hopelessness and despair, and an exaggerated response to minor stressors. This heightened response may impair immune functions.

Studies of Type A and C personalities suggest that expressing your emotions is beneficial but that habitually expressing exaggerated stress responses or hostility is unhealthy.

Researchers have also looked for personality traits that enable people to deal more successfully with stress. One such trait is *hardiness,* a particular form of optimism. People with a hardy personality view potential stressors as challenges and opportunities for growth and learning—not as burdens. They see fewer situations as stressful, and react less intensely to stress than nonhardy persons might. Hardy people are committed to their activities, have a sense of inner purpose and an inner locus of control, and feel at least partly in control of their lives.

The term *resilience* refers to personality traits associated with social and academic success in at-risk populations such as people from low-income families and those with mental or physical disabilities. Resilient people tend to set goals and face adversity through individual effort. There are three basic types of resilience, and each one determines how a person responds to stress:

QUESTIONS FOR CRITICAL THINKING AND REFLECTION

Think of the last time you faced a significant stressor. How did you respond? List the physical, emotional, and behavioral reactions you experienced. Did these responses help you deal with the stress, or did they interfere with your efforts to handle it?

- *Nonreactive resilience,* in which a person does not react to a stressor
- *Homeostatic resilience,* in which a person may react strongly but returns to baseline functioning quickly
- *Positive growth resilience,* in which a person learns and grows from the stress experience

Resilience is associated with emotional intelligence and violence prevention.

Can you do anything to change your personality traits and become more stress-resistant? It isn't likely. You can, however, change some of your typical behaviors and patterns of thinking, and develop positive techniques for coping with stressors. Strategies for successful stress management are described later in this chapter.

Cultural Background   Young adults from around the world come to America for a higher education; most students finish college with a greater appreciation for other cultures and worldviews. The clashing of cultures, however, can be a big source of stress for many students—especially when it leads to disrespectful treatment, harassment, or violence. It is important to remember that everyone's reaction

THINKING ABOUT THE ENVIRONMENT

Environmental problems—whether natural or man-made—can compound other sources of stress, such as working, commuting, or taking care of a family. Consider the environment where you live, attend school, or work. Do you live with any of the following?

- Smog or other pollutants, which make the air hard to breathe

- Crowding, which makes it difficult to move around

- Poverty, which limits your choices in many aspects of life

- Crime, which can make you feel unsafe or hypervigilant

If one or more environmental factors make life more stressful for you, look for resources in your community that can help. For example, public transportation may ease your commute while helping to reduce pollution in your town. For more information on the environment and environmental health, see Chapter 14.

to stress is influenced by his or her family and cultural background. Learning to accept and appreciate the cultural backgrounds of other people is both a mind-opening experience and a way to avoid stress over cultural differences.

Gender   Our **gender role**—the activities, abilities, and behaviors our culture expects of us based on our sex—can affect our experience of stress. Some behavior responses to stressors, such as crying or openly expressing anger, may be deemed more appropriate for one gender than the other.

Strict adherence to gender roles, however, can limit one's response to stress and can itself become a source of stress. Gender roles can also affect one's perception of a stressor. If a man derives most of his self-worth from his work, for example, retirement may be more stressful for him than for a woman whose self-image is based on several different roles.

See the box "Women, Men, and Stress" (p. 29) for more on gender and stress.

Experience   Past experiences can profoundly influence the evaluation of a potential stressor. Consider someone who has had a bad experience giving a speech in the past. He or she is much more likely to perceive an upcoming speech as stressful than someone who has had positive public speaking experiences.

STRESS AND HEALTH

According to the American Psychological Association, 77% of adult Americans reported stress-related health problems in 2007. The role of stress in health is complex, but evidence suggests that stress can increase vulnerability to many ailments. Several theories have been proposed to explain the relationship between stress and disease.

The General Adaptation Syndrome

The term **general adaptation syndrome (GAS)** describes what many believe is a universal and predictable response pattern to all stressors. As mentioned earlier, some stressors are pleasant (such as attending a party), but others are unpleasant (such as getting a bad grade). In the GAS theory, the stress triggered by a pleasant stressor is called **eustress;** stress brought on by an unpleasant stressor is called **distress.** The sequence of physical responses associated with GAS is the same for eustress and distress and occurs in three stages (Figure 2.3):

- *Alarm.* The alarm stage includes the complex sequence of events brought on by the fight-or-flight reaction. At this stage, the body is more susceptible to disease or injury because it is geared up to deal with a crisis. Someone in this stage may experience headaches, indigestion, anxiety, and disrupted eating or sleep patterns.
- *Resistance.* With continued stress, the body develops a new level of homeostasis in which it is more resistant

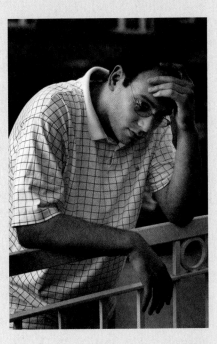

GENDER MATTERS

Women, Men, and Stress

connect

Men and women alike experience stress, but they experience it differently.

Women and Stress

Women are more likely than men to find themselves balancing multiple roles, such as those of student, spouse, and parent. Women who work outside the home still do most of the housework—although today's husbands are helping in greater numbers than previous generations did—and housework isn't limited to cleaning or doing laundry. For example, more than 60% of women make all decisions about their family's health care, including decisions about elderly parents. The combined pressures of home, workplace, and school can create very high stress levels.

Men and Stress

Men who fit a traditional male gender role may feel compelled to be in charge at all times. This may create tension in interpersonal situations and limit men's ability to build a support network. Such men may keenly feel the responsibility to support a family, which can compound existing pressures at home and work.

Perceptions of Stress

In late 2007, the American Psychological Association released the results of its annual "Stress in America" survey. The survey shows the different views American men and women have of their personal stress. Respondents said stress affects them in the following ways:

	Women	Men
Experience extreme stress	35%	28%
Stress has increased in past 5 years	50%	46%
Experience physical problems stemming from stress	82%	71%
Lose at least 1 hour of sleep nightly because of stress	24%	16%

The survey also shows that women are more likely than men to cope with stress through behaviors such as overeating or taking prescription medications.

Physiological Differences

Levels of testosterone (the primary male hormone, responsible for many masculine traits) increase from puberty onward, so men tend to have higher blood pressure than women of the same age. This factor contributes to greater wear on the male circulatory system, sometimes increasing a man's risk for cardiovascular disease. A part of the brain that regulates emotions, the amygdala, is sensitive to testosterone. This may be one reason that men are more likely than women to find certain situations (such as social interactions) to be stressful.

Conversely, women have higher levels of oxytocin (a hormone involved in social interaction and mood regulation) and are more likely to respond to stressors by seeking social support. This coping response may give women a longevity advantage over men by decreasing the risk of some stress-related disorders. It does not, however, free women from stress-related ailments, and women are more likely than men to suffer stress-related hypertensions, depression, and obesity.

---

to disease and injury than usual. In this stage, a person can cope with normal life and added stress.

• **Exhaustion.** The first two stages of GAS require a great deal of energy. If a stressor persists, or if several stressors occur in succession, general exhaustion sets in.

This is not the sort of exhaustion you feel after a long, busy day; rather, it's a life-threatening physiological state.

Allostatic Load

Although the GAS model is still viewed as a key conceptual contribution to the understanding of stress, some

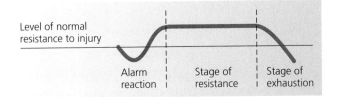

FIGURE 2.3 The general adaptation syndrome. During the alarm phase, a lower resistance to injury is evident. With continued stress, resistance to injury is actually enhanced. With prolonged exposure to repeated stressors, exhaustion sets in, with a return of low resistance levels seen during acute stress.

gender role A culturally expected pattern of behavior and attitudes determined by a person's sex.

general adaptation syndrome (GAS) A pattern of stress responses consisting of three stages: alarm, resistance, and exhaustion.

eustress Stress resulting from a pleasant stressor.

distress Stress resulting from an unpleasant stressor.

TERMS

aspects of it are outdated. For example, increased susceptibility to disease after repeated or prolonged stress is now thought to be due to the effects of the stress response itself rather than to a depletion of resources (exhaustion state). In particular, long-term overexposure to stress hormones such as cortisol has been linked with health problems. Further, although physical stress reactions promote homeostasis (resistance stage), they also have negative effects on the body.

The long-term wear and tear of the stress response is called the **allostatic load.** An individual's allostatic load is dependent on many factors, including genetics, life experiences, and emotional and behavioral responses to stressors. A high allostatic load may be due to frequent stressors, poor adaptation to common stressors, an inability to shut down the stress response, or imbalances in the stress response of different body systems. A high allostatic load is linked with heart disease, hypertension, obesity, and reduced brain and immune system functioning. In other words, when your allostatic load exceeds your ability to cope, you are more likely to get sick.

Psychoneuroimmunology

One of the most fruitful areas of current research into the relationship between stress and disease is **psychoneuroimmunology (PNI).** PNI is the study of the interactions among the nervous system, the endocrine system, and the immune system. The underlying premise of PNI is that stress, through the actions of the nervous and endocrine systems, impairs the immune system and thereby affects health.

A complex network of nerve and chemical connections exists between the nervous and endocrine systems and the immune system. In general, increased levels of cortisol are linked to a decreased number of immune system cells, or lymphocytes (see Chapter 13 for more on the immune system). Epinephrine appears to promote the release of lymphocytes but at the same time reduces their efficiency. Scientists have identified hormone-like substances called *neuropeptides* that appear to translate stressful emotions into biochemical events, some of which impact the immune system, providing a physical link between emotions and immune function.

Different types of stress may affect immunity in different ways. For instance, during acute stress (typically lasting between 5 and 100 minutes), white blood cells move into the skin, where they enhance the immune response. During a stressful event sequence, such as a personal trauma and the events that follow, however, there are typically no overall significant immune changes. Chronic (ongoing) stressors such as unemployment have negative effects on almost all functional measures of immunity. Chronic stress may cause prolonged secretion of cortisol and may accelerate the course of diseases that involve inflammation, including multiple sclerosis, heart disease, and type 2 diabetes.

Mood, personality, behavior, and immune functioning are intertwined. For example, people who are generally pessimistic may neglect the basics of health care, become passive when ill, and fail to engage in health-promoting behaviors. People who are depressed may reduce physical activity and social interaction, which may in turn affect the immune system and the cognitive appraisal of a stressor. Optimism, successful coping, and positive problem solving, on the other hand, may positively influence immunity.

Links Between Stress and Specific Conditions

Although much remains to be learned, it is clear that people who have unresolved chronic stress in their lives or who handle stressors poorly are at risk for a wide range of health problems. In the short term, the problem might be just a cold, a stiff neck, or a stomachache. Over the long term, the problems can be more severe—cardiovascular disease (CVD), high blood pressure, impaired immune function, or accelerated aging.

Cardiovascular Disease During the stress response, heart rate increases and blood vessels constrict, causing blood pressure to rise. Chronic high blood pressure is a major cause of atherosclerosis, a disease in which blood vessels become damaged and caked with fatty deposits. These deposits can block arteries, causing heart attacks and strokes.

Certain types of emotional responses may increase a person's risk of CVD. As described earlier, people who tend to react to situations with anger

QUESTIONS FOR CRITICAL THINKING AND REFLECTION
Have you ever been so stressed that you felt ill in some way? If so, what were your symptoms? How did you handle them? Did the experience affect the way you reacted to other stressful events?

TERMS

allostatic load The long-term negative impact of the stress response on the body.

psychoneuroimmunology (PNI) The study of the interactions among the nervous, endocrine, and immune systems.

Two-thirds of visits to family practitioners are due to stress-related issues.

—**American Academy of Family Physicians, 2007**

QUICK STATS

Stress and Your Brain

Like a computer that registers information in response to typing on a keyboard, your brain is able to respond to and store information about changes in your environment. Unlike a computer, your brain has the attribute of *plasticity*—it physically changes its structure and function in response to experience. Plasticity allows your brain to be altered by psychological stress.

Moderate stress enhances the ability to acquire and remember information, while high levels of acute stress can impair learning. For example, people can often remember minute details following a fender bender but can't recall the events surrounding a major car crash. Thus, it is good to be a little nervous before an exam—but not too nervous.

The effects of stress on brain form and function are apparent in

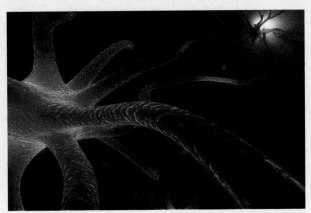

a structure called the *hippocampus*, which is involved in learning and memory. High levels of chronic stress cause brain cells (neurons) in the hippocampus to shrink in size or die, thus impairing learning and memory. New research in neuroscience has revealed that the hippocampus actually grows new neurons

during adulthood. However, stress acts to reduce new cell birth in the hippocampus, reducing the replacement of lost neurons. Together, these effects of stress result in fewer neurons and fewer connections between neurons in the hippocampus, thus decreasing the capacity for information processing.

People who are depressed or who suffer from post-traumatic stress disorder have higher levels of stress hormones in their bloodstream and smaller hippocampi than others. Even in the absence of a serious disorder, it is thought that the accumulation of stress effects across the life span can contribute to brain aging. Thus, the way you cope with stress can affect the way your brain works both immediately and over the long term.

and hostility are more likely to have heart attacks than are people with a less explosive, more trusting personality.

Psychological Problems The hormones and other chemicals released during the stress response cause emotional as well as physical changes (see the box "Stress and Your Brain"). Stress also activates the enzyme PKC, which influences the brain's prefrontal cortex. Excess PKC can negatively affect focus, judgment, and the ability to think clearly. Moreover, many stressors are inherently anxiety-producing, depressing, or both. Stress has been found to contribute to psychological problems such as depression, panic attacks, anxiety, eating disorders, and post-traumatic stress disorder (PTSD). PTSD, which afflicts war veterans, rape and child abuse survivors, and others who have suffered or witnessed severe trauma, is characterized by nightmares, flashbacks, and a diminished capacity to experience or express emotion.

Altered Functioning of the Immune System PNI research helps explain how stress affects the immune system. Some of the health problems linked to stress-related changes in immune function include vulnerability to colds and other infections, asthma and allergy attacks, susceptibility to cancer, and flare-ups of chronic diseases such as genital herpes and HIV infection.

Other Health Problems Many other health problems may be caused or worsened by excessive stress, including the following:

- Digestive problems such as stomachaches, diarrhea, constipation, irritable bowel syndrome, and ulcers
- Tension headaches and migraines (see the box "Headaches: A Common Symptom of Stress," on p. 32)
- Insomnia and fatigue
- Injuries, including on-the-job injuries caused by repetitive strain
- Menstrual irregularities, impotence, and pregnancy complications

COMMON SOURCES OF STRESS

Being able to recognize potential sources of stress is an important step in successfully managing the stress in your life.

Major Life Changes

Any major change in your life that requires adjustment and accommodation can be a source of stress. Early adulthood and the college years are associated with many significant changes, such as moving out of the family home. Even changes typically thought of as positive—graduation, job promotion, marriage—can be stressful.

Clusters of life changes, particularly those that are perceived negatively, may be linked to health problems in some people. Personality and coping skills, however, are important moderating influences. People with a strong

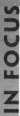

Headaches: A Common Symptom of Stress

More than 45 million Americans suffer from chronic, recurrent headaches. Headaches come in various types but are often grouped into three major categories: tension headaches, migraines, and cluster headaches. Other types of headaches have underlying organic causes, such as sinus congestion or infection.

Tension Headaches

Approximately 90% of all headaches are *tension headaches*, characterized by a dull, steady pain, usually on both sides of the head. It may feel as though a band of pressure is tightening around the head, and the pain may extend to the neck and shoulders. Acute tension headaches may last from hours to days, while chronic tension headaches may occur almost every day for months or even years.

Psychological stress, poor posture, and immobility are the leading causes of tension headaches. There is no cure, but the pain can sometimes be relieved with over-the-counter painkillers and with therapies such as massage, acupuncture, relaxation, hot or cold showers, and rest.

If your headaches are frequent, keep a diary with details about the events surrounding each one. If you can identify the stressors that are consistently associated with your headaches, you can begin to gain more control over the situation. If you suffer persistent tension headaches, you should consult your physician.

Migraines

Migraines typically progress through a series of stages lasting from several minutes to several days. They may produce a variety of symptoms, including throbbing pain that starts on one side of the head and may spread; heightened sensitivity to light; visual disturbances such as flashing lights; nausea; and fatigue. About 70% of migraine sufferers are women, and migraine headaches may have a genetic component.

Research suggests that people who get migraines may have abnormally excitable nerve cells in their brains. When triggered, these nerve cells send a wave of electrical activity throughout the brain, which in turn causes migraine symptoms. Potential triggers include menstruation, stress, fatigue, atmospheric changes, specific sounds or odors, and certain foods. The frequency of attacks varies from a few in a lifetime to several per week.

Keeping a headache journal can help a migraine sufferer identify headache triggers—the first step to avoiding them. In addition, many new treatments can help reduce the frequency, severity, and duration of migraines.

Cluster Headaches

Cluster headaches are extremely severe headaches that cause intense pain in and around one eye. They usually occur in clusters of one to three headaches each day over a period of weeks or

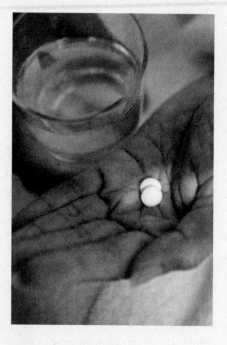

months, alternating with periods of remission in which no headaches occur. About 90% of people with cluster headaches are male.

There is no known cause or cure for cluster headaches, but a number of treatments are available. During cluster periods, it is important to refrain from smoking cigarettes and drinking alcohol, because these activities can trigger attacks.

For more information on treating headaches and when a headache may signal a serious illness, see Appendix B.

support network and a stress-resistant personality are less likely to become ill in response to life changes than people with fewer resources.

Daily Hassles

Although major life changes are undoubtedly stressful, they seldom occur regularly. Researchers have proposed that minor problems—life's daily hassles, such as losing your keys or wallet—can be an even greater source of stress because they occur much more often.

People who perceive hassles negatively are likely to experience a moderate stress response every time they are faced with one. Over time, this can take a significant toll on

health. Studies indicate that for some people, daily hassles contribute to a general decrease in overall wellness.

College Stressors

College is a time of major changes and minor hassles. For many students, college means being away from home and family for the first time. Nearly all students share stresses like the following:

• *Academic stress.* Exams, grades, and an endless workload await every college student but can be especially troublesome for young students just out of high school.

- *Interpersonal stress.* Most students are more than just students; they are also friends, children, employees, spouses, parents, and so on. Managing relationships while juggling the rigors of college life can be daunting, especially if some friends or family are less than supportive.
- *Time pressures.* Class schedules, assignments, and deadlines are an inescapable part of college life. But these time pressures can be drastically compounded for students who also have a job and/or family responsibilities.
- *Financial concerns.* The majority of college students need financial aid not just to cover the cost of tuition but to survive from day to day while in school. For many, college life isn't possible without a job, and the pressure to stay afloat financially competes with academic and other stressors.
- *Worries about the future.* As college life comes to an end, students face the reality of life after college. This means thinking about a career, choosing a place to live, and leaving the friends and routines of school behind.

As mentioned earlier, test anxiety is a source of stress for many students. To learn some proven techniques for overcoming test anxiety, see the Behavior Change Strategy at the end of this chapter.

Job-Related Stressors

Americans rate their jobs as a key source of stress in their lives. Tight schedules and overtime leave less time to exercise, socialize, and engage in other stress-proofing activities. More than one-third of Americans report that they always feel rushed, and nearly half say they would give up a day's pay for a day off. Worries about job performance, salary, and job security and interactions with bosses, co-workers, and customers can contribute to stress. High levels of job stress are also common for people who are left out of important decisions relating to their jobs. When workers are given the opportunity to shape how their jobs are performed, job satisfaction goes up and stress levels go down.

If job-related (or college-related) stress is severe or chronic, the result can be **burnout,** a state of physical, mental, and emotional exhaustion. Burnout occurs most often in highly motivated and driven individuals who come to feel that their work is not recognized or that they are not accomplishing their goals. People in the helping professions—teachers, social workers, caregivers, police officers, and so on—are also prone to burnout. For some people who suffer from burnout, a vacation or leave of absence may be appropriate. For others, a reduced work schedule, better communication with superiors, or a change in job goals may be necessary. Improving time-management skills can also help.

Nearly 40 million workdays are lost annually because of illness. Stress-related sleep disturbances, headaches, and damaged relationships are quick to arise and identify, but the effects of job stress on chronic diseases are harder to see because they take longer to develop. It's telling, however, that health care costs are nearly 50% greater for workers with high levels of stress.

Social Stressors

Social networks can be real or virtual. Both types can help improve your ability to deal with stress, but any social network can also become a stressor in itself.

Real Social Networks Although social support is a key buffer against stress, your interactions with others can themselves be a source of stress. The college years, in particular, can be a time of great change in interpersonal relationships. The larger community where you live can also act as a stressor.

Social stressors include prejudice and discrimination. You may feel stress as you try to relate to people of other ethnic or socioeconomic groups. If you are a member of a minority ethnic group, you may feel pressure to assimilate into mainstream society, or to spend as much time as possible with others who share your ethnicity or background. If English is not your first language, you may face the added burden of conducting daily activities in a language with which you are not comfortable. All these pressures can become significant sources of stress. (See the box "Diverse Populations, Discrimination, and Stress" on p. 34 for more information.)

Virtual Social Networks New technologies can potentially be time-savers because we don't have to go home or to the office to check our e-mail or phone messages, and we can make a call on a cell phone instead of jotting down notes to pass on at a later time. Telecommuting can ease the time pressures on people who find it necessary to work from home, such as parents with young children or people with disabilities.

Increased electronic interactivity, however, can also impinge on our personal space, waste time, and cause stress. On a typical day, for example, you may check for e-mail or voice mail several times, only to find no messages waiting for you. When messages are there, you may often find that some of them are of little or no value. If you are "always on" (that is, always available by voice or text messaging), some friends or colleagues may think it's all right to contact you any time, even if you're in class or trying to work. The convenience of staying electronically connected, therefore, comes at a price.

burnout A state of physical, mental, and emotional exhaustion.

Diverse Populations, Discrimination, and Stress

Stress Is universal, but in diverse multi-ethnic and multicultural nations such as the United States, some groups face special stressors and have higher-than-average rates of stress-related physical and emotional problems. These groups include ethnic minorities, the poor, those with disabilities, and those with atypical sexual orientations.

Discrimination occurs when people act according to their prejudices—biased, negative attitudes toward some group. Blatant examples are painting a swastika on a Jewish studies house or defacing a sculpture depicting a same-sex couple holding hands. More subtle examples are when an African American student notices that white shopkeepers in a mostly white college town tend to keep a close eye on him; a male-to-female transgender individual is treated with less respect by her professors and peers; a student using a wheelchair finds no accessible bathrooms; or an obese woman overhears remarks about eating and self-control.

Recent immigrants to the United States have to learn to live in a new society. This requires a balance between assimilating and changing to be like the majority, and maintaining a connection to their own culture, language, and religion. The process of acculturation is generally stressful, especially when the person's background is radically different from that of the people he or she is now living among. Parental expectations generate stress if they are too high or too low. If too high, the child may work too hard in an attempt to succeed at everything; if too low, the child may not work hard enough to succeed at anything.

Both immigrants and minorities that have lived for generations in the United States can face job- and school-related stressors because of stereotypes and discrimination. They may make less money in comparable jobs with comparable levels of education and may find it more difficult to achieve leadership positions. However, on a positive note, many who experience hardship, disability, or prejudice develop effective, goal-directed

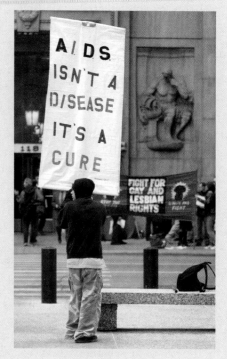

coping skills and are successful at overcoming obstacles and managing the stress they face.

Other Stressors

Have you tried to eat at a restaurant where the food was great, but the atmosphere was so noisy that it put you on edge? This is an example of an environmental stress—a condition or event in the physical environment that causes stress.

Like the noisy atmosphere of some restaurants, many environmental stressors are mere inconveniences that are easy to avoid. Others, such as pollen or construction noise, may be an unavoidable daily source of stress. For those who live in poor or violent neighborhoods or in a war-torn country, environmental stressors can be major stressors (see the box "Coping After Violence on Campus" on p. 35).

Some stressors are found not in our environment but within ourselves. We pressure ourselves to reach goals and

continuously evaluate our progress and performance. Setting goals and striving to reach them can enhance self-esteem if the goals are reasonable. Unrealistic expectations, however, can be a significant source of stress and can damage self-esteem. Other internal stressors are physical and emotional states such as illness and exhaustion; these can be both a cause and an effect of unmanaged stress.

MANAGING STRESS

You can control the stress in your life by taking the following steps:

- Shore up your support system.
- Improve your communication skills.
- Develop healthy exercise, eating, and sleeping habits.
- Learn to identify and moderate individual stressors.

The effort required is well worth the time. People who manage stress effectively not only are healthier but have more time to enjoy life and accomplish goals.

Social Support

The ability to share fears, frustrations, and joys makes life richer. Having the support of friends and family members seems to contribute to the well-being of body and mind.

QUESTIONS FOR CRITICAL THINKING AND REFLECTION

What are the top two or three stressors in your life right now? Are they new to your life—as part of your college experience—or are they stressors you've experienced in the past? Do they include both positive and negative experiences (eustress and distress)?

Coping After Violence on the Campus

Stories of violence on American campuses have become all-too familiar:

• In March 2008, an Auburn University student died from gunshot wounds sustained during a robbery. One day later, a University of North Carolina student was killed while being robbed in Chapel Hill, N.C.

• On February 14, 2008, a former Northern Illinois University student walked into one of the school's lecture halls and fatally shot five students before killing himself. Gunfire injured at least 16 other people.

• Just a few days earlier, a student at Louisiana Technical College in Baton Rouge shot two other students to death, then killed herself as classmates watched in horror.

• On April 16, 2007, a student killed 28 students and 5 teachers and injured 29 others during two attacks at Virginia Polytechnic Institute and State University (Virginia Tech). The attacker was acting out fantasies of revenge in a drama that held the nation's attention for weeks.

School shootings are not uniquely American events. They have also occurred at schools in Germany (2003) and Finland (2007)—both countries where access to guns is much more tightly controlled than in the United States.

People react to news of school violence in different ways, depending on their proximity to the event and its recency. In the case of school massacres,

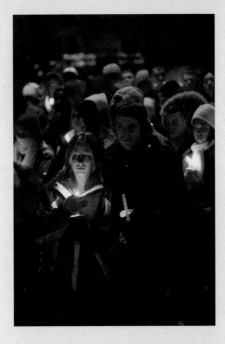

people far from the site may suffer emotional reactions simply from watching endless coverage on television.

Responses to violence or reports of violence include disbelief, shock, fear, anger, resentment, anxiety, mood swings, irritability, sadness, depression, panic, guilt, apathy, feelings of isolation or powerlessness, and many of the symptoms of excess stress. Most of those affected return to normal after a few weeks or months, but a few go on to develop post-traumatic stress disorder (PTSD), a more serious condition.

In the case of the Virginia Tech shootings, the school and community mobi-

lized quickly to respond to the expected surge in behavioral health needs generated by the attack. Hotline calls and emergency room visits increased dramatically, especially during the second and third weeks following the shootings. Information sources and support groups were established for people grieving the loss of friends, family, neighbors, or colleagues. Volunteers contacted each family that was directly affected by the shootings to offer help in making arrangements and other services.

If you are affected by a disastrous event such as a school shooting or terrorist attack, take these steps:

• Be sure that you have the best information about what happened, whether a continuing risk is present, and what you can do to avoid it. That information may be posted on Web sites or on local radio or TV stations.

• Don't expose yourself to so much media coverage that you begin to feel overwhelmed by it.

• Take care of yourself. Use the stress-relief techniques discussed in this chapter.

• Share your feelings and concerns with others. Be a supportive listener.

• If you feel able, help others in any way you can, such as by volunteering to work with victims.

• If you feel emotionally distressed days or weeks after the event, consider asking for professional help.

Social support can provide a critical counterbalance to the stress in our lives. Give yourself time to develop and maintain a network of people you can count on for emotional support, feedback, and nurturing. If you believe you don't have enough social support, consider becoming a volunteer to help build your network of friends and to enhance your spiritual wellness.

Communication

Communicating in an assertive way that respects the rights of others—while protecting your own rights—can prevent potentially stressful situations from getting out of control. Better communication skills can help everyone form and maintain healthy relationships. If you typically suppress your feelings, you might want to take an asser-

tiveness training course that can help you identify and change your patterns of communication. If you have trouble controlling your anger, you may benefit from learning anger management strategies.

Exercise

Exercise helps maintain a healthy body and mind and even stimulates the birth of new brain cells. Regular physical activity can also reduce many of the negative effects of stress. Consider the following examples:

• Taking a long walk can help decrease anxiety and blood pressure.

• A brisk 10-minute walk can leave you feeling more relaxed and energetic for up to 2 hours.

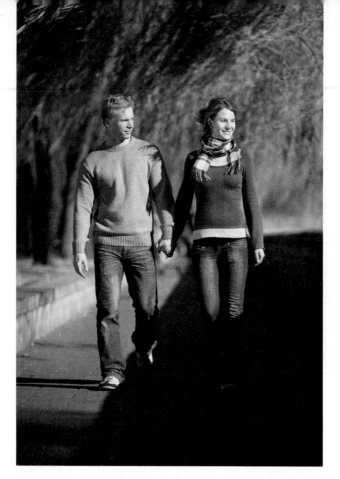

Exercise—even light activity—can be an effective antidote to stress.

Nutrition

A healthy diet gives you an energy bank to draw from whenever you experience stress. Eating wisely also can enhance your feelings of self-control and self-esteem. Learning the principles of sound nutrition is easy, and sensible eating habits rapidly become second nature when practiced regularly.

While your diet has an effect on the way your body handles stress, the reverse is also true. Excess stress can negatively affect the way you eat. Many people, for example, respond to stress by overeating; other people skip meals or stop eating altogether during stressful periods. Both responses are not only ineffective (they don't address the causes of stress), but potentially unhealthy.

Sleep

Most adults need 7–9 hours of sleep every night to stay healthy and perform their best. Getting enough sleep isn't just good for you physically; adequate sleep also improves mood, fosters feelings of competence and self-worth, enhances mental functioning, and supports emotional functioning.

How Sleep Works   Sleep occurs in two phases: **rapid eye movement (REM) sleep** and **non-rapid eye movement (NREM) sleep.** A sleeper goes through several cycles of NREM and REM sleep each night.

NREM sleep actually includes four stages of successively deeper sleep. As you move through these stages of sleep, a variety of physiological changes occur, including the following:

- Blood pressure drops.
- Respiration and heart rates slow.
- Body temperature declines.
- Growth hormone is released.
- Brain wave patterns become slow and even.

During REM sleep, dreams occur. REM sleep is characterized by the rapid movement of the eyes under closed eyelids. Heart rate, blood pressure, and breathing rate rise, and brain activity increases to levels equal to or greater than those during waking hours. Muscles in the limbs relax completely, resulting in a temporary paralysis. (This total relaxation may prevent you from acting out your dreams while you're asleep.)

Sleep and Stress   Stress hormone levels in the bloodstream vary throughout the day and are related to sleep patterns. Peak concentrations occur in the early morning, followed by a slow decline during the day and evening (Figure 2.4, p. 37). Concentrations return to peak levels during the final stages of sleep and in the early morning hours. Stress hormone levels are low during NREM sleep and increase during REM sleep. With each successive

- People who exercise regularly react with milder physical stress responses before, during, and after exposure to stressors.

- In a study, people who took three brisk 45-minute walks each week for 3 months reported that they perceived fewer daily hassles. Their sense of wellness also increased.

These findings should not be surprising, because the stress response mobilizes energy resources and readies the body for physical emergencies. If you experience stress and do not physically exert yourself, you are not completing the energy cycle. You may not be able to exercise while your daily stressors occur—during class, for example, or while sitting in a traffic jam—but you can be active at other times of the day. Physical activity allows you to expend the nervous energy you have built up and trains your body to more readily achieve homeostasis following stressful situations.

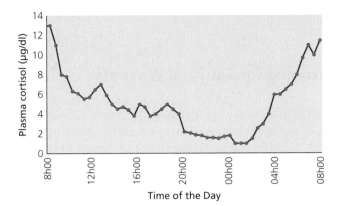

FIGURE 2.4 Changing levels of stress hormones in the bloodstream. Stress hormones, such as cortisol, fluctuate throughout the day and night and reach a high level during the last stages of sleep.

SOURCE: Palma B. D., et al. 2008. *Immune Outcomes of Sleep Disorders: The Hypothalamic-Pituitary-Adrenal Axis as a Modulatory Factor, Revista Brasileiro de Psiquiatria,* vol. 29 suppl., Figure 3. 1 São Paulo May 2007.

sleep cycle during the night, REM sleep lasts a little longer. This increase in REM sleep duration with each sleep cycle may underlie the progressive increase in circulating stress hormones during the final stages of sleep.

Even though stress hormones are released during sleep, it is the *lack* of sleep that has the greatest impact on stress. In someone who is suffering from **sleep deprivation** (not getting enough sleep over time), mental and physical processes steadily deteriorate. A sleep-deprived person experiences headaches, feels irritable, is unable to concentrate, and is more prone to forgetfulness. Poor-quality sleep has long been associated with stress and depression. A small 2008 study of female college students further associated sleep deprivation with an increased risk of suicide.

Acute sleep deprivation slows the daytime decline in stress hormones, so evening levels are higher than normal. A decrease in total sleep time also causes an increase in the level of stress hormones. Together, these changes may cause an increase in stress hormone levels throughout the day and may contribute to physical and mental exhaustion. Extreme sleep deprivation can lead to hallucinations and other psychotic symptoms, as well as to a significant increase in heart attack risk.

Sleep Problems According to the National Sleep Foundation's 2008 Sleep in America Poll, adults sleep an average of 6 hours and 40 minutes per night. (Compare this to the recommended 7–9 hours per night.) Although many of us can attribute the lack of sleep to long work days and family responsibilities, as many as 70 million Americans suffer from chronic sleep disorders—medical conditions that prevent them from sleeping well.

According to the Institute of Medicine, more than 50% of adults have trouble falling asleep or staying asleep—a condition called **insomnia.** The most common causes of insomnia are lifestyle factors, such as high caffeine or alco-

hol intake before bedtime; medical problems, such as a breathing disorder; and stress. About 75% of people who suffer from chronic insomnia report some stressful life event at the onset of their sleeping problems.

Another type of chronic sleep problem, called **sleep apnea,** occurs when a person stops breathing while asleep. Apnea can be caused by a number of factors, but it typically results when the soft tissue at the back of the mouth (such as the tongue or soft palate) "collapses" during sleep, blocking the airway. When breathing is interrupted, so is sleep, as the sleeper awakens repeatedly throughout the night to begin breathing again. In most cases, this occurs without the sleeper's even being aware of it. However, the disruption to sleep can be significant, and over time acute sleep deprivation can result from apnea. There are several treatments for apnea, including the use of medications, a special apparatus that helps keep the airway open during sleep, and surgery.

Time Management

Learning to manage your time can be crucial to coping with everyday stressors. Overcommitment, procrastination, and even boredom are significant stressors for many people. Along with gaining control of nutrition and exercise to maintain a healthy energy balance, time management is an important element in a wellness program. Try these strategies for improving your time-management skills:

- *Set priorities.* Divide your tasks into three groups: essential, important, and trivial. Focus on the first two, and ignore the third.
- *Schedule tasks for peak efficiency.* You've undoubtedly noticed you're most productive at certain times of

rapid eye movement (REM) sleep The portion of the sleep cycle during which dreaming occurs.

non-rapid eye movement (non-REM) sleep The portion of the sleep cycle that involves deep sleep; non-REM sleep includes four states of successively deeper sleep.

sleep deprivation A lack of sleep over a period of time.

insomnia A sleep problem involving the inability to fall or stay asleep; affects more than 50% of adults.

sleep apnea The interruption of normal breathing during sleep.

TERMS

the day (or night). Schedule as many of your tasks for those hours as you can, and stick to your schedule.

• **Set realistic goals and write them down.** Attainable goals spur you on. Impossible goals, by definition, cause frustration and failure. Fully commit yourself to achieving your goals by putting them in writing.

• **Budget enough time.** For each project you undertake, calculate how long it will take to complete. Then tack on another 10–15%, or even 25%, as a buffer.

• **Break up long-term goals into short-term ones.** Instead of waiting for or relying on large blocks of time, use short amounts of time to start a project or keep it moving.

• **Visualize the achievement of your goals.** By mentally rehearsing your performance of a task, you will be able to reach your goal more smoothly.

• **Keep track of the tasks you put off.** Analyze the reasons you procrastinate. If the task is difficult or unpleasant, look for ways to make it easier or more fun. For example, if you find the readings for one of your classes particularly difficult, choose an especially nice setting for your reading, and then reward yourself each time you complete a section or chapter.

• **Consider doing your least-favorite tasks first.** Once you have the most unpleasant ones out of the way, you can work on the tasks you enjoy more.

• **Consolidate tasks when possible.** For example, try walking to the store so that you run your errands and exercise in the same block of time.

• **Identify quick transitional tasks.** Keep a list of 5- to 10-minute tasks you can do while waiting or between other tasks, such as watering your plants, doing the dishes, or checking a homework assignment.

• **Delegate responsibility.** Asking for help when you have too much to do is no cop-out; it's good time management. Just don't delegate the jobs you know you should do yourself.

• **Say no when necessary.** If the demands made on you don't seem reasonable, say no—tactfully, but without guilt or apology.

• **Give yourself a break.** Allow time for play—free, unstructured time when you can ignore the clock. Don't consider this a waste of time. Play renews you and enables you to work more efficiently.

• **Avoid your personal "time sinks."** You can probably identify your own time sinks—activities like watching television, surfing the Internet, or talking on the phone that consistently use up more time than you anticipate and put you behind schedule. Some days, it may be best to avoid problematic activities altogether; for example, if you have a big paper due, don't sit down for a 5-minute TV break if it is likely to turn into a 2-hour break. Try a 5-minute walk if you need to clear your head.

• **Stop thinking or talking about what you're going to do, and just do it!** Sometimes the best solution for procrastination is to stop waiting for the right moment and just get started. You will probably find that things are not as bad as you feared, and your momentum will keep you going.

Striving for Spiritual Wellness

Spiritual wellness is associated with greater coping skills and higher levels of overall wellness. It is a very personal wellness component, and there are many ways to develop it. Researchers have linked spiritual wellness to longer life expectancy, reduced risk of disease, faster recovery, and improved emotional health.

Spirituality provides an ethical path to personal fulfillment that includes connectedness with self, others, and a higher power or larger reality. Spiritual wellness can make you more aware of your personal values and can help clarify them. Without an awareness of personal values, you might be driven by immediate desires and the passing demands of others. Living according to values means considering your options carefully before making a choice, choosing between options without succumbing to outside pressures that oppose your values, and making a choice and acting on it rather than doing nothing.

Confiding in Yourself Through Writing

Keeping a diary is analogous to confiding in others, except that you are confiding in yourself. This form of coping with severe stress may be especially helpful for those who are shy or introverted and find it difficult to open up to others. Although writing about traumatic and stressful events may have a short-term negative effect on mood, over the long term, stress is reduced and positive changes in health occur. A key to promoting health and well-being through journaling is to write about your emotional responses to stressful events. Set aside a special time each day or week to write down your feelings about stressful events in your life.

49,382 agencies need help from volunteers.

—The United Way, 2008

Cognitive Techniques

Some stressors arise in our own minds. Ideas, beliefs, perceptions, and patterns of thinking can add to our stress level. Each of the following techniques can help you change unhealthy thought patterns to ones that will help you cope with stress. As with any skill, mastering these techniques takes practice and patience.

Think and Act Constructively Think back to the worries you had last week. How many of them were needless? Think about things you *can* control. Try to stand aside from the problem, consider the positive steps you can take to solve it, and then carry them out. Remember, if you can successfully predict that a stressor will occur, you can better control your response to it.

Take Control   A situation often feels more stressful if you feel you're not in control of it. Time may seem to be slipping away before a big exam, for example. Unexpected obstacles may appear in your path, throwing you off course. When you feel your environment is controlling you instead of the other way around, take charge! Concentrate on what is possible to control, and set realistic goals. Be confident of your ability to succeed.

Problem-Solve   Students with greater problem-solving abilities report easier adjustment to university life, higher motivation levels, lower stress levels, and higher grades. When you find yourself stewing over a problem, sit down with a piece of paper and do some problem solving. Try this approach:

1. Define the problem in one or two sentences.
2. Identify the causes of the problem.
3. Consider alternative solutions; don't just stop with the most obvious one.
4. Weigh positive and negative consequences for each alternative.
5. Make a decision—choose a solution.
6. Make a list of what you will need to do to act on your decision.
7. Begin to carry out your list; if you're unable to do that, temporarily turn to other things.
8. Evaluate the outcome and revise your approach if necessary.

Modify Your Expectations   Expectations are exhausting and restricting. The fewer expectations you have, the more you can live spontaneously and joyfully. The more you expect from others, the more often you will feel let down. And trying to meet the expectations others have of you is often futile.

Stay Positive   If you beat up on yourself—"Late for class again! You can't even cope with college! How do you expect to ever hold down a professional job?"—change your inner dialogue. Talk to yourself as you would to a child you love: "You're a smart, capable person. You've solved other problems; you'll handle this one. Tomorrow you'll simply schedule things so you get to class with a few minutes to spare."

Cultivate Your Sense of Humor   When it comes to stress, laughter may be the best medicine. Even a fleeting smile produces changes in your autonomic nervous system that can lift your spirits. And a few minutes of belly laughing can be as invigorating as brisk exercise. Hearty

laughter elevates your heart rate, aids digestion, eases pain, and triggers the release of endorphins and other pleasurable and stimulating chemicals in the brain. After a good laugh, your muscles go slack; your pulse and blood pressure dip below normal. You are relaxed. Cultivate the ability to laugh at yourself, and you'll have a handy and instantly effective stress reliever.

Focus on What's Important   A major source of stress is trying to store too much data. Forget unimportant details (they will usually be self-evident) and organize important information. One technique you can try is to "chunk" the important material into categories. If your next exam covers three chapters from your textbook, consider each chapter a chunk of information. Then break down each chunk into its three or four most important features. Create a mental outline that allows you to trace your way from the most general category down to the most specific details. This technique can be applied to managing daily responsibilities as well.

Relaxation Techniques

The **relaxation response** is a physiological state characterized by a feeling of warmth and quiet mental alertness. This is the opposite of the fight-or-flight reaction. When the relaxation response is triggered by a relaxation technique, heart rate, breathing, and metabolism slow down. Blood pressure and oxygen consumption decrease. At the same time, blood flow to the brain and skin increases, and brain waves shift from an alert beta rhythm to a relaxed alpha rhythm. Practiced regularly, relaxation techniques can counteract the debilitating effects of stress.

Progressive Relaxation   Unlike most of the others, this simple method requires no imagination, willpower, or self-suggestion. You simply tense, and then relax, the muscles in your body, group by group. The technique, also known as deep muscle relaxation, helps you become aware of the muscle tension that occurs when you're under stress. When you consciously relax those muscles, other systems of the body get the message and ease up on the stress response.

Start, for example, with your right fist. Inhale as you tense it. Exhale as you relax it. Repeat. Next, contract and relax your right upper arm. Repeat. Do the same with your left arm. Then, beginning at your forehead and ending at your feet, contract and relax your other muscle groups. Repeat each contraction at least once, breathing in as you tense, breathing out as you relax. To speed up the process, tense and relax more muscles at one time—

relaxation response   A physiological state characterized by a feeling of warmth and quiet mental alertness.

TERMS

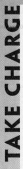

Meditation and the Relaxation Response

Here is a simple technique for eliciting the relaxation response.

The Basic Technique

1. Pick a word, phrase, or object to focus on. If you like, you can choose a word or phrase that has a deep meaning for you, but any word or phrase will work. Some meditators prefer to focus on their breathing.

2. Take a comfortable position in a quiet environment, and close your eyes if you're not focusing on an object.

3. Relax your muscles.

4. Breathe slowly and naturally. If you're using a focus word or phrase, silently repeat it each time you exhale. If you're using an object, focus on it as you breathe.

5. Keep a passive attitude. Disregard thoughts that drift in.

6. Continue for 10–20 minutes, once or twice a day.

7. After you've finished, sit quietly for a few minutes with your eyes first closed and then open. Then stand up.

Suggestions

• Allow relaxation to occur at its own pace; don't try to force it. Don't be surprised if you can't quiet your mind for more than a few seconds at a time; it's not a reason for anger or frustration. The more you ignore the intrusions, the easier doing so will become.

• If you want to time your session, peek at a watch or clock occasionally, but don't set a jarring alarm.

• The technique works best on an empty stomach, before a meal or about 2 hours after eating. Avoid times of day when you're tired—unless you want to fall asleep.

• Although you'll feel refreshed even after the first session, it may take a month or more to get noticeable results. Be patient. Eventually the relaxation response will become so natural that it will occur spontaneously, or on demand, when you sit quietly for a few moments.

---

both arms simultaneously, for instance. With practice, you'll be able to relax very quickly and effectively by clenching and releasing only your fists.

Visualization Also known as *imagery*, **visualization** lets you daydream without guilt. Next time you feel stressed, close your eyes. Imagine yourself floating on a cloud, sitting on a mountaintop, or lying in a meadow. Involve all your senses; imagine the sounds, the smells, and the other sensations that would be part of the scene. Your body will respond as if your imagery were real. An alternative: Close your eyes and imagine a deep purple light filling your body. Now change the color into a soothing gold. As the color lightens, so should your distress.

Visualization can also be used to rehearse for an upcoming event and enhance performance. By experiencing an event ahead of time in your mind, you can practice coping with any difficulties that may arise. Think positively, and you can "psych yourself up" for a successful experience.

Meditation The need to periodically stop our incessant mental chatter is so great that, from ancient times, hundreds of forms of **meditation** have developed in cultures all over the world. Meditation is a way of telling the

visualization A technique for promoting relaxation or improving performance that involves creating or re-creating vivid mental pictures of a place or an experience; also called *imagery*.

meditation A technique for quieting the mind by focusing on a particular word, object (such as a candle flame), or process (such as breathing).

mind to be quiet for a while, and it is potentially useful for reducing stress. According to a 2008 study, college students who learned how to use meditation for stress management were able to significantly reduce their daily stress levels. Further, those students found it easier to forgive others for perceived wrongdoings and spent less time focusing on negative thoughts.

Meditation helps you tune out the world temporarily, removing you from both internal and external sources of stress. The "thinker" takes time out to become the "observer"—calmly attentive, without analyzing, judging, comparing, or rationalizing. Regular practice of this quiet awareness will subtly carry over into your daily life, encouraging physical and emotional balance no matter what confronts you. For a step-by-step description of a basic meditation technique, see the box "Meditation and the Relaxation Response."

Another form of meditation, known as *mindfulness meditation,* involves paying attention to physical sensations, perceptions, thoughts, and imagery. Instead of focusing on a word or object to quiet the mind, you observe thoughts that occur without evaluating or judging them. Development of this ability requires regular practice but may eventually result in a more objective view of one's perceptions. It is believed that a greater understanding of one's moment-to-moment thought processes (mindful awareness) provides a richer and more vital sense of life and improves coping. Studies also suggest that people who rate high in mindfulness are less anxious and better able to deal with stress; among people with specific health problems, mindfulness can provide substantial benefits.

Deep Breathing Your breathing pattern is closely tied to your stress level. Deep, slow breathing is associated

40 CHAPTER 2 STRESS: THE CONSTANT CHALLENGE

Breathing for Relaxation

Controlled breathing can do more than just help you relax. It can also help control pain, anxiety, and other conditions that lead to or are related to stress. There are many methods of controlled breathing. Two of the most popular are belly breathing and tension-release breathing.

Belly Breathing

1. Lie on your back and relax.
2. Place one hand on your chest and the other on your abdomen. Your hands will help you gauge your breathing.
3. Take in a slow, deep breath through your nose and into your belly. Your abdomen should rise significantly (check with your hand); your chest should rise only slightly. Focus on filling your abdomen with air.
4. Exhale through your mouth, gently pushing out the air from your abdomen.

Tension-Release Breathing

1. Lie down or sit in a chair and get comfortable.
2. Take a slow, deep breath into your abdomen. Inhale through your nose. Try to visualize the air moving to every part of your body. As you breathe in, say to yourself, "Breathe in relaxation."
3. Exhale through your mouth. Visualize tension leaving your body. Say to yourself, "Breathe out tension."

There are many variations on these techniques. For example, sit in a chair and raise your arms, shoulders, and chin as you inhale; lower them as you exhale. Or slowly count to 4 as you inhale, then again as you exhale.

Many yoga experts suggest breathing rhythmically, in time with your own heartbeat. Relax and listen closely for the sensation of your heart beating, or monitor your pulse while you breathe. As you inhale, count to 4 or 8 in time with your heartbeat, then repeat the count as you exhale. Breathing in time with soothing music can work well, too.

Experts suggest inhaling through the nose and exhaling through the mouth. Breathe slowly, deeply, and gently. To focus on breathing gently, imagine a candle burning a few inches in front of you. Try to exhale softly enough to make the candle's flame flicker, not hard enough to blow it out.

Practice is important, too. Perform your chosen breathing exercise two or more times daily, for 5–10 minutes per session.

---

with relaxation. Rapid, shallow, often irregular breathing occurs during the stress response. With practice, you can learn to slow and quiet your breathing pattern, thereby also quieting your mind and relaxing your body. Breathing techniques can be used for on-the-spot tension relief as well as for long-term stress reduction.

The primary goal of many breathing exercises is to change your breathing pattern from chest breathing to diaphragmatic ("belly") breathing. For instructions on how to perform diaphragmatic breathing, refer to the box "Breathing for Relaxation."

Yoga Hatha yoga, the most common yoga style practiced in the United States, emphasizes physical balance and breath control. It integrates components of flexibility, muscular strength and endurance, and muscle relaxation; it also sometimes serves as a preliminary to meditation. A session of yoga typically involves a series of postures, each held for a few seconds to several minutes, which involve stretching and balance and coordinated breathing. Yoga can induce the relaxation response and promote body awareness and flexibility. If you are in-

terested in trying yoga, it's best to take a class from an experienced instructor.

Tai chi This martial art (in Chinese, *taijiquan*) is a system of self-defense that incorporates philosophical concepts from Taoism and Confucianism. In addition

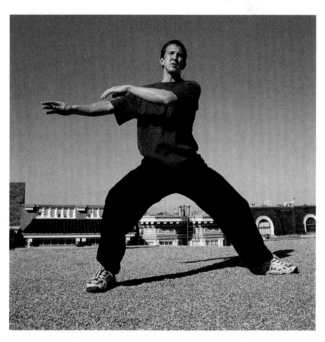

Taijiquan is one of many techniques for inducing the relaxation response.

to self-defense, tai chi aims to bring the body into balance and harmony to promote health and spiritual growth. It teaches practitioners to remain calm and centered, to conserve and concentrate energy, and to manipulate force by becoming part of it—by "going with the flow." Tai chi is considered the gentlest of the martial arts. Instead of quick and powerful movements, tai chi consists of a series of slow, fluid, elegant movements, which reinforce the idea of moving *with* rather than *against* the stressors of everyday life. As with yoga, it's best to start tai chi with a class from an experienced instructor.

Listening to Music Listening to music is another method of inducing relaxation. It can influence pulse, blood pressure, and the electrical activity of muscles. Exposure to soothing music leads to reduced levels of the stress hormone cortisol and causes changes in the electrical activity in the brain. To experience the stress-management benefits of music yourself, set aside a time to listen. Choose music that you enjoy and that makes you feel relaxed.

Other relaxation techniques include biofeedback, massage, hypnosis and self-hypnosis, and autogenic training. To learn more about these and other techniques for inducing the relaxation response, refer to For More Information at the end of the chapter.

Counterproductive Coping Strategies

College is a time when you'll learn to adapt to new and challenging situations and gain skills that will last a lifetime. It is also a time when many people develop habits, in response to stress, that are counterproductive and unhealthy. Such habits can last well beyond graduation.

Tobacco Use Cigarettes and other tobacco products contain nicotine, a chemical that enhances the actions of neurotransmitters. Nicotine can make you feel relaxed and even increase your ability to concentrate, but it is highly addictive, and nicotine dependence itself is considered a psychological disorder. Cigarette smoke also contains substances that cause heart disease, stroke, lung cancer, and emphysema. These negative consequences far outweigh any beneficial effects, and tobacco use should be avoided. The easiest thing to do is to not start.

Use of Alcohol and Other Drugs Having a few drinks might make you feel temporarily at ease, and drinking until you're intoxicated may help you forget your current stressors. However, using alcohol to deal with stress places you at risk for all the short-term and long-term problems associated with alcohol abuse. It also does nothing to address the actual causes of stress in your life. Although moderate alcohol consumption may have potential health benefits for some people, many college students have patterns of drinking that detract from wellness.

Using other psychoactive drugs to cope with stress is also usually counterproductive:

- Caffeine raises cortisol levels and blood pressure and can make you feel more stressed; caffeine also disrupts sleep. Other stimulants, such as amphetamine, can activate the stress response, and they affect the same areas of the brain that are involved in regulating the stress response.
- Marijuana use is relatively common among college students, who report that they smoke marijuana in an effort to induce relaxation and for "mind expansion." Use of marijuana causes a brief period of euphoria and decreased short-term memory and attentional abilities. Physiological effects clearly show that marijuana use doesn't cause relaxation; in fact, some neurochemicals in marijuana act to enhance the stress response, and getting high on a regular basis can elicit panic attacks. To compound this, withdrawal from marijuana may also be associated with an increase in circulating stress hormones.
- Opioids such as morphine and heroin can mimic the effects of your body's natural painkillers and act to reduce anxiety. However, tolerance to opioids develops quickly, and many users become dependent.

Unhealthy Eating Habits Eating is psychologically rewarding. The feelings of satiation and sedation that follow eating produce a relaxed state. However, regular use of eating as a means of coping with stress may lead to unhealthy eating habits. In fact, a 2006 survey by the American Psychological Association revealed that about 25% of Americans use food as a means of coping with stress or anxiety. These "comfort eaters" are twice as likely to be obese as average Americans.

CREATING A PERSONAL PLAN FOR MANAGING STRESS

What are the most important sources of stress in your life? Are you coping successfully with these stressors? No single strategy or program for managing stress will work for everyone, but you can use the principles of behavior management described in Chapter 1 to tailor a plan specifically to your needs.

Identifying Stressors

Before you can learn to manage the stressors in your life, you have to identify them. Many experts recommend

Stress Journal		Date 9-1 8-09
Time	Stressor	Reaction/Coping Strategy
7:45 AM	Tara wouldn't get out of the shower	Yelled at her, started an argument
8:35 AM	Late for class	Slouched in back of room; chewed my nails
11:55 AM	Dad called to discuss credit card debt	Cried, skipped lunch and went out to smoke with Greg
5:30 PM	Power outage at dorm, couldn't study	Took a walk with Tara, made up for arguing this morning, then went to library to study
7:45 PM	Ed called, asked to borrow money	Stayed calm, put down phone and counted to 10, then explained that he already owes me $50.
8:30 PM	Ed called, angry, said he wanted to break up	Argued on phone, then went out with Tara for a drink

FIGURE 2.5 A sample stress journal.
Tracking stressful events and reactions can help you understand how you normally cope with stress.

keeping a stress journal for a week or two (see Figure 2.5). Each time you feel or express a stress response, record the time and the circumstances in your journal. Note what you were doing at the time, what you were thinking or feeling, and the outcome of your response.

After keeping your journal for a few weeks, you should be able to identify your key stressors and spot patterns in how you respond to them. Take note of the people, places, events, and patterns of thought and behavior that cause you the most stress. You may notice, for example, that mornings are usually the most stressful part of your day. Or you may discover that when you're angry at your roommate, you're apt to respond with behaviors that only make matters worse. Keeping a journal allows you to be analytical about what produces the most stress in your life and fills in where your conscious memory fails you.

Designing Your Plan

Once you've identified the key stressors in your life, choose the stress reduction techniques that will work best for you and create an action plan for change. Finding a buddy to work with you can make the process more fun and increase your chances of success. Some experts recommend drawing up a formal contract with yourself.

Whether or not you complete a contract, it's important to design rewards into your plan. You might treat yourself to a special breakfast in a favorite restaurant on the weekend (as long as you eat a nutritious breakfast every weekday morning). It's also important to evaluate your plan regularly and redesign it as your needs change. Under times of increased stress, for example, you might want to focus on good eating, exercise, and relaxation habits. Over time, your new stress-management skills will be-

come almost automatic. You'll feel better, accomplish more, and reduce your risk of disease.

Getting Help

If the techniques discussed so far don't provide you with enough relief from the stress in your life, you might want to learn more about specific areas you wish to work on. Excellent self-help guides can be found in bookstores or

TIPS FOR TODAY AND THE FUTURE
For the stress you can't avoid, develop a range of stress-management techniques and strategies.

RIGHT NOW YOU CAN
- Practice deep breathing for 5–10 minutes.
- Visualize a relaxing, peaceful place and imagine yourself experiencing it as vividly as possible. Stay there as long as you can.
- Do some stretching exercises.
- Get out your datebook and schedule what you'll be doing the rest of today and tomorrow. Pencil in a short walk and a conversation with a friend.

IN THE FUTURE YOU CAN
- Take a class or workshop that can help you overcome a source of stress, such as one in assertiveness training or time management.
- Find a way to build relaxing time into every day. Just 15 minutes of meditation, stretching, or massage can induce the relaxation response.

Dealing with Test Anxiety

Are you a person who doesn't perform as well as you should on tests? Do you find that anxiety interferes with your ability to study effectively before the test and to think clearly in the test situation? If so, you may be experiencing test anxiety—an ineffective response to a stressful situation that can be replaced with more effective responses. If test anxiety is a problem for you, try some of the following strategies:

■ Before the test, find out everything you can about it—its format, the material to be covered, the grading criteria. Ask the instructor for practice materials. Study in advance; don't just cram the night before. Avoid all-nighters.

■ Devise a study plan. This might include forming a study group with one or more classmates or outlining what you will study, when, where, and for how long. Generate your own questions and answer them.

■ In the actual test situation, sit away from possible distractions, listen carefully to instructions, and ask for clarification if you don't understand a direction.

■ During the test, answer the easiest questions first. If you don't know an answer and there is no penalty for incorrect answers, guess. If there are several questions you have difficulty answering, review the ones you have already handled. Figure out approximately how much time you have to cover each question.

■ For math problems, try to estimate the answer before doing the precise calculations.

■ For true-false questions, look for qualifiers such as *always* and *never*. Such questions are likely to be false.

■ For essay questions, look for key words in the question that indicate what the instructor is looking for in the answer. Develop a brief outline of your answer, sketching out what you will cover. Stick to your outline, and keep track of the time you're spending on your answer. Don't get caught with unanswered questions when time is up.

■ Remain calm and focused throughout the test. Don't let negative thoughts rattle you. Avoid worrying about past performance, how others are doing, or the negative consequences of a poor test grade. If you start to become nervous, take some deep breaths and relax your muscles completely for a minute or so.

The best way to counter test anxiety is with successful test-taking experiences. The more times you succeed, the more your test anxiety will recede. If you find that these methods aren't sufficient to get your anxiety under control, you may want to seek professional help.

---

the library. Additional resources are listed in the For More Information section at the end of the chapter.

Your student health center or student affairs office can tell you whether your campus has a peer counseling program. Such programs are usually staffed by volunteer students with special training that emphasizes maintaining confidentiality. Peer counselors can guide you to other campus or community resources or can simply provide understanding. Support groups and short-term psychotherapy can also be tremendously helpful in dealing with stress-related problems.

SUMMARY

• When confronted with a stressor, the body undergoes a set of physical changes known as the fight-or-flight reaction. The sympathetic nervous system and endocrine system act on many targets in the body to prepare it for action.

• Emotional and behavioral responses to stressors vary among individuals. Ineffective responses increase stress but can be moderated or changed.

• Factors that influence emotional and behavioral responses to stressors include personality, cultural background, gender, and past experiences.

• The general adaptation syndrome (GAS) has three stages: alarm, resistance, and exhaustion.

• A high allostatic load characterized by prolonged or repeated exposure to stress hormones can increase a person's risk of health problems.

• Psychoneuroimmunology (PNI) looks at how the physiological changes of the stress response affect the immune system and thereby increase the risk of illness.

• Health problems linked to stress include CVD, colds and other infections, asthma and allergies, cancer, flare-ups of chronic diseases, psychological problems, digestive problems, headaches, insomnia, and injuries.

• A cluster of major life events that require adjustment and accommodation can lead to increased stress and an increased risk of health problems. Minor daily hassles increase stress if they are perceived negatively.

• Sources of stress associated with college may be academic, interpersonal, time-related, or financial pressures.

• Job-related stress is common, particularly for employees who have little control over decisions relating to their jobs. If stress is severe or prolonged, burnout may occur.

• New and changing relationships, prejudice, and discrimination are examples of interpersonal and social stressors.

- Social support systems help buffer people against the effects of stress and make illness less likely. Good communication skills foster healthy relationships.

- Exercise, nutrition, sleep, and time management are wellness behaviors that reduce stress and increase energy.

- Cognitive techniques for managing stress involve developing new and healthy patterns of thinking, such as practicing problem solving, monitoring self-talk, and cultivating a sense of humor.

- The relaxation response is the opposite of the fight-or-flight reaction. Techniques that trigger it, including progressive relaxation, imagery, meditation, and deep breathing, counteract the effects of chronic stress. Counterproductive coping strategies include smoking, drinking, and unhealthy eating.

- A successful individualized plan for coping with stress begins with the use of a stress journal or log to identify and study stressors and inappropriate behavioral responses. Completing a contract and recruiting a buddy can help your stress-management plan succeed.

- Additional help in dealing with stress is available from self-help books, peer counseling, support groups, and psychotherapy.

FOR MORE INFORMATION

BOOKS

Blonna, R. 2007. *Coping with Stress in a Changing World.* 4th ed. New York: McGraw-Hill. *A comprehensive guide to stress management that includes separate chapters on college stressors and spirituality.*

Greenberg, J. 2009. *Comprehensive Stress Management.* 11th ed. New York: McGraw-Hill. *Provides a clear explanation of the physical, psychological, sociological, and spiritual aspects of stress and offers numerous stress-management techniques.*

Kabat-Zinn, J. 2006. *Coming to Our Senses: Healing Ourselves and the World Through Mindfulness.* New York: Hyperion. *Explores the connections among mindfulness, health, physical, and spiritual well-being.*

Pennebaker, J. W. 2004. *Writing to Heal: A Guided Journal for Recovering from Trauma and Emotional Upheaval.* Oakland, Calif.: New Harbinger Press. *Provides information about using journaling to cope with stress.*

Sapolsky, R. M. 2004. *Why Zebras Don't Get Ulcers,* 3rd ed. New York: Henry Holt. *A scientific guide to stress, stress-related diseases, and coping.*

Seaward, B. L. 2006. *Managing Stress: Principles and Strategies for Health and Well-Being,* 5th ed. Boston: Jones and Bartlett. *A comprehensive textbook for college students.*

ORGANIZATIONS AND WEB SITES

American Psychiatric Association: Healthy Minds, Healthy Lives. Provides information on mental wellness developed especially for college students.

http://www.healthyminds.org/collegementalhealth.cfm
American Psychological Association. Provides information on stress management and psychological disorders.
http://www.apa.org; http://apahelpcenter.org
Association for Applied Psychophysiology and Biofeedback. Provides information about biofeedback and referrals to certified biofeedback practitioners.
http://www.aapb.org
Benson-Henry Institute for Mind Body Medicine. Provides information about stress-management and relaxation techniques.
http://www.mbmi.org
Medical Basis for Stress. Includes information on recognizing stress and on the physiological basis of stress, self-assessments for stress levels, and techniques for managing stress.
http://www.teachhealth.com
National Institute for Occupational Safety and Health (NIOSH). Provides information and links on job stress.
http://www.cdc.gov/niosh/topics/stress
National Institute of Mental Health (NIMH). Publishes informative brochures about stress and stress management as well as other aspects of mental health.
http://www.nimh.nih.gov
National Sleep Foundation. Provides information about sleep and how to overcome sleep problems such as insomnia and jet lag.
http://www.sleepfoundation.org
Student Counseling Virtual Pamphlet Collection. Links to online pamphlets from student counseling centers; topics include stress, sleep, and time management.
http://counseling.uchicago.edu/resources/virtualpamphlets/

SELECTED BIBLIOGRAPHY

American College Health Association. 2007. *American College Health Association—National College Health Assessment (ACHA—NCHA) 2007 Web Summary* (http://www.acha-ncha.org/data_highlights.html; retrieved December 27, 2008).

American Psychological Association. 2005. *The different kinds of stress* (http://www.apahelpcenter.org/articles/article.php?id=21; retrieved December 27, 2008).

American Psychological Association. 2005. *Learning to Deal with Stress* (http://helping.apa.org/articles/article.php?id=71; retrieved December 27, 2008).

American Psychological Association. 2006. *Hispanics and Stress* (http://apahelpcenter.mediaroom.com/flie.php/110/Executive+Summary+English+FINAL.pdf; retrieved December 27, 2008).

American Psychological Association. 2007. *Stress in America* (http://apahelpcenter.mediaroom.com/file.php/138/Stress+in+America+REPORT+FINAL.doc; retrieved December 27, 2008).

Ano, G. G., and E. B. Vasconcelles. 2005. Religious coping and psychological adjustment to stress: A meta-analysis. *Journal of Clinical Psychology* 61(4): 461–480.

Centers for Disease Control. 2005. *Coping with a Traumatic Event: Information for the Public* (http://www.bt.cdc.gov/masscasualties/copingpub.asp; retrieved December 27, 2008).

Cohen, S., W. J. Doyle, and A. Baum. 2006. Socioeconomic status is associated with stress hormones. *Psychosomatic Medicine* 68(3): 414–420.

Constantine, M. G., S. Okazaki, and S. O. Utsey. 2004. Self-concealment, social self-efficacy, acculturative stress, and depression in African, Asian, and Latin American international college students. *American Journal of Orthopsychiatry* 74(3): 230–241.

Frequent headaches, hidden dangers. 2006. *Consumer Reports on Health,* June.

Grossman, P., et al. 2004. Mindfulness-based stress reduction and health benefits: A meta analysis. *Journal of Psychosomatic Research* 57(1): 35–43.

Headaches. 2006. *Journal of the American Medical Association* 295(19): 2320.

How stress can make you forgetful, age faster. 2005. *Tufts University Health & Nutrition Letter,* February, 1.

Institute of Medicine Committee on Sleep Medicine and Research. 2006. *Sleep Disorders and Sleep Deprivation: An Unmet Public Health Problem,* ed. H. R. Colton and B. M. Altevogt. Washington, D.C. National Academies Press.

Lauderdale, D. S., et al. 2006. Objectively measured sleep characteristics among early-middle-aged adults: The CARDIA study. *American Journal of Epidemiology* 164(1): 17–18.

MacGeorge, Erina L., et al. 2004. Stress, social support, and health among college students after September 11, 2001. *Journal of College Student Development* 45(6): 655–670.

Mayo Foundation for Medical Education and Research. 2005. *Stress: Why you have it and how it hurts your health.* (http://www.mayoclinic. com/health/stress/SR00001; retrieved December 27, 2008).

Meier-Ewert, H. K., et al. 2004. Effect of sleep loss on C-reactive protein, an inflammatory marker of cardiovascular risk. *Journal of the American College of Cardiology* 43: 678–683.

Melamed, S., et al. 2004. Association of fear of terror with low-grade inflammation among apparently healthy employed adults. *Psychosomatic Medicine* 66(4): 484–491.

National Mental Health Association. 2006. *Coping with disaster: Tips for college students on coping with war and terrorism.* (http://www.nmha.org/reassurance/collegeWarCoping.cfm; retrieved December 27, 2008).

Nordboe, D. J., et al. 2007. Immediate Behavioral Health Response to the Virginia Tech Shootings. *Disaster Medicine and Public Health Preparedness* 1(Suppl. 1.): S31–S32.

Sax, L. J., et al. 2006. *The American Freshman: National Norms for Fall* 2005. Los Angeles: UCLA Higher Education Research Institute.

Segerstrom, S. C., and G. E. Miller. 2004. Psychological stress and the human immune system: A meta-analytic study of 30 years of inquiry. *Psychological Bulletin* 130(4): 601–630.

Stambor, Z. 2006. Stressed out nation. *Monitor on Psychology* 37(4) (http://www.apa.org/monitor/apr06/nation.html; retrieved December 27, 2008).

Steptoe, A., et al. 2004. Loneliness and neuroendocrine, cardiovascular, and inflammatory stress responses in middle-aged men and women. *Psychoneuroendocrinology* 29(5): 593–611.

Wetter, D. W., et al. 2004. Prevalence and predictors of transitions in smoking behavior among college students. *Health Psychology* 23(2): 168–177.

Wittstein, I. S., et al. 2005. Neurohumoral features of myocardial stunning due to sudden emotional stress. *New England Journal of Medicine* 352(6): 539–548.

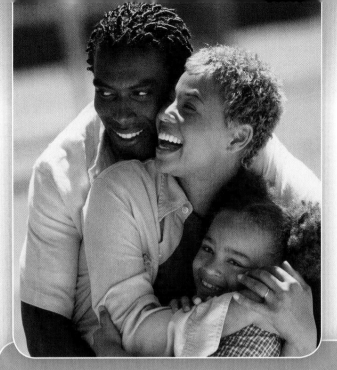

LOOKING AHEAD>>>>>

AFTER READING THIS CHAPTER, YOU SHOULD BE ABLE TO:

- Describe what it means to be psychologically healthy
- Explain how to develop and maintain a positive self-concept and healthy self-esteem
- Discuss the importance of an optimistic outlook, good communication skills, and constructive approaches to dealing with loneliness and anger
- Describe common psychological disorders
- List the warning signs of suicide
- Describe the different types of help available for psychological problems

PSYCHOLOGICAL HEALTH

3

Psychological health (or *mental health*) contributes to every dimension of wellness. It can be very difficult to maintain emotional, social, or even physical wellness if you are not psychologically healthy.

Psychological health, however, is a broad concept—one that is as difficult to define as it is important to understand. That is why the first section of this chapter is devoted to explaining what psychological health is and is not. The rest of the chapter discusses a number of common psychological problems, their symptoms, and their treatments.

If life doesn't bring you the pleasure or happiness you think it should, or if you believe you should be functioning at a higher level, you should know that there are ways of getting help. This chapter will show you how.

DEFINING PSYCHOLOGICAL HEALTH

Psychological health can be defined either negatively as the absence of sickness or positively as the presence of wellness. The narrow, negative definition has two advantages: It concentrates attention on the worst problems and on the people most in need, and it avoids value judgments about the best way to lead our lives. If we think of everyone who is not severely mentally disturbed as being mentally healthy, however, we end up ignoring common problems that can be addressed. Finally, freedom from disorders is only one factor in psychological wellness.

Self-Actualization

A positive definition—psychological health as the presence of wellness—is a more ambitious outlook that encourages us to fulfill our own potential.

During the 1960s, Abraham Maslow described such an ideal of mental health in his book *Toward a Psychology of Being*. According to Maslow, there is a *hierarchy of needs*, listed here in order of decreasing importance (Figure 3.1):

- Physiological needs
- Safety

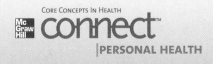

CORE CONCEPTS IN HEALTH

http://www.mcgrawhillconnect.com/personalhealth

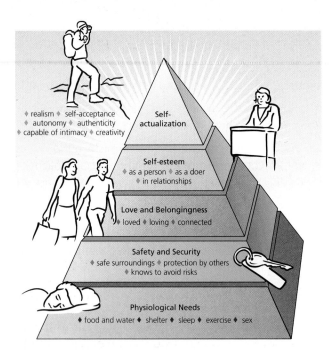

FIGURE 3.1 Maslow's hierarchy of needs.
SOURCE: Maslow, A. 1970. *Motivation and Personality,* 2nd ed. New York: Harper & Row.

- Being loved
- Maintaining self-esteem
- Self-actualization

When urgent (life-sustaining) needs—such as the need for food and water—are satisfied, less basic needs take priority. Most of us are well fed and feel reasonably safe, so we are driven by higher motives. Maslow's conclusions were based on his study of a group of visibly successful people who seemed to have lived, or be living, at their fullest. He stated that these people had achieved **self-actualization;** they had fulfilled a good measure of their human potential. Maslow suggested that self-actualized people all share certain qualities:

- *Realism.* Self-actualized people are realistic: They know the difference between what is real and what they want. As a result, they can cope with the world as it exists without demanding that it be different; they know what they can and cannot change. Just as important, realistic people accept evidence that contradicts what they want to believe. If evidence is strong enough, they adapt their belief systems accordingly.
- *Acceptance.* Psychologically healthy people accept themselves as they are. Self-acceptance requires a positive **self-concept,** or *self-image*—a positive but realistic perception of oneself. Similarly, psychological health requires an appropriately high but realistic level of **self-esteem.** People with healthy self-esteem value themselves as people; they feel good about themselves and are likely to live up to their positive self-image and enjoy successes

that in turn reinforce these good feelings. Self-acceptance also means being tolerant of one's own imperfections, an ability that makes it easier to accept the imperfections of others.

- *Autonomy.* Psychologically healthy people are *autonomous*, meaning they can direct themselves, acting independently of their social environment. **Autonomy** is more than physical independence; it is social, emotional, and intellectual independence, as well. Autonomous people are **inner-directed,** finding guidance from within, from their own rules and values. They have an internal locus of control and a high level of self-efficacy (see Chapter 1). By contrast, **other-directed** people often act only in response to what they feel as external pressure from others. Instead of speaking their true feelings, for example, other-directed people are more inclined to say what they believe will make other people happy.
- *Authenticity.* Autonomous people are not afraid to be themselves; sometimes, their capacity for being "real" may give them a certain childlike quality. They respond in a genuine, spontaneous way to whatever happens, without pretense or self-consciousness. Such people do not worry about being judged by others just for being themselves. This quality of genuineness is sometimes called **authenticity.**
- *Capacity for intimacy.* Healthy people can be physically and emotionally intimate. They are able to share their feelings and thoughts without fear of rejection. A psychologically healthy person is open to the pleasure of physical contact and the satisfaction of being close to others—but without being afraid of the risks involved in intimacy, such as the risk of having one's feelings hurt. (Chapters 4 and 5 discuss intimacy in more detail.)
- *Creativity.* Psychologically healthy people continually look at the world with renewed appreciation. Such appreciation can inform one's creativity, which helps explain why so many mentally healthy people are creative. They may not be great poets or painters, but they live their everyday lives in creative ways. Creative people seem to see more and to be open to new experiences; they don't fear the unknown or avoid uncertainty.

Self-actualization is an ideal to strive for. Rather than dwelling on the past, we need to concentrate on meeting current challenges in ways that lead to long-term mental

QUESTIONS FOR CRITICAL THINKING AND REFLECTION
Have you ever had a reason to feel concerned about your own psychological health? If so, what was the reason? Did your concern lead you to talk to someone about the issue, or to seek professional help? If you did, what was the outcome, and how do you feel about it now?

wellness. We must not consider ourselves failures if we do not achieve our full potential in every way or at every moment.

What Psychological Health Is Not

Psychological health is not the same as psychological **normality.** Being mentally normal simply means being close to average. We can define normal body temperature because a few degrees above or below this temperature means physical sickness. But your ideas and attitudes can vary tremendously without your losing efficiency or feeling emotional distress. In fact, psychological diversity—with the wide range of ideas, lifestyles, and attitudes it brings about—is a valuable asset to society.

Never seeking help for personal problems does not prove you are psychologically healthy, any more than seeking help proves you are mentally ill. Unhappy people may avoid seeking help for many reasons, and severely disturbed people may not even realize they need help.

Further, we can't say people are "mentally ill" or "mentally healthy" based solely on the presence or absence of symptoms. Consider the symptom of anxiety, for example. Anxiety can help you face a problem and solve it before it becomes too big. Someone who shows no anxiety may be refusing to recognize problems or to do anything about them. A person who is anxious for good reason is likely to be judged more psychologically healthy in the long run than someone who is inappropriately calm.

Finally, we cannot judge psychological health from the way people look. All too often, a person who seems to be OK and even happy suddenly takes his or her own life. Usually, such people lack close friends who might have known their desperation. At an early age, we learn to conceal our feelings and even to lie about them. We may believe that our complaints put unfair demands on others. While suffering in silence may sometimes be a virtue, it can also prevent one from getting help.

75% of all people who intend to commit suicide warn a family member or friend of their intention

—American Foundation for Suicide Prevention, 2008

QUICK STATS

MEETING LIFE'S CHALLENGES

Life is full of challenges—large and small. Everyone, regardless of heredity and family influences, must learn to cope successfully with new situations and new people.

Growing Up Psychologically

Our responses to life's challenges influence the development of our personality and identity.

96% of college students identified their parents as role models.

—Oregon State University/Texas A&M University Survey, 2006

QUICK STATS

Developing an Adult Identity

A primary task beginning in adolescence is the development of an adult identity: a unified sense of self, characterized by attitudes, beliefs, and ways of acting that are genuinely one's own. People with adult identities know who they are, what they are capable of, what roles they play, and their place among their peers. They have a sense of their own uniqueness but also appreciate what they have in common with others. They view themselves realistically and can assess their strengths and weaknesses without relying on the opinions of others. Achieving an identity also means that one can form intimate relationships with others while maintaining a strong sense of self.

Our identities evolve as we interact with the world and make choices about what we'd like to do and whom we'd like to model ourselves after. Developing an adult identity is particularly challenging in a heterogeneous, secular, and relatively affluent society like ours, in which many roles are possible, many choices are tolerated, and ample time is allowed for experimenting and making up one's mind.

psychological health Mental health, defined either negatively as the absence of illness or positively as the presence of wellness.

self-actualization The highest level of growth in Maslow's hierarchy.

self-concept The ideas, feelings, and perceptions one has about oneself; also called *self-image.*

self-esteem Satisfaction and confidence in oneself; the valuing of oneself as a person.

autonomy Independence; the sense of being self-directed.

inner-directed Guided in behavior by an inner set of rules and values.

other-directed Guided in behavior by the values and expectations of others.

authenticity Genuineness.

normality The psychological characteristics attributed to the majority of people in a population at a given time.

TERMS

Early identities are often modeled after parents—or the opposite of parents, in rebellion against what they represent. Over time, peers, rock stars, sports heroes, and religious figures are added to the list of possible models. In high school and college, people often join cliques that assert a certain identity, such as the "jocks," the "brains," or the "slackers." Although much of an identity is internal—a way of viewing oneself and the world—certain aspects of it can be external, such as styles of talking and dressing, ornaments like earrings, and hairstyles.

Early identities are rarely permanent. A student who works for good grades and approval one year can turn into a dropout devoted to hard rock and wild parties a year later. At some point, however, most of us adopt a more stable, individual identity that ties together the experiences of childhood and the expectations and aspirations of adulthood. However, we don't suddenly assume our final identity and never change after that. Life is more interesting for people who continue evolving into more distinct individuals, rather than being rigidly controlled by their pasts. Identity reflects a lifelong process, and it changes as a person develops new relationships and roles.

Developing an adult identity is an important part of psychological wellness. Without a personal identity, we begin to feel confused about who we are; this situation is called an **identity crisis**. Until we have "found ourselves," we cannot have much self-esteem, because a self is not firmly in place.

Developing Intimacy   Learning to live intimately with others and finding a productive role for yourself in society are other tasks of adulthood—to be able to love and work. People with established identities can form intimate relationships and sexual unions characterized by sharing, open communication, long-term commitment, and love. Those who lack a firm sense of self may have difficulty establishing relationships because they feel overwhelmed by closeness and the needs of another person. As a result, they experience only short-term, superficial relationships with others and may remain isolated.

Developing Values and Purpose in Your Life   Values are criteria for judging what is good and bad; they underlie our moral decisions and behavior. The first morality of the young child is to consider "good" to mean what brings immediate and tangible rewards, and "bad," whatever results in punishment. An older child will explain right and wrong in terms of authority figures and rules. But the final stage of moral development, one that not everyone attains, is being able to conceive of right and wrong in more abstract terms such as justice and virtue.

As adults we need to assess how far we have evolved morally and what values we actually have adopted. Without an awareness of our personal values, our lives may be hurriedly driven forward by immediate desires and the passing demands of others. Living according to values means doing the following:

- Considering your options carefully before making a choice
- Choosing between options without succumbing to outside pressures that oppose your values
- Making a choice and acting on it rather than doing nothing

Your actions and how you justify them proclaim to others what you stand for.

Achieving Healthy Self-Esteem

Having a healthy level of self-esteem means regarding your self, which includes all aspects of your identity, as good, competent, and worthy of love. It is a critical component of wellness.

Developing a Positive Self-Concept   Ideally, a positive self-concept begins in childhood, based on experiences both within the family and outside it. Children need to develop a sense of being loved and being able to give love and to accomplish their goals. If they feel rejected or neglected by their parents, they may fail to

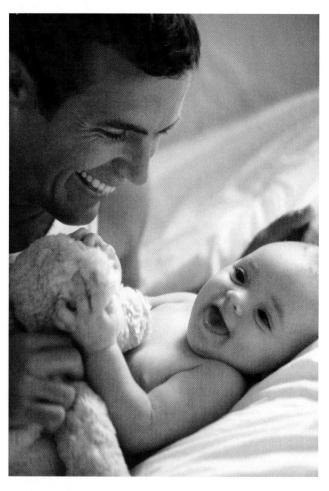

A positive self-concept begins in infancy. Knowing that he's loved and valued by his parents gives this baby a solid basis for lifelong psychological health.

develop feelings of self-worth. They may grow to have a negative concept of themselves.

Another component of self-concept is *integration*. An integrated self-concept is one that you have made for yourself—not someone else's image of you or a mask that doesn't quite fit. Important building blocks of self-concept are the personality characteristics and mannerisms of parents, which children may adopt without realizing it. Later, they may be surprised to find themselves acting like one of their parents. Eventually, such building blocks should be reshaped and integrated into a new, individual personality.

A further aspect of self-concept is *stability*. Stability depends on the integration of the self and its freedom from contradictions. People who have gotten mixed messages about themselves from parents and friends may have contradictory self-images, which defy integration and make them vulnerable to shifting levels of self-esteem. At times they regard themselves as entirely good, capable, and lovable—an ideal self—and at other times they see themselves as entirely bad, incompetent, and unworthy of love. Neither of these extreme self-concepts allow people to see themselves or others realistically, and their relationships with other people are filled with misunderstandings and ultimately with conflict.

Meeting Challenges to Self-Esteem   As an adult, you sometimes run into situations that challenge your self-concept. People you care about may tell you they don't love you or feel loved by you, for example, or your attempts to accomplish a goal may end in failure.

You can react to such challenges in several ways. The best approach is to acknowledge that something has gone wrong and try again, adjusting your goals to your abilities without radically revising your self-concept. Less productive responses are denying that anything went wrong and blaming someone else. These attitudes may preserve your self-concept temporarily, but in the long run they keep you from meeting the challenge.

The worst reaction is to develop a lasting negative self-concept in which you feel bad, unloved, and ineffective—in other words, to become demoralized. Instead of coping, the demoralized person gives up, reinforcing the negative self-concept and setting in motion a cycle of bad self-concept and failure. In people who are genetically predisposed to depression, demoralization can progress to additional symptoms, which are discussed later in the chapter.

One method for fighting demoralization is to recognize and test the negative thoughts and assumptions you may have about yourself and others. Try to note exactly when an unpleasant emotion—feeling worthless, wanting to give up, feeling depressed—occurs or gets worse, to identify the events or daydreams that trigger that emotion, and to observe whatever thoughts come into your head just before or during the emotional experience. It is helpful to keep a daily journal about such events.

People who are demoralized tend to use all-or-nothing thinking. They overgeneralize from negative events. They

overlook the positive and jump to negative conclusions, minimizing their own successes and magnifying the successes of others. They take responsibility for unfortunate situations that are not their fault, then jump to more negative conclusions and more unfounded overgeneralizations. Patterns of thinking that make events seem worse than they are in reality are called **cognitive distortions.**

When you react to a situation, an important piece of that reaction is your **self-talk**—the statements you make to yourself inside your own mind. Rational thinking and self-talk will not only help get you through the situation without feeling upset, but will also help you avoid damaging your own self-concept.

In your own fight against demoralization, it may be hard to think of a rational response until hours or days after the event that upset you. Responding rationally can be especially hard when you are having an argument with someone else, which is why people often say things they don't mean in the heat of the moment or develop hurt feelings even when the other person had no intention of hurting them.

Once you get used to noticing the way your mind works, however, you may be able to catch yourself thinking negatively and change the process before it goes too far. This approach to controlling your reactions is not the same as positive thinking—which means substituting a positive thought for a negative one. Instead, you simply try to make your thoughts as logical and accurate as possible, based on the facts of the situation as you know them, and not on snap judgments or conclusions that may turn out to be false.

Demoralized people can be tenacious about their negative beliefs—so tenacious that they make their beliefs come true in a self-fulfilling prophesy. For example, if you conclude that you are so boring that no one will like you anyway, you may decide not to bother socializing. This behavior could make the negative belief become a reality.

For additional tips on changing distorted, negative ways of thinking, see the box "Realistic Self-Talk."

Being Less Defensive

Sometimes our wishes come into conflict with people around us or with our conscience, and we become

---

identity crisis   Internal confusion about who one is.

values   Criteria for judging what is good and bad, which underlie one's moral decisions and behavior.

cognitive distortion   A pattern of negative thinking that makes events seem worse than they are.

self-talk   The statements a person makes to himself or herself.

TERMS

Realistic Self-Talk

Do your patterns of thinking make events seem worse than they truly are? Do negative beliefs about yourself become self-fulfilling prophecies? Substituting realistic self-talk for negative self-talk can help you build and maintain self-esteem and cope better with the challenges in your life. Here are some examples of common types of distorted, negative self-talk, along with suggestions for more accurate and rational responses.

Cognitive Distortion	Negative Self-Talk	Realistic Self-Talk
Focusing on negatives	School is so discouraging—nothing but one hassle after another.	School is pretty challenging and has its difficulties, but there certainly are rewards. It's really a mixture of good and bad.
Expecting the worst	Why would my boss want to meet with me this afternoon if not to fire me?	I wonder why my boss wants to meet with me. I guess I'll just have to wait and see.
Overgeneralizing	(After getting a poor grade on a paper) Just as I thought—I'm incompetent at everything.	I'll start working on the next paper earlier. That way, if I run into problems, I'll have time to consult with the TA.
Minimizing	I won the speech contest, but none of the other speakers was very good. I wouldn't have done as well against stiffer competition.	It may not have been the best speech I'll ever give, but it was good enough to win the contest. I'm really improving as a speaker.
Blaming others	I wouldn't have eaten so much last night if my friends hadn't insisted on going to that restaurant.	I overdid it last night. Next time I'll make different choices.
Expecting perfection	I should have scored 100% on this test. I can't believe I missed that one problem through a careless mistake.	Too bad I missed one problem through carelessness, but overall I did very well on this test. Next time I'll be more careful.
Believing you're the cause of everything	Sarah seems so depressed today. I wish I hadn't had that argument with her yesterday; it must have really upset her.	I wish I had handled the argument better, and in the future I'll try to. But I don't know if Sarah's behavior is related to what I said or even if she's depressed. In any case, I'm not responsible for how Sarah feels or acts; only she can take responsibility for that.
Thinking in black and white	I've got to score 10 points in the game today. Otherwise, I don't belong on the team.	I'm a good player or else I wouldn't be on the team. I'll play my best—that's all I can do.
Magnifying events	They went to a movie without me. I thought we were friends, but I guess I was wrong.	I'm disappointed they didn't ask me to the movie, but it doesn't mean our friendship is over. It's not that big a deal.

SOURCE: Adapted from Schafer, W. *Stress Management for Wellness*, 4th ed. Copyright © 2000 Wadsworth, a part of Cengage Learning, Inc. Reproduced by permission. www.cengage.com/permissions.

frustrated and anxious. If we cannot resolve the conflict by changing the external situation, we try to resolve the conflict internally by rearranging our thoughts and feelings. Some standard **defense mechanisms** are listed in Table 3.1. The drawback of many of these coping mechanisms is that they succeed temporarily, but make finding ultimate solutions much harder.

Recognizing your own defense mechanisms can be difficult, because they've probably become habits, occurring unconsciously. But we each have some inkling about how our mind operates. By remembering the details of conflict situations you have been in, you may be able to figure out which defense mechanisms you used in successful or unsuccessful attempts to cope. Try to look at yourself as an objective, outside observer would and analyze your thoughts and behavior in a psychologically stressful situation from the past. Having insight into what strategies you typically use can lead to new, less defensive and more effective ways of coping in the future.

Being Optimistic

Many psychologists believe that pessimism is not just a symptom of everyday depression but an important root cause, as well. Pessimists not only expect repeated failure and rejection but also accept it as deserved. Pessimists do not see themselves as capable of success, and they irrationally dismiss any evidence of their own accomplishments. This negative point of view is learned, typically at a young age from parents and other authority figures. But as an optimist would tell you, that means it also has the potential to be unlearned.

Psychologist Martin Seligman points out that we are more used to refuting negative statements, such as "The

Table 3.1	Defense and Coping Mechanisms	
Mechanism	**Description**	**Example**
Projection	Reacting to unacceptable inner impulses as if they were from outside the self	A student who dislikes his roommate feels that the roommate dislikes him.
Repression	Expelling from awareness an unpleasant feeling, idea, or memory	The child of an alcoholic, neglectful father remembers him as a giving, loving person.
Denial	Refusing to acknowledge to yourself what you really know to be true	A person believes that smoking cigarettes won't harm her because she's young and healthy.
Passive-aggressive behavior	Expressing hostility toward someone by being covertly uncooperative or passive	A person tells a coworker, with whom she competes for project assignments, that she'll help him with a report but then never follows through.
Displacement	Shifting one's feelings about a person to another person	A student who is angry with one of his professors returns home and yells at one of his housemates.
Rationalization	Giving a false, acceptable reason when the real reason is unacceptable	A shy young man decides not to attend a dorm party, telling himself he'd be bored.
Substitution	Deliberately replacing a frustrating goal with one that is more attainable	A student having a difficult time passing courses in chemistry decides to change his major from biology to economics.
Humor	Finding something funny in unpleasant situations	A student whose bicycle has been stolen thinks how surprised the thief will be when he or she starts downhill and discovers the brakes don't work.

problem is going to last forever and ruin everything, and it's all my fault," when they come from a jealous rival rather than from our own mind. But refuting such negative self-talk is exactly what a pessimist must learn to do in order to avoid chronic unhappiness. Pessimists must first recognize and then dispute the false, negative predictions they generate about themselves.

Maintaining Honest Communication

Another important area of psychological functioning is communicating honestly with others. It can be very frustrating for us and for people around us if we cannot express what we want and feel. Others can hardly respond to our needs if they don't know what those needs are. We must recognize what we want to communicate and then express it clearly. For example, how do you feel about going to the party instead of a movie? Do you care if your roommate talks on the phone late into the night?

Some people know what they want others to do but don't state it clearly because they fear denial of the request, which they interpret as personal rejection. Such people might benefit from **assertiveness** training: learning to insist on their rights and to bargain for what they want. Assertiveness includes being able to say no or yes depending on the situation.

Dealing with Loneliness

It can be hard to strike the right balance between being alone and being with others. Some people are motivated to socialize by a fear of being alone—not the best reason

to spend time with others. If you discover how to be happy by yourself, you'll be better able to cope with periods when you're forced to be alone—for example, when you've just broken off a romantic relationship or when your usual friends are away on vacation.

Unhappiness with being alone may come from interpreting it as a sign of rejection—that others are not interested in spending time with you. Before you reach such a conclusion, be sure that you give others a real chance to get to know you. Examine your patterns of thinking: You may harbor unrealistic expectations about other people—for example, that everyone you meet must like you and, if they don't, you must be terribly flawed.

If you decide that you're not spending enough time with people, take action to change the situation. College life provides many opportunities to meet people. If you're shy, you may have to push yourself to join a group. Look for something you've enjoyed in the past or in which you have a genuine interest.

defense mechanism A mental mechanism for coping with conflict or anxiety.

assertiveness Expression that is forceful but not hostile.

TERMS

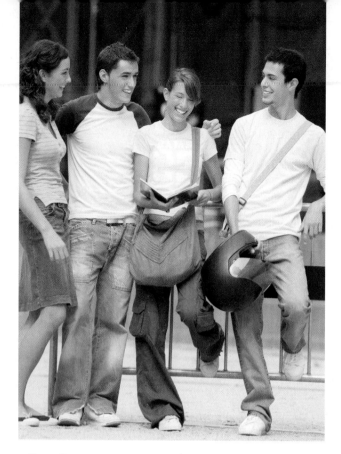

College offers many antidotes to loneliness, in the forms of clubs, organized activities, sports, and just hanging out with friends.

Dealing with Anger

Common wisdom holds that expressing anger is beneficial for psychological and physical health. However, recent studies have questioned this idea by showing that overtly hostile people seem to be at higher risk for heart attacks. Angry words or actions don't contribute to psychological wellness if they damage relationships or produce feelings of guilt or loss of control. Perhaps the best way to resolve this contradiction is to distinguish between a gratuitous expression of anger and a reasonable level of self-assertiveness.

At one extreme are people who never express anger or any opinion that might offend others, even when their own rights and needs are being jeopardized. If you have trouble expressing your anger, consider training in assertiveness and appropriate expressions of anger to help you learn to express yourself constructively.

QUESTIONS FOR CRITICAL THINKING AND REFLECTION

Think about the last time you were truly angry. What triggered your anger? How did you express it? Do you typically handle your anger in the same manner? How appropriate does your anger-management technique seem?

At the other extreme are people whose anger is explosive or misdirected—a condition called *intermittent explosive disorder (IED)*. IED is often accompanied by depression or another disorder. Explosive anger or rage, like a child's tantrum, renders individuals temporarily unable to think straight or to act in their own best interest. During an IED episode, a person may lash out uncontrollably, hurting someone else or destroying property. Anyone who expresses anger this way should seek professional help.

Managing Your Own Anger   If you feel explosive anger coming on, consider the following two strategies to head it off.

First, try to *reframe* what you're thinking at that moment. You'll be less angry at another person if there is a possibility that his or her behavior was not intentionally directed against you. Imagine that another driver suddenly cuts in front of you. You would certainly be angry if you knew the other driver did it on purpose, but you probably would be less angry if you knew he simply did not see you. You might be even less upset if you consider that there may be other mitigating factors—for example, that the other driver was involved in an urgent situation of his own. If you're angry because you've just been criticized, avoid mentally replaying scenes from the past when you received similar unjust criticisms. Think about what is happening now, and try to act differently than in the past—less defensively and more analytically.

Second, until you're able to change your thinking, try to *distract* yourself. Use the old trick of counting to 10 before you respond, or start concentrating on your breathing. If needed, take a longer cooling-off period by leaving the situation until your anger has subsided. This does not mean that you should permanently avoid the issues and people who make you angry. When you've had a chance to think more clearly about the matter, return to it.

Dealing with Anger in Other People   Anger can be infectious and disruptive to cooperation and communication. If someone you're with becomes very angry, respond "asymmetrically" by reacting not with anger but with calm. Try to validate the other person by acknowledging that he or she has some reason to be angry. This does not mean apologizing if you don't think you're to blame, or accepting verbal abuse, which is always inappropriate. Try to focus on solving the problem by allowing the person to explain why he or she is so angry and what can be done to alleviate the situation. Finally, if the person cannot be calmed, it may be best to disengage, at least temporarily. After a time-out, a rational problem-solving approach may be more successful.

PSYCHOLOGICAL DISORDERS

All of us have felt anxious at times, and in dealing with the anxiety we may have avoided doing something that

Table 3.2 Prevalence of Selected Psychological Disorders Among Americans

Disorder	Men		Women	
	Lifetime Prevalence (%)	Past Year Prevalence (%)	Lifetime Prevalence (%)	Past Year Prevalence (%)
Anxiety disorders				
Simple phobia	6.7	4.4	15.7	13.2
Social phobia	11.1	6.6	15.5	9.1
Panic disorder	2.0	1.3	5.0	3.2
Generalized anxiety disorder	3.6	2.0	6.6	4.3
Obsessive-compulsive disorder	1.7	0.5	2.8	0.8
Post-traumatic stress disorder	5.0	1.5	10.4	3.5
Mood disorders				
Major depressive episode	12.0	5.5	20.4	7.7
Manic episode	1.6	1.4	1.7	1.3
Schizophrenia and related disorders	1.0	0.8	0.5	0.4
Dementia	Depends on life expectancy	6.4 (age >=65)	Depends on life expectancy	5.7 (age >=65)

NOTE: Rates of the prevalence of dementia are highly dependent on how much impairment is considered dementia and on the age range of the population.

SOURCES: Kessler, R. C., et al. 2003. The epidemiology of major depressive disorder: Results from the National Comorbidity Survey Replication (NCS-R). *Journal of the American Medical Association* 289(23): 3095–3105; U.S. Department of Health and Human Services. 1999. *Mental Health: A Report of the Surgeon General.* Rockville, Md.: DHHS; Kessler, R. C., et al. 1995. Posttraumatic stress disorder in the National Comorbidity Survey. *Archives of General Psychiatry* 52(12): 1048–1060; Kessler, R. C., et al. 1994. Lifetime and 12-month prevalence of DSM-III-R psychiatric disorders in the United States. *Archives of General Psychiatry* 51(1): 8–19; Ferri, C. P., et al. 2005. Global prevalence of dementia: A Delphi consensus. *Lancet* 366: 2112–2117; Kukull, W. A., et al. 2002. Dementia and Alzheimer disease incidence. *Archives of Neurology* 59(Nov.): 1737–1776.

we wanted to do or should have done. Most of us have had periods of feeling down when we became pessimistic, less energetic, and less able to enjoy life. Many of us have been bothered at times by irrational thoughts or odd feelings. Such feelings and thoughts can be normal responses to the ordinary challenges of life, but when emotions or irrational thoughts start to interfere with daily activities and rob us of our peace of mind, they can be considered symptoms of a psychological disorder. (Table 3.2 shows the likelihood of these disorders occurring during one's lifetime and during the past year.)

Psychological disorders are generally the result of many factors. Genetic differences, which underlie differences in how the brain processes information and experience, are known to play an important role, especially in certain disorders. However, exactly which genes are involved, and how they alter the structure and chemistry of the brain, is still under study. Learning and life events are important, too: Identical twins often don't have the same psychological disorders in spite of having identical genes. Some people

26.2% of adult Americans suffer from a diagnosable psychological disorder.

—National Institute of Mental Health, 2008

have been exposed to more traumatic events than others, leading either to greater vulnerability to future traumas or, conversely, to the development of better coping skills. Further, what your parents, peers, and others have taught you strongly influences your level of self-esteem and how you deal with frightening or depressing life events (see the box "Ethnicity, Culture, and Psychological Disorders," p. 56).

→ Anxiety Disorders

Fear is a basic and useful emotion. Its value for our ancestors' survival cannot be overestimated; for modern humans, it provides motivation for self-protection and for learning to cope with new or potentially dangerous environmental or social situations. Only when fear is out of proportion to real danger can it be considered a problem. **Anxiety** is another word for fear, especially a feeling of fear that is not in response to any definite threat. Only when anxiety is experienced almost daily or in life situations that recur and cannot be avoided can anxiety be called a disorder.

→**anxiety** A feeling of fear that is not directed toward any definite threat.

TERMS

Ethnicity, Culture, and Psychological Disorders

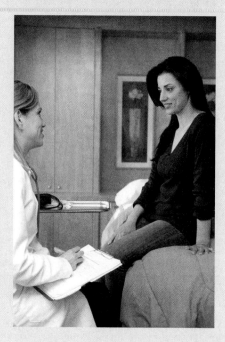

connect™

Psychological disorders differ in incidence and symptoms across cultures and ethnic groups around the world. This variability is usually attributable to cultural differences—factors such as how symptoms are interpreted and communicated, whether treatment is sought, and whether a social stigma is attached to a particular symptom or disorder.

Expression of Symptoms

People from different cultures or groups may manifest or describe symptoms differently. Consider the following examples:

- In Japan, people with social phobia may be more distressed about the imagined harm their social clumsiness causes to others than about their own embarrassment.

- Older African Americans may express depression in atypical ways—for example, denying depression by taking on a multitude of extra tasks.

- Somatization, the indirect reporting of psychological distress through non-specific physical symptoms, is more prevalent among African Americans, Puerto Ricans, and Chinese Americans.

- Schizophrenia may manifest with different delusions depending on the local culture.

Differing Attitudes

It is relatively easy for Americans of northern European descent to regard an emotional problem as psychological in nature and to therefore accept a psychological treatment. For other groups, symptoms of psychological distress may be viewed as a spiritual problem, best dealt with by religious figures.

People from some groups may have little hesitation about communicating intimate, personal problems to professional care providers. However, for others, particularly men and members of certain ethnic groups, loss of emotional control may be seen as a weakness.

In addition, the use of mental health services is viewed negatively in many cultures; this stigma may partly account for the fact that African Americans and Asian American/Pacific Islanders are only about half as likely as whites to use any type of mental health service.

Assimilation

One of the largest immigrant groups in the United States is from Mexico. Surprisingly, surveys show that these immigrants are psychologically healthier than their own children born in the United States. Mexican, Cuban, and Puerto Rican Hispanics in this country come from a culture where family bonds are valued and divorce is rare. As they assimilate and begin using English exclusively, however, these family bonds tend to weaken, but less so for Cubans than for Puerto Ricans or Mexicans. With assimilation, the incidence of anxiety, depression, and substance abuse increases.

Biological Risk Factors

Biology can also play a role in the differences seen among patients of different ethnic groups. For example, psychotropic drugs are broken down in the body by a specific enzyme known as CYP2C19. Reduction of the activity of this enzyme is caused by two mutations, one of which appears to be found only in Asian populations. These "poor metabolizers" are very sensitive to medications that

are broken down by this enzyme. The percentage of poor metabolizers among Asians is about 20%; among Latinos, about 5%; and among whites, 3%. Asian patients thus tend to have more adverse reactions to the doses of drugs standardized principally on white patients in the United States.

SOURCE: Alegria, M., et al. 2007. Understanding differences in past year psychiatric disorders for Latinos living in the US. *Social Science & Medicine* 65(2): 214–230; Kleinman, A. 2004. Culture and depression. *New England Journal of Medicine* 351(10): 951–953; Kirmayer, L. J. 2001. Cultural variations in the clinical presentation of depression and anxiety: Implications for diagnosis and treatment. *Journal of Clinical Psychiatry* 62 (Suppl. 13): 22–28; Lin, K. M. 2001. Biological differences in depression and anxiety across races and ethnic groups. *Journal of Clinical Psychiatry* 62 (Suppl. 13): 13–19.

Simple Phobia The most common and most understandable anxiety disorder, **simple,** or **specific, phobia** is a fear of something definite like lightning or a particular animal or location. Examples of commonly feared animals are snakes, spiders, and dogs; frightening locations are often high places or enclosed spaces. Sometimes, but not always, these fears originate in bad experiences, such as being bitten by a snake.

Social Phobia The 15 million Americans with **social phobia** fear humiliation or embarrassment while being

observed by others. Fear of speaking in public is perhaps the most common phobia of this kind. Extremely shy people can have social fears that extend to almost all social situations (see the box "Shyness" on p. 57).

Panic Disorder People with **panic disorder** experience sudden unexpected surges in anxiety, accompanied by symptoms such as rapid and strong heartbeat, shortness of breath, loss of physical equilibrium, and a feeling of losing mental control. Such attacks usually begin in one's early twenties and can lead to a fear of being in

Shyness

Shyness is a form of social anxiety, a fear of what others will think of one's behavior or appearance. Physical signs include a rapid heartbeat, a nervous stomach, sweating, cold and clammy hands, blushing, dry mouth, a lump in the throat, and trembling muscles. Shy people are often excessively self-critical, and their self-talk can be very negative. Their feelings of self-consciousness, embarrassment, and unworthiness can be overwhelming.

To avoid situations that make them anxious, shy people may refrain from making eye contact or speaking up in public. They may shun social gatherings and avoid college courses or job promotions that demand interpersonal interaction or public speaking.

Shyness is not the same thing as being introverted. Introverts prefer solitude to society. Shy people often long to be more outgoing, but their own negative thoughts prevent them from enjoying the social interaction they desire.

The consequences of severe shyness can include social isolation, loneliness, and lost personal and professional opportunities. Very shy people also have high rates of other anxiety and mood disorders and of substance abuse.

Shyness may be partly inherited. But for shyness, as for many health concerns, biology is not destiny. Many shy children outgrow their shyness, just as others acquire it later in life. Clearly, other factors are involved. The type of attachment between a child and his or her caregiver is important, as are parenting styles. Peo-

ple's experiences during critical developmental transitions, such as starting school and entering adolescence, have also been linked to shyness. For adults, the precipitating factor may be an event such as divorce or the loss of a job.

Shyness is very common, with 40–50% of Americans describing themselves as shy. However, only about 7–13% of adults are so shy that their condition interferes seriously with daily life. Recent surveys indicate that shyness rates may be rising in the United States. With the advent of technologies such as ATM machines, video games, voice mail, faxes, and e-mail, the opportunities for face-to-face interaction are diminishing. Electronic media can be a wonderful way for shy people to communicate, but they can also allow us to hide from social interaction. In fact, one study found that greater use of the Internet was associated with a decline in participants' communication with family members, a reduction in the size of their social circles, and an increase in levels of depression and loneliness.

Shyness is often undiagnosed, but help is available. Shyness classes, assertiveness training groups, and public speaking clinics are available (see the Behavior Change Strategy at the end of the chapter). For the seriously shy, effective treatments include cognitive-behavioral therapy and antidepressant drugs.

If you're shy, try to remember that shyness is widespread and that there are worse fates. Some degree of shyness has an upside. Shy people tend to be gentle,

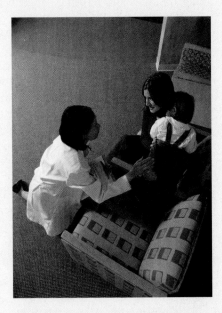

supportive, kind, and sensitive; they are often exceptional listeners. People who think carefully before they speak or act are less likely to hurt the feelings of others. Shyness may also facilitate cooperation. For any group or society to function well, a variety of roles is required, and there is a place for quieter, more reflective individuals.

SOURCE: American Psychological Association. 2007. *Painful Shyness in Children and Adults* (http://www.apahelpcenter.org/featuredtopics/feature.php?id=5; retrieved December 29, 2008); Ebeling-Witte, S., et al. 2007. Shyness, Internet use, and personality. *Cyberpsychology and Behavior* 10(5): 713–716; Rosenthal, J., et al. 2007. Beyond shy: When to suspect social anxiety disorder. *Journal of Family Practice* 56(5): 369–374.

crowds or closed places or of driving or flying. Sufferers fear that a panic attack will occur in a situation from which escape is difficult (such as while in an elevator), where the attack could be incapacitating and result in a dangerous or embarrassing loss of control (such as while driving a car or shopping), or where no medical help would be available if needed (such as when a person is alone away from home). Fears such as these lead to avoidance of situations that might cause trouble. The fears and avoidance may spread to a large variety of situations until a person is virtually housebound, a condition called **agoraphobia**.

Generalized Anxiety Disorder

A basic reaction to future threats is to worry about them. **Generalized anxiety disorder (GAD)** is a diagnosis given to people whose

simple (specific) phobia A persistent and excessive fear of a specific object, activity, or situation.

social phobia An excessive fear of being observed in public; speaking in public is the most common example.

panic disorder A syndrome of severe anxiety attacks accompanied by physical symptoms.

agoraphobia An anxiety disorder characterized by fear of being alone away from help and avoidance of many different places and situations; in extreme cases, a fear of leaving home. From the Greek for "fear of the public market."

generalized anxiety disorder (GAD) An anxiety disorder characterized by excessive, uncontrollable worry about all kinds of things and anxiety in many situations.

worries have taken on a life of their own, pushing out other thoughts and refusing banishment by any effort of will. The topics of the worrying are ordinary concerns: Will I be able to pass the exam next Friday? Where will I get money to get my car fixed?

The GAD sufferer's worrying is not completely unjustified—after all, thinking about problems can result in solving them. But this kind of thinking seems to just go around in circles, and the more you try to stop it, the more you feel at its mercy. The end result is a persistent feeling of nervousness, often accompanied by depression.

Obsessive-Compulsive Disorder The diagnosis of **obsessive-compulsive disorder (OCD)** is given to people with obsessions or compulsions or both.

• **Obsessions** are recurrent, unwanted thoughts or impulses. Unlike the worries of GAD, they are not ordinary concerns but improbable fears such as of suddenly committing an antisocial act or of having been contaminated by germs.

• **Compulsions** are repetitive, difficult-to-resist actions usually associated with obsessions. A common compulsion is hand washing, associated with an obsessive fear of contamination by dirt. Other compulsions are counting and repeatedly checking whether something has been done—for example, whether a door has been locked or a stove turned off.

People with OCD feel anxious, out of control, and embarrassed. Their rituals can occupy much of their time and make them inefficient at work and difficult to live with.

Post-Traumatic Stress Disorder People who suffer from **post-traumatic stress disorder (PTSD)** are reacting to severely traumatic events (events that produce a sense of terror and helplessness) such as physical violence to oneself or loved ones. Trauma occurs in personal assaults (rape, military combat), natural disasters (floods, hurricanes), and tragedies like fires and airplane or car crashes.

Symptoms include reexperiencing the trauma in dreams and in intrusive memories, trying to avoid anything associated with the trauma, and numbing of feelings. Hyperarousal, sleep disturbances, and other symptoms of anxiety and depression also commonly occur. Such symptoms can last months or even years.

The terrorist attacks on September 11, 2001, brought PTSD into the spotlight. Among those affected were survivors, rescue workers, passersby, residents of Manhattan in general, and to some extent, television viewers around the world who saw countless repeated images of the devastation. An estimated 150,000 New Yorkers suffered PTSD following the attacks; some were still experiencing symptoms 5 years later. Hurricane Katrina had a similarly devastating effect; in one survey, 19% of police officers and 22% of firefighters in the Gulf Coast states reported symptoms of PTSD. Soldiers wounded in combat are also at risk for PTSD; among soldiers wounded in Iraq or Afghanistan, rates of PTSD increased during the first year after the injury, suggesting that the emotional impact deepens with time. When symptoms persist, and when daily functioning is disrupted, professional help is needed.

Treating Anxiety Disorders Therapies for anxiety disorders range from medication to psychological interventions concentrating on a person's thoughts and behavior. Both drug treatments and cognitive-behavioral therapies are effective in panic disorder, OCD, and GAD. Simple phobias are best treated without drugs.

Mood Disorders

Daily, temporary mood changes typically don't affect our overall emotional state or level of wellness. A person with a **mood disorder**, however, experiences emotional disturbances that are intense and persistent enough to affect normal functioning. The two most common mood disorders are depression and bipolar disorder.

Depression The National Institutes of Health estimates that **depression** strikes nearly 10% of Americans annually, making it the most common mood disorder. Depression affects the young as well as adults; nearly 50% of college students report depression severe enough to hinder their daily functioning. Depression tends to be more severe

and persistent in blacks than in people of other races. Despite this, less than 50% of blacks affected by depression receive treatment for it.

Depression takes different forms but usually involves demoralization and can include the following:

• A feeling of sadness and hopelessness
• Loss of pleasure in doing usual activities
• Poor appetite and weight loss
• Insomnia or disturbed sleep
• Restlessness or, alternatively, fatigue
• Thoughts of worthlessness and guilt
• Trouble concentrating or making decisions
• Thoughts of death or suicide

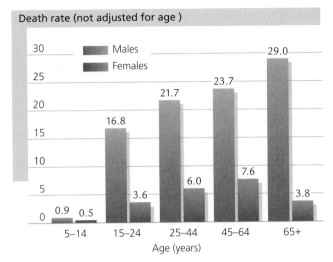

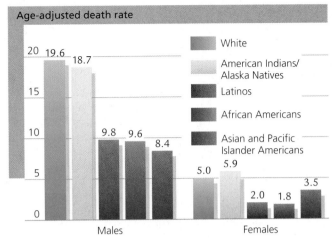

(a) Suicide rate by age and gender

(b) Suicide rate by ethnicity and gender (all ages)

VITAL STATISTICS

FIGURE 3.2   Rates of suicide per 100,000 people in the United States.   The rate of suicide varies by gender, age, and ethnicity. Rates are higher among men than women at all ages and are higher among whites compared to other groups. White men over age 65 have the highest rates of suicide. The age-adjusted national suicide rate is 10.9 per 100,000 people. These statistics are complete through 2004.

SOURCE: National Center for Health Statistics. 2007. *Health, United States, 2007*. Hyattsville, Md.: National Center for Health Statistics.

A person experiencing depression may not have all of these symptoms. Sometimes instead of poor appetite and insomnia, the opposite occurs—eating too much and sleeping too long. (Depression may contribute to weight gain in young women.) People can have most of the symptoms of depression without feeling depressed, although they usually experience a loss of interest or pleasure in things.

In major depression, symptoms are often severe; a diagnosis of *dysthymic disorder* may be applied to people who experience persistent symptoms of mild or moderate depression for 2 years or longer. In some cases, depression is a clear-cut reaction to specific events, such as the loss of a loved one or failing in school or work, whereas in other cases no trigger event is obvious.

RECOGNIZING THE WARNING SIGNS OF SUICIDE   One of the principal dangers of severe depression is suicide. Although a suicide attempt can occur unpredictably and unaccompanied by depression, the chances are greater if symptoms are numerous and severe. Additional warning signs of suicide include the following:

- Expressing the wish to be dead or revealing contemplated methods
- Increasing social withdrawal and isolation
- A sudden, inexplicable lightening of mood (which can mean the person has decided to commit suicide)

Certain risk factors increase the likelihood of suicide:

- A history of previous attempts
- A suicide by a family member or friend
- Readily available means, such as guns or pills
- A history of substance abuse or eating disorders
- Serious medical problems

In the United States, men have much higher suicide rates than women; white men over age 65 have the highest suicide rate (Figure 3.2). Whites and Native Americans

obsessive-compulsive disorder (OCD)   An anxiety disorder characterized by uncontrollable, recurring thoughts and the performing of senseless rituals.

obsession   A recurrent, irrational, unwanted thought or impulse.

compulsion   An irrational, repetitive, forced action, usually associated with an obsession.

post-traumatic stress disorder (PTSD)   An anxiety disorder characterized by reliving traumatic events through dreams, flashbacks, and hallucinations.

mood disorder   An emotional disturbance that is intense and persistent enough to affect normal function; two common types of mood disorders are depression and bipolar disorder.

depression   A mood disorder characterized by loss of interest, sadness, hopelessness, loss of appetite, disturbed sleep, and other physical symptoms.

Depression, Anxiety, and Gender

The common belief that females are more emotional than males has both a positive and a negative side. On the one hand, women are thought to express positive emotions more clearly than men, especially those related to sympathy and caring. On the other hand, women are more prone to negative emotions such as depression and worry.

One of the defining characteristics of a psychiatric disorder is that it interferes with daily activities and the ability to live a happy life. Thus, the higher incidence of anxiety and mood disorders in women is convincing evidence that they are more likely to suffer from emotional distress than are men.

Anxiety Disorders

Panic disorder is more than twice as common in women as in men, whereas obsessive-compulsive disorder occurs in men and women at about the same rate. In population surveys, social anxiety disorder is more common in women than in men, but men are more likely to seek treatment for it—perhaps because men are more likely to find it a barrier to success in white-collar jobs. In some surveys, PTSD is more common in women, but the incidence of PTSD depends on the incidence of traumatic events, which varies in different environments. Men are more often exposed to military combat, and women to rape. Trauma from motor vehicle crashes is a fairly common cause of PTSD in both sexes.

Depression and Suicide

Over their lifetimes, about 20% of women and 12% of men have serious depression. When women are depressed, they are more likely than men to experience guilt, anxiety, increased appetite and weight gain, and increased sleep. When women take antidepressants, they may need a lower dose than men;

at the same dosage, blood levels of medication tend to be higher in women. An issue for women who may become pregnant is whether antidepressants can harm a fetus or newborn. The best evidence indicates that the most frequently prescribed types of antidepressants do not cause birth defects, although some studies have reported withdrawal symptoms in some newborns whose mothers used certain antidepressants.

Although suicidal behavior is strongly associated with depression, and depression is more prevalent in women, many more men than women commit suicide. Overall, about three times as many women as men attempt suicide, but women's attempts are less likely to be lethal. In the United States, 60% of male suicides involve firearms.

Underlying Factors

Why women have more anxiety and depression than men is a matter of debate. Some experts think much of the difference is due to reporting bias: Women are more willing to admit to experiencing negative emotions, being stressed, or having difficulty coping. Women may also be more likely to seek treatment.

Other experts point to biologically based sex differences, particularly in the level and action of hormones. Greater anxiety and depression in women compared with men is most pronounced between puberty and menopause, when female hormones are most active. However, this period of life is also the time in which women's social roles and expectations may be the most different from those of men. Women may put more emphasis on relationships in determining self-esteem, so the deterioration of a relationship is a cause of depression that can hit women harder than men. In addition, culturally determined gender roles are more likely to place women in situations where they have less control

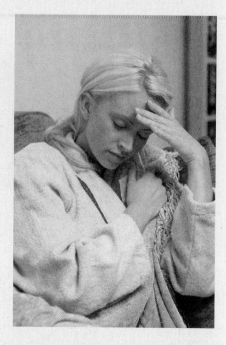

over key life decisions, and lack of autonomy is associated with depression.

The higher suicide rate among young men may relate to gender norms and expectations that men assert independence and physical prowess—sometimes expressed in risky, dangerous, and potentially self-destructive behavior. Such behavior, often involving drugs and alcohol and resulting in motor vehicle crashes, occurs more often in young people who later commit suicide. Even when suicidal intention is never expressed, suicidal impulses are often suspected of contributing to sudden deaths in this age group.

SOURCES: Sanz, E. J., et al. 2005. Selective serotonin reuptake inhibitors in pregnant women and neonatal withdrawal syndrome. *Lancet* 365(9458): 482–487; Kessler, R. C. 2003. Epidemiology of women and depression. *Journal of Affective Disorders* 74: 5–13; World Health Organization. 2002. *Gender and Mental Health.* Geneva: World Health Organization; Pigott, T. A. 1999. Gender differences in the epidemiology and treatment of anxiety disorders. *Journal of Clinical Psychiatry* 60(Suppl. 18): 4–15.

have higher rates than most other groups, but rates among blacks have been rising. Women attempt three times as many suicides as men, yet men succeed at more than three times the rate of women (see the box "Depression, Anxiety, and Gender"). Suicide rates among adolescents and young adults and among adults over 65 have been falling for the last two decades.

Sometimes mistaken for suicide attempts are acts of *self-injury*, including cutting, burning, hitting, and other forms of self-inflicted harm. The prevalence of self-injury is estimated at 3–4% in the general population but is higher in adolescents, especially females. In a 2007 study, 25% of college-age females surveyed said they had injured themselves intentionally. A maladaptive coping strategy, self-injury is believed to provide relief from unbearable psychological distress or pain, perhaps through the release of endorphins. A variety of psychotherapeutic interventions can help people who injure themselves. Whatever the reason behind it, however, self-harm should be taken very seriously because it may signal an increased risk for suicide. According to a 2007 British study, young persons who purposely hurt themselves were much more likely to commit suicide than the general population.

HELPING YOURSELF OR A FRIEND   If you are severely depressed or know someone who is, expert help from a mental health professional is essential. Don't be afraid to discuss the possibility of suicide with someone you fear is suicidal. You won't give them an idea they haven't already thought of. Asking direct questions is the best way to determine whether someone seriously intends to commit suicide. Encourage your friend to talk and to take positive steps to improve his or her situation.

Most communities have emergency help available, often in the form of a hotline telephone counseling service run by a suicide prevention agency (check the yellow pages). If you feel there is an immediate danger of suicide, do not leave the person alone. Call for help or take him or her to an emergency room.

TREATING DEPRESSION   Although treatments are highly effective, only about 35% of people who suffer from depression currently seek treatment. Treatment for depression depends on its severity and on whether the depressed person is suicidal. The best initial treatment for moderate to severe depression is probably a combination of drug therapy and psychotherapy. Newer prescription antidepressants work well, although they may take several weeks to take effect, and patients may need to try multiple medications before finding one that works well. Therefore, when suicidal impulses are strong, hospitalization may be necessary.

Antidepressants work by affecting key neurotransmitters in the brain, including serotonin. The herbal supplement St. John's wort may also affect serotonin levels, but it is not subject to the same testing and regulation as prescription medications (see the box "Alternative Remedies for Depression" on p. 62). Anyone who may be suffering from depression should seek a medical evaluation rather than self-treating with supplements.

Electroconvulsive therapy (ECT) is effective for severe depression when other approaches have failed, including medications and other electronic therapies such as magnetic stimulation. In ECT, an epileptic-like seizure is induced by an electrical impulse transmitted through electrodes placed on the head. Patients are given an anesthetic and a muscle relaxant to reduce anxiety and prevent injuries associated with seizures. A typical course of ECT includes three treatments per week for 2 to 4 weeks.

One type of depression is treated by having sufferers sit with eyes open in front of a bright light source every morning. These patients have **seasonal affective disorder (SAD)**; their depression worsens during winter months as the number of hours of daylight diminishes, then improves with the spring and summer. The American Psychiatric Association estimates that 10–20% of Americans suffer symptoms that may be linked to SAD. SAD is more common among people who live at higher latitudes, where there are fewer hours of light in winter. Light therapy may work by extending the perceived length of the day and thus convincing the brain that it is summertime even during the winter months.

Mania and Bipolar Disorder   People who experience **mania**, a less common feature of mood disorders, are restless, have a lot of energy, need little sleep, and often talk nonstop. They may devote themselves to fantastic projects and spend more money than they can afford. Many manic people swing between manic and depressive states, a syndrome called **bipolar disorder** because of the

THINKING ABOUT THE ENVIRONMENT

Depressive disorders such as SAD are triggered by environmental factors such as the long nights and gray skies of winter or job schedules that require one to work at night and sleep during the day. Anxiety disorders such as social phobia can be greatly compounded by living or working in a crowded area where one must deal with many other people.

If an environmental factor adds to your depression or anxiety, look for resources in your community that can help. For example, counseling can help with social anxiety, and inexpensive light treatments can relieve seasonal depression for some people. For more information on the environment and environmental health, see Chapter 14.

electroconvulsive therapy (ECT)   The use of electric shock to induce brief, generalized seizures; used in the treatment of selected psychological disorders.

seasonal affective disorder (SAD)   A mood disorder characterized by seasonal depression, usually occurring in winter, when there is less daylight.

mania   A mood disorder characterized by excessive elation, irritability, talkativeness, inflated self-esteem, and expansiveness.

bipolar disorder   A mental illness characterized by alternating periods of depression and mania.

TERMS

Alternative Remedies for Depression

Mainstream therapies for depression include medications accepted as safe and effective by government regulatory agencies, certain psychotherapies, and light therapy in the case of seasonal affective disorder. Yet, in surveys, 20% of people in the United States who suffer from depression report using unconventional therapies such as acupuncture, body movement therapy, homeopathy, qigong, faith healing, or herbs or other "natural" substances. With the exception of one herb, St. John's wort (*Hypericum perforatum*), these therapies have not been shown to be effective in double-blind placebo-controlled trials. Such trials are the only scientific way to show that a treatment has healing power beyond that of a **placebo.** (See Chapter 20 for more on different types of medical research studies.)

St. John's wort, a flowering plant that grows as a weed in the United States, has been reputed to have curative properties since the time of Hippocrates in ancient Greece. Modern pharmacological studies confirm that its active ingredients produce a number of biochemical and physiological changes in animals, although it's still unclear exactly how these changes might affect depression. Data from a number of studies suggest that St. John's wort could benefit people with mild to moderate depression, but concerns have been raised about the adequacy of those trials. Recently, two carefully designed trials were conducted on St. John's wort. In one, 375 mild to moderately depressed patients were randomly assigned to receive either a placebo or an extract of St. John's wort; the extract was statistically more effective than the placebo and did not have more side effects. In the other trial, 340 depressed patients were given either St. John's wort, a placebo, or sertraline, a prescription antidepressant. In that study, St. John's wort was no more effective than the placebo—but neither was sertraline. Because many other studies have shown sertraline to have better results than a placebo, this result casts doubt as to whether the study methods were sensitive enough to detect an antidepressant effect. In any case, consumers are left without a definitive answer on the effectiveness of St. John's wort.

An advantage of St. John's wort is that it causes fewer adverse effects than conventional antidepressants. In data from three studies including about 600 depressed patients, the herb produced no more adverse effects than did the placebo. There was no evidence of sedation, gastrointestinal disturbances, or other side effects associated with other antidepressants. However, the safety of St. John's wort in pregnancy has not been established, and it may interact with, and reduce the effectiveness of, certain medications, including oral contraceptives and some medications for treating heart disease, depression, HIV infections, and seizures.

One reason for the popularity of an herb for depression is that it doesn't require a prescription or any kind of contact with a physician or a therapist; for those who are not members of a generous health care plan, an herbal remedy may also be less expensive than a prescription antidepressant. On the other hand, people suffering from depression *should* seek professional advice and not try to get along entirely with self-diagnosis and self-help. If you are depressed enough to contemplate taking St. John's wort, you need to make an appointment to talk to a professional about your depression.

Bear in mind that St. John's wort does not work for everyone, and no expert advocates it for severe depression. Also, because herbal products are classified as dietary supplements, they are not scrutinized by the regulatory agencies that oversee prescription drugs. Thus, consumers have no guarantee that the product contains the herbs and dosages listed on the label.

SOURCES: Trautmann-Sponsel, R. D., and A. Dienel. 2004. Safety of Hypericum extract in mildly to moderately depressed outpatients: A review based on data from three randomized, placebo-controlled trials. *Journal of Affective Disorders* 82(2): 303–307; Lecrubier, Y., et al. 2002. Efficacy of St. John's wort extract WS 5570 in major depression: A double-blind, placebo-controlled trial. *American Journal of Psychiatry* 159(8): 1361–1366; Hypericum Depression Trial Study Group. 2002. Effect of *Hypericum perforatum* (St. John's wort) in major depressive disorder: A randomized controlled trial. *Journal of the American Medical Association* 287(14): 1807–1814; Shelton, R. C., et al. 2001. Effectiveness of St. John's wort in major depression. *Journal of the American Medical Association* 285 (15): 1978–1986.

two opposite poles of mood. Bipolar disorder affects men and women equally. Tranquilizers are used to treat individual manic episodes, while special drugs such as the salt lithium carbonate taken daily can prevent future mood swings. Anticonvulsants (used to prevent epileptic seizures) are also prescribed to stabilize moods; examples are Tegretol (carbamazepine) and Lamictal (lamotrigene).

Schizophrenia

Schizophrenia can be severe and debilitating or quite mild and hardly noticeable. Although people are capable of diagnosing their own depression, they usually don't diagnose their own schizophrenia, because they often can't see that anything is wrong. This disorder is not rare;

placebo A chemically inactive substance that a patient believes is an effective medical therapy for his or her condition. To help evaluate a therapy, medical researchers compare the effects of a particular therapy with the effects of a placebo. The "placebo effect" occurs when a patient responds to a placebo as if it were an active drug.

schizophrenia A psychological disorder that involves a disturbance in thinking and in perceiving reality.

QUESTIONS FOR CRITICAL THINKING AND REFLECTION

Have you ever wondered if you were depressed? Try to recall your situation at the time. How did you feel, and what do you think brought about those feelings? What, if anything, did you do to bring about change and to feel better?

Antidepressant Use in Young People

On September 14, 2004, a Food and Drug Administration (FDA) advisory committee recommended a warning label for antidepressant drugs based on evidence that their use increases the risk of suicidal thinking and behavior in children and adolescents.

Effectiveness

Drug treatment for depression is part of a success story in which people take seriously symptoms of depression and hints of suicidal thinking in children and teens. Over the past decade, the suicide rate among adolescents has fallen. Many factors have contributed to the decline, including stricter gun laws that make it harder for young people to get guns. Drug treatment has also been considered a key factor in the decline in suicide rates.

A 2005 review of reported childhood depression cases showed that between 1995 and 2002 the number of pediatric psychotherapy sessions declined significantly while prescriptions for antidepressants rose. Most of those prescriptions were for drugs that had not been approved for use in children. To date, only one drug—fluoxetine (Prozac)—has been approved for use specifically in children and teens. Studies have found that fluoxetine causes a greater improvement than a placebo, but the combination of drug therapy and cognitive-behavioral therapy is more beneficial than either treatment alone. The placebo effect, in which people improve while taking pills containing inactive compounds, is significant in studies of depression and can exceed 30%—meaning almost a third of people receiving a placebo experience an improvement in their symptoms.

Many antidepressants other than fluoxetine, especially other SSRIs, are also prescribed to young people, but these other drugs haven't been shown to be effective for that age group. Unpublished research data indicates that some SSRIs are *not* effective in children and teens or are only slightly more effective than a placebo.

Safety

The problem associated with SSRIs is the possibility that they increase the risk of suicide in some young people, particularly in the period immediately following the start of medication use. When study results were pooled, researchers found that in the short term, about 2–3% of users have an increased risk of suicidal thoughts and actions beyond the risk inherent from depression itself.

Researchers aren't exactly sure what causes this effect. One theory is that SSRIs reverse the lethargy associated with depression more quickly than they relieve the depression itself, giving users the energy to contemplate suicide in the interim. Antidepressants may work differently on the brains of young people than on the brains of adults, so there may be as yet unidentified effects.

In October 2004, the FDA published a public health advisory about using antidepressants in children and teens. It emphasizes that young people who take antidepressants should be monitored closely, especially when starting a new medication or changing the dosage of a drug. The FDA told manufacturers to revise the labeling of their products to include a boxed warning and expanded warning statements.

Depression is a serious illness that can increase the risk of suicide, and mental health professionals and patients must balance the risks of doing nothing against the potential risks and benefits of different types of treatments. These points were emphasized by the American Academy of Child and Adolescent Psychiatry in response to the FDA advisory.

The result of the FDA advisory was a reduction of more than 20% in the number of SSRI prescriptions for this age group. Along with this reduction in prescriptions was a 15% increase in the group's suicide rate. An advisory about antidepressants in children and adolescents was issued in the Netherlands at

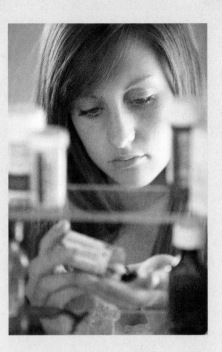

about the same time, with the same result: SSRI prescriptions dropped but the suicide rate increased. These statistics do not prove a cause-effect relationship but certainly are a reason for concern. For some young people, psychological treatment for depression may not have been a practical alternative to medication, because it was not available or not accepted.

SOURCES: Gibbons, R. D. 2007. Early evidence on the effects of regulators' suicidality warnings on SSRI prescriptions and suicide in children and adolescents. *American Journal of Psychiatry* 164(9): 1356–1363; Newman, T. B. 2004. Treating depression in children: A black-box warning for antidepressants in children? *New England Journal of Medicine* 351(16): 1595–1598; Brent, D. A. 2004. Treating depression in children: Antidepressants and pediatric depression—the risk of doing nothing. *New England Journal of Medicine* 351(16): 1598–1601; Treatment for Adolescents with Depression Study (TADS) Team. 2004. Fluoxetine, cognitive-behavioral therapy, and their combination for adolescents with depression. *Journal of the American Medical Association* 292(7): 807–820; Stafford, R. S., et al. 2005. Depression treatment during outpatient visits by U.S. children and adolescents. *Journal of Adolescent Health* 37(6): 434–442.

in fact, 1 in every 100 people has a schizophrenic episode sometime in his or her lifetime, most commonly starting in adolescence.

Scientists are uncertain about the exact causes of schizophrenia. Researchers have identified possible chemical and

structural differences in the brains of people with the disorder as well as several genes that appear to increase risk. Schizophrenia is likely caused by a combination of genes and environmental factors that occur during pregnancy and development. For example, children born to older fathers have higher rates of schizophrenia, as do children with pre-natal exposure to certain infections or medications.

Some general characteristics of schizophrenia include the following:

- *Disorganized thoughts.* Thoughts may be expressed in a vague or confusing way.

- *Inappropriate emotions.* Emotions may be either absent or strong but inappropriate.

- *Delusions.* People with delusions—firmly held false beliefs—may think that their minds are controlled by outside forces, that people can read their minds, that they are great personages like Jesus Christ or the president of the United States, or that they are being persecuted by a group such as the CIA.

- *Auditory hallucinations.* Schizophrenic people may hear voices when no one is present.

- *Deteriorating social and work functioning.* Social with-drawal and increasingly poor performance at school or work may be so gradual that they are hardly noticed at first.

None of these characteristics is invariably present. Some schizophrenic people are quite logical except on the subject of their delusions. Others show disorganized thoughts but no delusions or hallucinations.

A schizophrenic person needs help from a mental health professional. Suicide is a risk in schizophrenia, and expert treatment can reduce that risk and minimize the social consequences of the illness by shortening the period when symptoms are active. The key element in treatment is regular medication. At times medication is like insulin for diabetes—it makes the difference between being able to function or not. Sometimes hospitalization is tempo-rarily required to relieve family and friends.

GETTING HELP

Knowing when self-help or professional help is required for mental health problems is usually not as difficult as knowing how to start or which professional to choose.

Self-Help

If you have a personal problem to solve, a smart way to begin is by finding out what you can do on your own. Some problems are specifically addressed in this book. Behavioral and some cognitive ap-proaches are es-pecially useful for helping yourself. They all involve becoming more aware of self-defeating actions

and ideas and combating them in some way: by being more assertive; by communicating honestly; by raising your self-esteem by counteracting negative thoughts, people, and actions that undermine it; and by confronting, rather than avoiding, the things you fear. Get more information by see-ing what books are available in the psychology or self-help sections of libraries and bookstores, but be selective. Watch out for self-help books making fantastic claims that deviate from mainstream approaches.

Some people find it helpful to express their feelings in a journal. Grappling with a painful experience in this way provides an emotional release and can help you develop more constructive ways of dealing with similar situations in the future. Research indicates that using a journal this way can improve physical as well as emotional wellness.

For some people, religious belief and practice may pro-mote psychological health. Religious organizations provide a social network and a supportive community, and religious practices, such as prayer and meditation, offer a path for personal change and transformation.

Peer Counseling and Support Groups

Sharing your concerns with others is another helpful way of dealing with psychological health challenges. Just be-ing able to share what's troubling you with an accepting, empathetic person can bring relief. Comparing notes with people who have problems similar to yours can give you new ideas about coping.

Many colleges offer peer counseling through a health center or through the psychology or education depart-ment. Peer counseling is usually done by volunteer stu-dents who have received special training that emphasizes confidentiality. Peer counselors may steer you toward an appropriate campus or community resource or simply offer a sympathetic ear.

Many self-help groups work on the principle of bringing together people with similar problems to share their experiences and support one another. Support groups are typically organized around a specific prob-lem, such as eating disorders or substance abuse. Self-help groups may be listed in the phone book or the campus newspaper.

Professional Help

Sometimes self-help or talking to nonprofessionals is not enough. More objective, more expert, or more discreet help is needed. Many people have trouble accepting the need for professional help, and often those who most need help are the most unwilling to get it. You may someday find yourself having to overcome your own reluctance, or that of a friend, about seeking help.

Determining the Need for Professional Help In some cases, professional help is optional. Some people are interested in improving their psychological health in a general way by going into individual or group therapy to learn more about themselves and how to interact with others. Clearly, seeking professional help for these reasons is a matter of individual choice. In some situations, such as friction among family members or between partners, professional help can mean the difference between a painful divorce and a satisfying relationship.

Following are some strong indications that you or someone you know needs professional help:

- If depression, anxiety, or other emotional problems begin to interfere seriously with school or work performance or in getting along with others
- If suicide is attempted or is seriously considered (refer to the warning signs earlier in the chapter)
- If symptoms such as hallucinations, delusions, incoherent speech, or loss of memory occur
- If alcohol or drugs are used to the extent that they impair normal functioning during much of the week, if finding or taking drugs occupies much of the week, or if reducing their dosage leads to psychological or physiological withdrawal symptoms

Types of Psychotherapy   There are several approaches to treating psychological disorders:

- *Pharmacological therapy* is based on the premise that the mind's activity depends on an organic structure, the brain, whose composition is genetically determined. Pharmacological therapy relies on a wide variety of prescription medications to treat psychological disorders, but often in combination with one or more other therapies.
- *Behavioral therapy* focuses on current behavior patterns. The goal is to help the patient replace unhealthy, maladaptive behaviors with more positive ones. Shaping one's environment is a key part of this therapy. Behavioral therapy is often used to treat phobias and other anxiety disorders. For example, a person might be exposed to a feared object or situation in gradual stages in order to overcome an irrational fear of it.
- *Cognitive therapy* emphasizes the effect of ideas on behavior and feeling. People in cognitive therapy are taught to notice their unrealistic thoughts and to substitute more realistic ones. Cognitive and behavioral therapies are frequently combined. For exam-

ple, treatment of social anxiety might include gradual exposure to a feared situation like a party along with practice in identifying and changing unrealistic, negative self-talk.

- *Psychodynamic therapy* emphasizes the role of the past and of unconscious thoughts and impulses in shaping present behavior. Uncovering feelings and building self-awareness are common therapy goals.

Although these types of therapies may be described as distinctive orientations, most therapists offer a variety of approaches. Multiple therapies may be combined in various ways to meet the needs of a given patient's disorder or needs.

Choosing a Mental Health Professional   Mental health workers belong to several different professions and have different roles. Psychiatrists are medical doctors. They are experts in deciding whether a medical disease lies behind psychological symptoms, and they are usually involved in treatment if medication or hospitalization is required. Clinical psychologists typically hold a Ph.D. degree; they are often experts in behavioral and cognitive therapies. Other mental health workers include social workers, licensed counselors, and clergy with special training in pastoral counseling. In hospitals and clinics, various mental health professionals may join together in treatment teams.

TIPS FOR TODAY AND THE FUTURE
Most of life's psychological challenges can be met with self-help and everyday skills. You can take many steps to maintain your mental health.

RIGHT NOW YOU CAN
- Take a serious look at how you've been feeling recently. If you have any feelings that are especially hard to handle, consider how you can get help with them.
- Think of the way in which you are most creative (an important part of self-actualization), whether it's in music, art, or whatever you enjoy. Try to focus at least an hour each week on this activity.
- Review the list of defense mechanisms in Table 3.2. Have you used any of them recently or consistently over time? Think of a situation in which you used one of those mechanisms and determine how you could have coped with it differently.

IN THE FUTURE YOU CAN
- Write 100 positive adjectives that describe you. This exercise may take several days to complete. Post your list in a place where you will see it often.
- Record your reactions to upsetting events in your life. Are your reactions and self-talk typically negative or neutral? Decide whether you are satisfied with your reactions and if they are healthy.

QUESTIONS FOR CRITICAL THINKING AND REFLECTION
Have you ever thought professional psychological counseling or therapy might be appropriate for yourself or a loved one? What circumstances made you think this? Did you or your loved one seek professional help? What was the outcome?

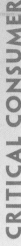

Choosing and Evaluating Mental Health Professionals

College students are usually in a good position to find convenient, affordable mental health care. Larger schools typically have both health services that employ psychiatrists and psychologists and counseling centers staffed by professionals and student peer counselors. Resources in the community may include a school of medicine, a hospital, and a variety of professionals who work independently. Although independent practitioners are listed in the telephone book, it's a good idea to get recommendations from physicians, clergy, friends who have been in therapy, or community agencies rather than pick a name at random.

Financial considerations are also important. Find out how much different services will cost and what your health insurance will cover. If you're not adequately covered by a health plan, don't let that stop you from getting help; investigate low-cost alternatives. City, county, and state governments often support mental health clinics for those who can afford to pay little or nothing for treatment. Some on-campus services may be free or offered at very little cost.

The cost of treatment is linked to how many therapy sessions will be needed, which in turn depends on the type of therapy and the nature of the problem. Psychological therapies focusing on specific problems may require eight or ten sessions at weekly intervals. Therapies aiming for psychological awareness and personality change can last months or years.

Deciding whether a therapist is right for you will require meeting the therapist in person. Before or during your first meeting, find out about the therapist's background and training:

• Does she or he have a degree from an appropriate professional school and a state license to practice?

• Has she or he had experience treating people with problems similar to yours?

• How much will therapy cost?

You have a right to know the answers to these questions and should not hesitate to ask them. After your initial meeting, evaluate your impressions:

• Does the therapist seem like a warm, intelligent person who would be able to help you and interested in doing so?

• Are you comfortable with the personality, values, and beliefs of the therapist?

• Is he or she willing to talk about the techniques in use? Do these techniques make sense to you?

If you answer yes to these questions, this therapist may be satisfactory for you. If you feel uncomfortable—and you're not in need of emergency care—it's worthwhile to set up one-time consultations with one or two others before you make up your mind. Take the time to find someone who feels right for you.

Later in your treatment, evaluate your progress:

• Are you being helped by the treatment?

• If you are displeased, is it because you aren't making progress, or because therapy is raising difficult, painful issues you don't want to deal with?

• Can you express dissatisfaction to your therapist? Such feedback can improve your treatment.

If you're convinced your therapy isn't working or is harmful, thank your therapist for her or his efforts, and find another.

For more on finding appropriate help, see the box "Choosing and Evaluating Mental Health Professionals."

SUMMARY

• Psychological health encompasses more than a single particular state of normality. Psychological diversity is valuable among groups of people.

• Defining psychological health as the presence of wellness means that to be healthy you must strive to fulfill your potential.

• Self-actualized people have high self-esteem and are realistic, inner-directed, authentic, capable of emotional intimacy, and creative.

• Crucial parts of psychological wellness include developing an adult identity, establishing intimate relationships, and developing values and purpose in life.

• A pessimistic outlook can be damaging; it can be overcome by developing more realistic self-talk.

• Honest communication requires recognizing what needs to be said and saying it clearly. Assertiveness enables people to insist on their rights and to participate in the give-and-take of good communication.

• People may be lonely if they haven't developed ways to be happy on their own or if they interpret being alone as a sign of rejection. Lonely people can take action to expand their social contacts.

• Dealing successfully with anger involves distinguishing between a reasonable level of assertiveness and gratuitous expressions of anger, heading off rage by reframing thoughts and distracting oneself, and responding to the anger of others with an asymmetrical, problem-solving orientation.

• People with psychological disorders have symptoms severe enough to interfere with daily living.

• Anxiety is a fear that is not directed toward any definite threat. Anxiety disorders include simple phobias, social phobias, panic disorder, generalized anxiety disorder, obsessive-compulsive disorder, and post-traumatic stress disorder.

• Depression is a common mood disorder; loss of interest or pleasure in things seems to be its most universal symptom. Severe depression carries a high risk of suicide, and suicidally depressed people need professional help.

• Symptoms of mania include exalted moods with unrealistically high self-esteem, little need for sleep, and rapid speech. Mood swings between mania and depression characterize bipolar disorder.

Dealing with Social Anxiety

Shyness is often the result of both high anxiety levels and lack of key social skills. To help overcome shyness, you need to learn to manage your fear of social situations and to develop social skills such as appropriate eye contact, initiating topics in conversations, and maintaining the flow of conversations by asking questions and making appropriate responses.

To reduce your anxiety in social situations, try some of the following strategies:

- Refocus your attention away from the stress reaction you're experiencing and toward the social task at hand. Your nervousness is much less visible than you think.

- Allow a warm-up period for new situations. Realize that you will feel more nervous at first, and take steps to relax and become more comfortable. Refer to the suggestions for deep breathing and other relaxation techniques in Chapter 2.

- If possible, take breaks during anxiety-producing situations. For example, if you're at a party, take a moment to visit the restroom or step outside. Alternate between speaking with good friends and striking up conversations with new acquaintances.

- Practice realistic self-talk. Replace your self-critical thoughts with more supportive ones: "No one else is perfect, and I don't have to be either." "It would have been good if I had a funny story to tell, but the conversation was interesting anyway."

Starting and maintaining conversations can be difficult for shy people, who may feel overwhelmed by their physical stress reaction. If small talk is a problem for you, try the following strategies:

- Introduce yourself early in the conversation. If you tend to forget names, repeat your new acquaintance's name to help fix it in your mind ("Nice to meet you, Amelia").

- Ask questions, and look for shared topics of interest. Simple, open-ended questions like "How's your presentation coming along?" or "How do you know our host?" encourage others to carry the conversation for a while and help bring forth a variety of subjects.

- Take turns talking, and elaborate on your answers. Simple yes and no answers don't move the conversation along. Try to relate something in your life—a course you're taking or a hobby you have—to something in the other person's life. Match self-disclosure with self-disclosure.

- Have something to say. Expand your mind and become knowledgeable about current events and local or campus news. If you have specialized knowledge about a topic, practice discussing it in ways that both beginners and experts can understand and appreciate.

- If you get stuck for something to say, try giving a compliment ("Great presentation!" or "I love your earrings.") or performing a social grace (pass the chips or get someone a drink).

- Be an active listener. Reward the other person with your full attention and with regular responses. Make frequent eye contact and maintain a relaxed but alert posture.

At first, your new behaviors will likely make you anxious. Don't give up—things *will* get easier. Create lots of opportunities to practice your new behaviors; your goal is to make them routine activities.

Eventually, you'll be able to sustain social interactions with comfort and enjoyment. If you find that social anxiety is a major problem for you and self-help techniques don't seem to work, consider looking into a shyness clinic or treatment program on your campus.

SOURCES: University of Texas at Dallas, Student Counseling Center. 2008 Update. *Self-Help: Overcoming Social Anxiety* (http://www.utdallas.edu/counseling/selfhelp/social-anxiety.html; retrieved December 29, 2008); Carducci, B. J. 2000. *Shyness: A Bold New Approach.* New York: Harper Paperbacks.

- Schizophrenia is characterized by disorganized thoughts, inappropriate emotions, delusions, auditory hallucinations, and deteriorating social and work performance.

- Help is available in a variety of forms, including self-help, peer counseling, support groups, and therapy with a mental health professional. For serious problems, professional help may be the most appropriate.

FOR MORE INFORMATION

BOOKS

Antony, M. M. 2008. *The Shyness & Social Anxiety Workbook: Proven, Step-by-Step Strategies for Overcoming Your Fear,* 2nd ed. Oakland, Calif.: New Harbinger. *Practical suggestions for fears of interacting with people you don't know.*

Grieco, R. 2009. *The Other Depression: Bipolar Disorder.* New York: Routledge. *Provides a complete introduction to bipolar disorder, its symptoms, and its current treatments.*

Jenkins, J., D. Keltner, and K. Oatley. 2006. *Understanding Emotions.* 2nd ed. Oxford: Blackwell. *A comprehensive guide to emotions, including current research on the neuroscience of emotions, evolutionary and cultural approaches to emotion, and the expression and communication of emotions.*

Nathan, P. E., and J. M. Gorman. 2007. *A Guide to Treatments That Work,* 3rd ed. New York: Oxford University Press. *A balanced and comprehensive report on various treatments for psychological disorders.*

Seligman, M. E. 2006. *Learned Optimism: How to Change Your Mind and Your Life* (Vintage Reprint Edition). New York: Vintage. *Introduces methods for overcoming feelings of helplessness and building a positive self-image that can contribute to emotional well-being.*

Thase, M. E., and S. S. Lang. 2006. *Beating the Blues: New Approaches to Overcoming Dysthymia and Chronic Mild Depression.* New York:

Oxford University Press. *Describes strategies for changing negative thinking patterns that lead to discouragement and pessimism; also discusses newer medications and alternative therapies.*

ORGANIZATIONS, HOTLINES, AND WEB SITES

American Association of Suicidology. Provides information about suicide and resources for people in crisis.

http://www.suicidology.org

Anxiety Disorders Association of America (ADAA). Provides information and resources related to anxiety disorders.

http://www.adaa.org

Depression and Bipolar Support Alliance (DBSA). Provides educational materials and information about support groups.

http://www.dbsalliance.org

Internet Mental Health. An encyclopedia of mental health information, including medical diagnostic criteria.

http://www.mentalhealth.com

Mental Health America. Provides consumer information on a variety of issues, including how to find help.

http://www.nmha.org

MindZone. Offers information on mental health issues specifically for teens.

http://www.copecaredeal.org

NAMI (National Alliance on Mental Illness). Provides information and support for people affected by mental illness.

800-950-NAMI (Help Line)

http://www.nami.org

National Hopeline Network. 24-hour hotline for people who are thinking about suicide or know someone who is; calls are routed to local crisis centers.

800-SUICIDE

http://www.hopeline.com

National Institute of Mental Health (NIMH). Provides helpful information about anxiety, depression, eating disorders, and other challenges to psychological health.

http://www.nimh.nih.gov

National Mental Health Information Center. A one-stop source for information and resources relating to mental health.

http://www.mentalhealth.org

SELECTED BIBLIOGRAPHY

Adams, R. E., and J. A. Boscarino. 2006. Predictors of PTSD and delayed PTSD after disaster: The impact of exposure and psychosocial resources. *The Journal of Nervous and Mental Disease* 194(7): 485–493.

American Psychiatric Association. 2000. *Diagnostic and Statistical Manual of Mental Disorders,* 4th ed., Text Revision *(DSM-IV-TR).* Washington, D.C.: American Psychiatric Association Press.

Antidepressants for children and adolescents: An update. 2006. *Harvard Mental Health Letter* 22(12): 4–5.

Avagianou, P. A., and M. Zafiropoulou. 2008. Parental bonding and depression: Personality as a mediating factor. *International Journal of Adolescent Medicine & Health* 20(3): 261–269.

Brenes, G. A., 2006. Age differences in the presentation of anxiety. *Aging and Mental Health* 10(3): 298–302.

Coryell, W. H. 2006. Clinical assessment of suicide risk in depressive disorder. *CNS Spectrums* 11(6): 455–461.

Eranti, S., et al. 2007. A randomized, controlled trial with 6-month follow-up of repetitive transcranial magnetic stimulation and electroconvulsive therapy for severe depression. *American Journal of Psychiatry* 164(1): 73–81.

Favaro, A., et al. 2007. Self-injurious behavior in a community sample of young women: Relationship with childhood abuse and other types of self-damaging behaviors. *Journal of Clinical Psychiatry* 68(1): 122–131.

Fazel, S., and M. Grann. 2006. The population impact of severe mental illness on violent crime. *American Journal of Psychiatry* 163(8): 1397–1403.

Forty, L., et al. 2009. Polarity at illness onset in bipolar I disorder and clinical course of illness. *Bipolar Disorders* 11(1): 82–88.

Hamilton, B. E., et al. 2007. Annual Summary of Vital Statistics: 2005. *Pediatrics* 119(2): 345–360.

Healy, D. 2006. Did regulators fail over selective serotonin reuptake inhibitors? *British Medical Journal* 333: 92–95.

Hettema, J. M., et al. 2006. A population-based twin study of the relationship between neuroticism and internalizing disorders. *American Journal of Psychiatry* 163(5): 857–864.

Jones, S. H., and G. Burrell-Hodgson. 2008. Cognitive-behavioral treatment of first diagnosis bipolar disorder. *Clinical Psychology & Psychotherapy* 15(6): 367–377.

Kasper, S., et al. 2006. Superior efficacy of St. John's wort extract WS(R) 5570 compared to placebo in patients with major depression: A randomized, double-blind, placebo-controlled, multi-center trial. *BMC Medicine* 4(1): 14.

Kendler, K. S., J. Myers, and C. A. Prescott. 2005. Sex differences in the relationship between social support and risk for major depression: A longitudinal study of opposite-sex twin pairs. *American Journal of Psychiatry* 162(2): 250–256.

Licinio, J., and M. L. Wong. 2005. Opinion: Depression, antidepressants and suicidality: A critical appraisal. *Nature Reviews: Drug Discovery* 4(2): 165–171.

Lin, Y. R., et al. 2008. Evaluation of assertiveness training for psychiatric patients. *Journal of Clinical Nursing* 17(21): 2875–2883.

McGirr, A., et al. 2006. An examination of DSM-IV depressive symptoms and risk for suicide completion in major depressive disorder: A psychological autopsy study. *Journal of Affective Disorders,* 17 July.

Nemeroff, C. B. 2006. The burden of severe depression: A review of diagnostic challenges and treatment alternatives. *Journal of Psychiatric Research,* 25 July [Epub ahead of print].

Ozer, D. J., and V. Benet-Martinez. 2006. Personality and prediction of consequential outcomes. *Annual Review of Psychology* 57: 401–421.

Rothwell, J. D. 2009. *In the Company of Others: An Introduction to Communication,* 3rd ed. New York: McGraw-Hill.

Saewyc, E. M., and R. Tonkin. 2008. Surveying adolescents: Focusing on positive development. *Pediatrics & Child Health* 13(1): 43–47.

Schatzberg, A. F., J. O. Cole, and C. DeBattista. 2007. *Manual of Clinical Psychopharmacology,* 6th ed. Washington, D.C.: American Psychiatric Publishing.

Simon, G. E., and J. Savarino. 2007. Suicide attempts among patients starting depression treatment with medications or psychotherapy. *American Journal of Psychiatry* 164(7): 1029–1034.

Simon, G. 2009. Collaborative care for mood disorders. *Current Opinion in Psychiatry.* 22(1): 37–41.

Singh, N. N., et al. 2007. Individuals with mental illness can control their aggressive behavior through mindfulness training. *Behavior Modification* 31(3): 313–328.

Verhaak, P. F., et al. 2009. Receiving treatment for common mental disorders. *General Hospital Psychiatry* 31(1): 46–55.

Williams, D., et al. 2007. Prevalence and distribution of major depressive disorder in African Americans, Caribbean blacks, and non-Hispanic whites. *Archives of General Psychiatry* 64: 305–315.

Zarit, S. H., and J. M. Zarit. 2006. *Mental Disorders in Older Adults: Fundamentals of Assessment and Treatment,* 2nd ed. New York: Guilford Press.

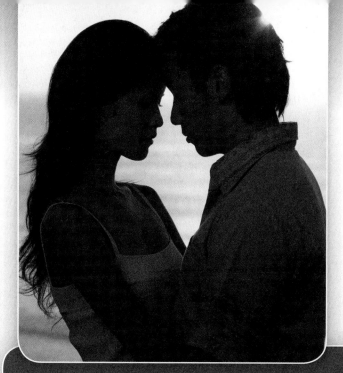

LOOKING AHEAD >>>>>

**AFTER READING THIS CHAPTER,
YOU SHOULD BE ABLE TO:**

- Explain the qualities that help people develop intimate relationships

- Describe different types of love relationships and the stages they often go through

- Identify common challenges of forming and maintaining intimate relationships

- Explain some elements of healthy and productive communication

- List some characteristics of successful families and some potential problems families face

INTIMATE RELATIONSHIPS AND COMMUNICATION

4

H uman beings need social relationships; we cannot thrive as solitary creatures. Nor could the human species survive if adults didn't cherish and support each other, if we didn't form strong mutual attachments with our infants, and if we didn't create families in which to raise children. Simply put, people need people.

Although people are held together in relationships by a variety of factors, the foundation of many relationships is the ability to both give and receive love. Love in its many forms—romantic, passionate, platonic, parental—is the wellspring from which much of life's meaning and delight flows. In our culture, it binds us together as partners, parents, children, and friends.

Just as important, we also need to develop a healthy relationship to ourselves, which includes the ability to self-soothe, to regulate our emotions, and to be alone with ourselves at times.

DEVELOPING INTIMATE RELATIONSHIPS

People who develop successful intimate relationships believe in themselves and in the people around them. They are willing to give of themselves—to share their ideas, feelings, time, needs—and to accept what others want to give them.

Self-Concept and Self-Esteem

The principal element that we all bring to our relationships is our *selves*. To have successful relationships, we must first accept and feel good about ourselves. A positive self-concept and a healthy level of self-esteem help us love and respect others.

As discussed in Chapter 3, the roots of our identity and sense of self can be found in childhood, in the relationships

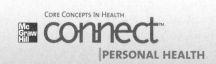

CORE CONCEPTS IN HEALTH
McGraw Hill connect™
| PERSONAL HEALTH

http://www.mcgrawhillconnect.com/personalhealth

we had with our parents and other family members. As adults, we probably have a sense that we're basically lovable, worthwhile people and that we can trust others if, as babies and children, we experienced the following:

- We felt loved, valued, and respected.
- Adults responded to our needs in a reasonably appropriate way.
- They gave us the freedom to explore and develop a sense of being separate individuals.

Gender Role   Another thing we learn in early childhood is *gender role*—the activities, abilities, and characteristics our culture deems appropriate for us based on whether we're male or female. In our society, men have traditionally been expected to work and provide for their families; to be aggressive, competitive, and power-oriented; and to use thinking and logic to solve problems. Women have been expected to take care of home and children; to be cooperative, supportive, and nurturing; and to approach life emotionally and intuitively. Although much more egalitarian gender roles are emerging in our society, the stereotypes we absorb in childhood tend to be deeply ingrained.

Attachment   Our ways of relating to others are also rooted in childhood. Some researchers have suggested that our adult styles of loving may be based on the style of **attachment** we established in infancy with our mother, father, siblings, or other primary caregiver. According to this view, people who are secure in their intimate relationships probably had a secure, trusting, mutually satisfying attachment to their mother, father, or other parenting figure. As adults, they find it relatively easy to get close to others. They don't worry about being abandoned or having someone get too close to them. They feel that other people like them and are generally well-intentioned.

People who are clinging and dependent in their relationships may have had an "anxious/ambivalent" attachment, in which a parent's inconsistent responses made them unsure that their needs would be met. As adults, they worry about whether their partners really love them and will stay with them. They tend to feel that others don't want to get as close as they do. They want to merge completely with another person, which sometimes scares others away.

People who seem to run from relationships may have had an "anxious/avoidant" attachment, in which a parent's inappropriate responses made them want to escape from his or her sphere of influence. As adults, they feel uncomfortable being close to others. They're distrustful

and fearful of becoming dependent. Their partners usually want more intimacy than they do.

Even if people's earliest experiences and relationships were less than ideal, however, they can still establish satisfying relationships in adulthood. In fact, relationships in adolescence and adulthood give us a golden opportunity to work on and through unresolved issues and conflicts from the past. After all, very few people have perfect parents and perfect siblings, and no one grows up without experiencing some sort of personal pain and conflict.

People can be resilient and flexible. They have the capacity to change their ideas, beliefs, and behavior patterns. They can learn ways to raise their self-esteem; they can become more trusting, accepting, and appreciative of others; and they can acquire the communication and conflict-resolution skills required for maintaining successful relationships. Although it helps to have a good start in life, it may be even more important to begin again, right from where you are. Most important is to be accepting and kind to ourselves as we are in the present and do our best to grow and develop emotionally.

Friendship

The first relationships we form outside the family are friendships. The friendships we form in childhood are important in our development; through them we learn about tolerance, sharing, and trust. Friendships usually include most or all of the following characteristics:

- *Companionship.* Friends are usually relaxed and happy in each other's company. They typically have common values and interests and make plans to spend time together.
- *Respect.* Friends have a basic respect for each other's humanity and individuality. Good friends respect each other's feelings and opinions and work to resolve their differences without demeaning or insulting each other. They also show their respect by being honest with each other (see the box "Being a Good Friend").
- *Acceptance.* Friends feel free to be themselves and express their feelings without fear of ridicule or criticism.
- *Help.* Sharing time, energy, and even material goods is important to friendship. Friends know they can rely on each other in times of need.
- *Trust.* Friends are secure in the knowledge that they will not intentionally hurt each other.
- *Loyalty.* Friends can count on each other. They stand up for each other in both word and deed.
- *Mutuality.* Friends retain their individual identities, but close friendships are characterized by a sense of mutuality—"what affects you affects me." Friends share the ups and downs in each other's lives.

TERMS

attachment   The emotional tie between an infant and his or her caregiver or between two people in an intimate relationship.

Being a Good Friend

How to Make Friends

• Find people with interests similar to your own. Join a club, participate in sports, do volunteer work, or join a discussion group to meet people with common interests.

• Be a good listener. Take a genuine interest in people. Solicit their opinions, and take time to listen to their problems and ideas.

• Take risks. If you meet someone interesting, ask him or her to join you for a meal or an event you would both enjoy.

How to Be a Good Friend

• Be trustworthy. Honor all confidences, and don't talk about your friend behind his or her back.

• Tell your friend about yourself. Self-disclosure—letting your friend know about your real concerns and joys—signals trust.

• Be supportive and kind. Be there when your friend is going through a rough time. Don't criticize your friend or offer unsolicited advice.

• Develop your capacity for intimacy. Intimate relationships are genuine, spontaneous, and caring.

• Don't expect perfection. Like any relationship, your friendship may go through difficult times. Talk through conflicts as they arise.

• Don't brag or boast excessively.

• Share past experiences, difficulties, and successes.

• Be altruistic; that is, be generous without expecting anything in return.

Table 4.1	Average Number of Confidants: 1985 and 2004	
	Americans with This Number of Confidants	
Number	**1985**	**2004**
0	10.0%	24.6%
1	15.0	19.0
2	16.2	19.2
3	20.3	16.9
4	14.8	8.8
5	18.2	6.5
6 or more	5.4	4.9

SOURCE: McPherson, M., et al. 2006. Social isolation in America: Changes in the core discussion networks over two decades. *American Sociological Review* 71: 353–375.

• *Reciprocity.* Friendships are reciprocal. There is give-and-take between friends and the feeling that both share joys and burdens more or less equally over time.

As important as friendships are, however, the average American's social circle is shrinking—to the point that nearly 25% of Americans say they have no one they want to confide in (Table 4.1). In 2006, sociologists from Duke University and the University of Arizona released details of a study confirming the issue. According to the study, Americans have fewer close friends than ever before. Most have only two friends they consider close enough to discuss problems with.

Love, Sex, and Intimacy

Love is one of the most basic and profound human emotions. It is a powerful force in all our intimate relationships. Love encompasses opposites: affection and anger, excitement and boredom, stability and change, bonds and freedom. Love does not give us perfect happiness, but it does give our lives meaning.

For most people, love, sex, and commitment are closely linked ideals in intimate relationships. Love reflects the positive factors that draw people together and sustain them in a relationship. It includes trust, caring, respect, loyalty, interest in the other, and concern for the other's well-being. Sex brings excitement and passion to the relationship. It intensifies the relationship and adds fascination and pleasure.

> **15%–18%** of married people will have an affair during their marriage.
>
> —**National Opinion Research Center, 2006**

Commitment, the determination to continue, reflects the stable factors that help maintain the relationship. Responsibility, reliability, and faithfulness are characteristics of commitment. Although love, sex, and commitment are related, they are not necessarily connected. One can exist without the others. Despite the various "faces" of love, sex, and commitment, most of us long for a special relationship that contains them all.

Other elements can be identified as features of love, such as euphoria, preoccupation with the loved one, idealization or devaluation of the loved one, and so on, but these tend to be temporary. These characteristics may include **infatuation**, which will fade or deepen into something more substantial. As relationships progress, the central aspects of love and commitment take on more importance.

Men and women tend to have different views of the relationship between love (or intimacy) and sex (or passion). Numerous studies have found that men can separate love from sex rather easily, although many men find that their most erotic sexual experiences occur in the context of a love relationship. Women generally view sex from the point of view of a relationship. Some people believe you can have satisfying sex without love—with friends, acquaintances, or strangers. Although sex with love is an important norm in our culture, it is frequently disregarded in practice, as the high incidence of extrarelational affairs attests.

The Pleasure and Pain of Love   The experience of intense love has confused and tormented lovers throughout history. They live in a tumultuous state of excitement, subject to wildly fluctuating feelings of joy and despair. They lose their appetite, can't sleep, and can think of nothing but the loved one. Is this happiness? Misery? Or both?

The contradictory nature of passionate love can be understood by recognizing that human emotions have two components: physiological arousal and an emotional explanation for the arousal. Love is just one of many emotions accompanied by physiological arousal; numerous unpleasant ones can also generate arousal, such as fear, rejection, frustration, and challenge. Although experiences like attraction and sexual desire are pleasant, extreme excitement is similar to fear and is unpleasant. For this reason, passionate love may be too intense to enjoy. Over time, the physical intensity and excitement tend to diminish. When this happens, pleasure may actually increase.

The Transformation of Love   All human relationships change over time, and love relationships are no exception. At first, love is likely to be characterized by high levels of passion and rapidly increasing intimacy. After a while, passion decreases as we become habituated to it and to the person. The diminishing of romance or passionate love is often experienced as a crisis in a relationship. If a more lasting love fails to emerge, the relationship will likely break up.

Unlike passion, however, commitment does not necessarily diminish over time. When intensity diminishes, partners often discover a more enduring love. They can now move from absorption in each other to a relationship

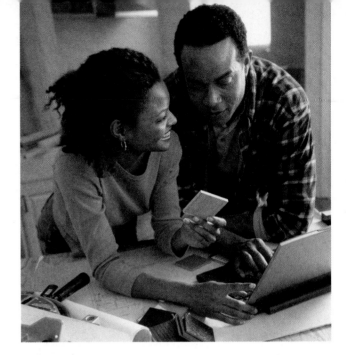

Although passion and physical intimacy often decline with time, other aspects of a relationship—such as commitment—tend to grow as the relationship matures.

that includes external goals and projects, friends, and family. In this kind of intimate, more secure love, satisfaction comes not just from the relationship itself but also from achieving other creative goals, such as work or child rearing. The key to successful relationships is in transforming passion into an intimate love, based on closeness, caring, and the promise of a shared future.

Challenges in Relationships

Many people believe that love naturally makes an intimate relationship easy to begin and maintain, but in fact, obstacles arise and challenges occur. Even in the best of circumstances, a loving relationship will be tested. Individuals bring to a relationship diverse needs and wants, some of which emerge only at times of change or stress.

Honesty and Openness   It's usually best to be yourself from the start to give both you and your potential partner a chance to find out if you are comfortable with each other's beliefs, interests, and lifestyles. Getting close to another person by sharing thoughts and feelings is emotionally risky, but it is necessary for a relationship to deepen. Take your time, and self-disclose at a slow but steady rate—one that doesn't make you

15.5% of college students say that relationship problems affect their academic performance.

—American College Health Association, 2007

TERMS

infatuation   An idealizing, obsessive attraction, characterized by a high degree of physical arousal.

feel too vulnerable or your partner too uncomfortable. Over time, you and your partner will learn more about each other and feel more comfortable sharing.

Unequal or Premature Commitment   Sometimes one person in an intimate partnership becomes more serious about the relationship than the other partner. In this situation, it can be very difficult to maintain a friendship without hurting the other person. Sometimes a couple makes a premature commitment, and then one of the partners has second thoughts and wants to break off the relationship. Sometimes both partners begin to realize that something is wrong, but each is afraid to tell the other. Most such problems can be dealt with only by honest and sensitive communication.

Unrealistic Expectations   Each partner brings hopes and expectations to a relationship, some of which may be unrealistic, unfair, and, ultimately, very damaging to the relationship. For example, if you believe that love will eliminate all of your problems, you may start to blame your partner for anything that goes wrong in your life. Other unrealistic expectations include the following:

- Expecting your partner to change.
- Assuming that your partner has all the same opinions, priorities, interests, and goals as you.
- Believing that a relationship will fulfill all of your personal, financial, intellectual, and social needs.

Competitiveness   If one partner always feels the strong need to compete and win, it can detract from the sense of connectedness, interdependence, equality, and mutuality between partners. The same can be said for a perfectionistic need to be right in every instance—to "win" every argument.

If competitiveness is a problem for you, ask yourself if your need to win is more important than your partner's feelings or the future of your relationship. Try noncompetitive activities or an activity where you are a beginner and your partner excels. Accept that your partner's views may be just as valid and important to your partner as your own views are to you.

Balancing Time Spent Together and Apart   You may enjoy time together with your partner, but you may also want to spend time alone or with other friends. If you or your partner interpret time apart as rejection or lack of commitment, it can damage a relationship. Talk with your partner about what time apart means and share your feelings about what you expect from the relationship in terms of time together. Consider your partner's feelings carefully, and try to reach a compromise that satisfies both of you.

Differences in expectations about time spent together can mirror differences in ideas about emotional closeness. Any romantic relationship involves giving up some degree of autonomy in order to develop an identity as a couple.

But remember that every person is unique and has different needs for distance and closeness in a relationship.

Jealousy   Jealousy is the angry, painful response to a partner's real, imagined, or likely involvement with a third person. Some people think that the existence of jealousy proves the existence of love, but jealousy is actually a sign of insecurity or possessiveness. In its irrational and extreme forms, jealousy can destroy a relationship by its insistent demands and attempts at control. Jealousy is a factor in precipitating violence in dating relationships among both high school and college students, and abusive spouses often use jealousy to justify their violence.

People with a healthy level of self-esteem are less likely to feel jealous. When jealousy occurs in a relationship, it's important for the partners to communicate clearly with each other about their feelings.

Supportiveness   Another key to successful relationships is the ability to ask for and give support. Partners need to know that they can count on each other during difficult times. If you are having trouble getting or giving the support that you or your partner needs, try some of

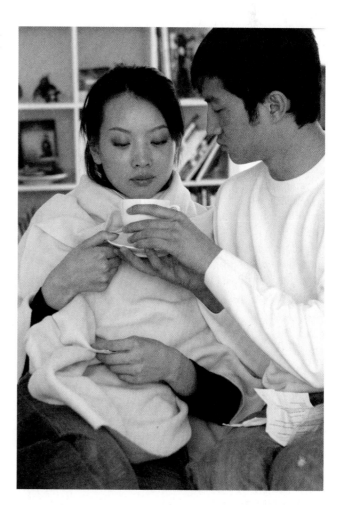

Supportiveness is a sign of commitment and compassion and is an important part of any healthy relationship.

Strategies for Enhancing Support in Relationships

- *Be aware of the importance of support.* Time and energy spent on support will help both you and your partner deal with stress and create a positive atmosphere that will help when differences or conflicts do occur.

- *Learn to ask for help from your partner.* Try different ways of asking for help and support from your partner and make note of which approaches work best for your relationship.

- *Help your partner the way she or he would like to be helped.* Some people prefer empathy and emotional support, whereas others like more practical help with problems.

- *Avoid negativity, especially when being asked for help.* Asking for help puts a person in a vulnerable position. If your partner asks for your aid, be gracious and supportive; don't use phrases like "I told you so" or "You should have just. . . ." Otherwise, your partner may learn not to ask for your help or support at all.

- *Make positive attributions.* If you're unsure about the reasons for your partner's behavior, give her or him the benefit of the doubt. For example, if your partner arrives for a date 30 minutes late and in a bad mood, assume it's because she or he had a bad day rather than attributing it to a character flaw or relationship problem. Offer appropriate support.

- *Help yourself.* Develop coping strategies for times your partner won't be available. These might include things you can do for yourself, such as going for a walk, or other people you can turn to for support.

- *Keep relationship problems separate.* Avoid bringing up relationship problems when you are offering or asking for help.

- *Avoid giving advice.* Immediately offering advice when asked for help implies that you are smarter or more capable than your partner at solving your partner's difficulty. Begin by providing emotional support and validating your partner's feelings. Then, if asked, help brainstorm solutions.

SOURCE: Plante, T., and K. Sullivan. 2000. *Getting Together and Staying Together: The Stanford Course on Intimate Relationships.* Bloomington, Ind.: 1st Books Library. Reprinted with permission of the author.

---

the suggestions in the box "Strategies for Enhancing Support in Relationships."

Unhealthy Relationships

Everyone should be able to recognize when a relationship is unhealthy. Relatively extreme examples of unhealthy relationships are those that are physically or emotionally abusive or that involve codependency; strategies for addressing these problems are presented in Chapters 7 and 16, respectively. Even relationships that are not abusive or codependent can still be unhealthy. If your relationship lacks love and respect and places little value on the time you and your partner have spent together, it may be time to get professional help or to end the partnership. Further, if your relationship is characterized by communication styles that include criticism, contempt, defensiveness, and withdrawal—despite real efforts to repair these destructive patterns—the relationship may not be salvageable. Spiritual leaders suggest that relationships are unhealthy when you feel that your sense of spontaneity, your potential for inner growth and joy, and your connection to your spiritual life is deadened. There are negative physical and mental consequences of being in an unhappy relationship; although breaking up is painful and difficult, it is ultimately better than living in a toxic relationship.

Ending a Relationship

Even when a couple starts out with the best of intentions, an intimate relationship may not last. Some breakups occur quickly following direct action by one or both partners, but many others occur over an extended period as the couple goes through a cycle of separating and reconciling.

Ending an intimate relationship is usually difficult and painful. Both partners may feel attacked and abandoned, but feelings of distress are likely to be more acute for the rejected partner. If you are involved in a breakup, the following suggestions may help make the ending easier:

- Give the relationship a fair chance before breaking up.
- Be fair and honest.
- Be tactful and compassionate.
- If you are the rejected person, give yourself time to resolve your anger and pain.
- Recognize the value in the experience.

Use the recovery period following a breakup for self-renewal. Redirect more of your attention to yourself, and reconnect with people and areas of your life that may have been neglected as a result of the relationship. Time will help heal the pain of the loss of the relationship.

QUESTIONS FOR CRITICAL THINKING AND REFLECTION

Have you ever ended an intimate relationship? If so, how did you handle it? How did you feel after the breakup? How did the breakup affect your former partner? Did the experience help you in other relationships? If so, in what way did it help?

COMMUNICATION

The key to developing and maintaining any type of intimate relationship is good communication.

Nonverbal Communication

Even when we're silent, we're communicating. We send messages when we look at someone or look away, lean forward or sit back, smile or frown. Especially important forms of nonverbal communication are touch, eye contact, and proximity. If someone we're talking to touches our hand or arm, looks into our eyes, and leans toward us when we talk, we get the message that the person is interested in us and cares about what we're saying. If a person keeps looking around the room while we're talking or takes a step backward, we get the impression the person is uninterested or wants to end the conversation.

The ability to interpret nonverbal messages correctly is important to the success of relationships. It's also important, when sending messages, to make sure our body language agrees with our words. When our verbal and nonverbal messages don't correspond, we send a mixed message.

Communication Skills

Three keys to good communication in relationships are self-disclosure, listening, and feedback.

• *Self-disclosure* involves revealing personal information that we ordinarily wouldn't reveal because of the risk involved. It usually increases feelings of closeness and moves the relationship to a deeper level of intimacy. Friends often disclose the most to each other, sharing feelings, experiences, hopes, and disappointments; married couples may share less because they think they already know everything about each other.

• *Listening,* the second key of good communication, is a rare skill. Good listening skills require that we spend more time and energy trying to fully understand another person's "story" and less time judging, evaluating, blaming, advising, analyzing, or trying to control. Empathy, warmth, respect, and genuineness are qualities of skillful listeners. Attentive listening encourages friends or partners to share more and, in turn, to be attentive listeners.

• *Feedback,* a constructive response to another's self-disclosure, is the third key to good communication. Giving positive feedback means acknowledging that the friend's or partner's feelings are valid—no matter how upsetting or troubling—and offering self-disclosure in response. Self-disclosure and feedback can open the door to change, whereas other responses block communication and change. (For tips on improving your skills, see the box "Guidelines for Effective Communication" on p. 76.)

Gender and Communication

Some of the difficulties people encounter in relationships can be traced to common gender differences in communication. Men and women generally approach conversation and communication differently. Men tend to use conversation in a *competitive* way, perhaps hoping to establish dominance in relationships. When male conversations are over, men often find themselves in a one-up or a one-down position. Women tend to use conversation in a more *affiliative* way, perhaps hoping to establish friendships. They negotiate various degrees of closeness, seeking to give and receive support. Men tend to talk more—though without disclosing more—and listen less. Women tend to use good listening skills such as eye contact, frequent nodding, focused attention, and asking relevant questions.

Even when a man and a woman are talking about the same subject, their unconscious goals may be very different. The woman may be looking for understanding and closeness, while the man may be trying to demonstrate his competence by giving advice and solving problems. Both styles are valid; the problem comes when differences in style result in poor communication and misunderstanding. See the box "Gender and Communication" on page 77 for more information.

Sometimes communication is not the problem in a relationship—the partners understand each other all too well. The problem is that they're unable or unwilling to change or compromise. Although good communication can't salvage a bad relationship, it does enable couples to see their differences and make more informed decisions.

Conflict and Conflict Resolution

Conflict is natural in intimate relationships. No matter how close two people become, they still remain separate individuals with their own needs, desires, past experiences, and ways of seeing the world. In fact, the closer the relationship, the more differences and the more opportunities for conflict there will be.

Conflict itself isn't dangerous to a relationship; in fact, it may indicate that the relationship is growing. But if it isn't handled in a constructive way, conflict can damage—and ultimately destroy—the relationship.

Conflict is often accompanied by anger—a natural emotion, but one that can be difficult to handle. If we express anger aggressively, we run the risk of creating distrust, fear, and distance; if we act it out without thinking things through, we can cause the conflict to escalate; if we

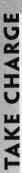

Guidelines for Effective Communication

Getting Started

• When you want to have a serious discussion with your partner, find an appropriate time and place. Choose a block of time when you will not be interrupted or rushed and a place that is private.

• Face your partner and maintain eye contact. Use nonverbal feedback to show that you are interested and involved in the communication process.

Being an Effective Speaker

• State your concern or issue as clearly as you can.

• Use "I" statements—statements about how *you* feel—rather than statements beginning with "You," which tell another person how you think he or she feels. When you use "I" statements, you are taking responsibility for your feelings. "You" statements are often blaming or accusatory and will probably get a defensive or resentful response. The statement "I feel unloved," for example, sends a clearer, less blaming message than the statement "You don't love me."

• Focus on a specific behavior rather than on the whole person. Be specific about the behavior you like or don't like. Avoid generalizations beginning with "You always" or "You never." Such statements make people feel defensive.

• Make constructive requests. Opening your request with "I would like" keeps the focus on your needs rather than your partner's supposed deficiencies.

• Avoid blaming, accusing, and belittling. Even if you are right, you have little to gain by putting your partner down. Studies have shown that when people feel criticized or attacked, they are less able to think rationally or solve problems constructively.

• Ask for action ahead of time, not after the fact. Tell your partner what you would like to have happen in the future; don't wait for him or her to blow it and then express anger or disappointment.

Being an Effective Listener

• Provide appropriate nonverbal feedback (nodding, smiling, making eye contact, and so on).

• Don't interrupt.

• Develop the skill of reflective listening. Don't judge, evaluate, analyze, or offer solutions (unless asked to do so). Your partner may just need to have you there in order to sort out feelings. By jumping in right away to "fix" the problem, you may actually be cutting off communication.

• Don't give unsolicited advice. Giving advice implies that you know more about what a person needs to do than he or she does; therefore, it often evokes anger or resentment.

• Clarify your understanding of what your partner is saying by restating it in your own words and asking if your understanding is correct. "I think you're saying that you would feel uncomfortable having dinner with my parents and that you'd prefer to meet them in a more casual setting. Is that right?" This type of specific feedback prevents misunderstandings and helps validate the speaker's feelings and message.

• Be sure you are really listening, not off somewhere in your mind rehearsing your reply. Try to tune in to your partner's feelings as well as the words.

• Let your partner know that you value what he or she is saying and want to understand. Respect for the other person is the cornerstone of effective communication.

---

suppress anger, it turns into resentment and hostility. The best way to handle anger in a relationship is to recognize it as a symptom of something that requires attention and needs to be changed. When angry, partners should exercise restraint so as not to become abusive. It is important to express anger skillfully and not in a way that is out of proportion to the issue at hand.

The sources of conflict for couples change over time but primarily revolve around the basic tasks of living together: dividing the housework, handling money, spending time together, and so on. Sexual interaction is also a source of disagreement for many couples.

The following strategies can be helpful when negotiating with a partner:

1. *Clarify the issue.* Take responsibility for thinking through your feelings and discovering what's really bothering you. Agree that one partner will speak first and have the chance to speak fully while the other listens. Then reverse the roles. Try to understand your partner's position fully by repeating what you've heard and asking questions to clarify or elicit more information. Agree to talk only about the topic at hand and not get distracted by other issues. Sum up what your partner has said.

2. *Find out what each person wants.* Ask your partner to express his or her desires. Don't assume you know what your partner wants and don't speak for him or her.

3. *Determine how you both can get what you want.* Brainstorm to generate a variety of options.

4. *Decide how to negotiate.* Work out a plan for change; for example, one partner will do one task and the other will do another task, or one partner will do a task in exchange for something he or she wants. Be willing to compromise, and avoid trying to "win."

5. *Solidify the agreements.* Go over the plan verbally and write it down, if necessary, to ensure that you both understand and agree to it.

Gender and Communication

GENDER MATTERS

From an early age, parents, teachers, and society send different messages to girls and boys regarding emotion. Boys learn to suppress and bury their feelings, especially fear and other emotions that make them feel vulnerable. Girls are encouraged to express and talk about their feelings.

These differences are further reinforced by peer groups. Gender segregation is already apparent in preschool and increases throughout middle childhood for most children. Boys and girls spend most of their time with peers of the same gender, and their communication styles are very different. For example, when conflict arises, girls tend to care more about preserving their relationships, and boys care more about maintaining the game they were playing.

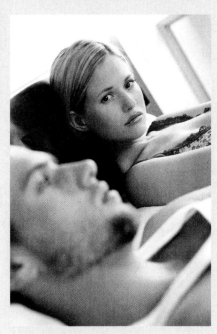

Research also shows that men have a more intense physiological response to certain emotions. In discussions around conflict, a man's blood pressure and heart rate rise higher and remain elevated longer. Part of the reason may be that a man's internal dialogue repeats upsetting thoughts (for example, "How could she say that? I can't take this!"). When anyone is physiologically or emotionally overwhelmed ("flooded"), productive communication is impossible.

A common pattern that arises between men and women is called "confront-withdraw." A woman approaches her male partner because she is upset and wants to talk about it. The man tries to calm her down, provides solutions he sees as rational, and/or withdraws. This response may make his partner even more upset and demanding, which causes the man to further shut down. Given what we know about gender differences, we might understand the man's response as one of self-protection, because he is entering territory that is both unknown and physically unpleasant.

In order to enjoy intimacy, men and women must work to better understand one another and develop a more compatible communication style.

Advice for Men

• When your partner raises an emotional topic, be aware of uncomfortable feelings and the desire to retreat.

• Do not run away (physically or emotionally)! Telling her to "calm down" will likely create the opposite response.

• Find a way to stay connected. This is the only way to deescalate the conflict.

• Empathize: Listen to what she is saying, and even if you disagree, communicate to her that you understand how she is feeling and where she is coming from. Often when a person feels genuinely heard, that is enough.

• Try not to think of her comments as personal attacks; instead, continue to empathize.

• You may need to calm yourself. Try taking long deep breaths, telling yourself that your partner needs to air her feelings, and remembering that she, too, wants the conflict to end.

• In some cases, a 20-minute break—during which you soothe yourself rather than think upsetting thoughts—can be helpful.

Advice for Women

• Try to be calm when approaching conflict; practice similar relaxation techniques to those described in "Advice for Men."

• Try to speak in ways that will not provoke defensiveness; complain rather than criticize, be specific, and use "I" statements.

• Try not to be critical of your partner's responses or his attempts to communicate.

• Be aware if he is withdrawing, and, if appropriate, help him to relax by using methods you have discussed previously.

SOURCE: Gottman, J. 1994. *Why Marriages Succeed or Fail . . . and How You Can Make Yours Last.* New York: Simon & Schuster.

?

QUESTIONS FOR CRITICAL THINKING AND REFLECTION

How do you handle conflict in your relationships? Do you fight intensely and then make up? Discuss, negotiate, and compromise? Avoid conflict altogether? Whatever your pattern of conflict resolution (or avoidance), where do you think you learned it? How effective is it for you? If it isn't working well, what ideas do you have for improvement?

6. *Review and renegotiate.* Decide on a time frame for trying out your plan, and set a time to discuss how it's working. Make adjustments as needed.

To resolve conflicts, partners have to feel safe in voicing disagreements. They have to trust that the discussion won't get out of control, that they won't be abandoned by the other, and that the partner won't take advantage of their vulnerability. Partners should follow some basic ground rules when they argue, such as avoiding ultimatums, resisting the urge to give the silent treatment, refusing to "hit below the belt," and not using sex to smooth over disagreements. When you argue, maintain a spirit of goodwill and avoid being harshly critical or contemptuous. If you and your partner find that you argue again and again over the same issue, it may be better to stop trying to resolve that problem and instead come to accept the differences between you.

PAIRING AND SINGLEHOOD

Although most people eventually marry or commit to a partner, everyone spends some time as a single person, and nearly all make some attempt, consciously or unconsciously, to find a partner. Intimate relationships are as important for singles as for couples.

Choosing a Partner

Most men and women select partners for long-term relationships through a fairly predictable process, although they may not be consciously aware of it. First attraction is based on easily observable characteristics: looks, dress, social status, and reciprocated interest. Most people pair with someone who:

- Lives in the same geographic area
- Is from a similar ethnic and socioeconomic background
- Has similar educational attainment
- Lives a similar lifestyle
- Is like them in terms of physical attraction

Once the euphoria of romantic love winds down, personality traits and behaviors become more significant factors in how the partners view each other. The emphasis shifts to basic values and future aspirations regarding career, family, and children. At some point, they decide whether the relationship feels viable and is worthy of their continued commitment.

Perhaps the most important question for potential mates to ask is, "How much do we have in common?" Although differences add interest to a relationship, similarities increase the chances of a relationship's success. Areas in which differences can affect a relationship include values, religion, ethnicity, attitudes toward sexuality and gender roles, socioeconomic status, familiarity with each other's culture, and interactions with the extended family (see the box "Interfaith and Intrafaith Partnerships" on p. 79). Acceptance and communication skills go a long way toward making a relationship work, no matter how different the partners.

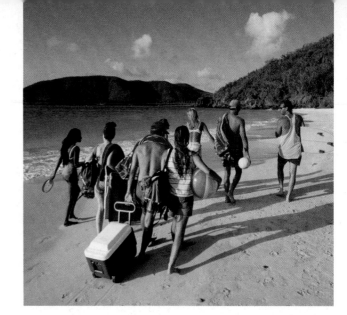

For many college students today, group activities have replaced dating as a way to meet and get to know potential partners.

Dating

Most Americans find romantic partners through some form of dating. Traditionally, in the male-female dating pattern, the man took the lead, initiating the date, while the woman waited to be called. In this pattern, casual dating might evolve into steady or exclusive dating, then engagement, and finally marriage. Although the American cultural norm is personal choice in courtship and mate selection, the popularity of dating services and online matchmaking suggests that many people want help finding a suitable partner (see the box "Online Relationships" on p. 80).

For many young people today, traditional dating has given way to a more casual form of getting together in groups. People go out in groups, rather than strictly as couples, and each person pays his or her way. A man and woman may begin to spend more time together, but often in the group context. If sexual involvement develops, it is more likely to be based on friendship, respect, and common interests than on expectations related to gender roles. In this model, mate selection may progress from getting together to living together to marriage.

Living Together

According to the U.S. Census Bureau, 4.9 million opposite-sex couples and 595,000 same-sex couples were living together in 2000. The Human Rights Campaign, however, estimates that the number of same-sex couples is closer to 1.6 million. Living together, or **cohabitation**, is one of the most rapid and dramatic social changes that has ever occurred in our society. It seems to be gaining acceptance as part of the normal mate-selection process. By age 30, about half of all men and women will have cohabited.

Living together provides many of the benefits of marriage: companionship; a setting for an enjoyable and mean-

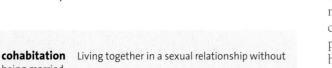

TERMS

cohabitation Living together in a sexual relationship without being married.

Interfaith and Intrafaith Partnerships

DIMENSIONS OF DIVERSITY

Interfaith marriage is common among Americans; for example, about 50% of Jews and 25% of Roman Catholics marry a partner of a different faith. There are many types of interfaith partnerships, including partners from (1) two completely different religions, (2) two religions with similar roots, (3) two divisions of the same religion, or (4) two denominations from the same religious division. The latter two are often called intrafaith partnerships.

Marrying someone of a different faith can broaden the partners' worldview and enrich their lives; however, it can also be a potential stressor and a challenge to a relationship. The impact of being an interfaith couple depends on how religious the partners are. There is no specifically correct way to address religious diversity in a partnership, but the following are some potential approaches.

Withdrawal: In some couples, both partners withdraw from their respective religions. Religious differences may be minimized, but the withdrawal may not last. If a partner was observant prior to the relationship, it is likely that she or he will want to become actively involved again. This often occurs with a significant life event such as the birth of a child or death of a parent.

Conversion: In many intrafaith couples, one partner converts to the religion of the other. Religious differences are decreased, but problems can occur if the partner who converts develops resentment, has difficulties with her or his family of origin, misses the old religion, or experiences feelings of guilt or betrayal.

Compromise: Some couples convert together to a new religion, possibly to a religion or denomination at a "midpoint" between their two religions. The couple may find a happy medium that is satisfying to both. However, both may experience the problems associated with conversion.

Multifaith: Some couples join both religions—formally or informally. They may alternate places of worship weekly or make other creative arrangements. The advantage of this pattern is that both partners maintain their religions and learn more about each other. Problems may arise if the religions have conflicting values or practices.

Ecumenical: In some relationships, partners merge their religions. They may combine the "best" of each or observe only the areas where the religions intersect. They may get the best of both worlds and/or discover that their religions have more in common than they thought. In some cases, however, the original religious institutions may condemn compromise.

Diversity: In some couples, each partner chooses to follow his or her own religion. If both partners are very religious, they do not then have to give up an important part of their lives. However, some partners consider this approach undesirable because it means more time spent apart.

Do Nothing: Some couples find no need to address religious differences because neither partner is observant or committed to a religion to an extent that it is a relationship challenge. They address specific issues if and when they arise.

Couples often handle their religious differences without a problem until they marry or have children. Planning an interfaith wedding can be fraught with unique stressors, such as differing rituals and the expectations of guests from different faiths. When children arrive, decisions may need to be made about issues such as baptism, circumcision, religious upbringing, and others.

To maintain a successful partnership, couples should communicate about religious issues before getting married and having children. Discuss the importance of your religions and religious needs. Consider ways that you can honor each other's religious traditions. Learn to discuss issues relating to religion and spirituality in ways to bring you closer together.

SOURCES: Robinson, B. A. 2007. *Inter-Faith Marriages* (http://www.religioustolerance.org/ifm_menu.htm; retrieved January 24, 2009); Robinson, B. A. 1999. *How Inter-Faith and Intra-Faith Couples Handle Religious Differences* (http://www .religioustolerance.org/ifm_diff.htm; retrieved January 24, 2009).

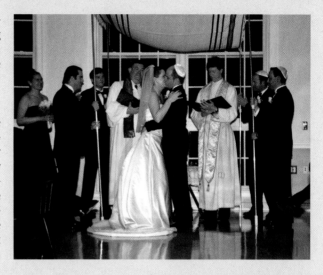

ingful relationship; the opportunity to develop greater intimacy through learning, compromising, and sharing; a satisfying sex life; and a way to save on living costs.

Living together has certain advantages over marriage. For one thing, it can give the partners a greater sense of autonomy. Not bound by the social rules and expectations that are part of the institution of marriage, partners may find it easier to keep their identity and more of their independence. Cohabitation doesn't incur the same obligations as marriage. If things don't work out, the partners may find it easier to leave a relationship that hasn't been legally sanctioned.

Roughly 50% of cohabitating couples get married.

—**National Institute of Child Health and Human Development, 2002**

QUICK STATS

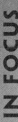

Online Relationships

Worldwide, tens of millions of people use the World Wide Web to network and to find friends and partners. Social networking Web sites like Friendster, Facebook, and MySpace offer a place for profiles, photos, blogs, music, videos, and e-mail to vast numbers of people, mostly teens and young adults, seeking to connect online.

Online dating sites and forums like Match.com are also popular, especially among those out of college who are seeking an intimate partner or an expanded circle of friends.

Connecting with people online has its advantages and its drawbacks. It allows people to communicate in a relaxed way, to try out different personas, and to share things they might not share with family or friends face-to-face. Many find that it offers a sense of privacy, safety, and comfort. It is easy to put yourself out there without too much investment—you can get to know someone from the comfort of your own home, set your own pace, and start and end the relationships at any time. With millions of singles using dating forums that allow them to outline exactly what they are seeking, the Internet can increase a person's chance of finding a good match.

There are drawbacks to meeting people online, however. People often misrepresent themselves, pretending to be very different—older or younger or even of a different sex—than they really are. Investing time and emotional resources in such relationships can be painful. There have also been a few instances in which online romances have become dangerous or even deadly (see Chapter 21 for information on cyberstalking).

Because people have greater freedom to reveal only what they want to, users should also be aware of a greater tendency to idealize online partners—setting themselves up for later disappointment. If you find that your online friend seems perfect, consider that a warning sign. Looking for partners online can become like shopping—the choices available may increase your tendency to search for perfection or find fault quickly, thereby keeping you from giving people a chance. Remember what is most important to you and keep your expectations realistic.

When looking for friends and partners online, you are also reducing an important and powerful source of information: chemistry and in-person intuition. Much of our communication is transmitted through body language and tone, which are not available online and cannot be fully captured even by Web cams. Trust your feelings regarding the process of the relationship. Are you revealing more than the other person? Is there a balance in the amount of time spent talking by each of you? Is the other person respecting your boundaries? Just as in real-life dating, online relationships require you to use common sense and to trust your instincts.

If you decide to pursue an online relationship, here are some strategies that can help you have a positive experience and stay safe:

• To improve your chances of meeting people interested in you as a person, avoid sexually oriented Web sites.

• Know what you are looking for as well as what you have to offer someone else. If you are looking for a relationship, make that fact clear. Find out the other person's situation and intentions.

• Many Web sites let users upload photos. Know, however, that your photo can be downloaded by anyone, distributed to other individuals or sites, and even altered. Don't post photos unless you are completely comfortable with the potential consequences.

• Don't give out personal information, including your real full name, school, or place of employment, until you feel sure that you are giving the information to someone who is trustworthy. Do not give anyone your address or phone number over the Internet.

• Consider setting up a second e-mail account for sending and receiving dating-related e-mails.

• If someone does not respond to a message, try not to take it personally. There are many reasons why a person may not pursue the connection. Do not send multiple messages to an unresponsive person; doing so could lead to an accusation of stalking. If someone stops responding to your messages, drop the interaction completely.

• Before deciding whether to meet an online friend in person, arrange to talk over the phone a few times.

• Don't agree to meet someone face-to-face unless you feel completely comfortable about it. Always meet initially in a very public place—a museum, a coffee shop, or a restaurant, not in private, and especially not at your home. Bring along a friend to further increase your safety, let a friend know where you will be, or plan to have a friend call you during the date.

If you pursue online relationships, don't let them interfere with your other interpersonal relationships and social activities. There can be an addictive element to online dating that can become unhealthy. To maximize your emotional and interpersonal wellness, use the Internet to widen your circle of friends, not shrink it.

But living together has some liabilities, too. In most cases, the legal protections of marriage are absent, such as health insurance benefits and property and inheritance rights. These considerations can be particularly serious if the couple has children, from either former relationships or the current one. Couples may feel social or family pressure to marry or otherwise change their living arrangements, especially if they have young children. The general trend, however, is toward legitimizing nonmarital partnerships; for example, some employers, communities, and states now extend benefits to unmarried domestic partners.

Although many people choose cohabitation as a kind of trial marriage, unmarried partnerships tend to be less stable than marriages. In a survey of women age 15–44 who had cohabited, fewer than half were still living—married (37%) or unmarried (10%)—with their first live-in partner, 34% had dissolved the relationship prior to marriage, and 21% had married and then divorced their partner. There is little evidence that cohabitation before marriage leads to happier or longer-lasting marriages; in fact, some studies have found slightly less marital satisfaction and slightly higher divorce rates among couples who had previously cohabited.

Same-Sex Partnerships

Regardless of **sexual orientation,** most people look for love in a close, satisfying, committed relationship. A person whose sexual orientation is lesbian, gay, or bisexual (LGB) may be involved in a **homosexual** (same-sex) relationship. Same-sex couples have many similarities with **heterosexual** couples (those who seek members of the opposite sex). According to one study, most gay men and lesbians have experienced at least one long-term relationship with a single partner. Like any intimate relationship, same-sex partnerships provide intimacy, passion, and security.

One difference between heterosexual and homosexual couples is that same-sex partnerships tend to be more egalitarian (equal) and less organized around traditional gender roles. Same-sex couples put greater emphasis on partnership than on role assignment. Domestic tasks are shared or split, and both partners usually support themselves financially.

Another difference between heterosexual and homosexual relationships is that same-sex partners often have to deal with societal hostility or ambivalence toward their relationship, in contrast to the societal approval and rights given to heterosexual couples (see the box "Same-Sex Marriage and Civil Unions" on page 82). *Homophobia,* fear or hatred of homosexuals, can be obvious, as in the case of violence or discrimination, or more subtle, such as how same-sex couples are portrayed in the media. Due to the impact of societal disapproval, community resources and support may be more important for same-sex couples as a source of identity and social support than they are for heterosexuals.

Singlehood

Despite the prevalence and popularity of marriage, a significant and growing number of adults in our society are unmarried—more than 110 million single individuals. The largest group of unmarried adults have never been married (Figure 4.1).

Several factors contribute to the growing number of single people. One is the changing view of singlehood, which is increasingly being viewed as a legitimate alternative to marriage. Education and career are delaying the age at which young people are marrying. The median age for marriage is now 27.1 years for men and 25.3 years for

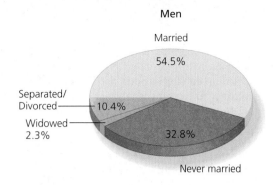

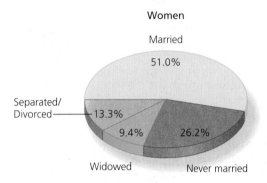

VITAL STATISTICS

FIGURE 4.1 Marital status of the U.S. population age 15 years and older.

SOURCE: U.S. Bureau of the Census. 2007. *America's Families and Living Arrangements, 2006* (http://www.census.gov/population/www/socdemo/hh-fam/cps2006.htm; retrieved January 21, 2009).

women. More young people are living with their parents as they complete their education, seek jobs, or strive for financial independence. Many other single people live together without being married. Gay people who would marry their partners if they were legally permitted to do so are counted among the single population. High divorce rates mean more singles, and people who have experienced divorce in their families may have more negative attitudes about marriage and more positive attitudes about singlehood.

Being single doesn't mean not having close relationships, however. Single people date, enjoy active and fulfilling

sexual orientation A consistent pattern of emotional and sexual attraction based on biological sex; it exists along a continuum that ranges from exclusive heterosexuality (attraction to people of the other sex) through bisexuality (attraction to people of both sexes) to exclusive homosexuality (attraction to people of one's own sex).

homosexual Emotional and sexual attraction to people of one's own sex.

heterosexual Emotional and sexual attraction to people of the other sex.

TERMS

Same-Sex Marriage and Civil Unions

Marriage is often viewed primarily as a social or religious institution, but it is in fact an institution defined by state and federal statutes that confer legal and economic rights and responsibilities. According to the U.S. General Accountability Office, there are more than 1000 federal laws in which a distinction is based on marriage. Marital status affects Social Security, federal tax status, Medicaid eligibility, inheritance, medical decision making, and many other aspects of life.

The push for legal recognition of same-sex partnerships began decades ago, but it was brought to the forefront of public debate beginning in the 1990s. Supporters of same-sex marriage rights, however, have met with stiff opposition at the state and federal levels.

The majority of states and the federal government have passed laws and amendments that effectively ban same-sex marriage. A federal law called the Defense of Marriage Act (DOMA), signed by President Clinton in 1996, defines marriage as the legal union between one man and one woman and refuses federal recognition of same-sex marriages. It also allows states to refuse to recognize same-sex marriages and civil unions performed in other states or countries. (Such action might otherwise be in violation of the U.S. Constitution's provision that each state will give "full faith and credit" to the laws of other states.)

In 2004, President Bush endorsed an amendment to the U.S. Constitution, the "Federal Marriage Amendment," that would permanently ban same-sex marriage and prevent expected future legal challenges to federal and state DOMAs. Under the proposed amendment, states would still be allowed to grant civil unions. The amendment was defeated in Congress in fall 2004 and again in summer 2006.

As of late 2008, the status of same-sex marriage and civil union laws was as follows in the United States:

- Most states had enacted their own mini-DOMAs and/or passed state constitutional amendments that ban same-sex marriages and, in some cases, civil unions. Most of these states further refuse to recognize same-sex marriages from other states.

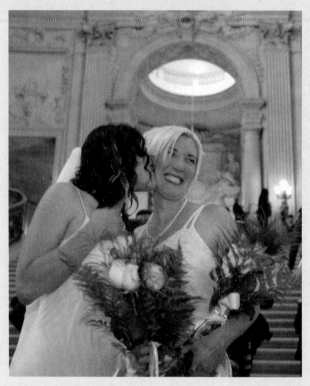

- Massachusetts began allowing same-sex marriages among its residents in 2006; same-sex non-residents cannot marry there. Connecticut legalized gay marriage in 2008.

- In 2008, Oregon granted domestic partners most of the same legal protections as marriage.

- Vermont, New Hampshire, and New Jersey all allow civil unions.

- The District of Columbia recognizes domestic partnerships. Similar types of recognition have been proposed in New York and Rhode Island, but the legislatures and courts in those states have not taken final action.

- Iowa has a DOMA, but it was overturned by a county judge in 2007. As of late 2008, the state was awaiting a decision on the issue by the Iowa Supreme Court.

- California enacted its own DOMA in 2000, but the state's Supreme Court overturned the act in 2008. After a few months of legalized same-sex marriages, California voters approved a constitutional amendment outlawing gay marriage. That amendment was immediately challenged in court.

What cases are made for and against civil union and same-sex marriage? Opponents put forth numerous arguments, including that the purpose of marriage is to procreate, that the Bible forbids same-sex unions, that homosexuals are seeking special rights, that it's bad for children and families, and that the majority of the population opposes such unions. The primary argument, however, is that same-sex marriage undermines the sanctity and validity of marriage as it is traditionally understood and thus undermines society. Rules and restrictions on who can marry preserve the value of the institution of marriage, according to this view. The underlying assumption of this position is that homosexual behavior is a choice and that people can change their orientation, though the process may be difficult.

Proponents of civil unions and same-sex marriage believe that sexual orientation is outside the control of the individual and results from genetic and environmental factors that create an unchangeable orientation. The issue of same-sex union is then seen as one of basic civil rights, in which a group is being denied rights—to publicly express their commitment to one another, to provide security for their children, and to receive the legal and economic benefits afforded to married heterosexual couples—on the basis of something as unalterable as skin color.

Both opponents and proponents of same-sex marriage point out that marriage is healthy for both men and women and is the main social institution promoting family values; both sides see this assertion as supportive of their position. What remains to be seen is how society in general is going to view same-sex marriage in the future—as a furthering of American values or as an attack on them.

social lives, and have a variety of sexual experiences and relationships. Other advantages of being single include more opportunities for personal and career development without concern for family obligations and more freedom and control in making life choices. Disadvantages include loneliness and a lack of companionship, as well as economic hardships (mainly for single women). Single men and women alike experience some discrimination and often are pressured to get married.

Nearly everyone has at least one episode of being single in adult life, whether prior to marriage, between marriages, following divorce or the death of a spouse, or for his or her entire life. How enjoyable and valuable this single time is depends on several factors, including how deliberately the person has chosen it; how satisfied the person is with his or her social relationships, standard of living, and job; how comfortable the person feels when alone; and how resourceful and energetic the person is about creating an interesting and fulfilling life.

MARRIAGE

The majority of Americans marry at some time in their life. Marriage continues to remain popular because it satisfies several basic needs. There are many important social, moral, economic, and political aspects of marriage, all of which have changed over the years. In the past, people married mainly for practical reasons, such as raising children or forming an economic unit. Today, people marry more for personal, emotional reasons.

Benefits of Marriage

The primary functions and benefits of marriage are those of any intimate relationship: affection, personal affirmation, companionship, sexual fulfillment, and emotional growth. Marriage also provides a setting in which to raise children, although an increasing number of couples choose to remain childless, and people can also choose to raise children without being married. Marriage is also important for providing for the future. By committing themselves to the relationship, people establish themselves with lifelong companions as well as some insurance for their later years.

Good marriages have been shown to have myriad positive effects on individuals' health (see the box "Are Intimate Relationships Good for Your Health?" on page 84).

Issues in Marriage

Although we might like to believe otherwise, love is not enough to make a successful marriage. Couples have to be strong and successful in their relationship before getting married, because relationship problems will be magnified rather than solved by marriage. The following relationship characteristics appear to be the best predictors of a happy marriage:

- The partners have realistic expectations about their relationship.
- Each feels good about the personality of the other.
- They communicate well.
- They have effective ways of resolving conflicts.
- They agree on religious/ethical values.
- They have an egalitarian role relationship.
- They have a good balance of individual versus joint interests and leisure activities.

Once married, couples must provide each other with emotional support, negotiate and establish marital roles, establish domestic and career priorities, handle their finances, make sexual adjustments, manage boundaries and relationships with their extended family, and participate in the larger community.

Marital roles and responsibilities have undergone profound changes in recent years. Many couples no longer accept traditional role assumptions, such as that the husband is solely responsible for supporting the family and the wife is solely responsible for domestic work. Today, many husbands share domestic tasks, and many wives work outside the home. In fact, over 50% of married women are in the labor force, including women with babies under 1 year of age. Although women still take most of the responsibility for home and children even when they work and although men still suffer more job-related stress and health problems than women do, the trend is toward an equalization of responsibilities.

The Role of Commitment

Coping with all these challenges requires that couples be committed to remaining in the relationship through its inevitable ups and downs. They need to be tolerant of each other's imperfections and keep their perspective and sense of humor. Commitment is based on conscious choice rather than on feelings, which, by their very nature, are transitory. Commitment is a promise of a shared future, a promise to be together, come what may. Commitment has become an important concept in recent years. To many people, commitment is a more important goal than living together or marriage.

Are Intimate Relationships Good for Your Health?

Findings suggest that there are intrinsic benefits to marriage. Married people, on average, live longer than unmarried people—whether single, divorced, or widowed—and they score higher on measures of mental health. They have a lower prevalence of headaches, low-back pain, inactivity, and psychological distress. Married people consistently report being happier than unmarried people.

The benefits of intimate relationships have been demonstrated for a range of conditions: People with strong social support are less likely to catch colds. They recover better from heart attacks, live longer with heart disease, and have higher survival rates for certain cancers. Among men with prostate cancer, those who are married live significantly longer than those who are single, divorced, or widowed. Women in satisfying marriages are less likely to develop risk factors associated with cardiovascular diseases than unmarried women or women in unhappy marriages. A 2006 study

found that people who never marry have a higher chance of dying prematurely than people who have been divorced, separated, or widowed.

What is it about social relationships that supports wellness? Some studies suggest that friends and partners may encourage and reinforce healthy habits, such as exercising, eating right, and seeing a physician when needed. In times of illness, a loving partner can provide both practical help (sometimes financial) and emotional support. Feeling loved, esteemed, and valued brings comfort at a time of vulnerability, reduces anxiety, and mitigates the damaging effects of stress and risks of social isolation.

Although good relationships may help the sick get better, bad relationships may have the opposite effect. The impact of relationship quality on the course of illness may be partly explained by effects of the immune system: A study of married couples whose fighting went beyond normal conflict and into

criticism and name-calling found them to have weaker immune responses than couples whose arguments were more civil. Hostile couples need more time for injuries to heal; their systems tend to contain higher levels of inflammatory agents, which have been linked to long-term illness. New research shows that high marital stress is linked with risky lifestyle choices and behaviors and non-adherence to medical regimens. Similarly, unhappy marriages are associated with risk factors for heart disease, such as depression, hostility, and anger.

Marriage, of course, isn't the only support system available. Whether married, in a committed partnership, or single, if you have supportive people in your life, you are likely to enjoy better physical and emotional health than if you feel isolated and alone. So when you start planning lifestyle changes to improve your health and well-being, don't forget to nurture your relationships with family and friends. Relationships are powerful medicine.

Separation and Divorce

People marrying today have a 50–55% chance of divorcing. The high rate of divorce in the United States reflects our extremely high expectations for emotional fulfillment and satisfaction in marriage (Figure 4.2). It also indicates that we no longer believe in the permanence of marriage.

The process of divorce usually begins with an emotional separation. Often one partner is unhappy and looks beyond the relationship for other forms of validation. Dissatisfaction increases until the unhappy partner decides he or she can no longer stay. Physical separation follows, although it may take some time for the relationship to be over emotionally.

Except for the death of a spouse or family member, divorce is the greatest stress-producing event in life. Research shows that divorced women are more likely to develop heart disease than married, remarried, or widowed women. Both men and women experience turmoil, depression, and lowered self-esteem during and after divorce. People expe-

QUICK STATS

Teens are twice as likely to abuse alcohol or other drugs if their parents are separated.

—*Pediatrics,* 2007

rience separation distress and loneliness for about a year and then begin a recovery period of 1–3 years. During this time they gradually construct a postdivorce identity, along with a new pattern of life. Most people are surprised by how long it takes to recover from divorce.

Children are especially vulnerable to the trauma of divorce, and sometimes counseling is appropriate to help them adjust to the changes in their lives. However, recent research has found that children who spend substantial time with both parents are usually better adjusted than those in sole custody arrangements and as well adjusted as their peers from intact families.

FAMILY LIFE

American families are very different today than they were even a few decades ago. Currently, about half of all families are based on a first marriage; almost one-third are headed by a single parent; the remainder are remarriages or involve some other arrangement. Despite the tremendous variation apparent in American families, certain patterns can still be discerned.

Becoming a Parent

Few new parents have any preparation for the job of parenting, yet they have to assume that role literally over-

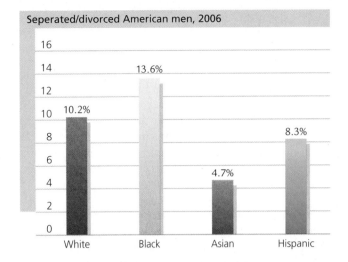

Seperated/divorced American men, 2006

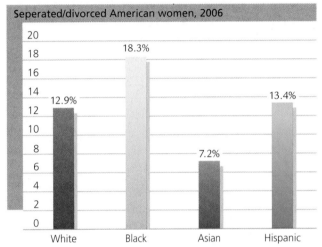

Seperated/divorced American women, 2006

FIGURE 4.2 Percentage of separated and divorced Americans, 2006.

SOURCE: U.S. Bureau of the Census. 2007. *America's Families and Living Arrangements, 2006* (http://www.census.gov/population/www/socdemo/hh-fam; retrieved January 21, 2009).

night. They have to learn quickly how to hold a baby, how to change it, how to feed it, how to interpret its cries. No wonder the birth of the first child is one of the most stressful transitions for any couple.

Even couples with an egalitarian relationship before their first child is born find that their marital roles become more traditional with the arrival of the new baby. The father becomes the primary provider and protector, and the mother becomes the primary nurturer. Most research indicates that mothers have to make greater changes in their lives than fathers do. Although men today spend more time caring for their infants than ever before, women still take the ultimate responsibility for the baby. In addition, women are usually the ones who make job changes; they may quit working or reduce their hours in order to stay home with the baby for several months or more, or they may try to juggle the multiple roles of mother, homemaker, and employer/employee and feel guilty that they never have enough time to do justice to any of these roles.

QUESTIONS FOR CRITICAL THINKING AND REFLECTION
How do you define "commitment" in a relationship? Is it simply a matter of staying faithful to a partner, or is there more? In your own relationships, what signs of commitment do you look for from your partner? What signs of commitment does your partner see in you?

Parenting

Sometimes being a parent is a source of unparalleled pleasure and pride—the first smile (at you), the first word, the first home run. But at other times parenting can seem like an overwhelming responsibility.

Parenting Styles Most parents worry about their ability to raise a healthy, responsible, and well-adjusted child. Parents may wonder about the long-term impact of each decision they make on their child's well-being and personality. According to parenting experts, no one action or decision (within limits) will determine a child's personality or development; instead, what is most important is the *parenting style,* or overall approach to parenting.

Research has revealed four general styles of parenting. The four styles vary primarily according to the levels of two characteristics of the parents:

- *Demandingness* encompasses the use of discipline and supervision, the expectation that children act responsibly and maturely, and the direct response to disobedience.

- *Responsiveness* refers to a parent's warmth and his or her intent to facilitate independence and self-confidence in a child by being supportive, connected, and understanding of the child's needs.

Most parents use a blend of the four general styles but tend toward one style.

AUTHORITARIAN *Authoritarian* parents are high in demandingness and low in responsiveness. They give orders and expect them to be obeyed, giving very little warmth or consideration to their children's special needs. They maintain a structured environment where the rules are explicit and set without input or discussion with the child. Children of authoritarian parents rate low on social competence, self-esteem, intellectual curiosity, spontaneity, and initiative. They perform fairly well in school and do not exhibit a lot of problem behavior; however, they have higher levels of depression.

AUTHORITATIVE *Authoritative* parents are high in both demandingness and responsiveness. They set clear boundaries and expectations, but they are also loving, supportive, and attuned to their children's needs. They are firm in

FAMILY LIFE **85**

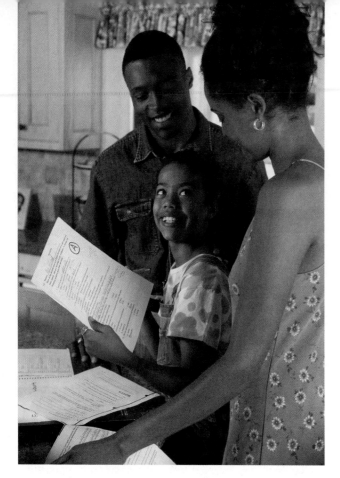

Setting clear boundaries, holding children to high expectations, and responding with warmth to children's needs are all positive parenting strategies.

their decisions but allow for a give-and-take in discussions with the intent of fostering independent thinking.

Both authoritarian and authoritative parents hold their children to high expectations. The difference is that authoritarian parents expect their children to follow their commands without question or comment and authoritative parents are more likely to explain their reasoning and allow children to express themselves. Research consistently shows that children of authoritative parents are the best adjusted and rate particularly high in social competence.

PERMISSIVE (OR INDULGENT) *Permissive* parents are high in responsiveness and low in demandingness. They do not expect their children to act maturely but instead allow them to follow their own impulses. They are very warm, patient, and accepting, and they are focused on not stifling their child's innate creativity. They use little discipline and are often nontraditional. Children of permissive parents have difficulty with impulse-control, are im-

mature, perform more poorly in school, have more problem behaviors, and take less responsibility for their actions. They also have higher self-esteem, better social skills, and lower levels of depression.

UNINVOLVED *Uninvolved* parents are low in both demandingness and responsiveness. They require little from their children and respond with little attention, frequency, or effort. In extreme cases, this style might reach the level of child neglect. Research has found that children of uninvolved parents perform worse in all areas measured compared with children of parents using the other styles.

Parenting and the Family Life Cycle Parenting that is responsive and demanding is the most beneficial for children. Providing a balance of firm limits and clear structure along with high levels of warmth, nurturance, and respect for the child's own special needs and temperament as well as her or his growing independence is the best predictor for raising a healthy child.

At each stage of the family life cycle, the relationship between parents and children changes. And with those changes come new challenges. The parents' primary responsibility to a small, helpless baby is to ensure its physical well-being around the clock. As babies grow into toddlers and begin to crawl and walk and talk, they begin to be able to take care of some of their own physical needs. For parents, the challenge at this stage is to strike a balance between giving children the freedom to explore and setting limits that will keep the children safe and secure. As children grow toward adolescence, parents need to give them increasing independence and gradually be willing to let them risk success or failure on their own.

Marital satisfaction for most couples tends to decline somewhat while the children are in school. Reasons include the financial and emotional pressures of a growing family and the increased job and community responsibilities of parents in their thirties, forties, and fifties. Once the last child has left home, marital satisfaction usually increases because the couple have time to enjoy each other once more.

Single Parents

According to the U.S. Census Bureau, about 28% of all children under 18 live with only one parent. In some single-parent families, the traditional family life cycle is reversed and the baby comes before the marriage. In these families, the single parent is usually a teenage mother; she may very well be black or Hispanic, and she may never get married or may not marry for several years. In 2006, about 56% of all black children were living with single parents, as were 29% of Hispanic children.

Economic difficulties are the primary problem for single mothers, especially for unmarried mothers who have not finished high school and have difficulty finding work. Divorced mothers usually experience a sharp drop in income the first few years on their own, but if they have job skills or education they usually can eventually support themselves and their children adequately. Other problems for single mothers are the often-conflicting demands of playing both father and mother and the difficulty of satisfying their own needs for adult companionship and affection.

Financial pressures are also a complaint of single fathers, but they do not experience them to the extent that single mothers do. Because they are likely to have less practice than mothers in juggling parental and professional roles, they may worry that they do not spend enough time with their children. Because single fatherhood is not as common as single motherhood, however, the men who choose it are likely to be stable, established, and strongly motivated to be with their children.

Research about the effect on children of growing up in a single-parent family is inconclusive. Evidence seems to indicate that these children tend to have less success in school and in their careers than children from two-parent families, but these effects may be associated more strongly with low educational attainment of the single parent than with the absence of the second parent. Two-parent families are not necessarily better if one of the parents spends little time relating to the children or is physically or emotionally abusive.

Stepfamilies

Single parenthood is usually a transitional stage: About three out of four divorced women and about four out of five divorced men will ultimately remarry. Rates are lower for widowed men and women, but overall, almost half the marriages in the United States are remarriages for the husband, the wife, or both. If either partner brings children from a previous marriage into the new family unit, a stepfamily (or "blended family") is formed.

Stepfamilies are significantly different from primary families and should not be expected to duplicate the emotions and relationships of a primary family. Research has shown that healthy stepfamilies are less cohesive and more adaptable than healthy primary families; they have a greater capacity to allow for individual differences and accept that biologically related family members will have emotionally closer relationships. Stepfamilies gradually gain more of a sense of being a family as they build a history of shared daily experiences and major life events.

Successful Families

Family life can be extremely challenging. A strong family is not a family without problems; it's a family that copes successfully with stress and crisis. Successful families are intentionally connected—members share experiences and meanings.

An excellent way to build strong family ties is to develop family rituals and routines—organized, repeated activities that have meaning for family members. Families with regular routines and rituals have healthier children, more satisfying marriages, and stronger family relationships. Some of the most common routines identified in research studies are dinnertime, a regular bedtime, and household chores; common rituals include birthdays, Christmas and other holidays, and Sunday activities. Family routines may even serve as protective factors, balancing out potential risk factors associated with single-parent families and families with divorce and remarriage. You may want to consider incorporating a regular family mealtime into your family routine, as it allows parents and children to develop closer relationships and leads to better parenting, healthier children, and better school performance.

Although there is tremendous variation in American families, researchers have proposed that six major qualities or themes appear in strong families:

1. *Commitment.* The family is very important to its members; sexual fidelity between partners is included in commitment.

2. *Appreciation.* Family members care about one another and express their appreciation. The home is a positive place for family members.

3. *Communication.* Family members spend time listening to one another and enjoying one another's company. They talk about disagreements and attempt to solve problems.

4. *Time together.* Family members do things together, often simple activities that don't cost money.

5. *Spiritual wellness.* The family promotes sharing, love, and compassion for other human beings.

6. *Coping with stress and crisis.* When faced with illness, death, marital conflict, or other crises, family members pull together, seek help, and use other coping strategies to meet the challenge.

It may surprise some people that members of strong families are often seen at counseling centers. They know that the smartest thing to do in some situations is to get help. Many resources are available for individuals and families seeking counseling; people can turn to physicians, clergy, marriage and family counselors, psychologists, or other trained professionals.

QUESTIONS FOR CRITICAL THINKING AND REFLECTION
Do you think of your own family as a "successful" family? Why or why not? Either way, what could you do to make your relationships in your family more successful? Are you comfortable talking to your family about these issues?

THINKING ABOUT THE ENVIRONMENT

Parents can instill a lifelong sense of environmental stewardship in their children by teaching them these simple habits:

- Recycle waste as much as possible.

- Purchase environmentally friendly products that are manufactured from recyclable materials.

- Turn off lights and appliances when they are not needed.

- Shop for locally grown foods that are raised through environmentally sustainable practices.

For more information on the environment, see Chapter 14.

TIPS FOR TODAY AND THE FUTURE

A balanced life includes ample time for nourishing relationships with friends, family, and intimate partners.

RIGHT NOW YOU CAN

- Seek out an acquaintance or a new friend and arrange a coffee date to get to know the person better.
- Call someone you love and tell him or her how important the relationship is to you. Don't wait for a crisis.

IN THE FUTURE YOU CAN

- Think about the conflicts you have had in the past with your close friends or loved ones and consider how you handled them. Decide whether your conflict-management methods were helpful or not. Using the suggestions in this chapter and Chapter 3, determine how you could better handle similar conflicts in the future.
- Think about your prospects as a parent. What kind of example have your parents set? How do you feel about having children in the future (if you don't have children already)? What can you do to prepare yourself to be a good parent?

SUMMARY

- Successful relationships begin with a positive sense of self and reasonably high self-esteem. Personal identity, gender roles, and styles of attachment are all rooted in childhood experiences.

- The characteristics of friendship include companionship, respect, acceptance, help, trust, loyalty, and reciprocity.

- Love, sex, and commitment are closely linked ideals in intimate relationships. Love includes trust, caring, respect, and loyalty. Sex brings excitement, fascination, and passion to the relationship.

- Common challenges in relationships relate to issues of self-disclosure, commitment, expectations, competitiveness, balancing time spent together and apart, and jealousy. Partners in successful relationships have strong communication skills and support each other in difficult times.

- The keys to good communication in relationships are self-disclosure, listening, and feedback.

- Conflict is inevitable in intimate relationships; partners need to have constructive ways to negotiate their differences.

- People usually choose partners like themselves. If partners are very different, acceptance and good communication skills are necessary to maintain the relationship.

- Most Americans find partners through dating or getting together in groups. Cohabitation is a growing social pattern that allows partners to get to know each other intimately without being married.

- Gay and lesbian partnerships are similar to heterosexual partnerships, with some differences. Partners often don't conform to traditional gender roles, and they may experience hostility or ambivalence rather than approval toward their partnership from society.

- Singlehood is a growing option in our society. Advantages include greater variety in sex partners and more freedom in making life decisions; disadvantages include loneliness and possible economic hardship, especially for single women.

- Marriage fulfills many functions for individuals and society. It can provide people with affection, affirmation, and sexual fulfillment; a context for child rearing; and the promise of lifelong companionship.

- Love isn't enough to ensure a successful marriage. Partners have to be realistic, feel good about each other, have communication and conflict-resolution skills, share values, and have a balance of individual and joint interests.

- When problems can't be worked out, people often separate and divorce. Divorce is traumatic for all involved, especially children, but the negative effects are usually balanced in time by positive ones.

- Four general parenting styles are authoritarian, authoritative, permissive, and uninvolved; the authoritative style is usually associated with the best outcomes.

- At each stage of the family life cycle, relationships change. Marital satisfaction may be lower during the child-rearing years and higher later.

- Many families today are single-parent families. Problems for single parents include economic difficulties, conflicting demands, and time pressures.

- Stepfamilies are formed when single, divorced, or widowed people remarry and create new family units. Stepfamilies gradually gain more of a sense of being a family as they build a history of shared experiences.

• Important qualities of successful families include commitment to the family, appreciation of family members, communication, time spent together, spiritual wellness, and effective methods of dealing with stress.

FOR MORE INFORMATION

For resources in your area, check your campus directory for a counseling center or peer counseling program, or check the agencies listed in the Mental Health section of the phone book.

BOOKS

Brooks, J. B. 2008. *The Process of Parenting,* 7th ed. New York: McGraw-Hill. *Demonstrates how parents and caregivers can translate their love and concern for children into effective parenting behavior.*

DeGenova, M. K., and F. P. Rice. 2006. *Intimate Relationships, Marriages, and Families,* 7th ed. New York: McGraw-Hill. *A comprehensive introduction to relationships.*

McKay, M., P. Fanning, and K. Paleg. 2007. *Couple Skills: Making Your Relationship Work,* 2nd rev. ed. New York: New Harbinger. *A comprehensive guide to improving communication, resolving conflict, and developing greater intimacy and commitment in relationships.*

Miller, R., D. Perlman, and S. S. Brehm. 2008. *Intimate Relationships,* 5th ed. New York: McGraw-Hill. *A balanced presentation of both the positive and the problematic aspects of intimate relationships.*

Olson, D., and J. DeFrain. 2007. *Marriages and Families: Intimacy, Diversity, and Strengths,* 6th ed. New York: McGraw-Hill. *A comprehensive introduction to relationships and families.*

ORGANIZATIONS AND WEB SITES

American Association for Marriage and Family Therapy. Provides information on a variety of relationship issues and referrals to therapists.
http://www.aamft.org

Association for Couples in Marriage Enrichment (ACME). An organization that promotes activities to strengthen marriage; a resource for books, tapes, and other materials.
http://www.bettermarriages.org

Conflict Resolution Information Source. Provides links to a broad range of Internet resources on conflict resolution. Information covers interpersonal, marriage, family, and other types of conflicts.
http://www.crinfo.org/

Family Education Network. Provides information about education, safety, health, and other family-related issues.
http://www.familyeducation.com

Gottman Institute. Includes tips and suggestions for relationships and parenting, including an online relationships quiz.
http://www.gottman.com

Life Innovations. Provides materials for premarital counseling and marital enrichment.
http://www.prepare-enrich.com

Parents Without Partners (PWP). Provides educational programs, literature, and support groups for single parents and their children. Search the online directory for a referral to a local chapter.
http://www.parentswithoutpartners.org

United States Census Bureau. Provides current statistics on births, marriages, and living arrangements.
http://www.census.gov

Yahoo/Lesbians, Gays, and Bisexuals. A Web site and search engine that contains many links to information and support for lesbians and gays.
http://dir.yahoo.com/society_and_culture/cultures_and_groups

See also the listings for Chapters 3 and 8.

SELECTED BIBLIOGRAPHY

Bookwala, J. 2005. The role of marital quality in physical health during the mature years. *Journal of Aging and Health* 17(1): 85–104.

Centers for Disease Control and Prevention. 2004. Marital status and health: United States, 1999–2002. *Advance Data from Vital and Health Statistics,* No. 351.

Christakis, N. A., et al. 2006. Mortality after hospitalization of a spouse. *New England Journal of Medicine* 354(7): 719–730.

Egelko, B. 2006. Fight over same-sex unions hits court in San Francisco. *San Francisco Chronicle,* 10 July.

Godoy, M. 2008. *NPR: Gay Marriage Laws Interactive Map* (http://www.npr.org/news/specials/gaymarriage/map; retrieved January 24, 2009).

Holt-Lunstad, J., W. Birmingham, and B. Q. Jones. 2008. Is there something unique about marriage? *Annals of Behavioral Medicine* 35(2): 239–244.

Human Rights Campaign. 2008. Relationship Recognition in the United States (http://www.hrc.org; retrieved January 24, 2009).

Human Rights Campaign. 2008. *Statewide Marriage Laws* (http://www.hrc.org; retrieved January 24, 2009).

Madden, M., and A. Lenhart. 2006. *Online Dating.* Washington, D.C.: Pew Internet & American Life Project.

McPherson, M., L. Smith-Lovin, and M. Brashears. 2006. Social isolation in America: Changes in core discussion networks over two decades. *American Sociological Review* 71: 353–375.

Medical memo: Marital stress and the heart. 2004. *Harvard Men's Health Watch,* May.

Mookadam, F., and H. M. Arthur. 2004. Social support and its relationship to morbidity and mortality after acute myocardial infarction: Systematic overview. *Archives of Internal Medicine* 164(14): 1514–1518.

Najib, A., et al. 2004. Regional brain activity in women grieving a romantic relationship breakup. *American Journal of Psychiatry* 161(12): 2245–2256.

National Conference of State Legislatures. 2008 Update. *Same Sex Marriage, Civil Unions and Domestic Partnerships* (http://www.ncsl.org/programs/cyf/samesex.htm; retrieved January 24, 2009).

Pleis, J. R., and M. Lethbridge-Cejku. 2007. Summary health statistics for U.S. adults: National Health Interview Survey, 2006. *Vital and Health Statistics* 10(235): 1–153.

Roisman, G. I., et al. 2008. Adult romantic relationships as contexts of human development: A multimethod comparison of same-sex couples with opposite-sex dating, engaged, and married dyads. *Developmental Psychology* 44(1): 91–101.

Schoen, R., et al. 2007. Family transitions in young adulthood. *Demography* 44(4): 807–820.

Strong, B., et al. 2005. *Human Sexuality: Diversity in Contemporary America,* 5th ed. New York: McGraw-Hill.

Wainright, J. L., S. T. Russell, and C. J. Patterson. 2004. Psychosocial adjustment, school outcomes, and romantic relationships of adolescents with same-sex parents. *Child Development* 75(6): 1886–1898.

Whisman, M. A., L. A. Uebelacker, and L. M. Weinstock. 2004. Psychopathology and marital satisfaction: The importance of evaluating both partners. *Journal of Consulting and Clinical Psychology* 72(5): 830–838.

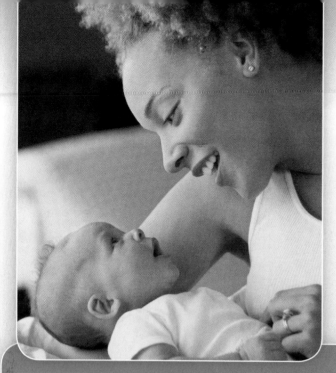

LOOKING AHEAD>>>>>

AFTER READING THIS CHAPTER, YOU SHOULD BE ABLE TO:

- Describe the structure and function of the female and male sex organs
- Explain the changes in sexual functioning that occur over the course of a person's life
- Describe the various ways human sexuality can be expressed
- Describe guidelines for safe, responsible sexual behavior
- Describe the physical and emotional changes a pregnant woman typically experiences
- Discuss the stages of fetal development
- List the important concepts of good prenatal care
- Outline the process of labor and delivery

SEXUALITY, PREGNANCY, AND CHILDBIRTH

5

Humans are sexual beings. Sexual activity is the source of our most intense physical pleasures, a central ingredient in many of our intimate emotional relationships, and the key to reproduction.

Sexuality is more than just sexual behavior. It is a complex, interacting group of inborn, biological characteristics and acquired behaviors people learn in the course of growing up in a particular family, community, and society. Sexuality includes biological sex (being biologically male or female), gender (masculine and feminine behaviors), sexual anatomy and physiology, sexual functioning and practices, and social and sexual interactions with others. Our individual sense of identity is powerfully influenced by our sexuality. We think of ourselves in fundamental ways as male or female; as heterosexual or homosexual; as single, attached, married, or divorced.

Basic information about the body, sexual functioning, and sexual behavior is vital to healthy adult life. Once we understand the facts, we have a better basis for making informed, responsible choices about our sexual activities.

SEXUAL ANATOMY

In spite of their different appearances, the sex organs of men and women arise from the same structures and fulfill similar functions. Each person has a pair of **gonads**; ovaries are the female gonads, and testes are the male gonads. The gonads produce **germ cells** and sex hormones. The germ cells are **ova** (eggs) in females and **sperm** in males. Ova and sperm are the basic units of reproduction; their union results in the creation of a new life.

Female Sex Organs

The external sex organs, or genitals, of the female are called the **vulva** (Figure 5.1). The *mons pubis*, a rounded mass of fatty tissue over the pubic bone, becomes covered with hair during puberty (biological maturation). Below it are two paired folds of skin called the labia majora (major lips) and the labia minora (minor lips). Enclosed within these folds are the clitoris, the opening of the urethra, and the opening of the vagina.

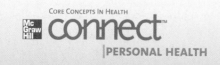

CORE CONCEPTS IN HEALTH

connect™

|PERSONAL HEALTH

http://www.mcgrawhillconnect.com/personalhealth

FIGURE 5.1 **The female sex organs.**

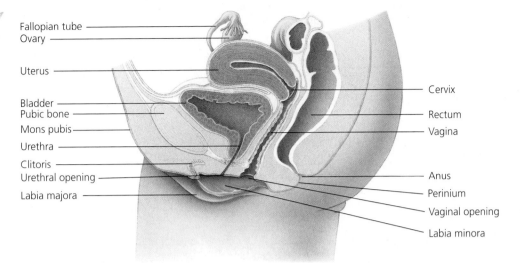

Fallopian tube
Ovary
Uterus
Bladder
Pubic bone
Mons pubis
Urethra
Clitoris
Urethral opening
Labia majora

Cervix
Rectum
Vagina
Anus
Perinium
Vaginal opening
Labia minora

The **clitoris** is highly sensitive to touch and plays an important role in female sexual arousal and orgasm. The clitoris consists of a shaft, glans, and spongy tissue that fills with blood during sexual excitement. The glans is the most sensitive part of the clitoris and is covered by the clitoral hood, or **prepuce,** which is formed from the upper portion of the labia minora.

The female **urethra** is a duct that leads directly from the urinary bladder to its opening between the clitoris and the opening of the vagina; it conducts urine from the bladder to the outside of the body. The female urethra is independent of the genitals.

The **vagina** is the passage that leads to the internal reproductive organs. It is the female structure for heterosexual sexual intercourse and also serves as the birth canal. Projecting into the upper part of the vagina is the **cervix,** which is the opening of the **uterus**—or *womb*—where a fertilized egg is implanted and grows into a **fetus.** A pair of **fallopian tubes** (or *oviducts*) extend from the top of the uterus. The end of each oviduct surrounds an **ovary** and guides the mature ovum down into the uterus after the egg exits the ovary.

Male Sex Organs

A man's external sex organs, or genitals, are the penis and the scrotum (Figure 5.2).

The **penis** consists of spongy tissue that becomes engorged with blood during sexual excitement, causing the organ to enlarge and become erect.

The **scrotum** is a pouch that contains a pair of sperm-producing male gonads, called **testes.** The scrotum maintains the testes at a temperature approximately 5°F below that of the rest of the body. The process of sperm production is extremely heat-sensitive. In hot temperatures the muscles in the scrotum relax, and the testes move away from the heat of the body.

TERMS

sexuality A dimension of personality shaped by biological, psychosocial, and cultural forces and concerning all aspects of sexual behavior.

gonads The primary reproductive organs that produce germ cells and sex hormones; the ovaries and testes.

germ cells Sperm and ova (eggs).

ovum A germ cell produced by a female, which combines with a male germ cell (sperm) to create a fetus; plural, *ova*. Also called an *egg*.

sperm A germ cell produced by a male, which combines with a female germ cell (ovum) to create a fetus.

vulva The external female genitals, or sex organs.

clitoris The highly sensitive female genital structure.

prepuce The foreskin of the clitoris or penis.

urethra The duct that carries urine from the bladder to the outside of the body.

vagina The passage leading from the female genitals to the internal reproductive organs; the birth canal.

cervix The end of the uterus opening toward the vagina.

uterus The hollow, thick-walled, muscular organ in which the fertilized egg develops; the womb.

fetus The developmental stage of a human from the 9th week after conception to the moment of birth.

fallopian tube A duct that guides a mature ovum from the ovary to the uterus. Also called an *oviduct*.

ovary One of two female reproductive glands that produce ova (eggs) and sex hormones; ovaries are the female gonads.

penis The male genital structure consisting of spongy tissue that becomes engorged with blood during sexual excitement.

scrotum The loose sac of skin and muscle fibers that contains the testes.

testis One of two male gonads, the site of sperm production; plural, *testes*. Also called *testicle*.

FIGURE 5.2 **The male sex organs.**

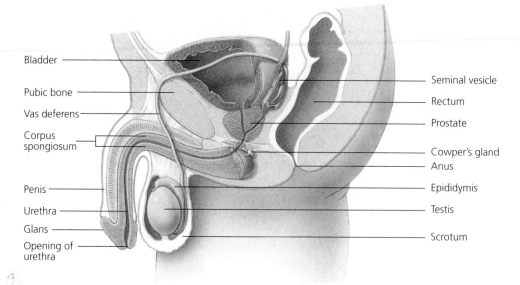

Bladder
Pubic bone
Vas deferens
Corpus spongiosum
Penis
Urethra
Glans
Opening of urethra

Seminal vesicle
Rectum
Prostate
Cowper's gland
Anus
Epididymis
Testis
Scrotum

Through the entire length of the penis runs the urethra, which can carry both urine and *semen,* the sperm-carrying fluid, to the opening at the tip of the penis. Although urine and semen share a common passage, they are prevented from mixing together by muscles that control their entry into the urethra. During its brief lifetime, a sperm takes the following route:

1. Sperm are produced inside a maze of tiny, tightly packed tubules within the testes. As they mature, sperm flow into a tube called the **epididymis,** which lies on the surface of each testis.

2. Sperm move from each epididymis into another tube called the **vas deferens,** which carries them upward into the abdominal cavity and through an organ called the **prostate gland.** This gland produces some of the fluid in semen, which helps transport and nourish the sperm.

3. The two *vasa deferentia* eventually merge into a pair of **seminal vesicles,** whose secretions provide nutrients for the semen.

4. On the final stage of their journey, sperm flow into the **ejaculatory ducts,** which join the urethra.

The **Cowper's glands** are two small structures flanking the urethra. During sexual arousal, these glands secrete a clear, preejaculatory fluid that appears at the tip of the penis. Pre-ejaculatory fluid may contain sperm, so withdrawal of the penis before ejaculation is not a reliable form of contraception.

Circumcision   The smooth, rounded tip of the penis is the highly sensitive **glans,** an important component in sexual arousal. The glans is partially covered by the foreskin, or prepuce, a retractable fold of skin that is removed by **circumcision** in about 60% of newborn males in the United States. Circumcision is performed for cultural, religious, and hygienic reasons, and rates of circumcision vary widely among different groups. Worldwide, the rate is about 30%.

The pros and cons of this simple procedure have been widely debated. Citing research findings, proponents argue that it promotes cleanliness and reduces the risk of urinary tract infections (UTIs) in newborns and the risk of sexually transmitted diseases (STDs), including HIV, later in life. STD education and the practice of abstinence or low-risk sexual behaviors have a far greater impact on the transmission of STDs than does circumcision. However, where safer sex practices are not adhered to, circumcision can have a protective effect. Recent studies in countries with high rates of HIV infection and AIDS have shown that circumcision can reduce the risk of acquiring HIV through heterosexual contact in men by as much as 60%.

Opponents of circumcision state that it is an unnecessary surgical procedure that causes pain and puts a baby at risk for complications. They also argue that circumcision reduces its sensitivity; research into this issue has been inconclusive.

The American Academy of Pediatrics (AAP) takes the position (opposed by some physicians) that although circumcision has potential medical benefits, the research is not sufficient to recommend the procedure routinely. When circumcision is performed, the AAP recommends that painkilling medication be provided.

QUICK STATS

20 million or more sperm per milliliter of semen is considered a normal sperm count.

—Mayo Clinic (www.mayoclinic.com), 2008

THINKING ABOUT THE ENVIRONMENT

Global studies indicate that sperm counts have dropped by as much as 50% in the past 30 years. Many researchers believe that exposure to toxic substances (such as lead, chemical pollutants, and radiation) may be the cause.

Of special interest is a class of chemicals called *endocrine disrupters*—substances found widely in the environment that mimic or interfere with the body's hormones. Endocrine disrupters may cause problems with reproduction, development, and fertility in humans; tests have linked these chemicals to reproductive problems in animals.

Endocrine disrupters may be found in plastics, detergents, food, toys, cosmetics, pesticides, and other everyday products. The U.S. Environmental Protection Agency is now creating a program to test for endocrine disruptors in certain substances.

For more information on the environment and health, see Chapter 14.

HORMONES AND THE REPRODUCTIVE LIFE CYCLE

Many cultural and personal factors help shape the expression of your sexuality, but biology also plays an important role. The sex hormones produced by the ovaries or testes have a major influence on the development and function of the reproductive system throughout life.

The sex hormones made by the testes are called **androgens,** the most important of which is *testosterone.* The female sex hormones, produced by the ovaries, belong to two groups: **estrogens** and **progestins,** the most important of which is *progesterone.* The ovaries also produce a small amount of testosterone. The cortex of the **adrenal glands** also produces androgens in both males and females.

The hormones produced by the testes, the ovaries, and the adrenal glands are regulated by the hormones of the **pituitary gland,** located at the base of the brain. This gland in turn is controlled by hormones produced by the **hypothalamus** in the brain.

Differentiation of the Embryo

The biological sex of an individual is determined by the fertilizing sperm at the time of conception. All human

QUESTIONS FOR CRITICAL THINKING AND REFLECTION

What are your personal views on circumcision? Who or what has influenced those opinions? Are the bases of your views primarily cultural, moral, or medical?

cells normally contain 23 pairs of chromosomes. In 22 of the pairs, the two partner chromosomes match. But in the twenty-third pair, the **sex chromosomes,** two configurations are possible. Individuals with two matching X chromosomes are female, and individuals with one X and one Y chromosome are male. Thus, at the time of conception, the genetic sex is established: Females are XX and males are XY.

Genetic sex dictates whether the undifferentiated gonads become ovaries or testes. If a Y chromosome is present, the gonads become testes; the testes will produce the male hormone **testosterone.** Testosterone circulates throughout the body and causes the undifferentiated reproductive structures to develop into male sex organs (penis, scrotum, and so on). If a Y chromosome is not

epididymis A storage duct for maturing sperm, located on the surface of each testis.

vas deferens A tube that carries sperm from the epididmyis through the prostate gland to the seminal vesicles; plural, *vasa deferentia.*

prostate gland An organ in the male reproductive system; produces some of the fluid in semen, which helps transport and nourish sperm.

seminal vesicle A tube leading from the vas deferens to the ejaculatory duct; secretes nutrients for the semen.

ejaculatory duct A tube that carries mature sperm to the urethra so they can exit the body upon ejaculation.

Cowper's gland In the male reproductive system, a small organ that produces preejaculatory fluid.

glans The rounded head of the penis or the clitoris.

circumcision Surgical removal of the foreskin of the penis.

androgens Male sex hormones produced by the testes in males and by the adrenal glands in both sexes.

estrogens A class of female sex hormones, produced by the ovaries, that bring about sexual maturation at puberty and maintain reproductive functions.

progestins A class of female sex hormones, produced by the ovaries, that sustain reproductive functions.

adrenal glands Endocrine glands, located over the kidneys, that produce androgens (among other hormones).

pituitary gland An endocrine gland at the base of the brain that produces follicle-stimulating hormone (FSH) and luteinizing hormone (LH), among others.

hypothalamus A region of the brain above the pituitary gland whose hormones control the secretions of the pituitary; also involved in the nervous control of sexual functions.

sex chromosomes The X and Y chromosomes, which determine an individual's biological sex.

testosterone The most important androgen (male sex hormone); stimulates an embryo to develop into a male and induces the development of male secondary sex characteristics during puberty.

present, there is no testosterone and the gonads become ovaries and the reproductive structures develop into female sex organs (clitoris, labia, and so on).

Female Sexual Maturation

Although humans are fully sexually differentiated at birth, the differences between males and females are accentuated at **puberty,** the period during which the reproductive system matures, secondary sex characteristics develop, and the bodies of males and females become more distinctive. The changes of puberty are induced by testosterone in males and estrogen and **progesterone** in females.

Physical Changes   The first sign of puberty in girls is breast development, followed by a rounding of the hips and buttocks. As the breasts develop, hair appears in the pubic region and later in the underarms. Shortly after the onset of breast development, girls show an increase in growth rate. Breast development usually begins between ages 8 and 13, and the time of rapid body growth occurs between ages 9 and 15.

The Menstrual Cycle   A major landmark of puberty for young women is the onset of the **menstrual cycle,** the monthly ovarian cycle that leads to menstruation (loss of blood and tissue lining the uterus) in the absence of pregnancy. The timing of **menarche** (the first *menstrual period*) varies with several factors, including ethnicity, genetics, and nutritional status. The current average age of menarche in the United States is around 12 and a half years of age, but it may also normally start several years earlier or later.

The day of the onset of bleeding is considered to be day 1 of the menstrual cycle. For the purposes of our discussion, a cycle of 28 days will be used; however, normal cycles vary in length from 21 to 35 days. The menstrual cycle consists of the following four phases (Figure 5.3):

1. Menses.   During **menses,** characterized by the menstrual flow, blood levels of hormones from the ovaries and the pituitary gland are relatively low. This phase of the cycle usually lasts from day 1 to about day 5.

2. Estrogenic Phase.   The estrogenic phase begins when the menstrual flow ceases and the pituitary gland begins to produce increasing amounts of follicle-stimulating hormone (FSH) and luteinizing hormone (LH). Under the influence of FSH, an egg-containing ovarian **follicle** begins to mature, producing increasingly higher amounts of estrogens. Stimulated by estrogen, the **endometrium,** the uterine lining, thickens with large numbers of blood vessels and uterine glands.

3. Ovulation.   A surge of a potent estrogen called *estradiol* from the follicle causes the pituitary to release a large burst of LH and a smaller amount of FSH. The high concentration of LH stimulates the developing follicle to re-

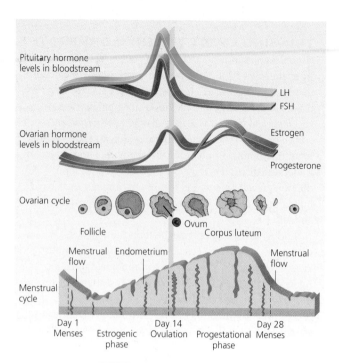

FIGURE 5.3   **The menstrual cycle.**

lease its ovum. This event is known as **ovulation.** After ovulation, the follicle is transformed into the **corpus luteum,** which produces progesterone and estrogen. Ovulation usually occurs about 14 days prior to the onset of menstrual flow.

4. Progestational Phase.   During the progestational phase of the cycle, the amount of progesterone secreted from the corpus luteum increases and remains high until the onset of the next menses. Under the influence of estrogen and progesterone, the endometrium continues to develop, readying itself to receive and nourish a fertilized ovum. When pregnancy occurs, the fertilized egg produces the hormone human chorionic gonadotropin (HCG), which maintains the corpus luteum. Thus, levels of ovarian hormones remain high and the uterine lining is preserved, preventing menses.

If pregnancy does not occur, the corpus luteum degenerates, and estrogen and progesterone levels gradually fall. Below certain hormonal levels, the endometrium can no longer be maintained, and it begins to slough off, initiating menses. As the levels of ovarian hormones fall, a slight rise in LH and FSH occurs, and a new menstrual cycle begins.

MENSTRUAL PROBLEMS   Menstruation is a normal biological process, but it may cause physical or psychological problems. **Dysmenorrhea** is characterized by cramps in the lower abdomen, backache, vomiting, nausea, a bloated feeling, diarrhea, and loss of appetite. Some of these symptoms can be attributed to uterine muscular contractions caused by chemicals called *prostaglandins.* Any drug that blocks the effects of prostaglandins, such as aspirin or ibuprofen, will usually alleviate some of the symptoms of dysmenorrhea.

Many women experience transient physical and emotional symptoms prior to the onset of their menstrual flow. Depending on their severity, these symptoms may be categorized along a continuum: **premenstrual tension, premenstrual syndrome (PMS)**, and **premenstrual dysphoric disorder (PMDD)**. Premenstrual tension symptoms are mild and may include negative mood changes and physical symptoms such as abdominal cramping and backache. More severe symptoms are classified as PMS; very severe symptoms that cause impairment in social functioning and work-related activities are classified as PMDD. All three conditions share a definite pattern: Symptoms appear prior to the onset of menses and disappear within a few days after the start of menstruation.

Symptoms associated with PMS and PMDD include physical changes such as breast tenderness, water retention (bloating), headache, and fatigue; insomnia or excessive sleep; appetite changes and food cravings; irritability, anger, and increased interpersonal conflict; mood swings; depression and sadness; anxiety and tearfulness; inability to concentrate; social withdrawal; and the sense that one is out of control or overwhelmed. PMDD is distinguished from PMS by the severity of symptoms, which in PMDD interfere significantly with work or school and with usual social activities and relationships.

Despite many research studies, the causes of PMS and PMDD are still unknown, and it is unclear why some women are more vulnerable than others. Most researchers feel that PMS is probably caused by a combination of hormonal, nutritional, and psychological factors.

Selective serotonin reuptake inhibitors (SSRIs), including Sarafem, Zoloft, Paxil, and Celexa, are the first-line treatment for PMDD. Until recently, women using SSRIs took the medication throughout the entire menstrual cycle, but it has now been shown that taking the medication during just the progestational phase of the cycle is similarly effective.

In 2006, the Yaz birth control pill was specifically approved by the FDA as a treatment for PMDD. A number of vitamins, minerals, and other dietary supplements have also been studied for PMS relief. Only one supplement, calcium, has been shown to provide relief in rigorous clinical studies; several others show promise, but more research is needed.

The following strategies provide relief for many women.

- *Limit salt intake.* Salt promotes water retention and bloating.

- *Exercise.* Women who exercise experience fewer symptoms before and after menstrual periods.

- *Don't use alcohol or tobacco.* Alcohol and tobacco may aggravate certain symptoms of PMS and PMDD.

- *Eat a nutritious diet.* Choose a low-fat diet rich in complex carbohydrates from vegetables, fruits, and whole-grains. Get enough calcium from calcium-rich foods and, if needed, supplements. Minimize your intake of sugar and caffeine, and avoid chocolate, which is rich in both.

- *Relax.* Try relaxation techniques during the premenstrual time.

If symptoms persist, keep a daily diary to track both the types of symptoms you experience and their severity, and see your physician for an evaluation.

Male Sexual Maturation

Reproductive maturation of boys occurs about 2 years later than that of girls; it usually begins at about age 10 or 11.

TERMS

puberty   The period of biological maturation during adolescence.

progesterone   The most important progestin (female sex hormone); induces the development of female secondary sex characteristics during puberty, regulates the menstrual cycle, and sustains pregnancy.

menstrual cycle   The monthly ovarian cycle, regulated by hormones; in the absence of pregnancy, menstruation occurs.

menarche   The first menstrual period, experienced by most young women at some point during adolescence.

menses   The portion of the menstrual cycle characterized by menstrual flow.

follicle   A saclike structure within the ovary, in which eggs (ova) mature.

endometrium   The lining of the uterus.

ovulation   The release of a mature egg (ovum) from an ovary.

corpus luteum   The part of the ovarian follicle left after ovulation, which secretes estrogen and progesterone during the second half of the menstrual cycle.

dysmenorrhea   Painful or problematic menstruation.

premenstrual tension   Mild physical and emotional changes associated with the time before the onset of menses; symptoms can include abdominal cramping and backache.

premenstrual syndrome (PMS)   A disorder characterized by physical discomfort, psychological distress, and behavioral changes that begin after ovulation and cease when menstruation begins.

premenstrual dysphoric disorder (PMDD)   Severe form of PMS, characterized by symptoms serious enough to interfere with work or school or with social activities and relationships.

Testicular growth is usually the first obvious sign of sexual maturity in boys. The penis also grows at this time, reaching adult size by about age 18. Pubic hair begins to develop after the genitals begin to increase in size, with underarm and facial hair gradually appearing. Hair on the chest, back, and abdomen increases later in development. The voice deepens as a result of the lengthening and thickening of the vocal chords. Boys grow taller for about 6 years after the first signs of puberty, with a very rapid period of growth about 2 years after puberty starts.

Aging and Human Sexuality

Changes in hormone production and sexual functioning occur as we age. As a woman approaches age 50, her ovaries gradually cease to function and she enters **menopause,** the cessation of menstruation. For some women, the associated drop in hormone production causes symptoms that are troublesome. The most common physical symptom of menopause is hot flashes, sensations of warmth rising to the face from the upper chest, with or without perspiration and chills. Other symptoms include headaches, dizziness, palpitations, and joint pains. Osteoporosis—decreasing bone density—can develop, making older women more vulnerable to fractures. Some menopausal women become moody, even markedly depressed, and they may also experience fatigue, irritability, and forgetfulness.

To alleviate the symptoms of menopause and reduce the risk of heart disease and osteoporosis, millions of women have been prescribed hormone therapy (HT), a regimen of hormones that includes estrogen and progesterone. In 2002, an ongoing study of HT involving more than 16,000 women was halted because the women taking HT for long periods suffered more strokes, heart attacks, and blood clots and had a higher incidence of breast cancer than women in the study taking a placebo. The positive findings from this study were a reduction in hip fractures and a reduced risk of colon cancer among the women taking HT. Many women who were taking HT stopped and many more never started as a result of the publicity surrounding the 2002 study. In 2007, analysis of data on breast cancer in the United States showed a decline in 2003 and 2004. Scientists reanalyzed the original 2002 data on HT and found that women who started HT close to the time of menopause tended to have a reduced risk of cardiovascular disease, while women who took HT several years after going through menopause had a higher risk of heart disease. As a result of these findings, women taking HT were advised to consult their health care providers about their personal risks and benefits.

Between the ages of 35 and 65, men experience a gradual decline in testosterone production resulting in the aging male syndrome, sometimes referred to as *male menopause* or *andropause.* Symptoms vary widely among men, but most men experience at least some of the following symptoms as they age: loss of muscle mass, increased fat mass, decreased sex drive, erectile problems, depressed

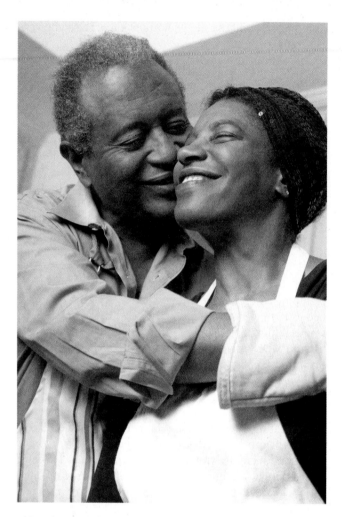

Although sexual physiology changes as people get older, many men and women readily adjust to these alterations.

mood, irritability, difficulties with concentration, increased urination, loss of bone mineral density, and sleep difficulties. In some cases, treatment with testosterone can help. While taking testosterone can be very harmful in young healthy men, older men with low testosterone levels may benefit from carefully prescribed testosterone treatment.

As women and men age, sexual activity can continue to be a source of pleasure and satisfaction for them. A recent study of sexuality in older Americans found that three-fourths of 57–64-year-olds were sexually active (defined as having at least one sexual partner in the last year). Half of those age 65–74, and about one-fourth of people age 75–85, remained sexually active.

SEXUAL FUNCTIONING

Sexual activity is based on stimulus and response. Erotic stimulation leads to sexual arousal (excitement), which may culminate in the intensely pleasurable experience of orgasm. But sexual activity should not be thought of only in terms of the sex organs. Responses to sexual stimulation involve not just the genitals but the entire body—and the mind as well.

Sexual Stimulation

Sexual excitement can come from many sources, both physical and psychological. Although physical stimuli have an obvious and direct effect, some people believe psychological stimuli—thoughts, fantasies, desires, perceptions—are even more powerfully erotic.

Physical Stimulation Physical stimulation comes through the senses: We are aroused by things we see, hear, taste, smell, and feel. The most obvious and effective physical stimulation is touching. Even though culturally defined practices vary and individual people have different preferences, most sexual encounters eventually involve some form of touching with hands, lips, and body surfaces. Kissing, caressing, fondling, and hugging are as much a part of sexual encounters as they are of expressing affection.

The most intense form of stimulation by touching involves the genitals. The clitoris and the glans of the penis are particularly sensitive to such stimulation. Other highly responsive areas include the vaginal opening, the nipples, the breasts, the insides of the thighs, the buttocks, the anal region, the scrotum, the lips, and the earlobes. Such sexually sensitive areas, or **erogenous zones,** are especially susceptible to sexual arousal for most people, most of the time. Often, though, what determines the response is not *what* is touched but how, for how long, and by whom. Under the right circumstances, touching any part of the body can cause sexual arousal.

Psychological Stimulation   Sexual arousal also has an important psychological component, regardless of the nature of the physical stimulation. Fantasies, ideas, memories of past experiences, and mood can all generate sexual excitement.

Arousal is also powerfully influenced by emotions. How you feel about a person and how the person feels about you matter tremendously in how sexually responsive you are likely to be. Even the most direct forms of physical stimulation carry emotional overtones. Kissing, caressing, and fondling express affection and caring. The emotional charge they give to a sexual interaction is at least as significant to sexual arousal as the purely physical stimulation achieved by touching.

The Sexual Response Cycle

Men and women respond physiologically with a predictable set of reactions, regardless of the nature of the stimulation.

Two physiological mechanisms explain most genital and bodily reactions during sexual arousal and orgasm. These mechanisms are vasocongestion and muscular tension. **Vasocongestion** is the engorgement of tissues that results when more blood flows into an organ than is flowing out. Thus, the penis becomes erect on the same principle that makes a garden hose become stiff when the water is turned on. Increased muscular tension culminates in rhythmical muscular contractions during orgasm.

Four phases characterize the sexual response cycle:

1. In the *excitement phase,* the penis becomes erect as its tissues become engorged with blood. The testes expand and are pulled upward within the scrotum. In women, the clitoris, labia, and vaginal walls are similarly engorged with blood and the vaginal walls become moist with lubricating fluid.

2. The *plateau phase* is an extension of the excitement phase. Reactions become more marked. In men, the penis becomes harder, and the testes become larger. In women, the lower part of the vagina swells, as its upper end expands and vaginal lubrication increases.

3. In the *orgasmic phase,* or **orgasm,** rhythmic contractions occur along the man's penis, urethra, prostate gland, seminal vesicles, and muscles in the pelvic and anal regions. These involuntary muscular contractions lead to the ejaculation of **semen,** which consists of sperm cells from the testes and secretions from the prostate gland and seminal vesicles. In women, contractions occur in the lower part of the vagina and in the uterus, as well as in the pelvic region and the anus.

QUESTIONS FOR CRITICAL THINKING AND REFLECTION
Think about your own experience as you matured sexually during puberty and adolescence. In what ways did these changes affect your life? How did they contribute to the person you are today?

---

menopause   The cessation of menstruation, occurring gradually around age 50.

erogenous zone   Any region of the body highly responsive to sexual stimulation.

vasocongestion   The accumulation of blood in tissues and organs.

orgasm   The discharge of accumulated sexual tension with characteristic genital and bodily manifestations and a subjective sensation of intense pleasure.

semen   Seminal fluid, consisting of sperm cells and secretions from the prostate gland and seminal vesicles.

4. In the *resolution phase,* all the changes initiated during the excitement phase are reversed. Excess blood drains from tissues, the muscles in the region relax, and the genital structures return to their unstimulated state.

More general physical reactions accompany the genital changes in both men and women. Beginning with the excitement phase, nipples become erect, the woman's breasts begin to swell, and in both sexes the skin of the chest becomes flushed; these changes are more marked in women. The heart rate doubles by the plateau phase, and respiration becomes faster. During orgasm, breathing becomes irregular and the person may moan or cry out. A feeling of warmth leads to increased sweating during the resolution phase. Deep relaxation and a sense of well-being pervade the body and the mind.

Male orgasm is marked by the ejaculation of semen. After ejaculation, men enter a *refractory period,* during which they cannot be restimulated to orgasm. Women do not have a refractory period, and immediate restimulation to orgasm is possible for some women.

Sexual Problems

Both physical and psychological factors can interfere with sexual functioning. Disturbances in sexual desire, performance, or satisfaction are referred to as **sexual dysfunctions.**

Common Sexual Health Problems   Some problems with sexual functioning are due to treatable or preventable infections or other sexual health problems. Conditions that affect women include the following:

• *Vaginitis,* inflammation of the vagina, is caused by a variety of organisms: *Candida* (yeast infection), *Trichomonas* (trichomoniasis), and the overgrowth of a variety of bacteria (bacterial vaginosis). Symptoms include vaginal discharge, vaginal irritation, and pain during intercourse.
• *Endometriosis* is the growth of endometrial tissue (tissue normally found lining the uterus) outside the uterus. Endometriosis can cause serious problems if left untreated because the endometrial tissue can scar and partially or

completely block the oviducts, causing infertility (difficulty conceiving) or sterility (the inability to conceive).
• *Pelvic inflammatory disease (PID)* is an infection of the uterus, oviducts, or ovaries caused when microorganisms spread to these areas from the vagina. Approximately 50–75% of PID cases are caused by sexually transmitted organisms associated with diseases such as gonorrhea and chlamydia. PID can cause scarring of the oviducts, resulting in infertility or sterility.

Sexual health problems that affect men include the following:

• *Prostatitis* is inflammation or infection of the prostate gland.
• *Testicular cancer* occurs most commonly in men in their twenties and thirties. A rare cancer, it has a very high cure rate if detected early.

Sexual Dysfunctions   The term *sexual dysfunction* encompasses disturbances in sexual desire, performance, or satisfaction. A wide variety of physical conditions and drugs may interfere with sexual functioning; psychological causes and problems in intimate relationships can be important factors in many cases.

COMMON SEXUAL DYSFUNCTIONS   Common sexual dysfunctions in men include **erectile dysfunction** (previously called *impotence*), the inability to have or maintain an erection sufficient for sexual intercourse; **premature ejaculation,** ejaculation before or just on penetration of the vagina or anus; and **retarded ejaculation,** the inability to ejaculate once an erection is achieved. Many men experience difficulty achieving an erection or ejaculating because of alcohol consumption, fatigue, or stress.

Female sexual problems generally involve either a lack of desire to have sex, the failure to become physically aroused even when sex is desired, the failure to have an orgasm (**orgasmic dysfunction**), or pain during sexual contact. All of these problems can have physical and psychological components. Many medical problems can influence a woman's desire and ability to respond sexually. Hormonal factors, especially menopause, also have a major influence. Psychological and social issues such as relationship difficulties, family stresses, depression, and past sexual trauma are all frequent causes of sexual dysfunction.

Many women experience orgasm but not during intercourse, or they experience orgasm during intercourse only if the clitoris is directly stimulated at the same time.

TERMS

sexual dysfunction   A disturbance in sexual desire, performance, or satisfaction.

erectile dysfunction   The inability to have or maintain an erection.

premature ejaculation   Involuntary orgasm before or shortly after the penis enters the vagina or anus; ejaculation that takes place sooner than desired.

retarded ejaculation   The inability to ejaculate when one wishes to during intercourse.

orgasmic dysfunction   The inability to experience orgasm.

Sex Enhancement Products

The search for substances that can enhance sexual function and pleasure probably began long before recorded history. Among the huge variety of herbal and animal concoctions that have been reputed to improve sexual function are ginseng, raw oysters, bear gallbladder, rhinoceros horn, and tiger penis. Although research has shown that none of these products works, people continue to sell these materials, sometimes at extremely high prices, to gullible buyers. The demand for exotic animal parts has contributed to the endangerment of some of these species.

Check your junk e-mail folder and it's likely to be full of advertisements for products that supposedly increase sexual prowess. Recently, a number of these products have been shown to contain potentially dangerous ingredients. For example, the Food and Drug Administration (FDA) has cautioned against many dietary supplements sold online as "all natural" sexual enhancement products under names such as Zimaxx, Libidus, Neophase, Nasutra, Vigor25, Actra-Rx, 4Evron, True Man, and Energy Max. These products have been shown to contain the same or very similar compounds as those found in prescription drugs for erectile dysfunction such as Viagra, despite their claims of being herbal or "all natural." No mention of these Viagra-like compounds is found on their labels, though many of them contain full- or even double-strength doses of these drugs.

The FDA is concerned that these falsely labeled products could have potentially dangerous or even lethal side effects, especially if they are taken by people who are being treated with heart drugs that contain nitrates. Nitrates are common compounds found in many drugs used to treat heart disease and high blood pressure. Nitrates cause blood vessels to dilate, as does Viagra. When the two types of drugs are used together, blood pressure can plummet, potentially resulting in fainting, falls, heart attacks, or strokes.

People with heart disease who take nitrates are usually instructed not to take Viagra-like medications, so they may be especially tempted to try sexual enhancement products that are marketed as "natural" or "herbal." Other types of nitrate compounds, such as amyl nitrate, are used as recreational drugs (sometimes called "poppers") and can be very dangerous when combined with Viagra-like drugs.

Another potentially dangerous group of products that are marketed for sexual enhancement online includes male sex hormones such as testosterone and DHEA (dehydroepiandrosterone). These hormones are potentially dangerous and should never be used without medical supervision. Side effects of male hormones include acne, testicular atrophy, infertility, enlarged breasts, baldness, and accelerated growth of preexisting prostate cancer. Nonprescription hormone products sold on the Internet are of particular concern because there is no guarantee of the actual strength or purity of the ingredients, or even whether the product contains any of the advertised hormone at all.

Another example of a potentially unsafe product sold on the Internet for sexual improvement is Yohimbine, an extract of tree bark. It is marketed as a dietary supplement for low libido, erectile dysfunction, and female sexual problems. These nonprescription forms of yohimbine are problematic because the FDA does not monitor dietary supplements for strength, purity, quality, effectiveness, or safety. A prescription form of Yohimbine (Yohimbine hydrochloride) is, like all prescription drugs, regulated by the FDA. Yohimbine can cause blood pressure changes and rapid and/or irregular heart beat.

Aggressive marketing of these sexual enhancement products on the Internet and television makes it likely that they will harm more and more people. Any product that purports to enhance sexual function, especially if it is sold online without medical supervision, should be viewed with healthy skepticism.

SOURCES: Many herbal sex pills carry hidden heart risk. 2007: *Sacramento Bee*, 13 November, A5; Mayo Clinic. 2006. *DHEA* (http://www.mayoclinic.com/health/dhea/NS_patient-dhea; retrieved January 29, 2009); Mayo Clinic. 2007. *Yohimbe* (http://www.mayoclinic.com/health/drug-information/DR601453; retrieved January 29, 2009); U.S. National Library of Medicine. 2006. *Yohimbe Bark Extract* (http://www.nlm.nih.gov/medlineplus/druginfo/natural/patient-yohimbe.html; retrieved January 29, 2009).

In general, the inability to experience orgasm under certain circumstances is a problem only if the woman considers it so.

TREATING SEXUAL DYSFUNCTION Most forms of sexual dysfunction are treatable. The first step is to have a physical examination to find a possible medical cause. Heart disease, diabetes, smoking, the use of alcohol or recreational drugs, and certain over-the-counter and prescription medications can all inhibit sexual response (see the box "Sex Enhancement Products").

Many treatments are available, particularly for erectile dysfunction. In 1998, Viagra (sildenafil citrate), the first-ever prescription pill for erectile dysfunction, was introduced. Since then, two other oral medications with actions similar to Viagra, Cialis (tadalafil) and Levitra (vardenafil),

have been approved by the FDA. All three work by enhancing the effects of nitric oxide, a chemical that relaxes smooth muscles in the penis. This increases the amount of blood flow and allows a natural erection to occur in response to sexual stimulation. The medications are generally safe for healthy men, but they should not be used by men who have a high risk of heart attack or stroke. They are effective in about 70% of users, but there are potential side effects, including headaches, indigestion, facial flushing, back pain, visual and hearing disturbances, and changes in blood pressure. Viagra, Cialis, and Levitra should never be taken by anyone who takes nitrate medication (usually prescribed for heart problems), and the recreational drugs amyl nitrate or nitrite (sometimes called "poppers") should never be combined with drugs for erectile dysfunction. The combination of nitrates and

Viagra-like drugs can cause a sudden potentially lethal drop in blood pressure.

Viagra use by men between the ages of 18 and 45 has risen dramatically—possibly due to use of the drug for recreational purposes. The drug may cut the refractory period in men who do not have erectile dysfunction; younger men may also be using it to cope with performance anxiety or the effects of other drugs, such as antidepressants.

Although Viagra is not approved by the FDA for use by women, a growing number of women are trying the drug. Research findings are mixed as to whether Viagra can increase sex drive and satisfaction levels in women. Recent studies have shown, however, that the drug can help women with sexual dysfunction caused by their use of antidepressant drugs.

Many people with no obvious physical disorder have sexual problems because of psychological and social issues. Too often, sexual difficulties are treated with drugs when nondrug strategies may be more appropriate. Psychosocial causes of dysfunction include troubled relationships, a lack of sexual skills, irrational attitudes and beliefs, anxiety, and psychosexual trauma, such as sexual abuse or rape. Many of these problems can be addressed by sex therapy.

Women who seek treatment for orgasmic dysfunction often have not learned what types of stimulation will excite them and bring them to orgasm. Most sex therapists treat this problem with **masturbation** (genital self-stimulation). Women are taught about their own anatomy and sexual responses and then are encouraged to experiment with masturbation until they experience orgasm.

SEXUAL BEHAVIOR

Many behaviors stem from sexual impulses, and sexual expression takes a variety of forms. Probably the most basic aspect of sexuality is reproduction. But sexual excitement and satisfaction are aspects of sexual behavior separate from reproduction. The intensely pleasurable sensations of arousal and orgasm are probably the strongest motivators for human sexual behavior. People are infinitely varied in the ways they seek to experience erotic pleasure (see the box "Sexual Decision Making").

→ Sexual Orientation

Sexual orientation is a consistent pattern of emotional and sexual attraction based on biological sex. It exists along a continuum that ranges from exclusive heterosexuality (attraction to people of the other sex) through bisexuality (attraction to people of both sexes) to exclusive homosexuality (attraction to people of one's own sex). The terms *straight* and *gay* are often used to refer to heterosexuals and homosexuals, respectively, and female homosexuals are also referred to as *lesbians.*

Sexual orientation involves feelings and self-concept, and individuals may or may not express their sexual orientation in their behavior. In national surveys, about 2–6% of men identify themselves as homosexuals and about 1.5% of women identify themselves as lesbians. Many theories try to account for the development of sexual orientation. At this time, most experts agree that sexual orientation results from multiple genetic, biological, cultural, social, and psychological factors.

So far, most studies on the origin of sexual orientation have focused on males. The factors that determine sexual orientation in women may be even more complex. Perhaps the most important message is that sexual orientation is most likely the result of the complex interaction of biological, psychological, and social factors, possibly different in the case of each individual.

Varieties of Human Sexual Behavior

Some sexual behaviors are aimed at self-stimulation only, whereas other practices involve interaction with a partner (see the box "Sexual Activity Among College Students" on p. 102). Some people choose not to express their sexuality at all.

Celibacy   Continuous abstention from sexual activities, termed **celibacy,** can be a conscious and deliberate choice, or it can be necessitated by circumstances. Health considerations and religious and moral beliefs may lead some people to celibacy, particularly until marriage or until an acceptable partner appears. Many people use the related term *abstinence* to refer to avoidance of just one sexual activity—intercourse.

Autoeroticism and Masturbation   The most common form of **autoeroticism** is **erotic fantasy,** creating imaginary experiences that range from fleeting thoughts to elaborate scenarios. Masturbation involves manually stimulating the genitals, rubbing them against objects, or

QUESTIONS FOR CRITICAL THINKING AND REFLECTION

If you are sexually active, would you consider using a product such as Viagra even if you didn't need it? Are you fully aware of the potential side effects of such products? In your opinion, would the potential benefits outweigh the risks?

Sexual Decision Making

Choosing to have sex can change a relationship as well as an individual's life. In making decisions about sexual activity, you owe it to yourself and your partner to think and talk honestly about your choices. Consider the following issues:

• *Your background, beliefs, and goals.* What are your religious, moral, and/or personal values regarding relationships and sex? What are your priorities at this time, and how will a sexual relationship fit into your goals and plans for the future? Are you physically, emotionally, and financially ready to accept the potential consequences of the choices you make?

• *Your relationship with your partner.* How do you feel about your partner and your relationship? Do you respect and trust each other? Do you feel comfortable talking about sexual issues, and

have you discussed contraception, pregnancy, and safer sex? How do you think having sex will affect your relationship and how you feel about yourself and your partner? What does having sex mean to each of you?

• *Your reasons for having sex.* What reasons do you have for moving into a sexual relationship? Are you being honest with yourself and your partner about this?

Personal decisions about sex should always be respected. You have the right to make your own choices and to do only what you feel comfortable with. When you make choices about sex based on self-respect, along with physical, emotional, and spiritual considerations, you'll be more likely to feel good about your decisions—now and in the future.

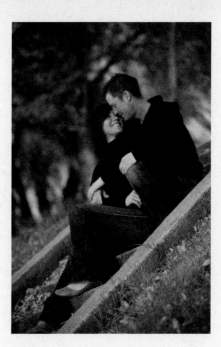

using stimulating devices such as vibrators. It may be used as a substitute for sexual intercourse or as part of sexual activity with a partner.

Touching and Foreplay   Touching is integral to sexual experiences, whether in the form of massage, kissing, fondling, or holding. Our entire body surface is a sensory organ, and touching almost anywhere can enhance intimacy and sexual arousal. Touching can convey a variety of messages, including affection, comfort, and a desire for further sexual contact.

During arousal, many men and women manually and orally stimulate each other by touching, stroking, and caressing their partner's genitals. Men and women vary greatly in their preferences for the type, pacing, and vigor of such **foreplay.** Working out the details to accommodate each other's pleasure is a key to enjoying these activities. Direct communication about preferences can enhance sexual pleasure and protect both partners from physical and psychological discomfort.

Oral-Genital Stimulation   Cunnilingus (the stimulation of the female genitals with the lips and tongue) and **fellatio** (the stimulation of the penis with the mouth) are common practices. Oral sex may be practiced either as part of foreplay or as a sex act culminating in orgasm. Although prevalence varies in different populations, 90% of men, 88% of women, and more than 50% of teens report that they have engaged in oral sex. Like all acts of sexual expression between two people, oral sex requires the cooperation and consent of both partners.

Anal Intercourse   About 10% of heterosexuals and 50% of homosexual males regularly practice anal stimulation and penetration by the penis or a finger. Because the anus is composed of delicate tissues that tear easily under such pressure, anal intercourse is one of the riskiest of sexual behaviors associated with the transmission of HIV and all other sexually transmitted infections. Anal intercourse is also associated with increased risk of anal cancer, hemorrhoids, anal fissures, prolapsed rectum, and fecal incontinence. The use of condoms is highly recommended for anyone engaging in anal sex.

Sexual Intercourse   For most adults, most of the time, **sexual intercourse** (*coitus*) is the ultimate sexual experience. The most common heterosexual practice is the man

masturbation   Self-stimulation for the purpose of sexual arousal and orgasm.

celibacy   Continuous abstention from sexual activity.

autoeroticism   Behavior aimed at sexual self-stimulation.

erotic fantasy   Sexually arousing thoughts and daydreams.

foreplay   Kissing, touching, and any form of oral or genital contact that stimulates people toward intercourse.

cunnilingus   Oral stimulation of the female genitals.

fellatio   Oral stimulation of the penis.

sexual intercourse   Sexual relations involving genital union; also called *coitus*, and also known as making love.

Sexual Activity Among College Students

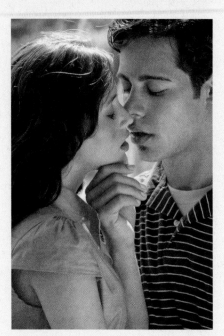

The popular perception of college students is that they are young, attractive, and highly sexually active. But how close are these stereotypes to reality? In a 2006 survey of nearly 95,000 college students, about one-third of the respondents said they had never had a sexual partner or were currently not sexually active. Of those students who reported having sex with a partner, the vast majority said they had only one partner. Only a small group—about 1 in 10 students—reported having had three or more sexual partners in the last year.

Students tend to grossly overestimate the sexual activity level of their peers, mirroring the popular perception of college students. In the survey, students guessed that their peers had more than twice as many sex partners as they actually did.

Slightly more than half of all students said they had not had sexual intercourse in the last 30 days. When asked what types of intercourse they engaged in, most sexually active students reported participating in either vaginal or oral intercourse. Anal intercourse was relatively rare, with only about 1 in 20 students reporting having had anal sex one or more times in the last month. Once again, students wildly overestimated the frequency of all types of intercourse among their fellow students; more than half of the students who were polled guessed that the typical student at their college was participating in anal sex, while in reality only a small minority of college students report having had anal sex.

Judging from the results of this large survey, condom use among college students is far from consistent. Only about 18% of students reported using a condom every time they had vaginal intercourse in the last month. Birth control pills were the most popular contraceptive, with condoms a close second. The vast majority of students do not use condoms when they engage in oral sex. When asked about condom use during anal sex—which is among the riskiest of all sexual behaviors in terms of acquiring a sexually transmitted disease—the majority of students who reported this activity did not use a condom the last time they had anal sex.

Among the college men polled in this study, 93% described themselves as heterosexual, as did 95% of women. About 4% of men identified themselves as gay and 1% of women identified themselves as lesbian. Another 2% of college men and 3% of women classified themselves as bisexual. Less than 1% of college students described themselves as transgendered.

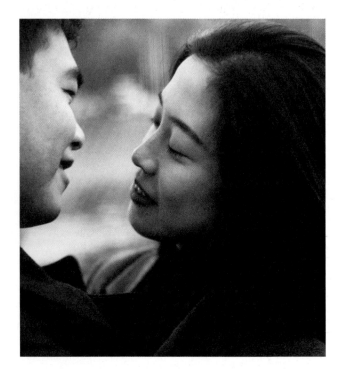

This couple's physical experiences together will be powerfully affected by their emotions, ideas, and values and by the quality of their relationship.

inserting his erect penis into the woman's dilated and lubricated vagina after sufficient arousal. Men and women engage in vaginal intercourse to fulfill both sexual and psychological needs. In a 2006 study by the National Center for Health Statistics, 87% of men age 15–44 and 98% of women in the same age group reported having had vaginal intercourse.

Atypical and Problematic Sexual Behaviors

In American culture, many kinds of sexual behavior are accepted. However, some types of sexual expression are considered harmful; they may be illegal, classified as

Sexsomnia: Sleep Disorders and Sex

A man accused of sexual assault claims he is not guilty of rape because he was sound asleep and completely unaware of his actions. Could he be telling the truth? Sleep experts say that such behavior while asleep is possible, although it is relatively uncommon.

Sexual arousal during sleep is normal and usually perfectly safe since it generally occurs during the rapid eye movement, or dreaming, phase of sleep when we are semiparalyzed. But some people have episodes of abnormal sleep in which they are able to perform complex physical activities without any awareness of what they are doing. They have no memory of these episodes once they are fully awake. This category of sleep disorder, called *parasomnia,* includes sleepwalk-

ing, sleep talking, sleep eating, sleep driving, and sleep sex.

Sexsomnia is a recently coined term for sleep sex disorder. Sleep researchers have observed this phenomenon in the laboratory and have correlated it with abnormal brain wave activity similar to that seen in other parasomnias. Sexsomnia has been in the news recently because several defendants in sexual assault cases have been acquitted when they were found to not be responsible for their actions due to sexsomnia. These cases have received considerable publicity, but it is important to remember that only a few cases of sexsomnia have been documented in medical literature and that the disorder is probably rather rare.

Another recent development that has brought attention to the disorder is the finding that popular sleep medications (called *sedative-hypnotic* drugs) seem to cause a phenomenon similar to the parasomnias in some people. There are reports of these people driving, making phone calls, and preparing and eating food while asleep. A few people report having sex while apparently asleep after taking these drugs.

As a result of these reports, the FDA has requested that the manufacturers of 13 sleep medications (including Ambien and Lunesta) include warnings about complex sleep behaviors on their labels. In addition, the FDA requested further clinical research into the potential side effects of these drugs.

SOURCES: Schenk, C. H., et al. 2007. Sleep and sex: What can go wrong? *Sleep* 30(6): 683–702; U.S. Food and Drug Administration. 2007. *FDA Requests Label Change for All Sleep Disorder Drug Products* (http://www.fda.gov/bbs/topics/news/2007/new01587.html; retrieved January 29, 2009).

mental disorders, or both. Because sexual behavior occurs on a continuum, it is sometimes difficult to differentiate a behavior that is simply atypical from one that is harmful (see the box "Sexsomnia: Sleep Disorders and Sex"). When attempting to evaluate an unusual sexual behavior, experts consider the issues of consent between partners and whether physical or psychological harm is done to the individual or to others.

The use of force and coercion in sexual relationships is one of the most serious problems in human interactions. The most extreme manifestation of **sexual coercion**—forcing a person to submit to another's sexual desires—is rape, but sexual coercion occurs in many subtler forms, such as sexual harassment.

Commercial Sex

Conflicting feelings about sexuality are apparent in the attitudes of Americans toward commercial sex: prostitution and sexually oriented materials in a variety of formats. Our society condemns sexually explicit material and prostitution, but it also provides their customers.

Pornography   Derived from the Greek word meaning "the writing of prostitutes," **pornography** (*porn*) is now often defined as obscene literature, art, or movies. A major problem in identifying pornographic material is that different people and communities have different opinions about what is obscene. Differing definitions of obscenity have led to many legal battles over potentially pornographic materi-

als. Currently, the sale and rental of pornographic materials is restricted so that only adults can legally obtain them; materials depicting children in sexual contexts are illegal in any format or setting.

Much of the debate about pornography focuses on whether it is harmful. Some people argue that adults who want to view pornographic materials in the privacy of their own homes should be allowed to do so. Others feel that the exposure to explicit sexual material can lead to delinquent or criminal behavior, such as rape or the sexual abuse of children. Currently, there is no reliable evidence that pornography by itself leads to violence or harmful sexual behavior, and debate is likely to continue.

Online Porn and Cybersex   The appearance of thousands of sexually oriented Web sites has expanded the number of people with access to pornography and has made it more difficult for authorities to enforce laws regarding porn. Of special concern is the increased availability of child pornography, which previously could be acquired only with great difficulty and at great legal risk. Online porn is now a multibillion-dollar industry.

TERMS

sexual coercion   The use of physical or psychological force or intimidation to make a person submit to sexual demands.

pornography   The explicit or obscene depiction of sexual activities in pictures, writing, or other material.

Hundreds of thousands of people also use the Internet to engage in **cybersex,** or *virtual sex.* Cybersex is erotic interaction between people who are communicating over a network such as the Internet; the participants are not in physical contact with each other. People who become addicted to cybersex or viewing online porn may become isolated and perform poorly at work or school. Their addiction may also have a negative impact on their interpersonal relationships.

Prostitution   The exchange of sexual services for money is **prostitution.** Prostitutes may be men, women, or children, and the buyer of a prostitute's services is nearly always a man. Except in parts of Nevada, prostitution is illegal in the United States. Most customers are white, middle-class, middle-aged, and married. Although they come from a wide variety of backgrounds, prostitutes are usually motivated to join the profession because of money.

AIDS is a major concern for prostitutes and their customers. Many prostitutes are injection drug users or are involved with men who are. The rate of HIV infection among prostitutes varies widely, but in some parts of the country it is as high as 25–50%.

Responsible Sexual Behavior

Healthy sexuality is an important part of adult life. It can be a source of pleasurable experiences and emotions and an important part of intimate partnerships. But sexual behavior also carries many responsibilities, as well as potential consequences such as pregnancy, STDs, and emotional changes in the relationship.

Open, Honest Communication   Each partner needs to clearly indicate what sexual involvement means to him or her. Does it mean love, fun, a permanent commitment, or

QUESTIONS FOR CRITICAL THINKING AND REFLECTION

If you are sexually active or plan to become active soon, how open have you been about communicating with your partner? Are you aware of your partner's feelings about sex and his or her comfort level with certain activities? Do you and your partner share the same views on contraception, STD prevention, and ethical issues about sex?

something else? The intentions of both partners should be clear. For strategies on talking about sexual issues with your partner, see the box "Communicating About Sexuality."

Agreed-On Sexual Activities   No one should pressure or coerce a partner. Sexual behaviors should be consistent with the sexual values, preferences, and comfort level of both partners. Everyone has the right to refuse sexual activity at any time.

Sexual Privacy   Intimate relationships involving sexual activity are based on trust, and that trust can be violated if partners reveal private information about the relationship to others. Sexual privacy also involves respecting other people—not engaging in activities in the presence of others that would make them uncomfortable.

Using Contraception   If pregnancy is not desired, contraception should be used during sexual intercourse. Both partners need to take responsibility for protecting against unwanted pregnancy. Partners should discuss contraception before sexual involvement begins.

Safer Sex   Both partners should be aware of and practice safer sex to guard against sexually transmitted diseases (STDs). Many sexual behaviors carry the risk of STDs, including HIV infection. Partners should be honest about their health and any medical conditions and work out a plan for protection.

Sober Sex   The use of alcohol or drugs in sexual situations increases the risk of unplanned, unprotected sexual activity. This is particularly true of young adults, many of whom engage in episodes of binge drinking during social events. Alcohol and drugs impair judgment and should not be used in association with sexual activity.

UNDERSTANDING FERTILITY

Conceiving a child is a highly complex process. Although many couples conceive readily, others can testify to the difficulties that can be encountered.

Communicating About Sexuality

To talk with your partner about sexuality, follow the general suggestions for effective communication given in Chapter 4. Getting started may be the most difficult part. Some people feel more comfortable if they begin by talking about talking—that is, initiating a discussion about why people are so uncomfortable talking about sexuality. Talking about sexual histories—how partners first learned about sex or how family and cultural background influenced sexual values and attitudes—is another way to get started. Reading about sex can also be a good beginning: Partners can read an article or book and then discuss their reactions.

Be honest about what you feel and what you want from your partner. Cultural and personal obstacles to discussing sexual subjects can be difficult to overcome, but self-disclosure is important for successful relationships. Research indicates that when one partner openly discusses attitudes and feelings, the other partner is more likely to do the same. If your partner seems hesitant to open up, try asking open-ended or either/or questions: "Where do you like to be touched?" or "Would you like to talk about this now or wait until later?"

If something is bothering you about your sexual relationship, choose a good time to initiate a discussion with your partner. Be specific and direct but also tactful. Focus on what you actually observe, rather than on what you think the behavior means. "You didn't touch or hug me when your friends were around" is an observation. "You're ashamed of me around your friends" is an inference about your partner's feelings. Try focusing on a specific behavior that concerns you rather than on the person as a whole—your partner can change behaviors but not his or her entire personality. For example, you could say "I'd like you to take a few minutes away from studying to kiss me" instead of "You're so caught up in your work, you never have time for me."

If you are going to make a statement that your partner may interpret as criticism, try mixing it with something positive: "I love spending time with you, but I feel annoyed when you. . . ." Similarly, if your partner says something that upsets you, don't lash back. An aggressive response may make you feel better in the short run, but it will not help the communication process or the quality of the relationship.

If you want to say no to some sexual activity, say no unequivocally. Don't send mixed messages. If you are afraid of hurting your partner's feelings, offer an alternative if it's appropriate: "I am uncomfortable with that. How about . . .?"

If you're in love, you may think that the sexual aspects of a relationship will work out magically without discussion. However, partners who never talk about sex deny themselves the opportunity to increase their closeness and improve their relationship.

→Conception

The process of conception involves the **fertilization** of an ovum (egg) from a woman by a sperm from a man. Every month during a woman's fertile years, her body prepares itself for conception and pregnancy. In one of her ovaries an egg matures and is released from its follicle. The egg, about the size of a pinpoint, travels through an oviduct, or fallopian tube, to the uterus in 3–4 days. The endometrium, or lining of the uterus, has already thickened for the implantation of a **fertilized egg**, or *zygote*. If the egg is not fertilized, it lasts about 24 hours and then disintegrates. It is expelled along with the uterine lining during menstruation.

Sperm cells are produced in the man's testes and ejaculated from his penis into the woman's vagina during sexual intercourse. Sperm cells are much smaller than eggs. The typical ejaculate contains millions of sperm, but only a few complete the journey through the uterus and up the fallopian tube to the egg.

Of those that reach the egg, only one will penetrate its hard outer layer. As sperm approach the egg, they release enzymes that soften this outer layer. Enzymes from hundreds of sperm must be released in order for the egg's outer layer to soften enough to allow one sperm cell to penetrate. The first sperm cell that bumps into a spot that is soft enough can swim into the egg cell. It then merges with the nucleus of the egg, and fertilization occurs. The sperm's tail, its means of locomotion, gets stuck in the outer membrane and drops off, leaving the sperm head inside the egg. The egg then releases a chemical that makes it impenetrable by other sperm.

The ovum carries the hereditary characteristics of the mother and her ancestors; sperm cells carry the hereditary characteristics of the father and his ancestors. Each parent cell—egg or sperm—contains 23 chromosomes, each of which contains **genes**, packages of chemical instructions for the developing baby. Genes provide the blueprint for a unique individual.

The usual course of events is that one egg and one sperm unite to produce one fertilized egg and one baby. But if the ovaries release two (or more) eggs during ovulation and if both eggs are fertilized, twins will develop. These twins will be no more alike than siblings from different pregnancies, because each will have come from a different fertilized egg. Twins who develop this way are referred to as **fraternal twins;** they may be the same sex or different sexes. About 70% of twins are fraternal. Twins can also develop from the division of a single fertilized egg into two cells that develop separately. Because these babies share all genetic material, they will be **identical twins.**

Infertility

Millions of couples have difficulty conceiving. **Infertility** is defined as the inability to conceive after trying for a year or more. It affects about 15% of the reproductive-age population of the United States.

Female Infertility   Female infertility usually results from one of two key causes—tubal blockage (40%) or failure to ovulate (40%). An additional 10% of cases of infertility are due to anatomical abnormalities, benign growths in the uterus, thyroid disease, and other uncommon conditions; the remaining 10% of cases are unexplained.

Blocked fallopian tubes are most commonly the result of pelvic inflammatory disease (PID), a serious complication of several sexually transmitted diseases. Each year, PID renders more than 100,000 American women infertile. More than 1 million cases of PID are treated each year, but physicians estimate that just as many may go untreated because of an absence of symptoms. Tubal blockages can also be caused by prior surgery or by endometriosis, which is typically treated with hormonal therapy and surgery.

Age impacts fertility; beginning at around age 30, a woman's fertility naturally begins to decline. Age is probably the main factor in ovulation failure. Exposure to toxic chemicals or radiation also appears to reduce fertility, as does cigarette smoking.

Male Infertility   Male factor infertility accounts for about 20% of infertile couples. The leading causes of male infertility can be divided into four main categories: hypothalamic pituitary disease or congenital disorders, testicular disease, disorders of sperm transport, and unexplained. Some acquired disorders of the testes can lead to infertility, such as damage from drug use, smoking, infection, or environmental toxins.

The sons of mothers who took DES may have increased sperm abnormalities and fertility problems. Studies have identified a link between infertility and overweight and obesity in men, although the mechanism responsible for the relationship was not clear.

Treating Infertility   The cause of infertility can be determined for about 85% of infertile couples. Most cases of infertility are treated with conventional medical therapies. Surgery can repair oviducts, clear up endometriosis, and correct anatomical problems in both men and women. Fertility drugs can help women ovulate, although they may cause multiple births. If these conventional treatments don't work, couples can turn to **assisted reproductive technology (ART)** techniques, as described in the following sections.

INTRAUTERINE INSEMINATION   Male infertility can sometimes be overcome by collecting and concentrating the man's sperm and introducing it by syringe into a woman's vagina or uterus, a procedure known as **artificial (intrauterine) insemination.** To increase the probability of success, the woman is often given fertility drugs to induce ovulation prior to the insemination procedure. The success rate is about 60–70%.

IVF, GIFT, AND ZIFT   Three related techniques involve removing mature eggs from a woman's ovary.

- In **in vitro fertilization (IVF),** the harvested eggs are mixed with sperm in a laboratory dish. If eggs are successfully fertilized, one or more of the resulting embryos are inserted into the woman's uterus. IVF is often used by women with blocked oviducts.

- In **gamete intrafallopian transfer (GIFT),** eggs and sperm are surgically placed into the fallopian tubes prior to fertilization.

TERMS

infertility   The inability to conceive after trying for a year or more.

assisted reproductive technology (ART)   Advanced medical techniques used to treat infertility.

artificial (intrauterine) insemination   The introduction of semen into the vagina by artificial means, usually by syringe.

in vitro fertilization (IVF)   Combining egg and sperm outside of the body and inserting the fertilized egg into the uterus.

gamete intrafallopian transfer (GIFT)   Surgically introducing eggs and sperm into the fallopian tube prior to fertilization.

zygote intrafallopian transfer (ZIFT)   Surgically introducing a fertilized egg into the fallopian tube.

trimester   One of the three 3-month periods of pregnancy.

human chorionic gonadotropin (HCG)   A hormone produced by the fertilized egg that can be detected in the urine or blood of the mother within a few weeks of conception.

- In **zygote intrafallopian transfer (ZIFT)**, eggs are fertilized outside the woman's body and surgically introduced into the oviducts after they begin to divide.

GIFT and ZIFT can be used by women who have at least one open fallopian tube. Variations on these three techniques are also becoming available.

SURROGATE MOTHERHOOD Surrogate motherhood involves a contract between an infertile couple and a fertile woman who agrees to carry a fetus. The surrogate mother agrees to be artificially inseminated by the father's sperm or to undergo IVF with the couple's embryo, to carry the baby to term, and to give it to the couple at birth. In return, the couple pays her for her services (typically around $50,000). There are thought to be several hundred births to surrogate mothers each year in the United States.

PREGNANCY

Pregnancy is usually discussed in terms of **trimesters**— three periods of about 3 months (or 13 weeks) each. During the first trimester, the mother experiences a few physical changes and some fairly common symptoms. During the second trimester, often the most peaceful time of pregnancy, the mother gains weight, looks noticeably pregnant, and may experience a general sense of well-being if she is happy about having a child. The third trimester is the hardest for the mother because she must breathe, digest, excrete, and circulate blood for herself and the growing fetus.

Pregnancy Tests

The earliest tests for pregnancy are chemical tests designed to detect the presence of **human chorionic gonadotropin (HCG),** a hormone produced by the implanted fertilized egg. These tests may be performed as early as 2 weeks after fertilization.

Home pregnancy tests can be very reliable, but the instructions must be followed carefully. If a home test done at the time of a missed menstrual period is negative, retesting after another week is recommended. In the first day or two following a missed period, the concentration of HCG may be too low to be detected by the test.

Changes in the Woman's Body

Hormonal changes begin as soon as the egg is fertilized, and for the next 9 months the woman's body nourishes the fetus and adjusts to its growth (Figure 5.4).

Early Signs and Symptoms Early recognition of pregnancy is important, especially for women with physical problems and nutritional deficiencies. The following symptoms are not absolute indications of pregnancy, but they are reasons to visit a gynecologist:

- *A missed menstrual period.* If an egg has been fertilized and implanted in the uterine wall, the endometrium is retained to nourish the embryo.
- *Slight bleeding.* Slight bleeding follows implantation of the fertilized egg in about 14% of pregnant women. Because this happens about the time a period is expected, the bleeding is sometimes mistaken for menstrual flow. It usually lasts only a few days.
- *Nausea.* About two-thirds of pregnant women feel nauseated, probably as a reaction to increased levels of progesterone and other hormones. Although this nausea is often called *morning sickness,* some women have it all day long. It frequently begins during the 6th week and disappears by the 12th week. In some cases, it lasts throughout the pregnancy.
- *Breast tenderness.* Some women experience breast tenderness, swelling, and tingling, usually described as different from the tenderness experienced before menstruation.
- *Increased urination.* Increased frequency of urination can occur soon after the missed period.
- *Sleepiness, fatigue, and emotional upset.* These symptoms result from hormonal changes.

The first reliable physical signs of pregnancy can be distinguished about 4 weeks after a woman misses her menstrual period. A softening of the uterus just above the cervix, called *Hegar's sign,* and other changes in the cervix and pelvis are apparent during a pelvic examination. The labia minora and the cervix may take on a purple color rather than their usual pink hue.

Continuing Changes in the Woman's Body During the first 3 months, the uterus enlarges to about three times its nonpregnant size, but it still cannot be felt in the abdomen. By the 4th month, it is large enough to make the abdomen protrude. By the 7th or 8th month, the uterus pushes up into the rib cage, which makes breathing slightly more difficult. The breasts enlarge and are sensitive; by week 8, they may tingle or throb. The pigmented area around the nipple, the areola, darkens and broadens.

Early in pregnancy, the muscles and ligaments attached to bones begin to soften and stretch. The joints between the pelvic bones loosen and spread, making it easier to

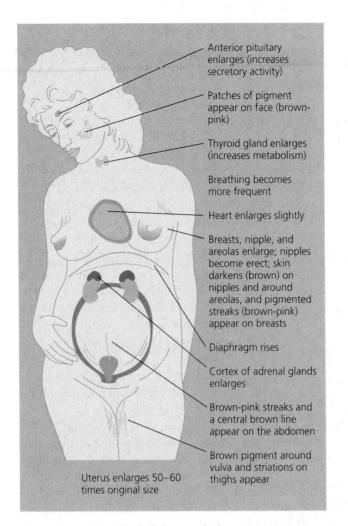

Anterior pituitary enlarges (increases secretory activity)

Patches of pigment appear on face (brown-pink)

Thyroid gland enlarges (increases metabolism)

Breathing becomes more frequent

Heart enlarges slightly

Breasts, nipple, and areolas enlarge; nipples become erect; skin darkens (brown) on nipples and around areolas, and pigmented streaks (brown-pink) appear on breasts

Diaphragm rises

Cortex of adrenal glands enlarges

Brown-pink streaks and a central brown line appear on the abdomen

Brown pigment around vulva and striations on thighs appear

Uterus enlarges 50–60 times original size

FIGURE 5.4 Physiological changes during pregnancy.

have a baby but harder to walk. The circulatory system becomes more efficient to accommodate the blood volume, which increases by 50%, and the heart pumps it more rapidly. The mother's lungs also become more efficient, and her rib cage widens to permit her to inhale up to 40% more air.

lightening   A process in which the uterus sinks down because the baby's head settles into the mother's pelvic area.

blastocyst   A stage of development, days 6–14, before the cell cluster becomes the embryo and placenta.

embryo   The stage of development between blastocyst and fetus; about weeks 2–8.

placenta   The organ through which the fetus receives nourishment and empties waste via the mother's circulatory system; after birth, the placenta is expelled from the uterus.

umbilical cord   The cord connecting the placenta and fetus, through which nutrients pass.

amniotic sac   A membranous pouch enclosing and protecting the fetus; also holds amniotic fluid.

The average weight gain during a healthy pregnancy is 27.5 pounds, although actual weight change varies with the individual. About 60% of the weight gain is directly related to the baby (such as the fetus and placenta); the rest accumulates over the woman's body as fluid and fat.

Changes During the Later Stages of Pregnancy   By the end of the 6th month, the increased needs of the fetus place a burden on the mother's lungs, heart, and kidneys. Her back may ache from the pressure of the baby's weight and from having to throw her shoulders back to keep her balance while standing. Her body retains more water, perhaps up to 3 extra quarts of fluid. Her legs, hands, ankles, or feet may swell, and she may be bothered by leg cramps, heartburn, or constipation. Despite discomfort, both her digestion and her metabolism are working at top efficiency.

The uterus prepares for childbirth with preliminary contractions, called *Braxton Hicks contractions*. Unlike true labor contractions, these are usually short, irregular, and painless. The mother may only be aware that at times her abdomen is hard to the touch. These contractions become more frequent and intense as the delivery date approaches.

In the 9th month, the baby settles into the pelvic bones, usually head down, fitting snugly. This process, called **lightening**, allows the uterus to sink down about 2 inches, producing a visible change in the mother's profile. Pelvic pressure increases, and pressure on the diaphragm lightens. Breathing becomes easier; urination becomes more frequent. Sometimes, after a first pregnancy, the baby doesn't settle down into the pelvis until labor begins.

The third trimester is the time of greatest physical stress during the pregnancy. A woman may find that her physical abilities are limited by her size. Because some women feel physically awkward and sexually unattractive, they may experience periods of depression. But many also feel a great deal of happy excitement and anticipation. The fetus may already be looked on as a member of the family, and both parents may begin talking to the fetus and interacting with it by patting the mother's belly. The upcoming birth will probably be a focus for both the woman and her partner (see the box "Pregnancy Tasks for Fathers").

Fetal Development

Now that we've seen what happens to the mother's body during pregnancy, let's consider the development of the fetus (Figure 5.5, p. 110).

The First Trimester   About 30 hours after the egg is fertilized, the cell divides, and this process of cell division repeats many times. As the cluster of cells drifts down the oviduct, several different kinds of cells emerge. The entire set of genetic instructions is passed to every cell, but each cell follows only certain instructions; if this were not the case, there would be no different organs or body parts. For example, all cells carry genes for hair color and eye

Pregnancy Tasks for Fathers

Before the Pregnancy

• *Consider your lifestyle and health habits.* A healthy lifestyle can help boost fertility and improve pregnancy outcome. Being too thin or too heavy may lower a man's sperm count, as may marijuana use. Men who smoke and drink have a lower concentration of sperm and a lower percentage of active sperm. Exposure to chemicals on the job may also affect pregnancy.

• *Check your budget, financial situation, and insurance status.* Make sure your finances are in order, and that you have as much life, health, and disability insurance as you can afford. See a financial planner for advice. Try putting away extra money every month now—both to practice living on a tighter budget and to actually save up for the baby.

• *Get any necessary health checks and genetic counseling.* See the discussion of potential health concerns in the section on "Preconception Care."

During the Pregnancy

• *Help your partner stay healthy during the pregnancy.* If you smoke, quit; secondhand smoke is dangerous for the developing fetus. Support your partner by making other lifestyle changes and/or joining her in any changes she's making; for example, drink nonalcoholic beverages, take walks with her, and get extra sleep.

• *Help around the home and with planning for the baby.* Help shop for necessi-ties, and help get your home ready for a baby. Pregnancy is hard work, so providing extra help with household chores and errands can be an important element of support. (Due to the risk of infection by toxoplasmosis, pregnant women should avoid handling cat litter; if you and your partner have a cat, emptying the litter box should be your job.)

• *Be involved.* Go to all the prenatal visits, birth preparation or education classes, hospital and nursery tours, and so on. Learn more about pregnancy, childbirth, and parenting by reading books, visiting Internet sites, and talking with other parents.

After the Baby Arrives

• *Help meet your baby's needs.* If your job allows, take parental leave to help with the new baby. Support the new mother by helping with baby care (feeding, diaper changes), laundry, shopping, and other chores. Take turns or join the mother when the baby needs care or feeding during the night; one survey found that more than half of fathers continue to sleep or pretend to be asleep when their babies cry during the night.

• *Support your partner, and reach out to others for help.* It is normal for a new mother to be tired and to experience mood changes, and some men also experience anxiety about their new role. Good communication between partners and help from supportive relatives and friends can help new parents adjust.

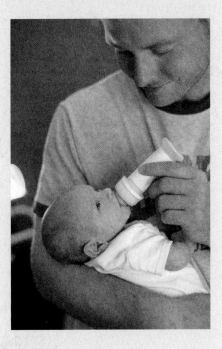

• *Give mom some time off.* A new mother needs time to recover from childbirth, even after she leaves the hospital or birthing center. This is especially true if the delivery was difficult, if a cesarean section was performed, or if an episiotomy was required. Aside from pitching in with daily chores, the father can aid the mother's recuperation by taking the baby for a few hours at a time. If the baby is being bottlefed, the dad may be able to take charge for a morning, an afternoon, or even the entire day.

---

color, but only the cells of the hair follicles and irises (of the eye) respond to that information.

On about the fourth day after fertilization, the cluster, now about 32–128 cells and hollow, arrives in the uterus; this is a **blastocyst.** On about the sixth or seventh day, the blastocyst attaches to the uterine wall, usually along the upper curve; over the next few days, it becomes firmly implanted and begins to draw nourishment from the endometrium, the uterine lining.

The blastocyst becomes an **embryo** by about the end of the 2nd week after fertilization. The inner cells of the blastocyst separate into three layers. One layer becomes inner body parts, the digestive and respiratory systems; the middle layer becomes muscle, bone, blood, kidneys, and sex glands; and the third layer becomes the skin, hair, and nervous tissue.

The outermost shell of cells becomes the **placenta, umbilical cord,** and **amniotic sac.** A network of blood vessels called *chorionic villi* eventually forms the placenta. The human placenta allows a two-way exchange of nutrients and waste materials between the mother and the fetus. The placenta brings oxygen and nutrients to the fetus and transports waste products out. The placenta does not provide a perfect barrier between the fetal circulation and the maternal circulation, however. Some blood cells

Up to 20% of pregnant woman have symptoms of major depression.

—**March of Dimes Foundation, 2007**

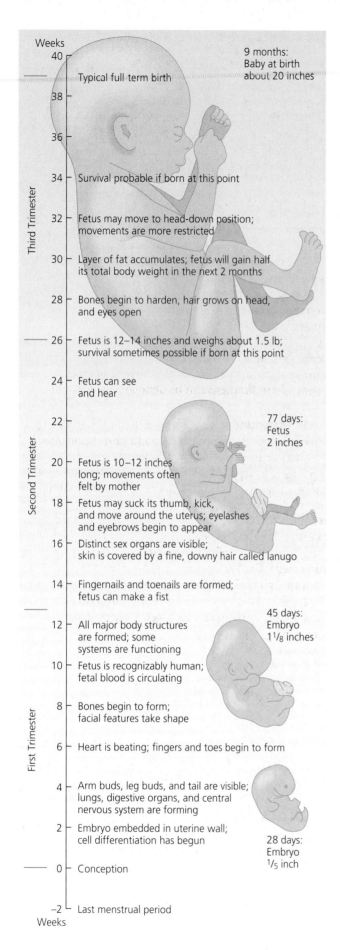

Weeks

40 — Typical full term birth

9 months:
Baby at birth
about 20 inches

38

36

34 — Survival probable if born at this point

32 — Fetus may move to head-down position;
movements are more restricted

30 — Layer of fat accumulates; fetus will gain half
its total body weight in the next 2 months

28 — Bones begin to harden, hair grows on head,
and eyes open

26 — Fetus is 12–14 inches and weighs about 1.5 lb;
survival sometimes possible if born at this point

24 — Fetus can see
and hear

22

77 days:
Fetus
2 inches

20 — Fetus is 10–12 inches
long; movements often
felt by mother

18 — Fetus may suck its thumb, kick,
and move around the uterus; eyelashes
and eyebrows begin to appear

16 — Distinct sex organs are visible;
skin is covered by a fine, downy hair called lanugo

14 — Fingernails and toenails are formed;
fetus can make a fist

12 — All major body structures
are formed; some
systems are functioning

45 days:
Embryo
1 1/8 inches

10 — Fetus is recognizably human;
fetal blood is circulating

8 — Bones begin to form;
facial features take shape

6 — Heart is beating; fingers and toes begin to form

4 — Arm buds, leg buds, and tail are visible;
lungs, digestive organs, and central
nervous system are forming

2 — Embryo embedded in uterine wall;
cell differentiation has begun

28 days:
Embryo
1/5 inch

0 — Conception

−2 — Last menstrual period
Weeks

Third Trimester

Second Trimester

First Trimester

FIGURE 5.5 A chronology of milestones in prenatal development.

are exchanged and certain substances, such as alcohol, pass freely from the maternal circulation through the placenta to the fetus.

The period between weeks 2 and 9 is a time of rapid differentiation and change. All the major body structures are formed during this time, including the heart, brain, liver, lungs, and sex organs; the eyes, nose, ears, arms, and legs also appear. Some organs begin to function—the heart begins to beat, and the liver starts producing blood cells. Because body structures are forming, the developing organism is vulnerable to damage from environmental influences such as drugs and infections.

By the end of the 2nd month, the brain sends out impulses that coordinate the functioning of other organs. The embryo is now a fetus, and most further changes will be in the size and refinement of working body parts. In the 3rd month, the fetus begins to be quite active. By the end of the first trimester, the fetus is about an inch long and weighs less than 1 ounce.

The Second Trimester To grow during the second trimester, to about 14 inches and 1.5 pounds, the fetus must have large amounts of food, oxygen, and water, which come from the mother through the placenta. All body systems are operating, and the fetal heartbeat can be heard with a stethoscope. The mother can detect fetal movements beginning in the 4th or 5th month. Against great odds, a fetus born prematurely at the end of the second trimester might survive.

The Third Trimester The fetus gains most of its birth weight during the last 3 months. Some of the weight is fatty tissue under the skin that insulates the fetus and supplies food. The fetus needs a great deal of calcium, iron, and nitrogen from the food the mother eats. Some 85% of the calcium and iron she consumes goes into the fetal bloodstream.

Although the fetus may live if it is born during the 7th month, it needs the fat layer acquired in the 8th month and time for the organs, especially the respiratory and digestive organs, to develop. It also needs the immunity supplied by the antibodies in the mother's blood during the final 3 months. The antibodies protect the fetus against many of the diseases to which she has acquired immunity. Breast milk can help the baby further resist infections because it also contains maternal antibodies.

Diagnosing Fetal Abnormalities About 3% of babies are born with a major birth defect. Information about the health and sex of a fetus can be obtained prior to birth through prenatal testing.

Ultrasonography (also called *ultrasound*) uses high-frequency sound waves to create a **sonogram,** or visual image, of the fetus in the uterus. Sonograms show the

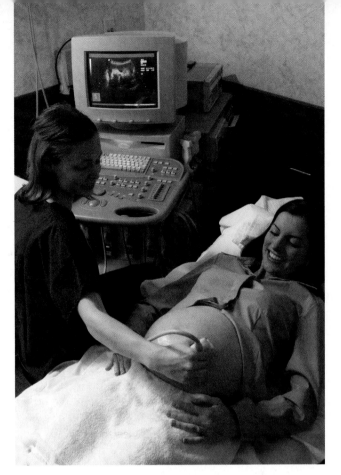

Ultrasonography provides information about the position, size, and physical condition of a fetus in the uterus.

position of the fetus, its size and gestational age, and the presence of certain anatomical problems. Sonograms can sometimes be used to determine the sex of the fetus. Sonograms are considered safe for a pregnant woman and the fetus, but the FDA advises against "keepsake" sonograms performed for no medical purpose.

Amniocentesis involves the removal of fluid from the uterus with a long, thin needle inserted through the abdominal wall. It is usually performed between 15 and 18 weeks into the pregnancy, although earlier amniocentesis is available. A genetic analysis of the fetal cells in the fluid can reveal the presence of chromosomal disorders, such as Down syndrome, and some genetic diseases, including Tay-Sachs disease (see the box "Ethnicity and Genetic Diseases" on p. 112). The sex of the fetus can also be determined.

Another prenatal test is **chorionic villus sampling (CVS)**, which can be performed earlier in pregnancy than amniocentesis, between weeks 10 and 12. This procedure involves removal through the cervix (by catheter) or abdomen (by needle) of a tiny section of chorionic villi, which contain fetal cells that then can be analyzed.

The **quadruple marker screen (QMS)** is a maternal blood test that can be used to help identify fetuses with neural tube defects, Down syndrome, and other anomalies. Blood is taken from the mother at 16–19 weeks of pregnancy and analyzed for four hormone levels—human chorionic gonadotropin (HCG), unconjugated estriol, alpha-fetoprotein (AFP), and inhibin-A. The hormone levels are compared to appropriate standards, and the results are used to estimate the probability that the fetus has particular anomalies. QMS is a screening test rather than a diagnostic test; in the case of abnormal QMS results, parents may choose further testing such as ultrasonography or amniocentesis.

A new first trimester screening test for Down syndrome combines ultrasound evaluation of nuchal translucency (the thickness of the back of the fetus's neck) with maternal blood testing. This test can be done between the 10th and 14th week of pregnancy. If results indicate an increased risk of abnormality, further diagnostic studies such as amniocentesis can be done for confirmation.

Fetal Programming Amniocentesis, CVS, and QMS look for chromosomal, genetic, and other anomalies that typically cause immediate problems. A new area of study known as *fetal programming theory* focuses on how conditions in the womb may influence the risk of adult diseases. For example, researchers have linked low birth weight to an increased risk of heart disease, high blood pressure, obesity, diabetes, and schizophrenia; high birth weight in female infants, however, has been linked to an increased risk of breast cancer in later life.

Although fetal programming theory is not yet embraced by all scientists, these studies emphasize that everything that occurs during pregnancy can have an impact on the developing fetus. In the future, people may be able to use information about their birth weight and other indicators of gestational conditions just as they can now use family history and genetic information—to alert them to special health risks and to help them improve their health.

TERMS

ultrasonography The use of high-frequency sound waves to view the fetus in the uterus; also known as *ultrasound*.

sonogram The visual image of the fetus produced by ultrasonography.

amniocentesis A process in which amniotic fluid is removed and analyzed to detect possible birth defects.

chorionic villus sampling (CVS) Surgical removal of a tiny section of chorionic villi to be analyzed for genetic defects.

quadruple marker screen (QMS) A measurement of four hormones, used to assess the risk of fetal abnormalities.

Genes carry the chemical instructions that determine the development of hundreds of individual traits, including disease risks, in every human being. Many traits and conditions involve multiple genes and environmental influences. Some diseases, however, can be traced to a mutation in a single gene.

Children inherit one set of genes from each parent. If only one copy of an abnormal gene is necessary to produce a disease, then it is called a *dominant* gene. Diseases caused by dominant genes seldom skip a generation; anyone who carries the gene will probably get the disease.

If two copies of an abnormal gene (one from each parent) are necessary for a disease to occur, then the gene is called *recessive*. Many diseases caused by recessive genes occur disproportionately in certain ethnic groups. Prospective parents who come from the same ethnic group can be tested for any recessive diseases that are known to occur in that group. If both parents are carriers, each of their children will have about a 25% chance of developing the disease.

The following list describes a few common conditions with proven genetic links in certain ethnic populations. If there is a history of any of these conditions in your family and you plan to have children, genetic tests and counseling can help assess the risk to your prospective offspring.

• *Sickle-cell disease* occurs in about 1 out of every 500 African American births and in 1 out of every 36,000 Hispanic American births, according to the CDC. In this disease, red blood cells, which carry oxygen to the body's tissues, change shape; the normally disc-shaped cells become sickle-shaped. The altered cells carry less oxygen and can block small blood vessels.

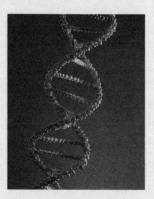

People who inherit one gene for sickle-cell disease (about 1 in 12 African Americans) experience only mild symptoms; those with two genes become severely, often fatally, ill.

If you are at risk for sickle-cell disease, you should take care to reduce stress and respond to minor infections, because red blood cells become sickle-shaped when the body is under stress. You should also have regular checkups and appropriate treatment, if required.

• *Hemochromatosis* ("iron overload") affects about 1 in 200 people. At highest risk are people of Northern European (especially Irish), Mediterranean, and Hispanic descent. In hemochromatosis, the body absorbs and stores up to ten times the normal amount of iron. Iron deposits form in the joints, liver, heart, and pancreas. If untreated, the disease can cause organ failure and death.

Early symptoms are often vague and include weakness, lethargy, darkening of the skin, and joint pain. Early detection and treatment are necessary to prevent damage. Treatment involves reducing iron stores by removing blood from the body (a process known as phlebotomy or "bloodletting").

• *Tay-Sachs disease*, another recessive disorder, occurs in about 1 in 3000 Jews of Eastern European ancestry. People with Tay-Sachs disease cannot properly metabolize fat. As a result, the brain and other nerve tissues deteriorate. Affected children show weakness in their movements and eventually develop blindness (by age 12–18 months) and seizures. This disease is fatal, and death usually occurs by age 6. No effective treatment is currently available.

• *Cystic fibrosis* occurs in 1 in 2500–3000 Caucasians; about 1 in 29 carries one copy of the cystic fibrosis gene. Because essential enzymes of the pancreas are deficient, the body cannot properly absorb nutrients. Thick mucus impairs functioning in the lungs and intestinal tracts of people with this disease. Cystic fibrosis is often fatal in early childhood, but treatments are increasingly effective in reducing symptoms and prolonging life. In some cases, symptoms do not appear until early adulthood.

• *Thalassemia* is a blood disease found most often among Italians, Greeks, and

to a lesser extent African Americans and Asians. When inherited from one parent, this form of anemia is mild; when two genes are present, the disease is severe and can cause fetal death.

Children with this condition require repeated blood transfusions, eventually resulting in a damaging iron buildup. New interventions, such as genetic engineering, bone marrow transplants, and chemicals that bind with excess iron and remove it from the body, offer promise. Transplantation of stem cells from the umbilical cord blood of an unaffected sibling or donor is already being used in some cases.

If you are at risk of carrying thalassemia, you should get regular checkups and monitor your health for symptoms, and learn ways to manage symptoms if they start to occur.

• *Lactose intolerance,* or intolerance to lactose-containing foods (primarily dairy products), is a common problem that often has a genetic component. In Europe and the United States, the prevalence is as high as 20% in Caucasians, 80–95% in Native Americans, 65–75% among Africans and African Americans, and 50% in Hispanics. The prevalence exceeds 90% in some populations in eastern Asia.

Clinical symptoms of lactose intolerance include diarrhea, abdominal pain, and flatulence after ingestion of milk or milk-containing products. These symptoms result from low intestinal lactase levels, which are commonly due to the reduced genetic expression of the enzyme lactase-phlorizin hydrolase. Genetically regulated reduction of lactase activity determined by racial or ethnic factors is the underlying mechanism of lactose malabsorption in healthy individuals.

If you suspect lactose intolerance, see your doctor for a lactose absorption test. In the absence of a correctable underlying disease, lactose malabsorption is treated by reducing lactose intake, finding alternatives to foods containing lactose, taking an enzyme substitute, and maintaining calcium and vitamin D intake.

Other health problems that have a hereditary component and that disproportionately affect certain ethnic groups include diabetes, osteoporosis, high blood pressure, alcoholism, and certain cancers. Later chapters discuss many of these links.

The Importance of Prenatal Care

Adequate prenatal care—as described in the following sections—is essential to the health of both mother and baby. All physicians recommend that women start getting regular prenatal checkups as soon as they become pregnant. Typically, this means one checkup per month during the first 8 months, then one checkup per week during the final month. About 84% of pregnant women begin receiving adequate prenatal care during the first trimester; about 3.5% wait until the last trimester or receive no prenatal care at all.

Regular Checkups   In the woman's first visit to her obstetrician, she will be asked for a detailed medical history of herself and her family. The physician or midwife will note any hereditary conditions that may assume increased significance during pregnancy. The tendency to develop gestational diabetes (diabetes during pregnancy only), for example, can be inherited; appropriate treatment during pregnancy reduces the risk of serious harm.

The woman is given a complete physical exam and is informed about appropriate diet. She returns for regular checkups throughout the pregnancy, during which her blood pressure and weight gain are measured, her urine is analyzed, and the size and position of the fetus are monitored.

Blood Tests   A blood sample is taken during the initial prenatal visit to determine blood type and detect possible anemia or Rh incompatibilities. The **Rh factor** is a blood protein. If an Rh-positive father and an Rh-negative mother conceive an Rh-positive baby, the baby's blood will be incompatible with the mother's. This condition is completely treatable with a serum called Rh-immune globulin, which destroys Rh-positive cells as they enter the mother's body and prevents her from forming antibodies to them. Blood may also be tested for evidence of hepatitis B, syphilis, rubella immunity, thyroid problems, and, with the mother's permission, HIV infection.

Prenatal Nutrition   A nutritious diet throughout pregnancy is essential for both the fetus and the mother. Not only does the baby get all its nutrients from the mother, but it also competes with her for nutrients not sufficiently available to meet both their needs. When a woman's diet is low in iron or calcium, the fetus receives most of it, and the mother may become deficient in the mineral. To meet the increased nutritional demands of her body, a pregnant woman shouldn't just eat more; she should make sure that her diet is nutritionally adequate.

Avoiding Drugs and Other Environmental Hazards

In addition to the food the mother eats, the drugs she takes and the chemicals she is exposed to affect the fetus. Everything the mother ingests may eventually reach the fetus in some proportion. Some drugs harm the fetus but not the mother because the fetus is in the process of developing and because the proper dose for the mother is a massive dose for the fetus.

During the first trimester, when the major body structures are rapidly forming, the fetus is extremely vulnerable to environmental factors such as viral infections, radiation, drugs, and other **teratogens,** any of which can cause **congenital malformations,** or birth defects. The most susceptible body parts are those growing most rapidly at the time of exposure. The rubella (German measles) virus, for example, can cause a congenital malformation of a delicate system such as the eyes or ears, leading to blindness or deafness, if exposure occurs during the first trimester, but it does no damage later in the pregnancy. Similarly, the drug thalidomide taken early in pregnancy prevents the formation of arms and legs in fetuses, but taken later, when limbs are already formed, it causes no damage. Other drugs can cause damage throughout prenatal development.

ALCOHOL   Alcohol is a potent teratogen. Getting drunk just one time during pregnancy may be enough to cause brain damage in a fetus. A high level of alcohol consumption during pregnancy is associated with miscarriages, stillbirths, and, in live babies, **fetal alcohol syndrome (FAS).** A baby born with FAS is likely to suffer from a small head and body size, unusual facial characteristics, congenital heart defects, defective joints, impaired vision, mental impairment, and abnormal behavior patterns. Researchers now doubt that any level of alcohol consumption is safe, and they recommend total abstinence during pregnancy.

> **Up to 1.5 in 1000** babies born in the United States have FAS.
>
> —CDC, 2006

TOBACCO   Smoking during pregnancy increases the risk of miscarriage, low birth weight, immune system impairment, and infant death; it may also cause genetic damage or physical deformations. If nicotine levels in a mother's bloodstream are high, fetal breathing rate and movement

Rh factor   A protein found in blood; Rh incompatibility between a mother and fetus can jeopardize the fetus's health.

teratogen   An agent or influence that causes physical defects in a developing fetus.

congenital malformation   A physical defect existing at the time of birth, either inherited or caused during gestation.

fetal alcohol syndrome (FAS)   A combination of birth defects caused by excessive alcohol consumption by the mother during pregnancy.

become more rapid; the fetus may also metabolize cancer-causing by-products of tobacco.

CAFFEINE Caffeine, a powerful stimulant, puts both mother and fetus under stress by raising the level of the hormone epinephrine. Caffeine also reduces the blood supply to the uterus. A pregnant woman should limit her caffeine intake to no more than the equivalent of two cups of coffee per day.

DRUGS Some prescription drugs, such as some blood pressure medications, can harm the fetus, so they should be used only under medical supervision. Many babies born to women who use antidepressants during pregnancy suffer withdrawal symptoms after birth. Recreational drugs, such as cocaine, are thought to increase the risk of major birth defects. Marijuana use may also interfere with fertility treatments, and methamphetamine use is associated with underweight babies.

STDS AND OTHER INFECTIONS Infections, including those that are sexually transmitted, are another serious problem for the fetus. Such infections can pose a threat before, during, and after birth. Rubella, syphilis, gonorrhea, hepatitis B, Group B streptococcus, herpes, and HIV are among the most dangerous infections for the fetus. Treatment of the mother or immunization of the baby just after birth can help prevent problems from many infections. Women at risk for HIV infection should be tested before or during pregnancy because early treatment can dramatically reduce the chance that the virus will be passed to the fetus; some experts advocate universal HIV screening for pregnant women.

Prenatal Activity and Exercise
Physical activity during pregnancy contributes to mental and physical wellness. Women can continue working at their jobs until late in their pregnancy, provided the work isn't so physically demanding that it jeopardizes their health. At the same time, pregnant women need more rest and sleep to maintain their own well-being and that of the fetus.

Regular moderate exercise during pregnancy appears to improve a woman's chance of an on-time delivery and may reduce the risk of pregnancy-related diabetes. A woman who exercised before becoming pregnant can often continue her program, with appropriate modifications to maintain her comfort and safety. A pregnant woman who hasn't been exercising and wants to start should first consult a physician.

The U.S. Department of Health and Human Services recommends 30 minutes of moderate exercise most days, unless physical complications prevent exercise. Regular cardiorespiratory endurance exercise is recommended. Walking, swimming, and stationary cycling are all good choices; more strenuous activities that could result in a fall are best delayed until after the birth.

Kegel exercises, to strengthen the pelvic floor muscles, are recommended for pregnant women. These exercises are performed by alternately contracting and releasing the muscles used to stop the flow of urine. Each contraction should be held for about 5 seconds. Kegel exercises should be done several times a day, for a total of about 50 repetitions daily.

Prenatal exercise classes are valuable because they teach exercises that tone the body muscles involved in birth, especially those of the abdomen, back, and legs.

Preparing for Birth
Childbirth classes are almost a routine part of the prenatal experience for both mothers and fathers these days. These classes typically teach the details of the birth process as well as relaxation techniques to help deal with the discomfort of labor and delivery. The mother learns and practices a variety of techniques so she will be able to choose what works best for her during labor when the time comes. The father typically acts as a coach, supporting his partner emotionally and helping her with her breathing and relaxing. He remains with her throughout labor and delivery, even when a cesarean section is performed.

Complications of Pregnancy and Pregnancy Loss

About 31% of mothers-to-be suffer complications during pregnancy. Some complications may prevent full-term development of the fetus or affect the health of the infant at birth. As discussed earlier in the chapter, exposure to harmful substances, such as alcohol or drugs, can harm the fetus. Other complications are caused by physiological problems or genetic abnormalities.

Ectopic Pregnancy
In an **ectopic pregnancy,** the fertilized egg implants and begins to develop outside of the uterus, usually in an oviduct (Figure 5.6).

Ectopic pregnancies usually occur because the fallopian tube is blocked, most often as a result of pelvic inflammatory disease; smoking also increases a woman's risk for ectopic pregnancy. The embryo may spontaneously abort, or the embryo and placenta may continue to expand until they rupture the oviduct. Sharp pain on one side of the abdomen or in the lower back, usually in about the 7th or 8th week, may signal an ectopic pregnancy, and there may be irregular bleeding.

An ectopic pregnancy is a medical emergency. Surgical removal of the embryo and the oviduct may be necessary to save the mother's life, although microsurgery can sometimes be used to repair the damaged oviduct. If diagnosed early, before the oviduct ruptures, ectopic pregnancy can often be successfully treated without surgery.

Spontaneous Abortion
A spontaneous abortion, or miscarriage, is the termination of pregnancy before the 20th week. About 15–20% of all clinically diagnosed pregnancies end in miscarriage, and many women have miscarriages without knowing they were pregnant. About

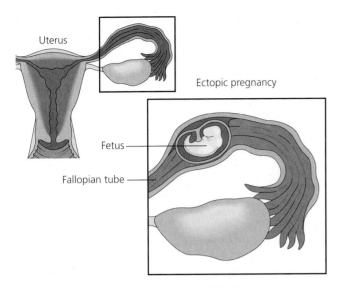

Uterus

Ectopic pregnancy

Fetus

Fallopian tube

FIGURE 5.6. Ectopic pregnancy in a fallopian tube.

30% of miscarriages occur before the 12th week of pregnancy. Most—about 60%—are due to chromosomal abnormalities in the fetus. Certain occupations that involve exposure to chemicals may increase the likelihood of a spontaneous abortion.

Stillbirth   The terms *fetal death, fetal demise, stillbirth,* and *stillborn* all refer to the delivery of a fetus that shows no signs of life. Risk factors for stillbirth include smoking, advanced maternal age, obesity, multiple gestations, and chronic disease. Risk for stillbirth is also correlated with race; black women have twice as many stillbirths as white women.

Preeclampsia   A disease unique to human pregnancy, **preeclampsia** is characterized by elevated blood pressure and the appearance of protein in the urine. Symptoms include headache, right upper-quadrant abdominal pain, vision changes (referred to as *scotomata*), and notable increased swelling and weight gain. If preeclampsia is untreated, patients can develop seizures, a condition called **eclampsia.** Other potential complications of preeclampsia are liver and kidney damage, bleeding, fetal growth restriction, and even fetal death.

Women with mild preeclampsia may be monitored closely as outpatients and placed on home bed rest. More severe cases may require hospitalization for close medical management and early delivery.

Placenta Previa   In **placenta previa,** the placenta either completely or partially covers the cervical opening, preventing the mother from delivering the baby vaginally. As a result, the baby must be delivered by cesarean section. Risk factors include prior cesarean delivery, multiple pregnancies, intrauterine surgery, smoking, multiple gestations, and advanced maternal age.

Placental Abruption   In **placental abruption,** a normally implanted placenta prematurely separates from the

uterine wall. Patients experience abdominal pain, vaginal bleeding, and uterine tenderness. The condition increases the risk of fetal death. The risk factors for developing a placental abruption are maternal age, tobacco smoking, cocaine use, multiple gestation, trauma, preeclampsia, hypertension, and preterm premature rupture of membranes.

Gestational Diabetes   During gestation, about 4% of all pregnant women develop **gestational diabetes (GDM)**, in which the body loses its ability to use insulin properly. In these women, diabetes occurs only during pregnancy. Women diagnosed with GDM have an increased risk of developing type 2 diabetes later in life. It is important to accurately diagnose and treat GDM as it can lead to preeclampsia, polyhydramnios (increased levels of amniotic fluid), large fetuses, birth trauma, operative deliveries, perinatal mortality, and neonatal metabolic complications.

Preterm Labor   When a pregnant woman goes into labor before the 37th week of gestation, she is said to undergo *preterm labor.* About 30–50% of preterm labors resolve themselves, with the pregnancy continuing to full term. In other cases, interventions may be required to delay labor and allow gestation to continue.

Labor Induction   If pregnancy continues well beyond the baby's due date, it may be necessary to induce labor artificially. This is one of the most common obstetrical procedures and is typically offered to pregnant women who have not delivered and are 7–14 days past their due date. Labor can be artificially induced in several ways.

Low Birth Weight and Premature Birth   A low-birth-weight (LBW) baby is one that weighs less than 5.5 pounds at birth. LBW babies may be **premature** (born before the 37th week of pregnancy) or full-term. Babies

ectopic pregnancy   A pregnancy in which the embryo develops outside of the uterus, usually in the fallopian tube.

preeclampsia   A condition of pregnancy characterized by high blood pressure and protein in the urine.

eclampsia   A severe, potentially life-threatening form of preeclampsia, characterized by seizures.

placenta previa   A complication of pregnancy in which the placenta covers the cervical opening, preventing the mother from delivering the baby vaginally.

placental abruption   A complication of pregnancy in which a normally implanted placenta prematurely separates from the uterine wall.

gestational diabetes (GDM)   A form of diabetes that occurs during pregnancy.

low birth weight (LBW)   Weighing less than 5.5 pounds at birth, often the result of prematurity.

premature   Born before the 37th week of pregnancy.

who are born small even though they're full-term are referred to as *small-for-date* or *small-for-gestational-age* babies. About half of all cases are related to teenage pregnancy, cigarette smoking, poor nutrition, and poor maternal health. Other maternal factors include drug use, stress, depression, and anxiety. Adequate prenatal care is the best way to prevent LBW.

Full-term LBW babies tend to have fewer problems than premature infants. Many of the premature infant's organs are not sufficiently developed. Even mild prematurity increases an infant's risk of dying in the first month or year of life. Premature infants are subject to respiratory problems, infections, and eating difficulties. As they get older, premature infants may have learning difficulties, behavior problems, and physical problems.

Infant Mortality The U.S. rate of **infant mortality,** the death of a child of less than 1 year of age, is near its lowest point ever; however, it remains far higher than that of most of the developed world. Poverty and inadequate health care are key causes.

Other causes of infant death are congenital problems, infectious diseases, and injuries. In **sudden infant death syndrome (SIDS),** an apparently healthy infant dies suddenly while sleeping. About 2250 infant deaths are attributed to SIDS each year. Research suggests that abnormalities in the brainstem, the part of the brain that regulates breathing, heart rate, and other basic functions, underline the risk for SIDS. Risk is greatly increased for infants with these innate differences if they are exposed to environmental risks, such as sleeping face down; being exposed to tobacco smoke, alcohol, or other drugs; or sleeping on a soft mattress or with fluffy bedding, pillows, or stuffed toys. Overbundling a baby or keeping a baby's room too warm also increases the risk of SIDS; because of this, SIDS deaths are more common in the colder months. Several studies have found that the use of a pacifier significantly reduces the risk of SIDS.

CHILDBIRTH

By the end of the 9th month of pregnancy, most women are tired of being pregnant; both parents are eager to start a new phase of their lives. Most couples find the actual process of birth to be an exciting and positive experience.

Choices in Childbirth

Many couples today can choose the type of practitioner and the environment they want for the birth of their child. A high-risk pregnancy is probably best handled by a specialist physician in a hospital with a nursery, but for low-risk births, many options are available.

Parents can choose to have their baby delivered by a physician or by a certified nurse-midwife. In the United States, most babies are delivered in hospitals or freestanding birth centers; in 2006, more than 25,000 babies were delivered at home. Many hospitals have introduced birth centers in response to criticism of traditional hospital routines. These centers provide a comfortable, emotionally supportive environment that is close to up-to-date medical equipment. It is important for prospective parents to discuss all aspects of labor and delivery with their physician or midwife beforehand, so they can learn what to expect and state their preferences.

Labor and Delivery

The birth process occurs in three stages (Figure 5.7, p. 117). **Labor** begins when hormonal changes in both the mother and the baby cause strong, rhythmic uterine **contractions** to begin. These contractions exert pressure on the cervix and cause the lengthwise muscles of the uterus to pull on the circular muscles around the cervix, causing effacement (thinning) and dilation (opening) of the cervix. The contractions also pressure the baby to descend into the mother's pelvis, if it hasn't already. The entire process of labor and delivery usually takes between 2 and 36 hours, depending on the size of the baby, the baby's position in the uterus, the size of the mother's pelvis, the strength of the uterine contractions, the number of prior deliveries, and other factors. The length of labor is generally shorter for second and subsequent births.

The First Stage of Labor The first stage of labor averages 13 hours for a first birth, although there is a wide variation among women. It begins with cervical effacement and dilation and continues until the cervix is completely dilated (10 centimeters). Contractions usually last about 30 seconds and occur every 15–20 minutes at first, more often later. The prepared mother relaxes as much as possible during these contractions to allow labor to proceed without being blocked by tension. Early in the first stage, a small amount of bleeding may occur as a plug of slightly bloody mucus that blocked the opening of the

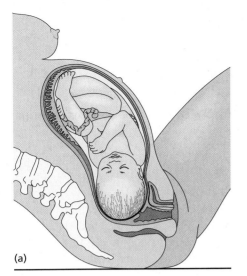

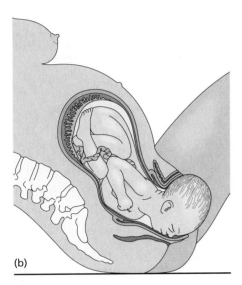

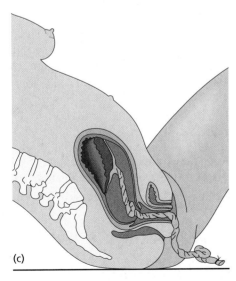

(a)

(b)

(c)

FIGURE 5.7 Birth: labor and delivery. (a) The first stage of labor; (b) the second stage of labor: delivery of the baby; (c) the third stage of labor: expulsion of the placenta.

cervix during pregnancy is expelled. In some women, the amniotic sac ruptures and the fluid rushes out; this is sometimes referred to as the "water breaking."

The last part of the first stage of labor, called **transition,** is characterized by strong and frequent contractions, much more intense than in the early stages of labor. Contractions may last 60–90 seconds and occur every 1–3 minutes. During transition the cervix opens completely, to a diameter of about 10 centimeters. The head of the fetus usually measures 9–10 centimeters; thus once the cervix has dilated completely, the head can pass through. Many women report that transition, which normally lasts about 30–60 minutes, is the most difficult part of labor.

The Second Stage of Labor   The second stage of labor begins with complete cervical dilation and ends with the delivery of the baby. The baby is slowly pushed down, through the bones of the pelvic ring, past the cervix, and into the vagina, which it stretches open. The mother bears down with the contractions to help push the baby down and out. The baby's back bends, the head turns to fit through the narrowest parts of the passageway, and the soft bones of the baby's skull move together and overlap as it is squeezed through the pelvis. When the top of the head appears at the vaginal opening, the baby is said to be crowning.

As the head of the baby emerges, the physician or midwife will remove any mucus from the mouth and nose, wipe the baby's face, and check to ensure that the umbilical cord is not around the neck. With a few more contractions, the baby's shoulders and body emerge. As the baby is squeezed through the pelvis, cervix, and vagina, the fluid in the lungs is forced out by the pressure on the baby's chest. Once this pressure is released as the baby emerges from the vagina, the chest expands and the lungs fill with air for the first time. The baby will still be connected to the mother via the umbilical cord, which is not cut until it stops pulsating. The baby will appear wet and often is covered with a cheesy substance. The baby's head may be oddly shaped at first, due to the molding of the soft plates of bone during birth, but it usually takes on a more rounded appearance within 24 hours.

TERMS

infant mortality   The death of a child less than 1 year of age.

sudden infant death syndrome (SIDS)   The sudden death of an apparently healthy infant during sleep.

labor   The act or process of giving birth to a child, expelling it with the placenta from the mother's body by means of uterine contractions.

contraction   Shortening of the muscles in the uterine wall, which causes effacement and dilation of the cervix and assists in expelling the fetus.

transition   The last part of the first stage of labor, during which the cervix becomes fully dilated; characterized by intense and frequent contractions.

The Third Stage of Labor In the third stage of labor, the uterus continues to contract until the placenta is expelled. This stage usually takes 5–30 minutes. It is important that the entire placenta be expelled; if part remains in the uterus, it may cause infection or bleeding. Breastfeeding soon after delivery helps control uterine bleeding because it stimulates the secretion of a hormone that makes the uterus contract.

The baby's physical condition is assessed with the **Apgar score,** a formalized system for assessing the baby's need for medical assistance. Heart rate, respiration, color, reflexes, and muscle tone are individually rated with a score of 0–2, and a total score between 0 and 10 is given at 1 and 5 minutes after birth. A score of 7–10 at 5 minutes is considered normal. Most newborns are also tested for 29 specific disorders, some of which are life-threatening. The American Academy of Pediatrics endorses these tests, but they are not routinely performed in every state.

Pain Relief During Labor and Delivery Women vary in how much pain they experience in childbirth. It is recommended that women and their partners learn about labor and what kinds of choices are available for pain relief. Childbirth preparation courses are a good place to start, and communicating with one's obstetrician or midwife is essential to assess the approaches that will be available. Breathing and relaxation techniques such as Lamaze or Bradley have been used effectively.

The most commonly employed medical intervention for pain relief is the epidural. This procedure involves placing a thin plastic catheter between the vertebrae in the lower back. Medication that reduces the transmission of pain signals to the brain is given through this catheter. Local anesthetic drugs are given in low concentration in order to minimize weakening of the leg muscles so that the mother can effectively push during the birth. The amount of medication given is quite low and does not accumulate in the baby or interfere with the baby's transition after birth. The mother is awake and is an active participant in the birth.

Women can also elect to have narcotics, such as fentanyl or demerol, given for pain relief during labor, but these medications usually provide less pain relief than the epidural and, if given shortly before the birth, can cause the baby to be less vigorous at birth.

Cesarean Deliveries In a **cesarean section,** the baby is removed through a surgical incision in the abdominal wall and uterus. Cesarean sections are necessary when a baby cannot be delivered vaginally—for example, if the baby's head is bigger than the mother's pelvic girdle or if the baby is in an unusual position. If the mother has a serious health condition such as high blood pressure, a cesarean may be safer for her than labor and a vaginal delivery. Cesareans are more common among women who are overweight or have diabetes. Other reasons for cesarean delivery include abnormal or difficult labor, fetal distress, and the presence of a dangerous infection like herpes that can be passed to the baby during delivery.

Repeat cesarean deliveries are also very common. About 90% of American women who have had one child by cesarean have subsequent children delivered the same way. Although the risk of complications from a vaginal delivery after a previous cesarean delivery is low, there is a small (1%) risk of serious complication to the mother and baby if the previous uterine scar opens during labor (uterine rupture). For this reason, women and their doctors may choose to deliver by elective repeat caesarean.

Like any major surgery, cesarean section carries some risk and should be performed only for valid medical reasons (not convenience). Women who have cesarean sections can remain conscious during the operation if they are given a regional anesthetic, and the father may be present.

The Postpartum Period

The **postpartum period,** a stage of about 3 months following childbirth, is a time of critical family adjustments. Parenthood begins literally overnight, and the transition can cause considerable stress.

Breastfeeding Currently, about 74% of mothers breastfeed their infants for a short time after delivery, up from about 10% in 1970. **Lactation,** the production of milk, begins about 3 days after childbirth. Prior to that time (sometimes as early as the second trimester), **colostrum** is secreted by the nipples. Colostrum contains antibodies that help protect the newborn from infectious diseases and is also high in protein.

Apgar score A formalized system for assessing a newborn's need for medical assistance.

cesarean section A surgical incision through the abdominal wall and uterus, performed to deliver a fetus.

postpartum period The period of about 3 months after delivering a baby.

lactation The production of milk.

colostrum A yellowish fluid secreted by the mammary glands around the time of childbirth until milk comes in, about the third day.

postpartum depression An emotional low that may be experienced by the mother following childbirth.

The American Academy of Pediatrics recommends breastfeeding exclusively for 6 months, then in combination with solid food until the baby is 1 year of age, and then for as long after that as a mother and baby desire. Currently, only 11% of U.S. mothers breast-feed exclusively for 6 months. Human milk is perfectly suited to the baby's nutritional needs and digestive capabilities, and it supplies the baby with antibodies. Breastfeeding decreases the incidence of infant ear infections, allergies, anemia, diarrhea, and bacterial meningitis. Preschoolers who were breastfed as babies are less likely to be overweight, and school-age children who were breastfed are less anxious and better able to cope with stress. Breastfeeding even has a beneficial effect on blood pressure and cholesterol levels later in life.

Breastfeeding is also beneficial to the mother. It contributes to postpregnancy weight loss and may reduce the risk of ovarian cancer, breast cancer, and postmenopausal hip fracture. For women who want to breast-feed but who have problems, help is available from support groups, books, or a lactation consultant.

However, bottlefeeding can also provide adequate nutrition, and both breastfeeding and bottlefeeding can be part of loving, secure parent-child relationships.

When a mother doesn't nurse, menstruation usually begins within about 10 weeks. However, ovulation—and pregnancy—can occur before menstruation returns, so breastfeeding is not a reliable contraceptive method.

Postpartum Depression   Many women experience fluctuating emotions during the postpartum period as hormone levels change. About 50–80% of new mothers experience "baby blues," characterized by episodes of sadness, weeping, anxiety, headache, sleep disturbances, and irritability. About 5–9% of new mothers experience **postpartum depression**, a more disabling syndrome characterized by despondency, mood swings, guilt, and occasional hostility. Rest, sharing feelings and concerns with others, and relying on supportive relatives and friends for assistance are usually helpful in dealing with mild cases of the baby blues or postpartum depression, which generally lasts only a few weeks. If the depression is serious, professional treatment may be needed.

Attachment   Another feature of the postpartum period is the development of attachment—the strong emotional tie that grows between the baby and the adult who cares for the baby. Parents can foster secure attachment relationships in the early weeks and months by responding sensitively to the baby's true needs. A secure attachment relationship helps the child develop and function well socially, emotionally, and mentally.

For most people, the arrival of a child provides a deep sense of joy and accomplishment. However, adjusting to parenthood requires effort and energy. Talking with friends and relatives about their experiences during the first few weeks or months with a baby can help prepare new parents for the period when the baby's needs may require all the energy that both parents have to expend. But the pleasures of nurturing a new baby are substantial, and many parents look back on this time as one of the most significant and joyful of their lives.

QUESTIONS FOR CRITICAL THINKING AND REFLECTION

If you are a woman, what are your views on labor and delivery options? If you have a child in the future, which facility, delivery, and pain management options do you think you would prefer? If you are a man, what are your views on participating in delivery? What role would you want to play?

TIPS FOR TODAY AND THE FUTURE

Wellness includes understanding your own sexuality and all its components. Preparation for being a parent begins long before pregnancy; it requires prospective parents to make responsible choices.

RIGHT NOW YOU CAN

- Deal with a sexual question or problem you may be avoiding. Unless you're sure it isn't a physical problem, see your physician.
- If you're in a sexual relationship, consider the information you and your partner have shared. Determine whether you know enough about one another to have a safe and healthy sexual relationship.
- Take time to think about whether you really want to have children. Cut through everyone else's expectations, which may stand in the way of making the decision that's best for you.
- Think of things your parents did that you liked when you were a child. Consider how you can do the same thing for your children.

IN THE FUTURE YOU CAN

- If you're in a sexual relationship or plan to begin one, open a dialog with your partner about sex. Make time to talk at length about the responsibilities and consequences of such a relationship.
- Make behavioral changes that can improve your prospects as a parent. For example, you may need to adopt healthier eating habits or start exercising more often.
- If you want to be a parent someday, start looking at the many sources of information on pregnancy, childbirth, and parenting. This is a good idea for anyone—man or woman—who plans to have a family.

SUMMARY

• The female external sex organs are called the vulva; the clitoris plays an important role in sexual arousal and orgasm. The vagina leads to the internal sex organs, including the uterus, oviducts, and ovaries.

• The male external sex organs are the penis and the scrotum; the glans of the penis is an important site of sexual arousal. Internal sexual structures include the testes, vas deferentia, seminal vesicles, and prostate gland.

• The menstrual cycle consists of four phases: menses, the estrogenic phase, ovulation, and the progestational phase.

• The ovaries gradually cease to function as women approach age 50 and enter menopause. The pattern of male sexual responses changes with age, and testosterone production gradually decreases.

• The sexual response cycle has four states: excitement, plateau, orgasm, and resolution.

• Physical and psychological problems can both interfere with sexual functioning. Treatment for sexual dysfunction should first address underlying medical conditions and then look at psychological problems.

• Human sexual behaviors include celibacy, erotic fantasy, masturbation, touching, cunnilingus, fellatio, anal intercourse, and vaginal intercourse.

• Responsible sexuality includes open communication, agreed-on sexual activities, sexual privacy, the use of contraception, safer sex practices, sober sex, and taking responsibility for consequences.

• Fertilization is a complex process culminating when a sperm penetrates the membrane of an egg released from the woman's ovary. Infertility affects about 10% of the reproductive-age population of the United States.

• During pregnancy, the uterus enlarges until it pushes up into the rib cage, the breasts enlarge, muscles and ligaments soften and stretch, and other body functions become more efficient.

• The fetal anatomy is almost completely formed in the first trimester of pregnancy, and is refined in the second; during the third trimester, the fetus grows and gains most of its weight.

• Prenatal tests include ultrasound, amniocentesis, chorionic villus sampling, and quadruple marker screening.

• Important elements of prenatal care include regular check-ups, good nutrition, avoiding drugs and other harmful environmental agents, and taking childbirth classes.

• Pregnancy usually proceeds without major complications. Problems that can occur include ectopic pregnancy, spontaneous abortion, and low birth weight.

• The first stage of labor begins with contractions that exert pressure on the cervix, causing effacement and dilation. The second stage begins with complete cervical dilation and ends when the baby emerges. The third stage of labor is expulsion of the placenta.

• During the postpartum period, the mother's body begins to return to its prepregnancy state and she may begin to breastfeed. Both mother and father must adjust to their new role as parents.

FOR MORE INFORMATION

BOOKS

Kelly, G.F. 2007. *Sexuality Today*, 9th ed. New York: McGraw-Hill. *An accessible approach that highlights cross-cultural examples, popular topics and issues, and case studies featuring college-age individuals.*

Lees, C., et al. 2007. *Pregnancy and Birth: Your Questions Answered.* London: Dorling Kindersley. *Answers hundreds of common questions about conception, pregnancy, and delivery.*

Omoto, A.M., and H.S. Kurtzman, eds. 2006. *Sexual Orientation and Mental Health: Examining Identity and Development in Lesbian, Gay, and Bisexual People.* Washington, D.C.: American Psychological Association. *Covers topics in mental health as well as sexual behavior, work satisfaction, and the well-being of children of same-sex couples.*

Wynbrandt, J. 2007. *Encyclopedia of Genetic Disorders and Birth Defects.* New York: Facts on File. *A detailed overview of many types of birth defects, both inherited and noninherited.*

Yarber, W., et al. 2010. *Human Sexuality: Diversity in Contemporary America,* 7th ed. New York: McGraw-Hill. *A comprehensive introduction to human sexuality.*

ORGANIZATIONS AND WEB SITES

American Association of Sex Educators, Counselors, and Therapists (AASECT). Certifies sex educators, counselors, and therapists and provides listings of local therapists dealing with sexual problems.
　　http://www.aasect.org

American College of Obstetricians and Gynecologists (ACOG). Provides written materials relating to many aspects of preconception care, pregnancy, and childbirth.
　　http://www.acog.org

American Society for Reproductive Medicine. Provides up-to-date information on all aspects of infertility.
　　http://www.asrm.org

Center for Young Women's Health. Includes information about topics such as menstruation, gynecological exames, eating disorders, body piercing, and sexual health.
　　http://www.youngwomenshealth.org

Centers for Disease Control and Prevention, National Center on Birth Defects and Developmental Disabilities. Provides information about a variety of topics related to birth defects, including fetal alcohol syndrome and the importance of folic acid.
　　http://www.cdc.gov/ncbddd

Health Resources and Services Administration (HRSA): Maternal and Child Health. Provides publications, videos, and other resources relating to maternal, infant, and family health.
　　http://www.ask.hrsa.gov/mch.cfm

International Council on Infertility Information Dissemination. Provides information on current research and treatments for infertility.

http://www.inciid.org

Kinsey Institute for Research in Sex, Gender, and Reproduction. One of the oldest and most respected institutions doing research on sexuality.

http://www.kinseyinstitute.org

The March of Dimes. Provides public education materials on many pregnancy-related topics, including birth defects.

http://www.marchofdimes.com

SELECTED BIBLIOGRAPHY

American Academy of Pediatrics Section on Breastfeeding. 2005. Breastfeeding and the use of human milk. *Pediatrics* 115 (2): 496–506.

American Academy of Pediatrics Task Force on Sudden Infant Death Syndrome. 2005. The Changing Concept of Sudden Infant Death Syndrome. *Pediatrics* 116 (5): 1245–1255.

American College Health Association. August 2007 Update. *American College Health Association-National College Health Assessment (ACHA-NCHA) Web Summary* (http://www.acha-ncha.org/data_highlights.html; retrieved January 29, 2009).

American Psychological Association. 2008. *Answers to Your Questions About Sexual Orientation and Homosexuality* (http://www.apa.org/topics/orientation.html; retrieved January 29, 2009).

Centers for Disease Control and Prevention. 2004. Teenagers in the United States: Sexual activity, contraceptive use, and childbearing, 2002. *Vital and Health Statistics* 23 (24).

Centers for Disease Control and Prevention. 2005. Percentage of never-married teens aged 15–19 years who reported ever having sexual intercourse, by sex and age group-United States, 1995 and 2002. *Morbidity and Mortality Weekly Report* 54 (30): 751.

Centers for Disease Control and Prevention. 2006. *Preconception Health and Care, 2006* (http://www.cdc.gov/ncbddd/preconception/documents/at-a-glance-4-11-06.pdf; retrieved January 29, 2009).

Centers for Disease Control and Prevention. 2007. Breastfeeding trends and updated national health objectives for exclusive breastfeeding-United States, birth years 2000–2004. *Morbidity and Mortality Weekly Report* 56 (30): 760–763.

Centers for Disease Control and Prevention. 2009. *2006 Assisted Reproductive Technology (ART) Success Rates: National Summary and Fertility Clinic Reports.* Atlanta: Centers for Disease Control and Prevention.

De Sutter, P. 2006. Rational diagnosis and treatment of infertility. *Best Practice & Research: Clinical Obstetrics & Gynaecology,* 9 June [epub].

Gades, N.M., et al. 2005. Association between smoking and erectile dysfunction: A population-based study. *American Journal of Epidemiology* 161 (4): 346–351.

Laumann, E.O., et al. 2005. Sexual problems among women and men aged 40–80 y: Prevalence and correlates identified in the Global Study of Sexual Attitudes and Behaviors. *International Journal of Impotence Research* 17 (1): 39–57.

Lee, J.M., et al. 2007. Weight status in young girls and the onset of puberty. *Pediatrics* 119 (3): 624–630.

Lindau, S.T., et al. 2007. A study of sexuality and health among older adults in the United States. *New England Journal of Medicine* 357 (8): 762–774.

National Center for Health Statistics. 2006. Fertility, contraception, and fatherhood: Data on men and women from Cycle 6 (2002) of the National Survey of Family Growth. Vital *Health Statistics* 23 (26).

National Center for Health Statistics. 2009. Births: Final data for 2006. *National Vital Statistics Report* 57 (7): 1–102.

National Center for Health Statistics. 2009. Births: Final data for 2006. *National Vital Statistics Reports* 57(7): 1–102.

National Institutes of Health. 2006. *NICHD Alerts Parents to Winter SIDS Risk and Updated AAP Recommendations* (http://www.nig.gov/news/pr/jan2006nichd-18.htm; retrieved August 5, 2006).

National Institutes of Health. 2007. *Decrease in Breast Cancer Rates Related to Reduction in Use of Hormone Replacement Therapy* (http://www.nih.gov/news/pr/apr2007/nci-18a.htm; retrieved January 27, 2009).

Pattenden, S., et al. 2006. Parental smoking and children's respiratory health: Independent effects of prenatal and postnatal exposure. *Tobacco Control* 15(4): 294–301.

Rossouw, J. E., et al. 2007. Postmenopausal hormone therapy and risk of cardiovascular disease by age and years since menopause. *Journal of the American Medical Association* 297(13): 1465–1477.

Scollan-Koliopoulos, M., et al. 2006. Gestational diabetes management: Guidelines to a healthy pregnancy. *Nurse Practitioner* 31(6): 14–23.

Stoll, B. J., et al. 2004. Neurodevelopmental and growth impairment among extremely low-birth-weight infants with neonatal infection. *Journal of the American Medical Association* 292(19): 2357–2365.

U.S. Department of Health and Human Services. 2007. *Aging Male Syndrome* (http://womenshealth.gov/mens/sexual/ams.cfm; retrieved January 27, 2009).

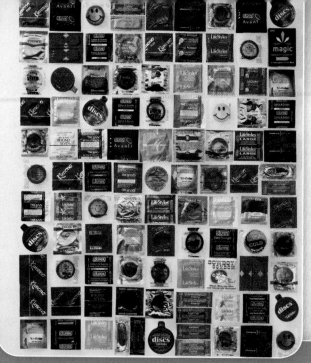

LOOKING AHEAD>>>>>

AFTER READING THIS CHAPTER, YOU SHOULD BE ABLE TO:

- Explain how contraceptives work and how to interpret information about a contraceptive method's effectiveness, risks, and benefits

- List the most popular contraceptives and discuss their advantages, disadvantages, and effectiveness

- Choose a method of contraception based on the needs of the user and the safety and effectiveness of the method

- Describe the history and current legal status of abortion in the United States

- Describe the methods of aboriton available in the United States

CONTRACEPTION AND ABORTION

6

People have always had a compelling interest in managing fertility and preventing unwanted pregnancies, a practice commonly known as **birth control.** Records dating to the fourth century B.C. describe the use of foods, herbs, drugs, douches, and sponges to prevent **conception,** which is the fusion of an ovum and sperm that creates a fertilized egg. Early attempts at **contraception** (blocking conception through the use of a device, substance, or method) were based on the same principle as many modern birth control methods.

Today, women and men can choose from many different types of **contraceptives** to avoid unwanted pregnancies. In addition to preventing pregnancy, many types of contraception play an important role in protecting against **sexually transmitted diseases (STDs).** Being informed about the realities and risks and making responsible decisions about sexual and contraceptive behavior are crucial components of lifelong wellness. Because many people's lives are severely affected by unplanned child rearing and because the option of abortion is becoming more re-

stricted, the problem of unplanned, unwanted pregnancies is serious.

PRINCIPLES OF CONTRACEPTION

There are many effective approaches to contraception, including the following:

- **Barrier methods** work by physically blocking the sperm from reaching the egg. Diaphragms, condoms, and several other methods are based on this principle.

- **Hormonal methods,** such as oral contraceptives (birth control pills), alter the biochemistry of the woman's body, preventing ovulation (the release of the egg) and producing changes that make it more difficult for the sperm to reach the egg if ovulation does occur.

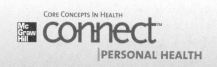

- **Natural methods** of contraception are based on the fact that egg and sperm have to be present at the same time if fertilization is to occur.
- **Surgical methods**—female and male sterilization—more or less permanently prevent transport of the sperm or eggs to the site of conception.

All contraceptive methods have advantages and disadvantages that make them appropriate for some people but not for others or the best choice at one period of life but not at another. Factors that affect the choice of method include effectiveness, convenience, cost, reversibility, side effects and risks, and protection against STDs. Later in this chapter, we help you sort through these factors to decide on the method that's best for you.

Contraceptive effectiveness is partly determined by the reliability of the method itself—the failure rate if it were always used exactly as directed ("perfect use"). Effectiveness is also determined by characteristics of the user, including fertility of the individual, frequency of intercourse, and how consistently and correctly the method is used. This "typical use" **contraceptive failure rate** is based on studies that directly measure the percentage of women experiencing an unintended pregnancy in the first year of contraceptive use. For example, the 8% failure rate of oral contraceptives means 8 out of 100 typical users will become pregnant in the first year. This failure rate is likely to be lower for women who are consistently careful in following instructions and higher for those who are frequently careless; the "perfect use" failure rate is 0.3%.

Another measure of effectiveness is the **continuation rate**—the percentage of people who continue to use the method after a specified period of time. This measure is important because many unintended pregnancies occur when a method is stopped and not immediately replaced with another. Thus, a contraceptive with a high continuation rate would be more effective at preventing pregnancy than one with a low continuation rate.

REVERSIBLE CONTRACEPTION

Reversibility is an extremely important consideration for young adults when they choose a contraceptive method, because most people either plan to have children or at least want to keep their options open until they're older.

QUESTIONS FOR CRITICAL THINKING AND REFLECTION

Prior to reading this section, how familiar were you with the principles of contraception? Did you know as much as you thought? Does this kind of information make you feel as though you should be more or less directly responsible for the contraceptive choices in your life?

Oral Contraceptives: The Pill

About a century ago, a researcher noted that ovulation does not occur during pregnancy. Further research revealed the hormonal mechanism: During pregnancy, the corpus luteum secretes progesterone and estrogen in amounts high enough to suppress ovulation. **Oral contraceptives (OCs),** or *birth control pills,* prevent ovulation by mimicking the hormonal activity of the corpus luteum. The active ingredients in OCs are estrogen and progestins, laboratory-made compounds that are closely related to progesterone.

In addition to preventing ovulation, the birth control pill has other backup contraceptive effects. It inhibits the movement of sperm by thickening the cervical mucus,

birth control   The practice of managing fertility and preventing unwanted pregnancies.

conception   The fusion of ovum and sperm, resulting in a fertilized egg, or *zygote.*

contraception   The prevention of conception through the use of a device, substance, or method.

contraceptive   Any agent or method that can prevent conception.

sexually transmitted disease (STD)   Any of several contagious diseases contracted through intimate sexual contact.

barrier method   A contraceptive that acts as a physical barrier, blocking the sperm from uniting with the egg.

hormonal method   A contraceptive that alters the biochemistry of a woman's body, preventing ovulation and making it more difficult for sperm to reach an egg if ovulation does occur.

natural method   An approach to contraception that does not use drugs or devices; requires avoiding intercourse during the period of the woman's menstrual cycle when an egg is likely to be present at the site of conception and the risk of pregnancy is greatest.

surgical method   Sterilization of a male or female, to permanently prevent the transport of sperm or eggs to the site of conception.

contraceptive failure rate   The percentage of women using a particular contraceptive method who experience an unintended pregnancy in the first year of use.

continuation rate   The percentage of people who continue to use a particular contraceptive after a specified period of time.

oral contraceptive (OC)   Any of various hormone compounds (estrogen and progestins) in pill form that prevent conception by preventing ovulation.

TERMS

alters the rate of ovum transport by means of its hormonal effects on the oviducts, and may prevent implantation by changing the lining of the uterus, in the unlikely event that a fertilized ovum reaches that area.

The most common type of OC is the *combination pill*. Each 1-month packet contains a 3-week supply of pills that combine varying types and amounts of estrogen and progestin. Most packets also include a 1-week supply of inactive pills to be taken following the hormone pills; others simply instruct the woman to take no pills at all for 1 week before starting the next cycle. During the week in which no hormones are taken, a light menstrual period occurs.

Newer use schedules include a variety of extended-cycle regimens. With the pills Seasonale and Seasonique, for example, a woman takes active pills for 84 consecutive days, then inactive pills for a week; this pattern reduces the number of menstrual periods from 13 per year to just 4 per year. With the pill Lybrel, active pills are taken indefinitely. This and other new OCs are specifically packaged for extended use. Other OCs with hormones similar to the prepackaged brands may be used in the same way. When taken without a break, Lybrel can stop a woman's monthly periods. Changing the menstrual cycle has not been linked with any major health risks, but more long-range research is needed.

Another, much less common, type of OC is the *minipill*, a small dose of a synthetic progesterone taken every day of the month. Because the minipill contains no estrogen, it has fewer side effects and health risks, but it is associated with more irregular bleeding patterns.

A woman is usually advised to start the first cycle of pills with a menstrual period to increase effectiveness and eliminate the possibility of unsuspected pregnancy. She must take each month's pills completely and according to instructions. Taking a few pills just prior to having sexual intercourse will not provide effective contraception. A backup method is recommended during the first week and any subsequent cycle in which the woman forgets to take any pills.

OC use was once linked to possible increased risks of heart attack and stroke. However, these risks have been substantially reduced by the use of lower-dosage pills (those with 50 micrograms or less of estrogen) and the identification of women at higher risk for complications.

Advantages   Oral contraceptives are very effective in preventing pregnancy. Nearly all unplanned pregnancies result because the pills were not taken as directed. The pill is relatively simple to use and does not hinder sexual spontaneity. Most women also enjoy the predictable regularity of periods, as well as the decrease in cramps and blood loss. For young women, the reversibility of the pill is especially important; **fertility**—the ability to reproduce—returns after the pill is discontinued (although not always immediately).

Medical advantages include a decreased incidence of benign breast disease, iron-deficiency anemia, pelvic inflammatory disease (PID), ectopic pregnancy, colon and rectal cancer, endometrial cancer (in the lining of the uterus), and ovarian cancer.

Disadvantages   Although oral contraceptives lower the risk of PID, they do not protect against HIV infection or other STDs in the lower reproductive tract. OCs have been associated with increased cervical chlamydia. Regular condom use is recommended for an OC user, unless she is in a long-term, mutually monogamous relationship with an uninfected partner.

The hormones in birth control pills influence all tissues of the body and can lead to a variety of disturbances. Symptoms of early pregnancy—morning nausea and swollen breasts, for example—may appear during the first few months of OC use. They usually disappear by the fourth cycle. Other side effects include depression, nervousness, changes in sex drive, dizziness, generalized headaches, migraine, bleeding between periods, and changes in the lining of the walls of the vagina, with an increase in clear or white vaginal discharge.

Serious side effects have been reported in a small number of women. These include blood clots, stroke, and heart attack, concentrated mostly in older women who smoke or have a history of circulatory disease. Recent studies have shown no increased risk of stroke or heart attack for healthy, young, nonsmoking women on lower-dosage pills. OC use is associated with little, if any, increase in breast cancer.

Birth control pills are not recommended for women with a history of blood clots (or a close family member with unexplained blood clots at an early age), heart disease or stroke, migraines with changes in vision, any form of cancer or liver tumor, or impaired liver function. Women with certain other health conditions or behaviors, including migraines without changes in vision, high blood pressure, cigarette smoking, and sickle-cell disease, require close monitoring.

When deciding whether to use OCs, each woman needs to weigh the benefits against the risks. To make an informed decision, she should seek the help of a health care professional. A woman can take several steps to decrease her risk from OC use:

1. Request a low-dosage pill. (OCs recommended for most new users contain 30–35 micrograms of estrogen.)

fertility   The ability to reproduce.

Pap test   A scraping of cells from the cervix for examination under a microscope to detect cancer.

2. Stop smoking.

3. Follow the dosage carefully and consistently.

4. Be alert to preliminary danger signals, which can be remembered with the word ACHES:

   Abdominal pain (severe)

   Chest pain (severe), cough, shortness of breath or sharp pain on breathing in

   Headaches (severe), dizziness, weakness, or numbness, especially if one-sided

   Eye problems (vision loss or blurring) and/or speech problems

   Severe leg pain (calf or thigh)

5. Have regular checkups to monitor blood pressure, weight, and urine, and have an annual examination of the thyroid, breasts, abdomen, and pelvis.

6. Have regular **Pap tests** to check for early cervical changes.

For most women, the known, directly associated risk of death from taking birth control pills is much lower than the risk of death from pregnancy (Table 6.1).

Effectiveness Oral contraceptive effectiveness varies substantially because it depends so much on individual factors. If taken exactly as directed, the failure rate of OCs is extremely low (0.3%). However, among average users, lapses such as forgetting to take a pill do occur, and a typical first-year failure rate is 8.7%. The continuation rate for OCs also varies; the average rate is 68% after 1 year.

Contraceptive Skin Patch

The contraceptive skin patch, Ortho Evra, is a thin, 1¾-inch square patch that slowly releases an estrogen and a progestin into the bloodstream. The patch prevents pregnancy in the same way as combination OCs. Each patch is worn continuously for 1 week and is replaced on the same day of the week for 3 consecutive weeks. The fourth week is patch-free, allowing a woman to have her menstrual period.

The patch can be worn on the upper outer arm, abdomen, buttocks, or upper torso (excluding the breasts); it is designed to stick to skin even during bathing or swimming. If a patch should fall off for more than a day, the FDA advises starting a new 4-week cycle of patches and using a backup method of contraception for the first week. Patches should be discarded according to the manufacturer's directions to avoid leakage of hormones into the environment.

Advantages With both perfect and typical use, the patch is as effective as OCs in preventing pregnancy. Compliance seems to be higher with the patch than with OCs, probably because the patch requires weekly instead of

Table 6.1	Contraceptive and Abortion Risks

Contraceptive Method	Risk of Death in Any Given Year
Oral contraceptives	
Nonsmoker	1 in 66,700
Age less than 35	1 in 200,000
Age 35–44	1 in 28,600
Heavy smoker (25 or more cigarettes/day)	1 in 1,700
Age less than 35	1 in 5,300
Age 35–44	1 in 700
IUDs	1 in 10,000,000
Barrier methods, spermicides	none
Fertility awareness methods, withdrawal	none
Sterilization	
Laparoscopic tubal ligation	1 in 38,500
Hysterectomy	1 in 1,600
Vasectomy	1 in 1,000,000
Legal abortion	
Before 9 weeks	1 in 262,800
9–12 weeks	1 in 100,100
13–15 weeks	1 in 34,400
After 15 weeks	1 in 10,200
Illegal abortion	1 in 3,000
Pregnancy and childbirth	1 in 10,000

SOURCE: Hatcher, R. A., et al. 2004. *Contraceptive Technology*, 18th rev. ed. New York: Ardent Media. Reprinted by permission of Ardent Media, Inc.

daily action. Medical benefits are likely to be comparable to those of OCs.

Disadvantages With patch use, additional measures must be taken to protect against STDs. Minor side effects are similar to those of OCs, although breast discomfort may be more common in patch users. Some women also experience skin irritation around the patch. More serious complications are thought to be similar to those of OCs, including an increased risk of side effects among women who smoke. However, because Ortho Evra exposes users to higher doses of estrogen than most OCs, patch use may further increase the risk of blood clots and other adverse effects.

Effectiveness With perfect use, the patch's failure rate is very low (0.3%) in the first year of use. The typical failure rate is assumed to be lower than the pill's 8.7%. The product appears to be less effective when used by women weighing more than 198 pounds.

Vaginal Contraceptive Ring

The NuvaRing is a vaginal ring that is molded with a mixture of progestin and estrogen. The 2-inch ring slowly

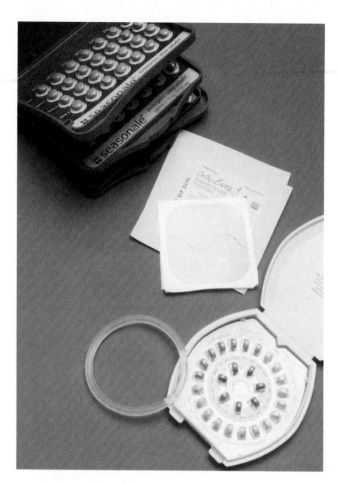

Reversible hormonal contraceptives are available in several forms. Shown here are the patch, the ring, and birth control pills.

Effectiveness As with the pill and patch, the perfect use failure rate is about 0.3% and the typical use failure rate is likely to be lower than the pill's 8.7%.

Contraceptive Implants

Contraceptive implants are placed under the skin of the upper arm and deliver a small but steady dose of progestin (a synthetic progesterone) over a period of years. One such implant, called Implanon, is a single implant that was approved for use in the United States in 2006. This device is effective for 3 years.

The progestins in implants have several contraceptive effects. They cause hormonal shifts that may inhibit ovulation and affect development of the uterine lining. The hormones also thicken the cervical mucus, inhibiting the movement of sperm. Finally, they may slow the transport of the egg through the fallopian tubes. Contraceptive implants are best suited for women who wish to have continuous and long-term protection against pregnancy.

Advantages Contraceptive implants are highly effective. After insertion of the implants, no further action is required; contraceptive effects are quickly reversed upon removal. Because implants, unlike the combination pill, contain no estrogen, they carry a lower risk of certain side effects, such as blood clots and other cardiovascular complications. The thickened cervical mucus resulting from implant use has a protective effect against PID.

Disadvantages Like the pill, an implant provides no protection against HIV infection and STDs in the lower reproductive tract. Although the implants are barely visible, their appearance may bother some women. The most common side effects of contraceptive implants are menstrual irregularities, including longer menstrual periods, spotting between periods, or having no bleeding at all. The menstrual cycle usually becomes more regular after 1 year of use. Less common side effects include headaches, weight gain, breast tenderness, nausea, acne, and mood swings. Cautions and more serious health concerns are similar to those associated with oral contraceptives but are less common.

Effectiveness The overall failure rate for Implanon is estimated at about 0.1%.

Injectable Contraceptives

Hormonal contraceptive injections were developed in the 1960s and are currently being used in at least 80 countries throughout the world. The first injectable contraceptive approved for use in the United States was Depo-Provera, which uses long-acting progestins. Injected into the arm or buttocks, Depo-Provera is usually given every 12 weeks, although it actually provides effective contraception for a few weeks beyond that. As another progestin-only

releases hormones and maintains blood hormone levels comparable to those found with OC use; it prevents pregnancy in the same way as OCs. A woman inserts the ring anytime during the first 5 days of her menstrual period and leaves it in place for 3 weeks. During the fourth week, which is ring-free, her next menstrual period occurs. A new ring is then inserted. Rings should be discarded according to the manufacturer's directions to avoid leakage of hormones into the environment. Backup contraception must be used for the first 7 days of the first ring use or if the ring has been removed for more than 3 hours during use.

Advantages The NuvaRing offers 1 month of protection with no daily or weekly action required. It does not require a fitting by a clinician, and exact placement in the vagina is not critical as it is with a diaphragm. Medical benefits are probably similar to those of OCs.

Disadvantages The NuvaRing gives no protection against STDs. Side effects are roughly comparable to those seen with OC use, except for a lower incidence of nausea and vomiting. Other side effects may include vaginal discharge, vaginitis, and vaginal irritation. Medical risks also are similar to those found with OC use.

contraceptive, it prevents pregnancy in the same ways as implants.

Advantages Injectable contraceptives are highly effective and require little action on the part of the user. Because the injections leave no trace and involve no ongoing supplies, injectables allow women almost total privacy in their decision to use contraception. Depo-Provera has no estrogen-related side effects; it requires only periodic injections rather than the minor surgical procedures of implant insertion and removal.

Disadvantages Injectable contraceptives provide no protection against HIV infection and STDs in the lower reproductive tract. A woman must visit a health care facility every 3 months to receive the injections. The side effects of Depo-Provera are similar to those of implants; menstrual irregularities are the most common, and after 1 year of using Depo-Provera many women have no menstrual bleeding at all. Weight gain is a common side effect. After discontinuing the use of Depo-Provera, women may experience temporary infertility for up to 12 months.

Reasons for not using Depo-Provera are similar to those for not using implants. Extended use of Depo-Provera is associated with decreased bone density, a risk factor for osteoporosis; women who use Depo-Provera are advised to do weight-bearing exercise and take 1000 mg of calcium daily. Women are advised to use Depo-Provera as a long-term contraceptive (longer than 2 years, for example) only if other methods are inadequate.

Effectiveness The perfect use failure rate is 0.3% for Depo-Provera. With typical use, the failure rate increases to 6.7% in the first year of use. The 1-year continuation rate for Depo-Provera is about 56%.

Emergency Contraception

Emergency contraception (EC) refers to postcoital methods—those used after unprotected sexual intercourse. An emergency contraceptive may be appropriate if a regularly used method has failed (for example, if a condom breaks) or if unprotected sex has occurred. Sometimes called the "morning-after pill," emergency contraceptives are designed only for emergency use and should not be relied on as a regular birth control method.

Until recently the most frequently used emergency contraceptive was a two-dose regimen of certain oral contraceptives. Postcoital pills appear to work primarily by inhibiting or delaying ovulation and by altering the transport of sperm and/or eggs; they do not affect a fertilized egg already implanted in the uterus.

Plan B is a newer product specifically designed for emergency contraception. Overall, Plan B reduces pregnancy risk by about 89%. It is most effective if initiated in the first 12 hours. Possible side effects are similar to those associated with the OC regimen and can include nausea, stomach pain, headache, dizziness, and breast tenderness.

In August 2006, the FDA approved the use of Plan B as an over-the-counter (OTC) drug for women age 18 and older. Prior to that time, it was available to all women by prescription and in some states directly from pharmacists. It remains a prescription drug for those under age 18. Plan B is stocked behind the counter because proof of age or a prescription is required to purchase it.

Easy access to emergency contraception is important because the sooner the drug is taken, the more effective it is. Some clinicians advise women to keep a package of emergency contraception on hand in case their regular contraception method fails. Research has found that ready access to emergency contraception does *not* lead to an increase in unprotected intercourse, unintended pregnancies, or STDs.

Despite FDA approval, not all physicians, hospitals, or pharmacists make emergency contraception available, even in cases of sexual assault. (See the box "Access to Emergency Contraception" for more information.) Increasingly, however, states are requiring pharmacies to carry Plan B. Call the Emergency Contraception Hotline (888-NOT-2-LATE) for more information about access.

Intrauterine devices, discussed in the next section, can also be used for emergency contraception: If inserted within 5 days of unprotected intercourse, they are even more effective than OCs.

The Intrauterine Device (IUD)

The **intrauterine device (IUD)** is a small plastic device placed in the uterus as a contraceptive. Two IUDs are now available in the United States: the Copper T-380A (also known as the ParaGard), which gives protection for up to 10 years, and the Levonorgestral IUD (Mirena), which releases small amounts of progestin and is effective for up to 5 years.

Researchers do not know exactly how IUDs prevent pregnancy. Current evidence suggests that they work primarily by preventing fertilization. IUDs may cause

emergency contraception A birth control method used after unprotected sexual intercourse has occurred.

intrauterine device (IUD) A plastic device inserted into the uterus as a contraceptive.

TERMS

Access to Emergency Contraception

Even though the FDA approved the emergency contraceptive drug Plan B for over-the-counter sale to adults in 2006, many women still have trouble getting emergency contraception (EC) when they need it most.

Soon after the start of Plan B sales, some pharmacists refused to dispense the drug, even to women who had a doctor's prescription for it. Most of these pharmacists—and in some cases, pharmacy management, physicians, and hospitals—claimed a moral or religious basis for declining to distribute Plan B. The drug, they contended, is more an abortifacient than a contraceptive, because it might interfere with the implantation of a fertilized egg in a woman's uterus.

As a result, women seeking emergency contraception found their requests being turned down by doctors, pharmacists, and even some emergency room staff. In most cases, the women have been able to obtain the drug from another medical professional, but many of them say the experience left them humiliated as well as inconvenienced.

The controversy over Plan B has raised an important but difficult question about the role of religious and moral beliefs among health care providers, especially pharmacists. That is, should a doctor or pharmacist be allowed to refuse treatment if he or she feels the treatment is immoral or contrary to his or her religious beliefs?

Many Plan B proponents contend that health care professionals who refuse to provide the drug are jeopardizing the physical and emotional health of patients. Proponents also argue the issue of fairness: If a pharmacy sells some types of contraceptives, such as condoms and standard birth control pills, then it should sell *all* forms of contraception, including EC. At the very least, say Plan B supporters, if pharmacists or doctors refuse to dispense the drug, they should be willing to direct patients to other professionals who will provide it.

According to the Guttmacher Institute, 16 states now require emergency room staff to provide emergency contraception to women who have been sexually assaulted; in 11 other states, EC must be made available on request to assault victims.

A few states have adopted legislation encouraging pharmacists to provide EC services; in nine states, for example, pharmacists can provide Plan B without a prescription under certain circumstances. Another two states require pharmacists to fill all valid prescriptions that are presented to them.

On the other hand, a few other states have placed restrictions on access to EC, and five states have regulations that specifically allow pharmacists or pharmacies to refuse to sell any kind of contraceptives, including EC.

A number of pharmacists have filed suits in several states to overturn regulations that require them to dispense Plan B; a few of these suits have been successful. Many experts believe that the rights of individual health care providers to deny certain services on religious grounds may ultimately prevail over a woman's right to receive emergency contraceptive services.

In 2007, the American College of Obstetricians and Gynecologists (ACOG) released a position statement on the issue of "conscientious refusal" to provide reproductive medical services. The group urged doctors who object to EC to give patients prior notice of their objections while continuing to give accurate medical information about health services such as contraception and abortion. When doctors refuse to perform the actual services, the ACOG urges them to refer patients to other doctors who are willing to provide them.

Women who have trouble getting EC may find help from organizations such as Planned Parenthood (http://www.plannedparenthood.org). Web sites such as Princeton University's Emergency Contraception site (http://ec.princeton.edu) enable visitors to search for EC providers by ZIP code.

---

biochemical changes in the uterus and affect the movement of sperm and eggs; although less likely, they may also interfere with implantation of fertilized eggs. Mirena slowly releases very small amounts of hormones, which impedes fertilization or implantation.

An IUD must be inserted and removed by a trained professional. The device is threaded into a sterile inserter, which is introduced through the cervix; a plunger pushes the IUD into the uterus. The threads protruding from the cervix are trimmed so that only 1–1½ inches remain in the upper vagina.

Advantages Intrauterine devices are highly reliable and are simple and convenient to use, requiring no attention except for a periodic check of the string position. They do not require the woman to anticipate or interrupt sexual activity. According to the American College of Obstetricians and Gynecologists, IUD use reduces the risk of developing endometrial cancer by as much as 40%. Usually IUDs have only localized side effects, and in the absence of complications they are considered a fully reversible contraceptive.

Disadvantages Heavy menstrual flow and bleeding and spotting between periods may occur, although with Mirena menstrual periods tend to become shorter and lighter over time. Another side effect is pain, particularly uterine cramps and backache, which seem to occur most

male condom A sheath, usually made of thin latex (synthetic rubber), that covers the penis during sexual intercourse; used for contraception and to prevent STDs.

ejaculation An abrupt discharge of semen from the penis after sexual stimulation.

spermicide A chemical agent that kills sperm.

often in women who have never been pregnant. Spontaneous expulsion of the IUD happens to 5–6% of women within the first year, most commonly during the first months after insertion.

A serious but rare complication of IUD use is pelvic inflammatory disease (PID). Most pelvic infections among IUD users occur shortly after insertion, are relatively mild, and can be treated successfully with antibiotics. However, early and adequate treatment is critical—a lingering infection can lead to tubal scarring and subsequent infertility.

Some physicians advise against the use of IUDs by young women who have never been pregnant because of the increased incidence of side effects in this group and the risk of infection with the possibility of subsequent infertility. Early IUD danger signals are abdominal pain, fever, chills, foul-smelling vaginal discharge, irregular menstrual periods, and other unusual vaginal bleeding. A change in string length should also be noted. An annual checkup is important and should include a Pap test and a blood check for anemia if menstrual flow has increased.

Effectiveness   The typical failure rate of IUDs during the first year of use is 0.6% for the ParaGard and 0.1% for Mirena. Effectiveness can be increased by periodically checking to see that the device is in place and by using a backup method for the first few months after IUD insertion. The continuation rate of IUDs is about 80% after 1 year of use.

Male Condoms

The **male condom** is a thin sheath designed to cover the penis during sexual intercourse. Most brands available in the United States are made of latex, although condoms made of polyurethane are also now available. Condoms prevent sperm from entering the vagina and provide protection against disease. Condom sales have increased dramatically in recent years, primarily because they are the only method that provides substantial protection against HIV infection as well as some protection against other STDs. At least one-third of all male condoms are bought by women. This figure will probably increase as more women become aware of the serious risks associated with STDs and assume the right to insist on condom use.

The man or his partner must put the condom on the penis before it is inserted into the vagina, because the small amounts of fluid that may be secreted unnoticed prior to **ejaculation** often contain sperm capable of causing pregnancy. The rolled-up condom is placed over the head of the erect penis and unrolled down to the base of the penis, leaving a half-inch space (without air) at the tip to collect semen (Figure 6.1). Some brands of condoms have a reservoir tip designed for this purpose. Uncircumcised men must first pull back the foreskin of the penis. Partners must be careful not to damage the condom with fingernails, rings, or other rough objects.

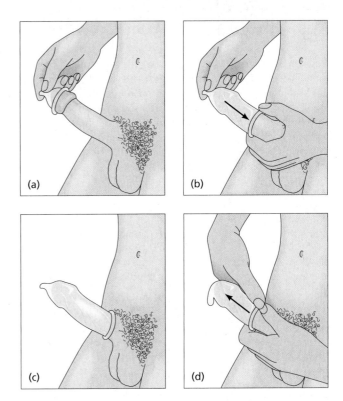

FIGURE 6.1   Use of the male condom.   (a) Place the rolled-up condom over the head of the erect penis. Hold the top half-inch of the condom (with air squeezed out) to leave room for semen. (b) While holding the tip, unroll the condom onto the penis. Gently smooth out any air bubbles. (c) Unroll the condom down to the base of the penis. (d) To avoid spilling semen after ejaculation, hold the condom around the base of the penis as the penis is withdrawn. Remove the condom away from your partner, taking care not to spill any semen.

Prelubricated condoms are available containing the **spermicide** nonoxynol-9, the same agent found in many of the contraceptive creams that women use. However, spermicidal condoms are no more effective than condoms without spermicide, even though they cost more. Furthermore, these condoms have been associated with urinary tract infections in women and, if they cause tissue irritation, an increased risk of HIV transmission.

If desired, users can lubricate their own condoms with contraceptive foam, creams, or jelly. If vaginal irritation occurs with these products, water-based preparations such as K-Y Jelly can be used. Any products that contain mineral or vegetable oil—including baby oil, many lotions, regular petroleum jelly, cooking oils (corn oil, shortening, butter, and so on), and some vaginal lubricants and anti-fungal or anti-itch creams—should never

Buying and Using Over-the-Counter Contraceptives

You can buy several types of contraceptives without a prescription. These have several advantages—they are readily accessible and relatively inexpensive, they are moderately effective at preventing pregnancy, and some offer some protection against HIV infection and other STDs. But like all methods, over-the-counter contraceptives work only if they are used correctly. The following guidelines can help you maximize the effectiveness of your method of choice.

Male Condoms

• *Buy latex condoms.* If you're allergic to latex, use a polyurethane condom or wear a lambskin condom under a latex one. Lambskin condoms provide no STD protection; polyurethane condoms are more likely to slip or break than latex. Spermicidal condoms provide no additional protection against pregnancy or STDs.

• *Buy and use condoms while they are fresh.* Packages have an expiration date or a manufacturing date. Don't use a condom after the expiration date or more than 5 years after the manufacturing date (2 years if it contains spermicide).

• *Try different styles and sizes.* Male condoms come in a variety of textures, colors, shapes, lubricants, and sizes. Shop around until you find a brand that's right for you. Condom widths and lengths vary by about 10–20%. A condom that is too tight may be uncomfortable and more likely to break; one that is too loose may slip off.

• *Use "thinner" condoms with caution.* Condoms advertised as "thinner" are often no thinner than others, and the thinnest ones tend to break more easily.

• *Don't remove the condom from an individual sealed wrapper until you're ready to use it.* Open the packet carefully. Don't use a condom if it's gummy, dried out, or discolored. Keep extra condoms on hand.

• *Store condoms correctly.* Don't leave condoms in extreme heat or cold, and don't carry them in a pocket wallet.

• *Use only water-based lubricants.* Never use oil-based lubricants like Vaseline or hand lotion, as they may cause a latex condom to break. Avoid oil-based vaginal products.

• *Use male condoms correctly* (see Figure 6.2). Use a new condom every time you have intercourse. Misuse is by far the leading reason that condoms fail.

• *Use emergency contraceptive pills if a condom slips or breaks.*

Female Condoms

• *Make sure your condom comes with the necessary supplies and information.* The FC female condom comes individually wrapped. With your condom, you should receive a leaflet containing instructions and a small bottle of additional lubricant.

• *Buy and use female condoms while they are fresh.* Check the expiration dates on the condom packet and the lubricant bottle.

• *Buy several condoms.* Buy one or more for practice before using one during sex. Have a backup in case you have a problem with insertion or use.

• *Read the leaflet instructions carefully.* Practice inserting the condom and checking that it's in the proper position.

• *Use the female condom correctly.* Make sure the penis is inserted into the pouch and that the outer ring is not pushed into the vagina. Add lubricant around the outer ring if needed.

• *Use emergency contraception pills if a condom slips or breaks.*

Contraceptive Sponges

• *Buy and use contraceptive sponges when they are fresh.* Check the expiration date on each package.

• *Read and follow the package instructions carefully.* Moisten the sponge with water and place high in the vagina.

• *Use each sponge only once.* The sponge may be left in place for up to 24 hours without the addition of spermicide for repeated intercourse.

Spermicides

• *Try different types of spermicides.* You may find one type easier or more convenient to use. Foams come in aerosol cans and are similar to shaving cream in consistency. Foams are thicker than creams, which are thicker than jellies. Foams, creams, and jellies usually require applicators; spermicidal suppositories and films do not.

• *Read and follow the package directions carefully.* Cans of foam must be shaken before use. Jellies and creams are often inserted with an applicator just outside the entrance to the cervix. Suppositories and film must be placed with a finger.

• *Pay close attention to the timing of use.* Follow the package instructions for inserting the spermicide at the appropriate time before intercourse actually occurs. Spermicides have a fairly narrow window of effectiveness. Be sure to also allow the recommended amount of time for suppositories and films to dissolve.

• *Use an additional full dose for each additional act of intercourse.*

• *Leave the spermicide in place for 8 hours after the last act of intercourse.*

• *Consider using spermicides with another form of birth control.* These include a condom, diaphragm, or cervical cap. Combined use provides greater protection against pregnancy.

Emergency Contraceptive Pills

Plan B pills are highly effective when taken soon after unprotected intercourse. If you are 18 or older, you can purchase Plan B over the counter. It is stocked behind the counter, so you will have to request it from the pharmacist and show proof of age. It is not available at convenience stores or other retail outlets where younger women might have access to it without a prescription. To maximize effectiveness, follow the instructions on the package carefully.

be used with latex condoms. Such products can cause latex to begin to disintegrate within 60 seconds, thus greatly increasing the chance of condom breakage. (Polyurethane is not affected by oil-based products.)

Advantages   Condoms are easy to purchase and are available without prescription or medical supervision (see the box "Buying and Using Over-the-Counter Contraceptives"). In addition to being free of medical side effects (other than occasional allergic reactions), latex condoms help protect against STDs. A recent study determined that condoms may also protect women from human papilloma virus (HPV), which causes cervical cancer. Condoms made of polyurethane are appropriate for people who are allergic to latex. However, they are more likely to slip or break than latex condoms, and therefore may give less protection against STDs and pregnancy. (Lambskin condoms permit the passage of HIV and other disease-causing organisms, so they can be used only for pregnancy prevention, not the prevention of STDs.) Except for abstinence, correct and consistent use of latex male condoms offers the most reliable available protection against the transmission of HIV.

Disadvantages   The most common complaints about condoms are that they diminish sensation and interfere with spontaneity. Some people find these drawbacks serious, but others consider them only minor disadvantages.

Effectiveness   In actual use, the failure rate of condoms varies considerably. First-year rates among typical users average about 17.4%. With perfect use, the first-year failure rate is about 2%. At least some pregnancies happen because the condom is carelessly removed after ejaculation. Some may also occur because of breakage or slippage, which may happen 1–2 times in every 100 instances of use for latex condoms and up to 10 times in every 100 instances for polyurethane condoms. Breakage is more common among inexperienced users. Other contributing factors include poorly fitting condoms, insufficient lubrication, excessively vigorous sex, and improper storage (because heat destroys rubber, latex condoms should not be stored for long periods in a wallet or a car's glove compartment). To help ensure quality, condoms should not be used past their expiration date or more than 5 years past their date of manufacture (2 years for those with spermicide).

If a condom breaks or is carelessly removed, the risk of pregnancy can be reduced somewhat by the immediate use of a vaginal spermicide. Some clinicians recommend keeping emergency contraceptive pills on hand.

Female Condoms

A female condom is a latex or polyurethane pouch that can be inserted into a woman's vagina. The female condom currently available is a disposable device that comes in one size and consists of a soft, loose-fitting polyure-thane sheath with two flexible rings. The ring at the closed end is inserted into the vagina and placed at the cervix much like a diaphragm. The ring at the open end remains outside the vagina. The walls of the condom protect the inside of the vagina.

The directions that accompany the condom should be followed closely. It can be inserted up to 8 hours before intercourse and should be used with the supplied lubricant or a spermicide to prevent penile irritation. As with male condoms, users need to take care not to tear the condom during insertion or removal. Following intercourse, the woman should remove the condom immediately, before standing up. By twisting and squeezing the outer ring, she can prevent the spilling of semen.

Advantages   Female condoms can be inserted before sexual activity and are thus less disruptive than male condoms. Because the outer part of the condom covers the area around the vaginal opening as well as the base of the penis during intercourse, it offers potentially better protection against genital warts or herpes. The polyurethane pouch can be used by people who are allergic to latex. And because polyurethane is thin and pliable, there is little loss of sensation. When used correctly, the female condom should theoretically provide protection against HIV transmission and STDs comparable to that of the latex male condom. However, in research involving typical users, the female condom was less effective in preventing both pregnancy and STDs. With careful instruction and practice, effectiveness can be improved.

Disadvantages   As with the traditional condom, interference with spontaneity is likely to be a common complaint. The outer ring, which hangs visibly outside the vagina, may be bothersome during foreplay. Female condoms, like male condoms, are made for one-time use. A single female condom costs about four times as much as a single male condom.

Effectiveness   The typical first-year failure rate of the female condom is 27%. Having Plan B available as a backup contraceptive is recommended.

The Diaphragm with Spermicide

The **diaphragm** is a dome-shaped cup of thin rubber stretched over a collapsible metal ring. When correctly used with spermicidal cream or jelly, the diaphragm covers the cervix, blocking sperm from entering the uterus.

Diaphragms are available only by prescription. Because of individual anatomical differences, a diaphragm must

diaphragm   A contraceptive device consisting of a flexible, dome-shaped cup that covers the cervix and prevents sperm from entering the uterus.

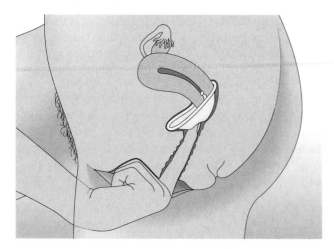

FIGURE 6.2   The diaphragm properly positioned.

be carefully fitted by a trained clinician to ensure both comfort and effectiveness. The fitting should be checked with each routine annual medical examination, as well as after childbirth, abortion, or a weight change of more than 10 pounds.

The woman spreads spermicidal jelly or cream on the diaphragm before inserting it and checking its placement (Figure 6.2). If more than 6 hours elapse between the time of insertion and the time of intercourse, additional spermicide must be applied. The diaphragm must be left in place for at least 6 hours after the last act of coitus to give the spermicide enough time to kill all the sperm. With repeated intercourse, a condom should be used for additional protection.

To remove the diaphragm, the woman simply hooks the front rim down from the pubic bone with one finger and pulls it out. She should wash it with mild soap and water, rinse it, pat it dry, and then examine it for holes or cracks. After inspecting the diaphragm, she should store it in its case.

Advantages   A diaphragm can be inserted up to 6 hours before intercourse. Its use can be limited to times of sexual activity only, and it allows for immediate and total

toxic shock syndrome (TSS)   A bacterial disease occasionally associated with tampon use and with diaphragm use; symptoms include weakness, cold and clammy hands, fever, nausea, and headache.

FemCap   A small flexible cup that fits over the cervix, to be used with spermicide.

sponge   A contraceptive device about 2 inches in diameter that fits over the cervix and acts as a barrier, spermicide, and seminal fluid absorbent.

reversibility. The diaphragm is free of medical side effects (other than rare allergic reactions). When used along with spermicidal jelly or cream, it offers significant protection against gonorrhea and possibly chlamydia, STDs that are transmitted only by semen and for which the cervix is the sole site of entry. Diaphragm use can also protect the cervix from semen infected with the human papillomavirus, which causes cervical cancer. However, the diaphragm is unlikely to protect against STDs that can be transmitted through vaginal or vulvar surfaces (in addition to the cervix), including HIV infection, genital herpes, and syphilis.

15% of contraceptive users employ two methods (such as a condom and diaphragm) at the same time.

—Guttmacher Institute, 2008

Disadvantages   Diaphragms must always be used with a spermicide, so a woman must keep both of these somewhat bulky supplies with her whenever she anticipates sexual activity. Diaphragms require extra attention, since they must be cleaned and stored with care to preserve their effectiveness. Some women cannot wear a diaphragm because of their vaginal or uterine anatomy or frequent bladder infections.

Diaphragms have also been associated with a slightly increased risk of **toxic shock syndrome (TSS),** an occasionally fatal bacterial infection. To reduce the risk of TSS, a woman should wash her hands carefully with soap and water before inserting or removing the diaphragm, should not use the diaphragm during menstruation or when abnormal vaginal discharge is present, and should never leave the device in place for more than 24 hours.

Effectiveness   With perfect use, the failure rate is about 6%. Typical failure rates are 16% during the first year of use. The main causes of failure are incorrect insertion, inconsistent use, and inaccurate fitting. If a diaphragm slips during intercourse, a woman may choose to use emergency contraception.

Lea's Shield

Lea's Shield is a one-size-fits-all diaphragm-like device, available by prescription. Made of silicone rubber, it can be used by women who are allergic to latex, and it is not damaged by petroleum-based products. The shield has a valve that allows the flow of air and fluids from the cervix as well as a loop that aids in insertion and removal. The device may be inserted at any time prior to intercourse, but should be left in place for 8 hours after last intercourse; it can be worn for up to 48 hours. Like the dia-

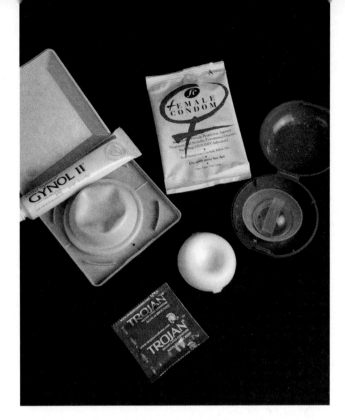

Many contraceptive methods work by blocking sperm from entering the cervix. Barrier methods pictured here are the diaphragm, the female condom, the male condom, the sponge, and the FemCap cervical cap.

phragm, it must be used with spermicide. Studies completed thus far have reported advantages, disadvantages, and failure rates similar to those of the diaphragm.

FemCap

FemCap, another barrier device, is a small flexible cup that fits snugly over the cervix and is held in place by suction. This cervical cap is a clear silicone cup with a brim around the dome to hold spermicide and trap sperm and a removal strap over the dome. It comes in three sizes and must be fitted by a trained clinician. It is used like a diaphragm, with a small amount of spermicide placed in the cup and on the brim before insertion.

Advantages Advantages of the cervical cap are similar to those associated with diaphragm use and include partial STD protection. It is an alternative for women who cannot use a diaphragm because of anatomical reasons or recurrent urinary tract infections. Because the cap fits tightly, it does not require backup condom use with repeated intercourse. It may be left in place for up to 48 hours.

Disadvantages Along with most of the disadvantages associated with the diaphragm, difficulty with insertion and removal is more common for cervical cap users. Because there may be a slightly increased risk of TSS with prolonged use, the cap should not be left in place for more than 48 hours.

Effectiveness Studies indicate that the average failure rate for the cervical cap is 16% for women who have never had a child and 32% for women who have had a child. Failure rates drop significantly with perfect use.

The Contraceptive Sponge

The **sponge** is a round, absorbent device about 2 inches in diameter with a polyester loop on one side (for removal) and a concave dimple on the other side, which helps it fit snugly over the cervix. The sponge is made of polyurethane and is presaturated with the same spermicide that is used in contraceptive creams and foams. The spermicide is activated when moistened with a small amount of water just before insertion. The sponge, which can be used only once, acts as a barrier, as a spermicide, and as a seminal fluid absorbent.

Advantages The sponge offers advantages similar to those of the diaphragm and cervical cap, including partial protection against some STDs. In addition, sponges can be obtained without a prescription or professional fitting, and they may be safely left in place for 24 hours without the addition of spermicide for repeated intercourse.

Disadvantages Reported disadvantages include difficulty with removal and an unpleasant odor if the sponge is left in place for more than 18 hours. Allergic reactions, such as irritation of the vagina, are more common with the sponge than with other spermicide products, probably because the overall dose contained in each sponge is significantly higher than that used with other methods. If irritation of the vaginal lining occurs, the risk of yeast infections and STDs (including HIV) may increase. Because the sponge has also been associated with toxic shock syndrome, the same precautions must be taken as described for diaphragm use.

Effectiveness The typical effectiveness of the sponge is the same as the diaphragm (16% failure rate during the first year of use) for women who have never experienced childbirth. For women who have had a child, however, sponges are significantly less effective than diaphragms.

Vaginal Spermicides

Spermicidal compounds developed for use with a diaphragm have been adapted for use without a diaphragm by combining them with a bulky base. Foams, creams, and jellies must be placed deep in the vagina near the cervical entrance and must be inserted no more than 60 minutes before intercourse. After an hour, their effectiveness is drastically reduced, and a new dose must be inserted.

The spermicidal suppository is small and easily inserted like a tampon; it is important to wait at least 15 minutes after insertion before having intercourse. The

Vaginal Contraceptive Film (VCF) is a paper-thin 2-inch square of film that contains spermicide. It is folded over one or two fingers and placed high in the vagina, as close to the cervix as possible.

Another application of spermicide is required before each repeated act of coitus. If the woman wants to **douche**, she should wait for at least 6 hours after the last intercourse to make sure that there has been time for the spermicide to kill all the sperm; douching is not recommended, however, because it can irritate vaginal tissue and increase the risk of various infections.

Advantages   The use of vaginal spermicides is relatively simple and can be limited to times of sexual activity. They are readily available in most drugstores and do not require a prescription or a pelvic examination. Spermicides allow for complete and immediate reversibility, and the only medical side effects are occasional allergic reactions. Vaginal spermicides may provide limited protection against some STDs but should never be used instead of condoms for reliable protection.

Disadvantages   When used alone, vaginal spermicides must be inserted shortly before intercourse, so their use may be seen as an annoying disruption. Spermicides can alter the balance of bacteria in the vagina and may increase the occurrence of yeast infections and urinary tract infections. Also, this method does not protect against gonorrhea, chlamydia, or HIV. Overuse of spermicides can irritate vaginal tissues; if this occurs, the risk of HIV transmission may increase.

Effectiveness   The typical failure rate is about 29% during the first year of use. Spermicide is generally recommended only in combination with other barrier methods or as a backup to other contraceptives. Plan B provides a better backup than spermicides, however.

Abstinence, Fertility Awareness, and Withdrawal

Millions of people throughout the world do not use any of the contraceptive methods described earlier, either because of religious conviction, cultural prohibitions, poverty, or lack of information and supplies. If they use any method at all, they are likely to use one of the following relatively "natural" methods.

Abstinence   The decision not to engage in sexual intercourse for a chosen period of time, or **abstinence,** has been practiced throughout history for a variety of reasons. Until relatively recently, many people abstained because they had no other contraceptive measures. Today, few American women rely on periodic abstinence as a contraceptive method. For those who do, other methods may simply seem unsuitable. Concern about possible side effects, STDs, and unwanted pregnancy may be factors. For others, the most important reason for choosing abstinence is a moral one, based on cultural or religious beliefs or strongly held personal values. Many people feel that sexual intercourse is appropriate only for married couples or for people in serious, committed relationships. Abstinence may also be considered the wisest choice in terms of one's emotional needs. A period of abstinence, for example, may be useful as a time to focus energies on other aspects of one's life.

Couples may choose abstinence to allow time for their relationship to grow. A period of abstinence allows partners to get to know each other better and to develop trust and respect for each other. Many couples who choose to abstain from sexual intercourse in the traditional sense turn to other mutually satisfying alternatives. These may include dancing, massage, hugging, kissing, petting, mutual masturbation, and oral-genital sex.

The Fertility Awareness Method   The basis for the **fertility awareness method (FAM)** is abstinence from coitus during the fertile phase of a woman's menstrual cycle. Ordinarily, only one egg is released by the ovaries each month, and it lives about 24 hours unless it is fertilized. Sperm deposited in the vagina may be capable of fertilizing an egg for up to 6–7 days, so conception can theoretically occur only during 8 days of any cycle. Predicting which 8 days is difficult; several methods can be used.

The *calendar method* is based on the knowledge that the average woman releases an egg 14–16 days before her next period begins. Few women menstruate with complete regularity, so a record of the menstrual cycle must be kept for 12 months, during which time some other method of contraception must be used. The first day of each period is counted as day 1. To determine the first fertile, or "unsafe," day of the cycle, subtract 18 from the number of days in the shortest cycle (Figure 6.3). To determine the last unsafe day of the cycle, subtract 11 from the number of days in the longest cycle.

A variation of the calendar method known as the Standard Days Method (SDM) can be used by women with regular menstrual cycles between 26 and 32 days long.

TERMS

douche   To apply a stream of water or other solutions to a body part or cavity such as the vagina; not a contraceptive technique.

abstinence   Avoidance of sexual intercourse; a method of contraception.

fertility awareness method (FAM)   A method of preventing conception based on avoiding intercourse during the fertile phase of a woman's cycle.

withdrawal   A method of contraception in which the man withdraws his penis from the vagina prior to ejaculation; also called *coitus interruptus*.

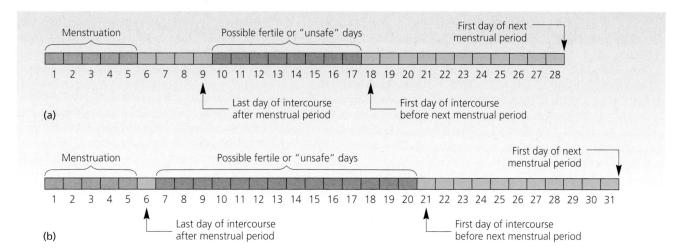

FIGURE 6.3 The fertility awareness method of contraception. This chart shows the safe and unsafe days for (a) a woman with a regular 28-day cycle and (b) a woman with an irregular cycle ranging from 25 to 31 days.

Couples must avoid unprotected intercourse on days 8 through 19 of the woman's cycle. Some women who use SDM use a string of color-coded beads to track their fertile days.

The *temperature method* is based on the knowledge that a woman's body temperature drops slightly just before ovulation and rises slightly after ovulation. A woman using the temperature method records her basal (resting) body temperature (BBT) every morning before getting out of bed and before eating or drinking anything. Once the temperature pattern is apparent (usually after about 3 months), the unsafe period for intercourse can be calculated as the interval from day 5 (day 1 is the first day of the period) until 3 days after the rise in BBT. To arrive at a shorter unsafe period, some women combine the calendar and temperature methods, calculating the first unsafe day from the shortest cycle of the calendar chart and the last unsafe day as the third day after a rise in BBT.

The *mucus method* (or Billings method) is based on changes in the cervical secretions throughout the menstrual cycle. During the estrogenic phase, cervical mucus increases and is clear and slippery. At the time of ovulation, some women can detect a slight change in the texture of the mucus and find that it is more likely to form an elastic thread when stretched between thumb and finger. After ovulation, these secretions become cloudy and sticky and decrease in quantity. Infertile, safe days are likely to occur during the relatively dry days just before and after menstruation. These additional clues have been found to be helpful by some couples who rely on the fertility awareness method.

FAM is not recommended for women who have very irregular cycles—about 15% of all menstruating women. Any woman for whom pregnancy would be a serious problem should not rely on FAM alone, because the failure rate is high—approximately 25% during the first year of use. FAM offers no protection against STDs.

Withdrawal In **withdrawal,** or *coitus interruptus,* the male removes his penis from the vagina just before he ejaculates. Withdrawal has a relatively high failure rate because the male has to overcome a powerful biological urge. In addition, because preejaculatory fluid may contain viable sperm, pregnancy can occur even if the man withdraws prior to ejaculation. Sexual pleasure is often affected because the man must remain in control and the sexual experience of both partners is interrupted.

The failure rate for typical use is about 18% in the first year. Men who are less experienced with sexual intercourse and withdrawal or who have difficulty in foretelling when ejaculation will occur have higher failure rates. Withdrawal does not protect against STDs.

> **4%** of women who practice some sort of contraception rely on withdrawal as their birth control method.
>
> —Guttmacher Institute, 2008

Combining Methods

Couples can choose to combine the preceding methods in a variety of ways, both to add STD protection and/or to increase contraceptive effectiveness. For example, condoms are strongly recommended along with OCs whenever there is a risk of STDs (Table 6.2). Foam may be added to condom use to increase protection against both STDs and pregnancy. For many couples, and especially for women, the added benefits far outweigh the extra effort and expense.

Table 6.3 summarizes the effectiveness of available contraceptive methods.

Table 6.2 Contraceptive Methods and STD Protection

Method	Level of Protection
Hormonal methods	Do not protect against HIV or STDs in lower reproductive tract; increase risk of cervical chlamydia; provide some protection against PID.
IUD	Does not protect against STDs; associated with PID in first month after insertion.
Latex or polyurethane male condom	Best method for protection against STDs (if used correctly); does not protect against infections from lesions that are not covered by the condom. (Lambskin condoms do not protect against STDs.)
Female condom	Theoretically should reduce the risk of STDs, but research results are not yet available.
Diaphragm, sponge, or cervical cap	Protects against cervical infections and PID. Diaphragms, sponges, and cervical caps should not be relied on for protection against HIV.
Spermicide	Modestly reduces the risk of some vaginal and cervical STDs; does not reduce the risk of HIV, chlamydia, or gonorrhea. If vaginal irritation occurs, infection risk may increase.
FAM	Does not protect against STDs.
Sterilization	Does not protect against STDs.
Abstinence	Complete protection against STDs (as long as all activities that involve the exchange of body fluids are avoided).

Table 6.3 Contraceptive Effectiveness

Method	First-Year Failure Rates	
	Typical Use	Perfect Use
Pill	8.7%	0.3%
Patch	8.0%	0.3%
Ring	8.0%	0.3%
Implant	1.0%	0.05%
Injectable (3-month)	6.7%	0.3%
ParaGard IUD	1.0%	0.6%
Mirena IUD	0.1%	0.1%
Male condom	17.4%	2.0%
Female condom	27.0%	5.0%
Diaphragm	16.0%	6.0%
Cervical cap		
Never had a child	16.0%	9.0%
Have had a child	32.0%	26.0%
Sponge		
Never had a child	16.0%	9.0%
Have had a child	32.0%	20.0%
Spermicides	29.0%	18.0%
Periodic abstinence	25.3%	
Withdrawal	18.4%	4.0%
Vasectomy	0.2%	0.1%
Tubal sterilization	0.7%	0.5%

SOURCE: Guttmacher Institute. 2008. *In Brief: Facts on Contraceptive Use.* New York: Guttmacher Institute.

QUESTIONS FOR CRITICAL THINKING AND REFLECTION

If you are sexually active, do you use any of the reversible methods described in the preceding sections? Based on the information given here, do you believe you are using your contraceptive perfectly, or in a way that increases your risk of an unintended pregnancy?

PERMANENT CONTRACEPTION: STERILIZATION

Sterilization is permanent, and it is highly effective at preventing pregnancy. At present it is the most commonly used method both in the United States and in the world. It is especially popular among couples who have been married 10 or more years and who have had all the children they intend to have. Sterilization does not protect against STDs.

An important consideration in choosing sterilization is that, in most cases, it cannot be reversed. Some couples choosing male sterilization store sperm to extend the option of childbearing.

Some studies indicate that male sterilization is preferable to female sterilization because the overall cost of a female procedure is about four times that of a male procedure and women are much more likely than men to experience both minor and major complications following the operation. Furthermore, feelings of regret seem to be somewhat more prevalent in women than in men after sterilization.

Male Sterilization: Vasectomy

The procedure for male sterilization, **vasectomy,** involves severing the vasa deferentia, two tiny ducts that transport sperm from the testes to the seminal vesicles. The testes continue to produce sperm, but the sperm are absorbed into the body. Because the testes contribute only about 10% of the total seminal fluid, the actual quantity of ejaculate is only slightly reduced. Hormone production from the testes continues with very little change, and secondary sex characteristics are not altered.

Vasectomy is ordinarily performed in a physician's office and takes about 30 minutes. A local anesthetic is injected into the skin of the scrotum near the vasa. Small incisions are made at the upper end of the scrotum where it joins the body, and the vas deferens on each side is exposed, severed, and tied off or sealed by electrocautery. Some doctors seal each of the vasa with a plastic clamp, which is the size of a grain of rice. The incisions are then closed with sutures, and a small dressing is applied. Pain and swelling are usually slight and can be relieved with ice compresses, aspirin, and the use of a scrotal support. Bleeding and infection occasionally develop but are usually easily treated.

Men can have sex again as soon as they feel no further discomfort, usually after about a week. Another method of contraception must be used for at least 3 months after vasectomy, however, because sperm produced before the operation may still be present in the semen. Microscopic examination of a semen sample can confirm that sperm are no longer present in the ejaculate.

Vasectomy is highly effective. In a small number of cases, a severed vas rejoins itself, so some physicians advise yearly examination of a semen sample. The overall failure rate for vasectomy is 0.2%. About one-half of vasectomy reversals are successful. In at least half of all men who have had vasectomies, the process of absorbing sperm (instead of ejaculating it) results in antisperm antibodies that may interfere with later fertility. The length of time between the vasectomy and the reversal surgery may also be an important predictor of reversal success.

Female Sterilization

The most common method of female sterilization involves severing or blocking the oviducts, thereby preventing eggs from reaching the uterus and sperm from entering the fallopian tubes. Ovulation and menstruation continue, but the unfertilized eggs are released into the abdominal cavity and absorbed. Although progesterone levels in the blood may decline slightly, hormone production by the ovaries and secondary sex characteristics are generally not affected.

Tubal sterilization (also called *tubal ligation*) is most commonly performed by a method called **laparoscopy.** A laparoscope, a tube containing a small light, is inserted through a small abdominal incision, and the surgeon looks through it to locate the fallopian tubes. Instruments are passed either through the laparoscope or through a second small incision, and the two fallopian tubes are sealed off with ties or staples or by electrocautery. General anesthesia is usually used. The operation takes about 15 minutes. Tubal sterilization can also be performed shortly after a vaginal delivery, or in the case of cesarean section immediately after the uterine incision is repaired.

Although tubal sterilization is somewhat riskier than vasectomy, with a rate of minor complications of about 6–11%, it is the more common procedure (see the box "Contraceptive Use Among American Women"). Potential problems include bowel injury, wound infection, and bleeding. Serious complications are rare, and the death rate is low. The failure rate for tubal sterilization is about 0.7%. When pregnancies occur, an increased percentage of them are ectopic. Because reversibility rates are low and the procedure is costly, female sterilization should be considered permanent.

A new female sterilization device called the Essure System consists of tiny springlike metallic implants that are inserted through the vagina and into the fallopian tubes, using a special catheter. Within several months, scar tissue forms over the implants, blocking the tubes.

In late 2007, the Food and Drug Administration's Obstetrics and Gynecology Devices Panel recommended FDA approval of a new method for blocking a woman's fallopian tubes. The procedure—potentially to be marketed under the commercial name Adiana—involves using a catheter to create small lesions just inside the entrance to each fallopian tube. A small device, the size of a grain of rice, is then placed in each tube. As the lesions heal, healthy new tissue grows on and around the device, eventually blocking the fallopian tube. Based on the manufacturer's studies, the FDA advisory panel estimated that Adiana's 1-year failure rate was about 1.1%.

sterilization Surgically altering the reproductive system to prevent pregnancy. Vasectomy is the procedure in males; tubal sterilization or hysterectomy is the procedure in females.

vasectomy The surgical severing of the ducts that carry sperm to the ejaculatory duct.

tubal sterilization Severing or blocking the oviducts to prevent eggs from reaching the uterus; also called *tubal ligation*.

laparoscopy Examining the internal organs by inserting a tube containing a small light through an abdominal incision.

TERMS

Contraceptive Use Among American Women

connect™

About 62 million women in the United States are in their childbearing years (15–44) and thus face decisions about contraception. About 62% of these women use some form of contraception. Most of the remaining 38% are either sterile, pregnant or trying to become pregnant, or not sexually active.

Only 7% of American women are fertile, sexually active, not seeking pregnancy, *and* not using contraceptives; this small group accounts for almost half of the 3 million unintended pregnancies that occur each year. The unintended pregnancies that occur among contraceptive users are usually the result of inconsistent or incorrect use of methods. For example, one-third of barrier method users report not using their method every time they have intercourse.

Oral contraceptives and female sterilization are the two most popular methods among American women (see figure). However, choice of contraceptive method and consistency of use vary with age, marital status, and other factors:

• *Age:* Sterilization is much more common among older women, particularly those who are over 35 years of age and/or who have had children. Young women in their teens and twenties are more likely to use the pill or condoms. Older

women, however, are more likely to use reversible methods consistently—they are less likely to miss pills and more likely to use barrier methods during every act of intercourse.

• *Marital status:* Women who are or were married have much higher rates of sterilization than women who have never been married. Those who have never been married have high rates of OC and condom usage.

• *Ethnicity:* Overall rates of contraceptive use and use of OCs are highest among white women. Female sterilization, implants, and injectables are more often used by African American women and Latinas, and IUD use is highest among Latinas. Condom use is highest among Asian American women and similar across other ethnic groups. Male sterilization is much more common among white men than among men of other ethnic groups.

• *Socioeconomic status and educational attainment:* Low socioeconomic status and low educational attainment are associated with high rates of female sterilization and low rates of pill and condom use. However, women who are poor or have low educational attainment and who use OCs have higher rates of consis-

tent use than women who are wealthier or have more education. About 20% of women age 15–44 lack adequate health insurance, increasing the cost and difficulty of obtaining contraceptives.

Some trends in contraceptive use may also reflect the differing priorities and experiences of women and men. For example, female sterilization is more expensive and carries greater health risks than male sterilization—yet it is more than twice as common. (Worldwide, female sterilization is more than four times as common as male sterilization.) This pattern may reflect culturally defined gender roles and the fact that women are more directly affected by unintended pregnancy. In surveys, women rate pregnancy prevention as the single most important factor when choosing a contraceptive method; in contrast, men rate STD prevention as equally important.

SOURCES: Frost, L. J., et al. 2007. Factors associated with contraceptive use and nonuse, United States, 2004. *Perspectives on Sexual and Reproductive Health* 39(2): 90–99; Guttmacher Institute. 2008. *In Brief: Facts on Contraceptive Use.* New York: Guttmacher Institute; Ryan, S., et al. 2007. Knowledge, perceptions, and motivations for contraception: Influence on teens' contraceptive consistency. *Youth & Society* 39(2) 182–208.

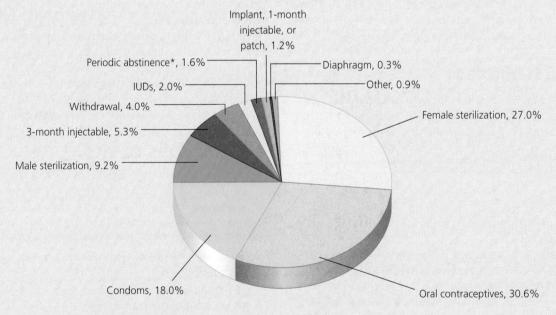

Contraceptive use among American women age 15–44 years.

*Includes women using either the calendar method or natural family planning.

Talking with a Partner About Contraception

Many people have a difficult time talking about contraception with a potential sex partner. How should you bring it up? And whose responsibility is it, anyway? Talking about the subject may be embarrassing at first, but imagine the possible consequences of *not* talking about it. An unintended pregnancy or a sexually transmitted disease could profoundly affect you for the rest of your life. Talking about contraception is one way of showing that you care about yourself, your partner, and your future.

Before you talk with your partner, explore your own thoughts and feelings. Find out the facts about different methods of contraception, and decide which one you think would be most appropriate for you. If you're nervous about having this discussion with your partner, it may help to practice with a friend.

Pick a good time to bring up the subject. Don't wait until you've started to have sex. A time when you're both feeling comfortable and relaxed will improve your chances of having a good discussion. Tell your partner what you know about contraception and how you feel about using it, and talk about what steps you both need to take to get and use a method you can live with. Listen to what your partner has to say, and try to understand his or her point of view. You may need to have more than one discussion, and it may take some time for both of you to feel comfortable with the subject. *But don't have sex until this issue is resolved.*

If you want your partner to be involved but he or she isn't interested in talking about contraception, or if he or she leaves all the responsibility for it up to you, consider whether this is really a person you want to be sexually involved with. If you decide to go ahead with the involvement, you may want to enlist the support of a friend, family member, or health care worker to help you make and implement decisions about contraception.

Hysterectomy, removal of the uterus, is the preferred method of sterilization for only a small number of women, usually those with preexisting menstrual problems.

WHICH CONTRACEPTIVE METHOD IS RIGHT FOR YOU?

Each person must consider many variables in deciding which method is most acceptable and appropriate for her or him. Key considerations include those listed here:

THINKING ABOUT THE ENVIRONMENT

Overpopulation is a key contributor to the global environmental crisis and is due in some part to the lack of contraception and family planning services in many parts of the world. In many central African nations, for example, less than 20% of the population use any type of contraception. The shortage of contraceptive services is a particular problem in undeveloped countries, where more than 30% of pregnancies are unplanned. In these regions, resources such as food, clean water, and fuel are already in short supply and serious environmental degradation has already occurred.

As populations grow—driven in large part by unplanned pregnancies—competition increases for scarce resources. In response to the problem of overpopulation, international organizations such as the World Health Organization and the United Nations are making efforts to increase global awareness of contraception and to make contraceptive methods more readily available.

1. *Health risks.* When considering any contraceptive method, determine whether it may pose a risk to your health. For example, IUDs are not recommended for young women without children because of an increased risk of pelvic infection and subsequent infertility. Hormonal methods should be used only after a clinical evaluation of your medical history. Other methods have only minor and local side effects. Talk with your physician about the potential health effects of different methods for you.

2. *The implications of an unplanned pregnancy.* Many teens and young adults fail to consider how their life would be affected by an unexpected pregnancy. When considering contraception (or deciding whether to have sex in the first place), think about the potential consequences of your choices.

3. *STD risk.* STDs are another potential consequence of sex. In fact, several activities besides vaginal intercourse (such as oral sex) can put you at risk for an STD. Condom use is of critical importance whenever any risk of STDs is present. This is especially true when you are not in an exclusive, long-term relationship or if you are a woman taking the pill, because cervical changes that occur during hormone use may increase vulnerability to certain diseases. Abstinence or activities that don't involve intercourse or any other exchange of body fluids can be a satisfactory alternative for some people.

hysterectomy Total or partial surgical removal of the uterus.

Men's Involvement in Contraception

What can be done to increase men's involvement in contraception? Health care professionals are taking the following approaches:

• Develop programs and campaigns that stress the importance of information, counseling, and medical care relating to sexual and reproductive matters from adolescence on. Men are less likely than women to seek regular checkups, but regular care for men would benefit men in their own right and both men and women as individuals, couples, and families.

• Recruit and train male health workers, who can be important advocates and role models for healthful behaviors. Expand educational material and clinical

programs that focus on male contraception and reproductive health.

• Focus on men as obstacles to women's contraceptive use and as an untapped group of potential users. Educate men about the ways in which stereotypical views of male or female sexuality can inhibit good reproductive health for both men and women. Stress the importance of shared responsibility.

• Develop educational and clinical programs specifically targeted at young men. Men in their early twenties are most likely to engage in risky sexual behaviors and to have adverse reproductive health outcomes. Surveys indicate that most men use a condom the first time they have intercourse, but condom use subsequently

declines—and there is much greater reliance on female contraceptive methods.

What can individuals do? Men can increase their participation in contraception in the following ways:

• Initiate and support communication regarding contraception and STD protection.

• Buy and use condoms whenever appropriate.

• Help pay contraceptive costs.

• Be available for shared responsibility in the resolution of an unintended pregnancy, should one occur.

---

4. *Convenience and comfort level.* The hormonal methods are generally ranked high in this category, unless there are negative side effects and health risks or forgetting to take pills is a problem for you. If this is the case for you, a vaginal ring may be a good alternative to the pill. Some people think condom use disrupts spontaneity and lowers penile sensitivity. (Creative approaches to condom use and improved quality can decrease these concerns.) The diaphragm, cervical cap, contraceptive sponge, female condom, and spermicides can be inserted before intercourse begins but are still considered a significant inconvenience by some.

5. *Type of relationship.* Barrier methods require more motivation and sense of responsibility from *each* partner than hormonal methods do. When the method depends on the cooperation of one's partner, assertiveness is necessary, no matter how difficult. This is especially true in new relationships, when condom use is most important. When sexual activity is infrequent, a barrier method may make more sense than an IUD or one of the hormonal methods.

6. *Ease and cost of obtaining and maintaining each method.* Investigate the costs of different methods. If you have insurance, find out if it covers any of the costs.

7. *Religious or philosophical beliefs.* For some, abstinence and/or FAM may be the only permissible contraceptive methods.

Whatever your needs, circumstances, or beliefs, *do* make a choice about contraception. Not choosing anything is the one method known *not* to work. This is an area in which taking charge of your health has immediate and profound implications for your future.

THE ABORTION ISSUE

Few issues are as complex and emotionally charged as abortion. In the United States, public attention has focused on the legal definition of abortion and the issue of restricting its practice. These far-reaching questions are important, but the most difficult aspects of abortion are personal—especially for women who must decide whether to have an abortion.

The word **abortion,** by strict definition, means the expulsion of an embryo or fetus from the uterus before it is

QUESTIONS FOR CRITICAL THINKING AND REFLECTION
What are the most important factors influencing your personal decisions about contraception? List these factors in order of their priority to you, and determine whether you have given each factor full consideration in choosing a contraceptive method.

sufficiently developed to survive. As commonly used, however, the term *abortion* refers only to those expulsions that are artificially induced by mechanical means or drugs. The term **miscarriage** is generally used when referring to a *spontaneous abortion*—one that occurs naturally with no causal intervention. In this chapter, *abortion* refers to a deliberately induced expulsion.

The History of Abortion in the United States

For more than two centuries, abortion policy in the United States followed English common law, which made the practice a crime only when performed after "quickening" (fetal movement that begins at about 20 weeks).

Opposition to abortion attracted little attention until the mid-1800s, when newspaper advertisements for abortion preparations became common and concern grew that women were using abortion as a means of birth control or to cover up extramarital activity. By the 1900s abortion was illegal in every state. These anti-abortion laws stayed in effect until the 1960s, when courts began to invalidate them on the grounds of constitutional vagueness and violation of the right to privacy (see the box "Key Abortion Decisions and Legislation").

Current Legal Status

In 1973, the U.S. Supreme Court made abortion legal in the landmark case of *Roe v. Wade*. To replace the restrictions most states still imposed at that time, the justices devised new standards to govern abortion decisions. They divided pregnancy into three parts, or trimesters, giving a woman less choice about abortion as her pregnancy advances toward full term.

In the first trimester, the abortion decision must be left to the judgment of the pregnant woman and her physician. During the second trimester, similar rights remain up to the point when the fetus becomes **viable**—that is, capable of surviving outside of the uterus. Today, most clinicians define this point as 24 weeks of gestation. When the fetus is considered viable, a state may regulate and even bar all abortions except those considered necessary to preserve the mother's life or health.

Although abortion remains legal throughout the United States, subsequent rulings by the Supreme Court allow states to regulate abortion throughout pregnancy as long as an "undue burden" is not imposed on women seeking the procedure. As a result, states have passed a variety of laws that have had the effect of reducing women's access to abortion. Between 1995 and 2006, the number of state laws restricting abortion more than quadrupled. For example:

- In 24 states where pre-abortion counseling is required, counseling must be followed by a waiting period before an abortion can be performed.

- In 34 states, parents must give consent or at least be notified before a minor can undergo an abortion.

- 36 states prohibit abortions after a specified point in pregnancy except in cases where the mother's life or health is endangered, where the pregnancy is the result of rape or incest, or where severe fetal abnormalities have been detected. These restrictions and their exceptions vary by state.

- In 32 states and the District of Columbia, the use of state funds for abortions is restricted except when the mother's life is in danger or the pregnancy is the result of rape or incest.

Currently, 36 states have laws prohibiting abortion after a certain point in pregnancy, with exceptions, and 17 states provide nonfederal public money to assist some poor women seeking medically necessary abortions. Concerns have been raised that a two-tiered system has been created—one for women with means and another for those without.

Public Opinion

Some people strongly identify exclusively with either the pro-life or the pro-choice stance, but many have moral beliefs that are a mixture of the two. Many people instinctively feel that the fetus gains increasing human value as a pregnancy advances. In this view, first-trimester abortion is acceptable but later-term abortion should be performed only when the mother's health is in jeopardy. Although the most vocal groups in the abortion debate tend to paint a black-and-white picture, the majority of Americans view abortion as a complex issue without any easy answers.

In general, U.S. public opinion on abortion seems to change depending on the specific situation. Many individuals approve of legal abortion as an option when destructive health or welfare consequences could result from continuing pregnancy, but they do not advocate abortion as a simple way out of an inconvenient situation. Overall, most adults in the United States approve of legal abortion and are opposed to overturning the basic right to abortion established in *Roe v. Wade* (Figure 6.4 on page 143). However, the amount of public support varies considerably depending on the circumstances surrounding the abortion request.

Personal Considerations

For the pregnant woman who is considering abortion, the usual legal and moral arguments may sound meaningless

Key Abortion Decisions and Legislation

1700s to mid-1800s Abortion is generally legal throughout the United States.

Mid-1800s to mid-1900s Abortion becomes illegal in all 50 states, with certain exceptions that vary by state (for example, to save the life of the mother). The federal Comstock Act of 1873 makes it illegal to distribute or possess information about, or devices or medications for, contraception or abortion.

1965 *Griswold v. Connecticut:* The Supreme Court overturns a law prohibiting use of contraceptives by married couples, stating that it violates the right of marital privacy guaranteed in the Bill of Rights.

1967–1973 Some states rewrite their abortion laws, including four states that repeal abortion bans.

1972 *Eisenstadt v. Baird:* The Supreme Court overturns a law banning distribution of contraceptives to unmarried adults, stating that the ban violates the equal protection clause of the constitution.

1973 *Roe v. Wade:* The Supreme Court strikes down a Texas law banning abortion and rules that abortion is encompassed within the constitutional right to privacy.

1976 *Planned Parenthood of Central Missouri v. Danforth:* The Supreme Court rules against a statute that requires married women to obtain their spouse's approval before having an abortion and requires minors to obtain written parental consent.

1980 *Harris v. McRae:* The Supreme Court upholds restrictions on Medicaid

funding for abortions except as needed to protect the life of the mother or in other special circumstances.

1986 *Thornburgh v. American College of Obstetricians and Gynecologists:* The Supreme Court strikes down a law requiring any woman seeking an abortion to receive a state-scripted lecture from her physician about potential risks and possible alternatives.

1989 *Webster v. Reproductive Health Services:* The Supreme Court upholds a state law prohibiting the use of public facilities for abortions that are not medically necessary and requiring physicians to do viability testing on fetuses of more than 20 weeks' gestation.

1991 *Rust v. Sullivan:* The Supreme Court rules that clinics receiving federal Title X (family planning) funding can be prohibited from counseling, referring, or providing information about abortions.

1992 *Planned Parenthood of Southeastern Pennsylvania v. Casey:* The Supreme Court upholds the *Roe* decision but allows states to restrict abortion access as long as the restrictions do not impose an undue burden on women seeking abortions. It upholds a provision requiring minors to obtain consent from one parent or a judge (judicial bypass) to obtain an abortion.

1994 Congress passes the Freedom of Access to Clinics Act, making it a crime to injure, intimidate, or interfere through threats, force, or physical obstruction with a woman's right to obtain reproductive health services, including abortion.

2000 The FDA approves mifepristone (RU-486), the abortion pill.

2000 *Stenberg v. Carhart:* The Supreme Court finds a Nebraska law banning partial-birth abortion unconstitutional because it lacks an exception for the health of the mother and imposes an undue burden on women seeking abortions.

2003 Congress passes and President Bush signs the Partial Birth Abortion Ban Act with no exception to the ban in cases of risk to a woman's health.

2004 The Partial Birth Abortion Ban Act is declared unconstitutional by federal judges in San Francisco, New York, and Lincoln, Nebraska. Also, the Freedom of Choice Act (FOCA) is introduced in the Senate. At the federal level, FOCA would prohibit state and federal government entities from denying or interfering with a woman's right to choose to bear a child, to terminate a pregnancy before viability, or to terminate a pregnancy after viability when termination is necessary to protect the mother's life or health.

2007 *Gonzales v. Carhart:* The Supreme Court upholds the Partial Birth Abortion Ban Act and imposes a nationwide ban on a rare but controversial abortion procedure, called intact dilation and extraction (intact D & E).

SOURCES: Cornell University Legal Information Institute. 2009. *U.S. Supreme Court Decisions* (http://supct.law.cornell.edu/supct/; retrieved February 3, 2009); CBS News. 2007. *Abortion Timeline* (http://www.cbsnews.com/htdocs/abortion/timeline.html; retrieved February 3, 2009); National Public Radio. 2003. *History of the Abortion Debate: Timeline of Significant Supreme Court Decisions* (http://www.npr.org/news/specials/roevwade/timeline.html; retrieved February 3, 2009). Planned Parenthood. 2008. *Abortion Issues.* (http://www.plannedparenthood.org/issues-action/abortion-issues-5946.html; retrieved February 3, 2009).

QUICK STATS

42% of Americans identify themselves as pro-life; 53% identify themselves as pro-choice.

—Gallup, Inc., 2008

as she attempts to weigh the many short- and long-term ramifications for all lives directly concerned. If she chooses abortion, can she accept that decision in terms of her own religious and moral beliefs? What are her long-range feelings likely to be regarding this decision? What are her partner's feelings regarding abortion, and how will she deal with his response?

For the woman who decides against abortion and chooses instead to continue the pregnancy, there are other questions. If she decides to raise the child herself, will she have the resources to do it well? Is a supportive, lasting relationship with her partner likely? If not, how does she feel about being a single parent?

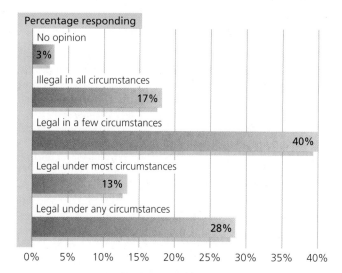

Percentage responding

No opinion
3%

Illegal in all circumstances
17%

Legal in a few circumstances
40%

Legal under most circumstances
13%

Legal under any circumstances
28%

0%   5%   10%   15%   20%   25%   30%   35%   40%

VITAL STATISTICS

FIGURE 6.4   Public opinion about abortion.

SOURCE: "Public Opinion About Abortion," from http://www.gallup.com/poll/
27628/Public-Divided-ProChoice-vs-ProLife-Abortion-Labels.aspx. Reprinted with
permission from Gallup, Inc.

If the pregnant woman considers adoption, she will have to try to predict what her emotional responses will be throughout the full-term pregnancy and the adoption process. What are her long-range feelings likely to be? What type of adoption would be most appropriate? (The box "The Adoption Option" addresses some of these questions.)

Abortion Statistics

Abortions are fairly common in the United States. Among American women, about 50% of all pregnancies are unintended; about 40% of such pregnancies end in abortion. About 22% of all pregnancies—wanted and unwanted—end in abortion, not including those that end in miscarriage. More than 45 million legal abortions were performed in the United States between 1973 and 2005.

After the Supreme Court's ruling in *Roe v. Wade,* the number of abortions rapidly increased in the United States (Figure 6.5). According to the Guttmacher Institute (a private organization that tracks statistics on contraception and abortion), nearly 750,000 abortions occurred in 1973; the number rose each year after that, until hitting a peak of 1.6 million in 1990. The number has steadily declined since then, with just over 1.2 million legal abortions reported in 2005, the most recent year for which data is available.

The number of late-term abortions has dropped over time, as well. In 2005, 89% of abortions occurred during the first 12 weeks (the first trimester) of pregnancy; about 1% were performed after the 20th week.

The Guttmacher Institute estimates that about 50% of American women will experience an unintended preg-

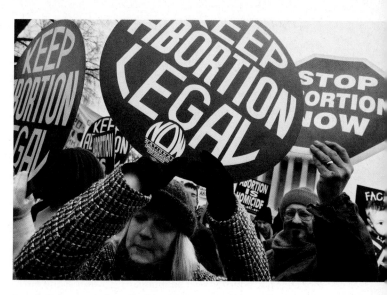

Pro-choice groups believe that the decision to end or continue a pregnancy is a personal matter. Pro-life groups oppose abortion on the basis of their belief that life begins at conception.

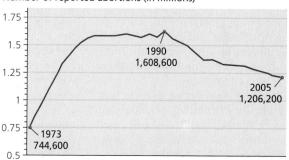

Number of reported abortions (in millions)

1.75

1.5

1.25

1

0.75

0.5

1990
1,608,600

2005
1,206,200

1973
744,600

VITAL STATISTICS

FIGURE 6.5   Number of reported abortions in the United States, 1973–2005.

SOURCE: Jones, R. K., et al. 2008. Abortion in the United States: Incidence and Access to Services, 2005. *Perspectives on Sexual and Reproductive Health* 40(1): 6–16.

nancy by age 45, and more than one-third will have an abortion. Based on national research, the majority of American women who get abortions share the following characteristics:

• Are under age 25

• Have previously given birth

• Have never been married

• Are poor

• Live in a metropolitan area

238 abortions were performed for every 1000 live births in the United States in 2004.

—CDC, 2008

QUICK STATS

The Adoption Option

Between 1952 and 1972, nearly 9% of unmarried pregnant women gave their children up for adoption; currently, however, less than 1% of women choose to place a child for adoption. This decline is probably due to a variety of factors, including increased rates of contraceptive use and an easing of the social stigma of single parenthood. The drop in adoption rates in the 1970s probably reflected an increase in the abortion rate following the 1973 legalization of abortion; however, since 1990 adoption rates have remained steady, while the abortion rate has declined, indicating that women are not choosing abortion over adoption.

If you are pregnant and considering adoption, make sure you explore all possibilities before you make a final choice. The decision to go through an unwanted pregnancy and then give the baby to another family is difficult and takes tremendous love, maturity, and courage. Adoption is permanent: The adoptive parents will raise your child and have legal authority for his or her welfare. Think about your life now and in the future as you weigh alternatives.

There are many people who can help you consider your options, including your partner, friends, family members, or a professional counselor at a crisis pregnancy center, a family planning clinic, or a family services, social services, or adoption agency. A counselor should always treat you with respect and be willing to discuss all your options with you—keeping the baby, having an abortion, or arranging an adoption.

There are two types of adoptions, confidential and open. In confidential adoption, the birth parents and the adoptive parents never know each other. Adoptive parents will be given any information, such as medical information, that they would need to help take care of the child. A later meeting between the child and birth parents is possible in confidential adoption, however, if the birth parents leave information with the agency or lawyer who handled the adoption and/or in a national adoption registry.

In an open adoption, the birth parents and adoptive parents know something about each other. There are different levels of openness, ranging from reading a brief description of prospective adoptive parents to meeting them and sharing full information. Birth parents may also be able to stay in touch with the family by visiting, calling, or writing.

In all states, you can work with a licensed child-placing (adoption) agency. In most, you can also work directly with an adopting couple or their attorney; this is called a private or independent adoption. Prospective adoptive parents can be located through personal ads, a physician, adoptive parent support groups, national matching services, and family members and friends.

You will also need to consider the reaction and rights of the birth father. A woman can choose to have an abortion without the consent or knowledge of the father, but once the baby is born, the father has certain rights. These rights vary from state to state but, at a minimum, most states require that the birth father be notified of the adoption.

As with abortion, there are emotional and physical risks associated with pregnancy, childbirth, and adoption. Throughout the adoption process, make sure that you have the help you need and that you carefully consider all your options. Deciding how to handle an unplanned pregnancy is important, and you have the power to make your own decisions.

SOURCES: Child Welfare Information Gateway. 2007. *Are You Pregnant and Thinking About Adoption?* (http://www.childwelfare.gov/pubs/f _pregna/index.cfm; retrieved February 3, 2009); Child Welfare Information Gateway. 2006. *Voluntary Relinquishment for Adoption: Numbers and Trends* (http://www.childwelfare.gov/pubs/s _place.cfm; retrieved February 3, 2009).

Black and Hispanic women are more likely to have an abortion than white women. This disparity is likely due to limited access to and funds for contraception. Figure 6.6 provides some more statistical information about American women who choose to have abortions.

Methods of Abortion

Abortion methods can be divided into two categories: surgical and medical. Surgical abortion is by far the most common, accounting for about 87% of all abortions performed in the United States in 2005. Medical abortion, in which one or more drugs are used to induce abortion, accounted for 13% of all U.S. abortions in 2005.

First developed in China in 1958, **suction curettage** (commonly known as *dilation and curettage*, or *D & C*) is the most common method for abortions performed from the 6th to the 12th week of pregnancy. It is used in about 90% of all abortions performed in the United States. The procedure can be done quickly, usually on an outpatient basis, and the risk of complications is small.

A sedative may be given, along with a local anesthetic. A speculum is inserted into the vagina, and the cervix is cleansed with a surgical solution. The cervix is dilated and a suction curette, a specially designed tube, is then inserted into the uterus. The curette is attached to the rubber tubing of an electric pump, and suction is applied.

QUESTIONS FOR CRITICAL THINKING AND REFLECTION

What are your views on abortion? How have these views been shaped throughout your life? Have you had any personal experience with abortion, or know someone who has? If so, how did this experience help to shape your views?

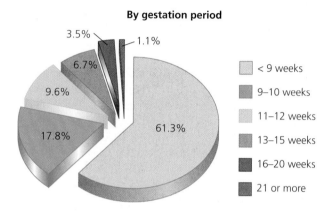

By woman's age

17%

50%

33%

19 and under

20–24

25 and over

By gestation period

3.5%

1.1%

6.7%

9.6%

17.8%

61.3%

< 9 weeks

9–10 weeks

11–12 weeks

13–15 weeks

16–20 weeks

21 or more

VITAL STATISTICS

FIGURE 6.6   Distribution of abortions by the woman's age and by the weeks of gestation: 2005.

SOURCE: Guttmacher Institute. 2008. *In Brief: Facts on Induced Abortion in the United States* (http://www.guttmacher.org/pubs/fb_induced_abortion.html; retrieved February 3, 2009).

In 20–30 seconds, the uterus is emptied. Moderate cramping is common during evacuation. To ensure that no fragments of tissue are left in the uterus, the doctor usually scrapes the uterine lining with a metal curette, an instrument with a spoonlike tip. The entire suction curettage procedure takes 5–10 minutes.

For more than 30 years, gynecologists have used **manual vacuum aspiration (MVA)** to manage incomplete abortions, for endometrial sampling in nonpregnant women, and for elective abortion. During this procedure, as in suction curettage, the woman receives a local anesthetic and her cervix is dilated. A plastic tube attached to a handheld syringe is inserted through the cervix and into the uterus. The syringe provides gentle suction, which empties the uterus.

MVA has several advantages over the traditional D & C. Manual vacuum aspiration may be used earlier in pregnancy, can be performed in the office, and does not require an electric pump or additional equipment. It is also significantly cheaper than suction curettage, does not re-

quire electricity, and can be performed by mid-level providers such as midwives and nurses. For these reasons, MVA is ideal for low-resource settings. A number of recent studies have shown that the two techniques have equivalent safety profiles and low rates of complications when done up to 10 weeks of gestation.

Multi-fetal (twin and higher multiple) pregnancies are associated with high fetal morbidity and mortality rates. **Multi-fetal pregnancy reduction (MFPR)** is a procedure that reduces the number of fetuses in a multiple pregnancy. It is usually performed during the first trimester. In the most common method of MFPR, the fetal heart is injected with potassium chloride. The dead fetus is then absorbed by the mother's body. Multi-fetal reduction reduces the risk of preterm delivery for the remaining fetus and improves maternal pregnancy outcomes.

Only about one in ten abortions is performed after the 12th week of pregnancy. The method most commonly used for abortion from 13 to 24 weeks of pregnancy is **dilation and evacuation (D & E)**. The cervix is opened using dilators, which gradually expand the cervix overnight. The next day, the uterus is emptied using surgical instruments and an aspirating machine.

Intact dilation and extraction (known controversially as *partial birth abortion*) is a surgical abortion wherein an intact fetus is removed from the uterus. Occasionally, the skull is collapsed after fetal limbs and body are delivered to allow it to pass more easily through the cervix. This procedure is performed only rarely, representing 0.17% of all abortions in the United States. Experts say that intact dilation and extraction can be useful when certain fetal anomalies are present, such as severe hydrocephalus (swelling of the fetus's head), and that the procedure may be the safest option for the mother in some circumstances. Intact dilation and extraction became illegal after the 2007 Supreme Court ruling in the case of *Gonzales v. Carhart*, even in situations where the mother's health may be in jeopardy.

Medical abortion is generally used in very early pregnancy, within 49 days of the last menstrual period. The

suction curettage   Removal of the embryo or fetus by means of suction; also called *dilation and curettage (D & C)*.

manual vacuum aspiration (MVA)   The vacuum aspiration of uterine contents shortly after a missed period using a handheld syringe.

multi-fetal pregnancy reduction (MFPR)   A method of abortion used to reduce the number of fetuses in a multiple-fetus pregnancy.

dilation and evacuation (D & E)   The method of abortion most commonly used between 13 and 24 weeks of pregnancy. Following dilation of the cervix, both vacuum aspiration and curettage instruments are used as needed.

intact dilation and extraction   A rarely used method of late-term abortion, wherein an intact fetus is removed from the uterus.

TERMS

combination of drugs that is given causes the embryo and products of conception to be passed out through the vagina, as in a natural miscarriage. Mifepristone, misoprostol, and methotrexate are three widely used drugs.

Medical abortion is generally safer than surgical abortion because it involves no anesthesia or surgical risks. Some women feel that medical abortion allows them to take more control of the procedure and gives them more privacy than a surgical abortion would. The major disadvantages are that the process takes days or even weeks to complete and that bleeding after the procedure is often heavier and lasts longer than with surgical abortion. Medical abortion also generally requires more clinic visits than surgical abortion. The cost to the patient is generally about the same.

Complications of Abortion

Along with questions regarding the actual procedure of abortion, many people have concerns about possible aftereffects. More information is gradually being gathered on this important subject.

Possible Physical Effects   The incidence of immediate problems following an abortion (infection, bleeding, trauma to the cervix or uterus, and incomplete abortion requiring repeat curettage) varies widely. The potential for problems is significantly reduced by a woman's good health, early timing of the abortion, use of the suction method, performance by a well-trained clinician, and the availability and use of prompt follow-up care.

Problems related to infection can be minimized through preabortion testing and treatment for gonorrhea, chlamydia, and other infections. Postabortion danger signs are fever above 100°F; abdominal pain or swelling, cramping, or backache, abdominal tenderness (to pressure), prolonged or heavy bleeding, foul-smelling vaginal discharge, vomiting or fainting, delay in resuming menstrual periods (6 weeks or more).

QUESTIONS FOR CRITICAL THINKING AND REFLECTION

What is your stand on the issue of late-term abortion? Do you feel it is never acceptable, or is it acceptable under certain circumstances? If so, what are those circumstances?

Some cramping and bleeding are an expected part of ending a pregnancy. In rare cases, life-threatening bleeding, infections, or other problems can occur following a miscarriage, surgical abortion, or medical abortion. Prompt medical attention should be sought if heavy bleeding, severe abdominal pain, or fever occurs.

Possible Psychological Effects   After an exhaustive review completed in 1988, the then surgeon general, C. Everett Koop, concluded that the available evidence failed to demonstrate either a negative or a positive long-term impact of abortion on mental health. More recent research has resulted in the same general conclusion. The frequency of any psychiatric diagnoses in women who have undergone an abortion procedure is no higher than in women with no such history.

TIPS FOR TODAY AND THE FUTURE

Your decisions about contraception are among the most important you will make in your life. You may never have to face an unintended pregnancy, but you should know what choices you would have, as well as where you stand on the issue of abortion.

RIGHT NOW YOU CAN

- Visualize the kind of life you want to have in the future. Does your vision include a family? If so, how far in the future do you see this happening? If you're sexually active now, are you confident that you're doing everything possible to prevent an unwanted pregnancy? Remember that no method of contraception is 100% effective.
- If you're sexually active, discuss your contraceptive method with your partner. Make sure you are using the method that works best for you.
- Work with your partner to choose a backup contraceptive method to use in case your primary method isn't effective enough.
- Examine your feelings about the possibility of becoming a parent, especially if it were to happen unintentionally.
- Consider your views on the morality of abortion, and whether it is acceptable under certain circumstances.

IN THE FUTURE YOU CAN

- Talk to your physician about contraception and get his or her advice on choosing the best method.
- Occasionally discuss your contraceptive method with your partner to make sure it continues to meet your needs. A change in health status or lifestyle may make a different form of contraception preferable in the future.
- If you are sexually active or plan to become sexually active, talk to your partner about abortion. Do you share similar views and feelings, or are they different? How would you resolve conflicts about this issue?

QUESTIONS FOR CRITICAL THINKING AND REFLECTION

Suppose you are in the position of lending support to a friend who has gone through an abortion. What sort of physical or emotional signals would you look for? What kind of support would you be willing to offer?

The psychological side effects of abortion, however, are less clearly defined than the physical ones. Responses vary and depend on the individual woman's psychological makeup, family background, current personal and social relationships, cultural attitudes, and many other factors. A woman who has specific goals with a somewhat structured life may be able to incorporate her decision to have an abortion as the unequivocally best and most acceptable course more easily than a woman who feels uncertain about her future.

Although many women experience great relief after an abortion and virtually no negative feelings, some go through a period of ambivalence. Along with relief, they often feel a mixture of other responses, such as guilt, regret, loss, sadness, and/or anger. For a woman who experiences psychological or emotional effects after an abortion, talking with a close friend or family member can be very helpful. Supportive people can help her feel positive about herself and her decision. Unresolved emotions may persist, and a woman should seek professional counseling.

SUMMARY

- The choice of contraceptive method depends on effectiveness, convenience, cost, reversibility, side effects and risk factors, and protection against STDs.

- Hormonal methods may include a combination of estrogen and progestins or progesterone alone. Hormones may be delivered via pills, patch, vaginal ring, implants, or injections. They prevent ovulation, inhibit the movement of sperm, and affect the uterine lining so that implantation is prevented.

- The most commonly used emergency contraceptives are two-dose regimens of OCs and Plan B, which is now available without a prescription to women 18 and older.

- IUDs may cause biochemical changes in the uterus, affect movement of sperm and eggs, or interfere with the implantation of the egg in the uterus.

- Male condoms are simple to use, immediately reversible, and provide STD protection; female condoms are available but are more difficult to use.

- The diaphragm, Lea's Shield, cervical cap, and contraceptive sponge cover the cervix and block sperm from entering; all are used with or contain spermicide.

- Vaginal spermicides come in the form of foams, creams, jellies, suppositories, and film.

- So-called natural methods include abstinence, withdrawal, and fertility awareness method (FAM).

- Vasectomy—male sterilization—involves severing the vasa deferentia. Female sterilization involves severing or blocking the oviducts.

- Issues to be considered in choosing a contraceptive include the individual health risks of each method, the implications of an unplanned pregnancy, STD risk, convenience and comfort level, type of relationship, the cost and ease of obtaining and maintaining each method, and religious or philosophical beliefs.

- The 1973 *Roe v. Wade* Supreme Court case devised new standards to govern abortion decisions; based on the trimesters of pregnancy, it limited a woman's choices as her pregnancy advanced.

- Although the Supreme Court continued to uphold its 1973 decision, later rulings gave states further power to regulate abortion.

- The controversy between pro-life and pro-choice viewpoints focuses on the issue of when life begins. Overall public opinion in the United States supports legal abortion in at least some circumstances and opposes overturning *Roe v. Wade*.

- Methods of abortion include suction curettage, manual vacuum aspiration, dilation and evacuation, and dilation and extraction.

- Physical complications following abortion can be minimized by overall good patient health, early timing, use of the suction method, a well-trained physician, and follow-up care. Psychological aftereffects of abortion vary with the individual.

FOR MORE INFORMATION

BOOKS

Alters, S. M., ed. 2008. *Abortion: An Eternal Social and Moral Issue.* Farmington Hills, Mich.: Gale Cengage. *A brief reference outlining legal, political, and ethical issues.*

Guillebaud, J. 2007. *Contraception Today,* 6th ed. London: Informa Healthcare. *A pocket guide popular with clinicians, but also useful to the layperson.*

Hatcher, R. A., et al. 2008. *Contraceptive Technology,* 19th ed. New York: Ardent Media. *A reliable source of up-to-date information on contraception.*

National Abortion and Reproductive Rights Action League Foundation. 2008. *Who Decides? A State-by-State Review of Abortion and Reproductive Rights.* Washington, D.C.: NARAL Foundation. *An in-depth annual review of the legal status of reproductive rights in the United States.*

Zieman, M., et al. 2007. *A Pocket Guide to Managing Contraception,* 2007–2009 ed. Tiger, Ga.: Bridging the Gap Foundation. *An easy-to-use, reliable source of contraceptive information.*

ORGANIZATIONS AND WEB SITES

Association of Reproductive Health Professionals. Offers educational materials about family planning, contraception, and other reproductive health issues; the Web site includes an interactive questionnaire to help people choose contraceptive methods.

    http://www.arhp.org

Emergency Contraception Web Site. Provides extensive information about emergency contraception; sponsored by the Office of Population Research at Princeton University.

    http://www.not-2-late.com

The Guttmacher Institute. A nonprofit institute for reproductive health research, policy analysis, and public education.

    http://www.agi-usa.org

It's Your Sex Life. Provides information about sexuality, relationships, contraceptives, and STDs; geared toward teenagers and young adults.

    http://www.itsyoursexlife.com

MedlinePlus: Abortion. Managed by the National Library of Medicine and the National Institutes of Health, this site provides a list of informational resources on various aspects of abortion.

    http://www.nlm.nih.gov/medlineplus/abortion.html

National Abortion and Reproductive Rights Action League. Provides information on the politics of the pro-choice movement. Also provides information on the abortion laws and politics in each state.

    http://www.naral.org

National Abortion Federation. Provides information and resources on the medical and political issues relating to abortion; managed by health care providers.

    http://www.prochoice.org

National Adoption Center. A national agency focused on finding adoptive homes for children with special needs or who are currently in foster care.

    http://www.adopt.org

National Right to Life Committee. Provides information on alternatives to abortion and the politics of the pro-life movement.

    http://www.nrlc.org

Planned Parenthood Federation of America. Provides information on family planning, contraception, and abortion and provides counseling services.

    http://www.plannedparenthood.org

SELECTED BIBLIOGRAPHY

Advance provision of emergency contraception for pregnancy prevention (full review). 2007. *Cochrane Database of Systematic Reviews* (2): CD005497.

Boonstra, H., et al. 2006. *Abortion in Women's Lives.* New York: Guttmacher Institute.

Broen, A. N., et al. 2006. Predictors of anxiety and depression following pregnancy termination: A longitudinal five-year follow-up study. *Acta Obstetricia et Gynecologica Scandinavica* 85(3): 317–323.

Brohet, R. M., et al. 2007. Oral contraceptives and breast cancer risk in the international BRCA 1/2 carrier cohort study: A report from EMBRACE, GENEPSO, GEO-HEBON, and the IBCCS Collaborating Group. *Journal of Clinical Oncology* 25(25): 3831–3836.

Burkman, R. T. 2007. Transdermal hormonal contraception: Benefits and risks. *American Journal of Obstetrics and Gynecology* 197(2): 134.e1–134.e6.

Chen A., et al. 2004. Mifepristone-induced early abortion and outcome of subsequent wanted pregnancy. *American Juornal of Epidemiology* 160(2): 110–117.

Coffee, A. L., et al. 2007. Long-term assessment of symptomatology and satisfaction of an extended oral contraceptive regimen. *Contraception* 75(6): 444–449.

Cohen, S. A. 2007. New Data on Abortion Incidence, Safety Illuminate Key Aspects of Worldwide Abortion Debate. *Guttmacher Policy Review* 10(4): 2–5.

Cook, L. A., et al. 2007. Vasectomy occlusion techniques for male sterilization. *Cochrane Database of Systematic Reviews,* 18 April (2): CD003991.

Frost, J. J., et al. 2007. Factors associated with contraceptive use and nonuse, United States, 2004. *Perspectives on Sexual and Reproductive Health* 39(2): 90–99.

Grimes, D. A. 2006. Estimation of pregnancy-related mortality risk by pregnancy outcome, United States, 1991 to 1999. *American Journal of Obstetrics and Gynecology* 194(1): 92–94.

Grimes, D. A., et al. 2006. Unsafe Abortion: The preventable pandemic. *Lancet* 368: 908–919.

Guttmacher Institute. 2008. *Facts on Induced Abortion in the United States.* (http://www.guttmacher.org/pubs/fb_induced_abortion.html; retrieved February 3, 2009).

Guttmacher Institute. 2009. *An Overview of Abortion Laws: State Policies in Brief* (http://www.guttmacher.org/statecenter/spibs/spib_OAL.pdf; retrieved February 3, 2009).

Ho, P. C. 2006. Women's perceptions on medical abortion. *Contraception* 74(1): 11–15.

International Planned Parenthood. 2007. *The Health Dangers of Unsafe Abortion* (http://www.ippf.org/en/Resources/Articles/The+health+dangers+of +unsafe+abortion.htm; retrieved February 3, 2009).

Isley, M. M., and A. Edelman. 2007. Contraceptive implants: An overview and update. *Obstetrics and Gynecology Clinics of North America* 34(1): 73–90.

Macaluso, M., et al. 2007. Efficacy of the male latex condom and of the female polyurethane condom as barriers to semen during intercourse: A randomized clinical trial. *American Journal of Epidemiology* 166(1): 88–96.

MacIsaac, L., and E. Espey. 2007. Intrauterine contraception: The pendulum swings back. *Obstetrics and Gynecology Clinics of North America* 34(1): 91–111.

Moreau, C., et al. 2007. Oral contraceptive tolerance: Does the type of pill matter? *Obstetrics and Gynecology* 109(6): 1277–1285.

Nettleman, M. D., et al. 2007. Reasons for unprotected intercourse: Analysis of the PRAMS survey. *Contraception* 75(5): 361–366.

Planned Parenthood. 2007. *Abortion After the First Trimester in the United States* (http://www.plannedparenthood.org/news-articles-press/politics-policy-issues/abortion-access/trimester-abortion-6140.htm; retrieved February 3, 2009).

Rocca, C. H., et al. 2007. Beyond access: Acceptability, use and nonuse of emergency contraception among young women. *American Journal of Obstetrics and Gynecology* 196(1): 29.e1–29.e6.

Roumen, F. J. 2007. The contraceptive vaginal ring compared with the combined oral contraceptive pill: A comprehensive review of randomized controlled trials. *Contraception* 75(6): 420–429.

Sit, D., et al. 2007. Psychiatric outcomes following medical and surgical abortion. *Human Reproduction* 22(3):878–884.

Swica, Y. 2007. The transdermal patch and the vaginal ring: Two novel methods of combined hormonal contraception. *Obstetrics and Gynecology Clinics of North America* 34(1): 31–42.

Westhoff, C. L., et al. 2007. Oral contraceptive discontinuation: Do side effects matter? *American Journal of Obstetrics and Gynecology* 196(4): 412.e1–412.e6; discussion 412.e6–412.e7.

Zurawin, R. K., and L. Ayensu-Coker. 2007. Innovations in contraception: A review. *Clinical Obstetrics and Gynecology* 50(2): 425–439.

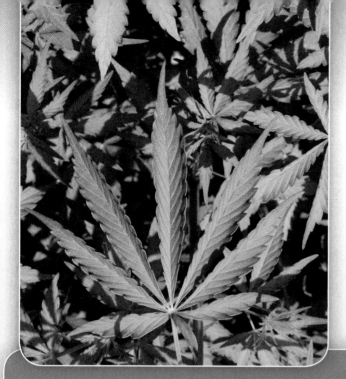

LOOKING AHEAD>>>>>

AFTER READING THIS CHAPTER, YOU SHOULD BE ABLE TO:

- Define and discuss the concepts of addictive behavior, substance abuse, and substance dependence

- Explain factors contributing to drug use and dependence

- List the major categories of psychoactive drugs and describe their effects, methods of use, and potential for abuse and dependence

- Discuss social issues related to psychoactive drug use and its prevention and treatment

- Evaluate the role of drugs and other addictive behaviors in your life and identify your risk factors for abuse or dependence

THE USE AND ABUSE OF PSYCHOACTIVE DRUGS

7

The use of **drugs** for both medical and social purposes is widespread in America (Table 7.1). Many people believe that every problem has or should have a chemical solution. For fatigue, many turn to caffeine; for insomnia, sleeping pills; for anxiety or boredom, alcohol or other recreational drugs. Advertisements, social pressures, and the human desire for quick solutions to life's difficult problems all contribute to the prevailing attitude that drugs can ease all pain. Unfortunately, using drugs can—and often does—have serious consequences.

The most serious consequences are abuse and **addiction.** The drugs most often associated with abuse are **psychoactive drugs**—those that alter a person's experiences or consciousness. In the short term, psychoactive drugs can cause **intoxication,** a state in which sometimes unpredictable physical and emotional changes occur. A person who is intoxicated may experience serious changes in physical functioning. His or her emotions and judgment may be affected in ways that lead to uncharacteristic and

unsafe behavior. In the long term, recurrent drug use can have profound physical, emotional, and social effects.

ADDICTIVE BEHAVIOR

Although addiction is most often associated with drug use, many experts now extend the concept of addiction to other behaviors. **Addictive behaviors** are habits that have gotten out of control, with resulting negative effects on a person's health.

What Is Addiction?

Historically, the term *addiction* was applied only when the habitual use of a drug produced chemical changes in the user's body. One such change is physical tolerance, in which the body adapts to a drug so that the initial dose no longer produces the original emotional or psychological effects. This process, caused by chemical changes, means

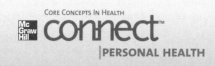

Table 7.1 — Nonmedical Drug Use Among Americans, 2007

	Percentage Using Substance in the Past 30 Days	
	College Students (age 18–25)	All Americans (age 12 and older)
Illicit Drugs	19.7	8.0
Tobacco (all forms)	41.8	28.6
Cigarettes	36.2	24.2
Smokeless tobacco	5.3	3.2
Cigars	11.8	5.4
Pipe tobacco	1.2	0.8
Alcohol	61.2	51.1
Binge alcohol use	41.8	23.3
Marijuana and hashish	16.4	5.8
Cocaine	1.7	0.8
Crack	0.2	0.2
Heroin	0.1	0.1
Methamphetamine	0.4	0.2
Hallucinogens	1.5	0.4
LSD	0.2	0.1
PCP	0.0	0.0
Ecstasy	0.7	0.2
Inhalants	0.4	0.2
Nonmedical use of psychotherapeutics	6.0	2.8
Pain relievers	4.6	2.1
OxyContin	0.5	0.1
Tranquilizers	1.7	0.7
Stimulants	1.1	0.4
Sedatives	0.2	0.1

SOURCE: Office of Applied Studies, Substance Abuse and Mental Health Services Administration. 2008. *Results from the 2007 National Survey on Drug Use and Health: National Findings* (http://oas.samhsa.gov/nsduh.htm; retrieved February 3, 2009).

the user has to take larger and larger doses of the drug to achieve the same high. The concept of addiction as a disease process, one based in brain chemistry rather than a moral failing, has led to many advances in the understanding and treatment of drug addiction.

As scientists have learned about addictive behaviors, they have been able to distinguish between different levels of addiction. In particular, the concepts of drug addiction and drug **habituation** have been defined over the past few decades to help explain how drug use impacts people's lives in different ways. These two terms are often differentiated as follows:

- *Drug addiction* is defined by four important characteristics: the compulsive desire for a drug, the need to increase the dosage associated with psychological and physical dependence, harmful effects to the individual, and harm to society.

- *Drug habituation* (or habit) is often considered to mean a lesser version of addiction. It is defined by the routine use of a drug without reaching the level of compulsion or increased need for greater dosage associated with drug addiction. Further, drug habituation is accompanied by psychological but not physical dependence.

Distinguishing among different levels of drug addiction is important for developing and implementing successful prevention and treatment strategies. These definitions, however, are under continual debate.

Some scientists think that other behaviors may share some of the chemistry of drug addiction. They suggest that activities like gambling, eating, exercising, and sex trigger the release of brain chemicals that cause a pleasurable rush in much the same way that psychoactive drugs do. The brain's own chemicals thus become the "drug" that can cause addiction. These theorists suggest that all addictions have a common mechanism in the brain. In this view, addiction is partly the result of our own natural wiring. This view does not mean that people are not responsible for their addictive behavior, however.

Characteristics of Addictive Behavior

Experts have identified some general characteristics typically associated with addictive behaviors:

- *Reinforcement.* Addictive behaviors are reinforcing. Some aspect of the behavior produces pleasurable physical and/or emotional states or relieves negative ones.

- *Compulsion or craving.* The individual feels a strong compulsion—a compelling need—to engage in the behavior, often accompanied by obsessive planning for the next opportunity to perform it.

- *Loss of control.* The individual loses control over the behavior and cannot block the impulse to do it.

- *Escalation.* Addiction often involves a pattern of escalation, in which more and more of a particular substance or activity is required to produce its desired effects.

- *Negative consequences.* The behavior continues despite serious negative consequences, such as problems with academic or job performance, personal relationships, and health; legal or financial troubles are also typical.

The Development of Addiction

An addiction often starts when a person does something to bring pleasure or avoid pain. The activity may be drinking a beer, using the Internet, playing the lottery, or going shopping. If it works, the person is likely to repeat it. He

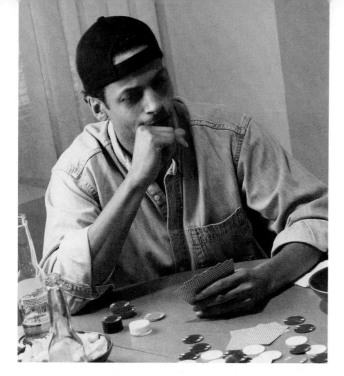

Many college students have gotten caught up in the poker craze. By some estimates, the number of college-age poker players has doubled in recent years.

or she becomes increasingly dependent on the behavior, and tolerance may develop—that is, the person needs more of the behavior to feel the same effect. Eventually, the behavior becomes a central focus of the person's life, and there is a deterioration in other areas, such as school performance or relationships. The behavior no longer brings pleasure, but it is necessary to avoid the pain of going without it. What started as a seemingly innocent way of feeling good can become a prison.

Although many common behaviors are potentially addictive, most people who engage in them do not develop problems. The reason lies in the combination of factors that are involved in the development of addiction, including personality, lifestyle, heredity, the social and physical environment, and the nature of the substance or behavior in question.

Characteristics of People with Addictions

The causes and course of an addiction are extremely varied, but people with addictions seem to share some characteristics. Many use a substance or activity as a substitute for healthier coping strategies. People vary in their ability to manage their lives, and those who have the most trouble dealing with stress and painful emotions may be more susceptible to addiction.

Some people may have a genetic predisposition to addiction to a particular substance; such predispositions may involve variations in brain chemistry. People with

addictive disorders usually have a distinct preference for a particular addictive behavior. They also often have problems with impulse control and self-regulation and tend to be risk takers.

Examples of Addictive Behaviors

Some behaviors that are not related to drugs can become addictive for some people.

Compulsive or Pathological Gambling Compulsive gamblers cannot control the urge to gamble, even in the face of financial and personal ruin. Most compulsive gamblers seek excitement even more than money. Increasingly larger bets are necessary to produce the desired level of excitement. When financial resources become strained, the person may lie or steal to pay off debts. The consequences of compulsive gambling are not just financial; the suicide rate of compulsive gamblers is 20 times higher than that of the general population.

The American Psychiatric Association (APA) recognizes pathological gambling as a mental disorder and lists ten characteristic behaviors, including preoccupation with gambling, unsuccessful efforts to cut back or quit, and lying to family members to conceal the extent of involvement with gambling. Gambling is often linked to other risky behaviors, and many compulsive gamblers also have drug and alcohol abuse problems.

In the United States, an estimated 1% of adults are compulsive (pathological) gamblers, and another 2% are

TERMS

drug Any chemical other than food intended to affect the structure or function of the body.

addiction Psychological or physical dependence on a substance or behavior, characterized by a compulsive desire and increasing need for the substance or behavior and by harm to the individual and/or society.

psychoactive drug A drug that can alter a person's consciousness or experience.

intoxication The state of being mentally affected by a chemical (literally, a state of being poisoned).

addictive behavior Any habit that has gotten out of control, resulting in a negative effect on one's health.

habituation Similar to addiction, involving the routine use of a substance, but without the level of compulsion or increasing need that characterizes addiction.

"problem gamblers." In a recent survey of more than 10,000 students from more than 100 colleges, 42% of students reported having gambled at least once in the past year, and about 3% reported gambling at least once a week.

Compulsive Exercising Compulsive exercising has been widely studied and is now recognized as a serious departure from normal behavior. It is often accompanied by more severe psychiatric disorders such as anorexia nervosa or bulimia. Traits frequently associated with compulsive exercising include an excessive preoccupation and dissatisfaction with body image, the use of laxatives or vomiting to lose weight, and the development of other obsessive-compulsive symptoms.

Experts don't completely agree on what frequency and intensity of physical activity constitute compulsive exercising. Many compulsive exercisers, however, get involved in physical activities that cause bodily harm. For example, research has shown that professional bodybuilders, when compared to recreational exercisers engaged in weight lifting, are often dissatisfied with muscle size. Because of the frequency and intensity of their workouts, some bodybuilders face an increased risk of injuries due to harmful weight-lifting practices.

Work Addiction The term *workaholic* is often used to describe individuals with an excessive preoccupation with work and work-related activities. Work addiction, however, is actually based on a set of symptoms, including: an intense work schedule, the inability to limit one's own work schedule, the inability to relax, even when away from work, and failed attempts at curtailing the intensity of work, (in some cases).

Someone suffering from work addiction is likely to neglect other areas of his or her life. For example, work addicts may tend to exercise less, spend less time with family and friends, and stay away from social activities.

Further, work addiction typically coincides with a well-known risk factor for cardiovascular disease—the Type A personality. Traits associated with Type A personality include competitiveness, ambition, drive, time urgency, restlessness, and hyperalertness.

Sex and Love Addiction Some researchers believe that the initial rush of arousal and erotic or romantic chemistry produces an effect in the brain comparable to that of taking amphetamines or morphine. After a time, the brain becomes desensitized, and the addict must then seek his or her next rush by pursuing a new partner. Behaviors associated with sex addiction include an extreme preoccupation with sex, a compulsion to have sex repeatedly within a short period of time, spending a great deal of time and energy looking for partners or engaging in sex, using sex as a means of relieving painful feelings, and suffering negative emotional, personal, and professional consequences as a result of sexual activities.

QUESTIONS FOR CRITICAL THINKING AND REFLECTION

Have you ever repeatedly or compulsively engaged in a behavior that had negative consequences? What was the behavior, and why did you continue? Did you ever worry that you were losing control? Were you able to bring the behavior under control?

Even therapists who challenge the concept of sex addiction recognize that some people become overly preoccupied with sex, cannot seem to control their sex drive, and act in potentially harmful ways in order to obtain satisfaction. This pattern of sexual behavior seems to meet the criteria for addictive behaviors discussed earlier.

Compulsive Buying or Shopping A compulsive buyer repeatedly gives in to the impulse to buy more than he or she needs or can afford. Compulsive spenders usually buy luxury items rather than daily necessities. They are usually distressed by their behavior and its social, personal, and financial consequences. Some experts link compulsive shopping with neglect or abuse during childhood; it also seems to be associated with eating disorders, depression, and bipolar disorder.

Internet Addiction Millions of Americans have become compulsive Internet users. Internet addicts skip important school, social, or recreational activities; they often spend their work time online, which has led many employers to adopt strict Internet usage policies. Despite negative financial, social, or academic consequences, compulsive Internet users don't feel able to stop. As with other addictive behaviors, online addicts may be using their behavior to alleviate stress or avoid painful emotions.

According to a 2006 study, 5–10% of the U.S. population may experience Internet addiction. Another study showed that Internet addicts spent an average of 38 hours online every week.

Other behaviors that can become addictive include eating, watching TV, and playing video games. Any substance or activity that becomes the focus of a person's life at the expense of other needs and interests can be damaging to health.

DRUG USE, ABUSE, AND DEPENDENCE

Drugs are chemicals other than food that are intended to affect the structure or function of the body. They include prescription medicines such as antibiotics and antidepressants; nonprescription or over-the-counter (OTC) substances such as alcohol, tobacco, and caffeine products; and illegal substances such as LSD and heroin.

Drug Abuse and Dependence

The APA's *Diagnostic and Statistical Manual of Mental Disorders* is the authoritative reference for defining all sorts of behavioral disorders, including those related to drugs. The APA has chosen not to use the term *addiction*, in part because it is so broad and has so many connotations. Instead, the APA refers to two forms of substance (drug) disorders: substance abuse and substance dependence. Both are maladaptive patterns of substance use that lead to significant impairment or distress. Although the APA's definitions are more precise and more directly related to drug use, they clearly encompass the general characteristics of addictive behavior described in the preceding section.

Abuse   As defined by the APA, **substance abuse** involves one or more of the following:

- Recurrent drug use, resulting in a failure to fulfill major responsibilities at work, school, or home
- Recurrent drug use in situations in which it is physically hazardous, such as before or while driving a car
- Recurrent drug-related legal problems
- Continued drug use despite persistent social or interpersonal problems caused or exacerbated by the effects of the drug

The pattern of use may be constant or intermittent, and **physical dependence** may or may not be present. For example, a person who smokes marijuana once a week and cuts classes because he or she is high is abusing marijuana, even though he or she is not physically dependent.

Dependence   Substance dependence is a more complex disorder and is what many people associate with the idea of addiction. The seven specific criteria the APA uses to diagnose substance dependence are listed below. The first two are associated with physical dependence; the final five are associated with compulsive use. To be considered dependent, one must experience a cluster of three or more of these symptoms during a 12-month period.

1. *Developing tolerance to the substance.* When a person requires increased amounts of a substance to achieve the desired effect or notices a markedly diminished effect with continued use of the same amount, he or she has developed **tolerance.**

2. *Experiencing withdrawal.* In an individual who has maintained prolonged, heavy use of a substance, a drop in its concentration within the body can result in unpleasant physical and cognitive **withdrawal** symptoms. For example, nausea, vomiting, and tremors are common for alcohol, opioids, and seda-

tives. Some drugs have no significant withdrawal symptoms.

3. *Taking the substance in larger amounts or over a longer period than was originally intended.*

4. *Expressing a persistent desire to cut down or regulate substance use.*

5. *Spending a great deal of time obtaining the substance, using the substance, or recovering from its effects.*

6. *Giving up or reducing important social, school, work, or recreational activities because of substance use.*

7. *Continuing to use the substance in spite of recognizing that it is contributing to a psychological or physical problem.*

If a drug-dependent person experiences either tolerance or withdrawal, he or she is considered physically dependent. However, not everyone who experiences tolerance or withdrawal is drug dependent and dependence can occur without a physical component, based solely on compulsive use.

Who Uses Drugs?

The use and abuse of drugs occur at all income and education levels, among all ethnic groups, and at all ages (see the box "Drug Use Among College Students"). Society is concerned with the casual or recreational use of illegal drugs because it is not really possible to know when drug use will lead to abuse or dependence. Some casual users

TERMS

substance abuse   A maladaptive pattern of using any substance that persists despite adverse social, psychological, or medical consequences. The pattern may be intermittent, with or without tolerance and physical dependence.

physical dependence   The result of physiological adaptation that occurs in response to the frequent presence of a drug; typically associated with tolerance and withdrawal.

substance dependence   A cluster of cognitive, behavioral, and physiological symptoms that occur in someone who continues to use a substance despite suffering significant substance-related problems, leading to significant impairment or distress; also known as *addiction.*

tolerance   Lower sensitivity to a drug so that a given dose no longer exerts the usual effect and larger doses are needed.

withdrawal   Physical and psychological symptoms that follow the interrupted use of a drug on which a user is physically dependent; symptoms may be mild or life-threatening.

Drug Use Among College Students

By some measures of substance abuse, double-digit prevalence is the defining characteristic of drug use on college campuses for certain drugs.

According to the most recent survey data from the Substance Abuse and Mental Health Services Administration (SAMHSA), 19.7% of young adults age 18–25 reported using an illicit drug in the past 30 days (see Table 7.1). This number represents a slight decline from 2005 and 2006. The same survey shows that past-month tobacco use decreased and binge drinking remained steady, while marijuana and cocaine use decreased slightly.

Other surveys show that recreational drug use is fairly common among college students. According to the 2007 American College Health Association—National College Health Assessment, more than 12% of college students reported using marijuana at least once in the past 30 days. Another 1.2% said they had used cocaine at least once in the past 30 days, and nearly 2% reported using amphetamines.

Family history, peer pressure, depression, anxiety, low self-esteem, and the dynamics of college life (for example, the drive to compete and distorted perception of drug use among peers) have been suggested as potential explanations for drug use among college students.

Excessive alcohol use often accompanies illicit drug use. In fact, the term AOD (Alcohol and Other Drug) has been developed to refer to this type of substance use among college students. Further, AOD use and depression and/or anxiety are generally recognized as coexisting conditions that require a comprehensive approach to prevention and treatment. Despite the growing awareness among college counselors and other health professionals who work with college students, it is not entirely clear whether anxiety and depression precede the onset of alcohol and drug use, or whether early pre-college exposure to alcohol and drug use exacerbates more serious psychiatric disorders by the time a student enters college. A third line of research suggests that AOD use, depression, and anxiety share common causes such as genetic predisposition and/or family history.

However, one aspect of drug use among college students remains clear: AOD use has dramatic consequences for the educational, family, and community life of students. Poor academic performance has been linked with AOD use. Further, driving while intoxicated remains one of the most dangerous outcomes associated with AOD use affecting families and communities.

---

develop substance-related problems; others do not. Some psychoactive drugs are more likely than others to lead to dependence (Table 7.2), but some users of even heroin or cocaine do not meet the APA's criteria for substance dependence.

It isn't possible to accurately predict which drug users will become abusers, but young people at a high risk of *trying* drugs share certain characteristics:

Table 7.2	Psychoactive Drugs and Their Potential for Producing Dependence	
	Potential for Dependence	
Drug	**Physical**	**Psychological**
Alcohol	Possible	Possible
Amphetamine	Possible	High
Barbiturates	High	Moderate
Chloral hydrate	Moderate	Moderate
Cocaine	Possible	High
Codeine	Moderate	Moderate
Crack cocaine	High	High
Hashish	Unknown	Moderate
Heroin	High	High
Ice (smoked methamphetamine)	High	High
LSD	None	Unknown
Marijuana	Unknown	Moderate
Methaqualone	High	High
Opium	High	High
PCP	Unknown	High
Psilocybin	None	Unknown

SOURCES: U.S. Department of Health and Human Services, Substance Abuse and Mental Health Services Administration. 2007. *Drugs of Abuse* (http://ncadi.samhsa.gov/govpubs/rop926; retrieved February 3, 2009); Beers, M. H., et al. 2006. *The Merck Manual of Diagnosis and Therapy*, 18th ed. New York: Wiley.

- *Being young.* People who start using drugs when they're very young have a greater risk of dependence and health consequences.

- *Being male.* Males are twice as likely as females to abuse illicit drugs (see the box "Gender Differences in Drug Use and Abuse").

- *Being a troubled adolescent.* Teens are more likely to try drugs if they have poor self-image or self-control, use tobacco, or suffer from certain mental or emotional problems.

- *Being a thrill-seeker.* A sense of invincibility is a factor in drug experimentation.

- *Being in a dysfunctional family.* A chaotic home life or parental abuse increases the risk of drug use. The same is true for children from a single-parent home or whose parents didn't complete high school.

- *Being in a peer group that accepts drug use.* Young people who are uninterested in school and earn poor grades are more likely to try drugs.

- *Being poor.* Young people who live in disadvantaged areas are more likely to be around drugs at a young age.

- *Dating young.* Adolescent girls who date boys two or more years older than themselves are more likely to use drugs.

Gender Differences in Drug Use and Abuse

GENDER MATTERS

Men are more likely than women to use, abuse, and be dependent on illicit drugs. Rates of use are similar in males and females age 12–17, but among those 18 and older, more men than women use drugs and have problems associated with drug use (see table). Men account for about 80% of arrests for drug abuse violations, 70% of admissions for treatment, and 65% of drug-related deaths.

There are also gender differences in why and how young people use drugs. Young males tend to use alcohol or drugs for sensation seeking or to enhance their social status, factors tied to culturally based gender roles. Young women tend to use drugs to improve mood, increase confidence, and reduce inhibitions. Boys are likelier to receive offers to use drugs in public settings, whereas girls are likelier to receive offers in a private place such as a friend's residence.

Despite overall lower rates of drug use, females may have unique biological vulnerabilities to certain drugs, and they may move more quickly from use to abuse. Major life transitions, including the physical and emotional changes as-

sociated with puberty, increase the risk of drug use and abuse for girls more so than for boys. Certain other drug abuse risk factors are also more common in female adolescents, including depression, low self-esteem, eating disorders, and a history of physical or sexual abuse.

Adolescent boys and girls share some protective factors relating to drug abuse, including positive family relationships and extracurricular activities; religious involvement is protective for both boys and girls but may be more protective for girls.

Among older men and women, marriage, children, and employment are associated with lower rates of drug abuse and dependence. Rates of drug abuse and dependence among married adults are less than half of those among unmarried adults. Similar patterns are seen in adults who live with children versus those who do not live with children and adults who are employed versus those who are unemployed.

	National Survey Results: Percent Reporting in Past Year	
	Males	**Females**
Illicit drug use*	17.4	11.6
Age 12–17	19.4	18.0
Age 18–25	37.2	29.1
Age 26 and older	13.5	7.9
Drove under the influence of an illicit drug	5.7	2.4
Illicit drug or alcohol abuse or dependence	12.5	5.7
Treatment for drug dependence	1.3	0.5

*Illicit drugs include marijuana/hashish, cocaine, heroin, hallucinogens, inhalants, and prescription-type psychotherapeutics used nonmedically.

SOURCE: Office of Applied Studies, Substance Abuse and Mental Health Services Administration. 2008. *Results from the 2007 National Survey on Drug Use and Health: National Findings* (http://oas.samhsa.gov/nsduh.htm; retrieved February 3, 2009).

What about people who *don't* use drugs? As a group, nonusers also share some characteristics. Not surprisingly, people who perceive drug use as risky and who disapprove of it are less likely to use drugs than those who believe otherwise. Drug use is also less common among people who have positive self-esteem and self-concept and who are assertive, independent thinkers who are not controlled by peer pressure. Self-control, social competence, optimism, academic achievement, and regular church attendance are also linked to lower rates of drug use. Home environments are also influential: Coming from a strong family, one that has a clear policy on drug use, is another characteristic of people who don't use drugs (see the box "Spirituality and Drug Abuse").

Why Do People Use Drugs?

Young people, especially those from middle-class backgrounds, are frequently drawn to drugs by the allure of the exciting and illegal. They may be curious, rebellious, or vulnerable to peer pressure. Young people may want to imitate adult models in their lives or in the movies. Most people who take illicit drugs do so experimentally, typically trying the drug one or more times but not continuing. The main factors in the initial choice of a drug are whether it is available and whether peers are using it.

Although some people use drugs because they have a desire to alter their mood or are seeking a spiritual experience, others are motivated primarily by a desire to escape boredom, anxiety, depression, feelings of worthlessness, or other distressing symptoms of psychological problems. They use drugs as a way to cope with the difficulties they are experiencing. The common practice in our society of seeking a drug solution to every problem is a factor in the widespread reliance on both illicit and prescription drugs.

For people living in poverty in the inner cities, many of these reasons for using drugs are magnified. The problems are more devastating, the need for escape more compelling. Furthermore, the buying and selling of drugs provide access to an unofficial, alternative economy that may seem like an opportunity for success.

Risk Factors for Dependence

Research indicates that some people may be born with certain characteristics of brain chemistry or metabolism that make them more vulnerable to drug dependence. Psychological risk factors for drug dependence include difficulty in controlling impulses and a strong need for excitement, stimulation, and immediate gratification. Feelings of rejection, hostility, aggression, anxiety, or depression are also

Spirituality and Drug Abuse

Although there are diverse religious viewpoints on drug use, many religions infer some link between psychoactive drugs and spirituality. Some religions use drugs in the quest for spiritual transcendence: American Indian, Polynesian, African, and other indigenous religions have used psychoactive drugs such as peyote, khat, alcohol, and hashish for expanding consciousness and developing personal spirituality. Other religions view psychoactive drugs as a threat to spirituality. In Islam, for example, the consumption of alcohol and certain other drugs is strictly forbidden.

In studies of American teens and adults, spiritual or religious involvement is generally associated with a lower risk of trying psychoactive drugs and, for those who do use drugs, a lower risk of heavy use and dependence. Possible reasons include the adoption of a strict code of behavior or set of principles that forbids drug use, the presence of a social support system for abstinence or mod-

eration, and the promotion of values that include avoidance of drug use.

The relationship between religious faith and avoidance of drug use appears to be even stronger in teens than in adults. Teens who attend 25 or more religious services per year are about half as likely to use illicit drugs as teens who attend services less frequently. Overall, people who spend time regularly engaging in spiritual practices such as prayer and transcendental meditation have lower rates of drug abuse.

People with current substance-abuse problems tend to have lower rates of religious affiliation and involvement and lower levels of spiritual wellness, characterized by a lack of a sense of meaning in life. One of the hallmarks of drug dependence is spending increasing amounts of time and energy obtaining and using drugs; such a pattern of behavior inevitably reduces the resources an individual puts toward developing physical, emotional, and spiritual wellness.

Among people in treatment for substance abuse, higher levels of religious faith and spirituality may contribute to the recovery process. A study of people recovering from alcohol or other drug abuse found that spirituality and religiousness were associated with increased coping skills, greater optimism about life, greater resilience to stress, and greater perceived social support. More research is needed to clarify the relationships among spirituality, religion, drug use, and recovery. Although behaviors such as prayer or meditation can be measured, it is more difficult to determine what such practices mean to the individual.

SOURCES: Brown, A. E., et al. 2006. Alcohol recovery and spirituality: Strangers, friends, or partners? *Southern Medical Journal* 99(6): 654–657; Substance Abuse and Mental Health Network. 2004. Religious beliefs and substance use among youths. *NSDUH Report*, January; Dunn, M. S. 2005. The relationship between religiosity, employment, and political beliefs on substance use among high school seniors. *Journal of Alcohol and Drug Education* 49(1): 73.

associated with drug dependence. People may turn to drugs to blot out their emotional pain. People with mental illnesses have a very high risk of substance dependence.

Other Risks of Drug Use

In 2005, 1.4 million emergency room visits were related to drug misuse or abuse.

Intoxication People who are under the influence of drugs—intoxicated—may act in uncharacteristic and unsafe ways because both their physical and mental functioning are impaired. They are more likely to be injured from a variety of causes, including falls, drowning, and automobile crashes; to engage in unsafe sex, increasing their risk for sexually transmitted diseases and unintended pregnancy; and to be involved in incidents of aggression and violence, including sexual assault.

Unexpected Side Effects Psychoactive drugs have many physical and psychological effects

beyond the alteration of consciousness. These effects range from nausea and constipation to paranoia, depression, and heart failure. Some drugs also carry the risk of fatal overdose.

Unknown Drug Constituents There is no quality control in the illegal drug market, so the composition, dosage, and toxicity of street drugs is highly variable. Studies indicate that half of all street drugs don't contain their promised primary ingredient; in some cases, a drug may be present in unsafe dosages or mixed with other drugs to boost the effects. Careless manufacturing practices can result in the presence of toxic contaminants.

Risks Associated with Injection Drug Use Many injection drug users (IDUs) share or reuse needles, syringes, and other injection equipment, which can easily become contaminated with the user's blood. Small amounts of blood can carry enough human immunodeficiency virus (HIV) and hepatitis C virus (HCV) to be infectious. In 2006, injection drug use accounted for about 13% of all new HIV/AIDS cases; many more were attributed to sexual contact with IDUs. Injection drug use also accounts for the majority of HCV infections.

The surest way to prevent diseases related to injection drug use is never to inject drugs. Syringe exchange programs (SEPs)—where IDUs can trade a used syringe for a new one—have been advocated to help slow the spread of

QUICK STATS

More than 4 million Americans have injected heroin, cocaine, or a stimulant at least once in their life.

—SAMHSA, 2008

HIV and reduce the rates and cost of other health problems associated with injection drug use. Getting people off drugs is clearly the best solution, but there are far more IDUs than treatment facilities can currently handle.

Legal Consequences Many psychoactive drugs are illegal, so using them can result in large fines and/or imprisonment. According to the Federal Bureau of Investigation (FBI), law enforcement officials made 1.8 million arrests for drug abuse violations (13% of all arrests) in 2007—more arrests than for any other offense that year.

HOW DRUGS AFFECT THE BODY

The same drug may affect different people differently or the same person in different ways under different circumstances. Beyond a fairly predictable general change in brain chemistry, the effects of a drug may vary depending on drug factors, user factors, and social factors.

Changes in Brain Chemistry

Once a psychoactive drug reaches the brain, it acts on one or more **neurotransmitters,** either increasing or decreasing their concentration and actions. Cocaine, for example, affects dopamine, a neurotransmitter thought to play a key role in the process of reinforcement—the brain's way of telling itself "That's good; do the same thing again." Heroin, nicotine, alcohol, and amphetamines also affect dopamine levels through their effects on the brain.

The duration of a drug's effect depends on many factors and may range from 5 minutes (crack cocaine) to 12 or more hours (LSD). As drugs circulate through the body, they are metabolized by the liver and eventually excreted by the kidneys in urine. Small amounts may also be eliminated in other ways, including in sweat, in breast milk, and via the lungs.

Drug Factors

When different drugs or dosages produce different effects, the differences are usually caused by one or more of five different drug factors:

1. The **pharmacological properties** of a drug are its overall effects on a person's body chemistry, behav-

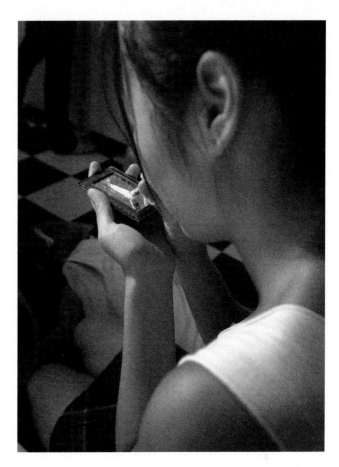

Method of use (or route of administration) is one variable in the overall effect of a drug on the body.

ior, and psychology. The pharmacological properties also include the amount of a drug required to exert various effects, the time course of these effects, and other characteristics, such as a drug's chemical composition.

2. The **dose-response function** is the relationship between the amount of drug taken and the type and intensity of the resulting effect. Many psychological effects of drugs reach a plateau in the dose-response function, so that increasing the dose does not increase the effect any further. With LSD, for example, the maximum changes in perception occur at a certain dose, and no further changes in perception take place if higher doses are taken. However, all drugs

neurotransmitter A brain chemical that transmits nerve impulses.

pharmacological properties The overall effects of a drug on a person's behavior, psychology, and chemistry.

dose-response function The relationship between the amount of a drug taken and the intensity and type of the resulting effect.

TERMS

have more than one effect, and the dose-response functions usually are different for different effects. This means that increasing the dose of any drug may begin to result in added effects, which are likely to be increasingly unpleasant or dangerous at high doses.

3. The **time-action function** is the relationship between the time elapsed since a drug was taken and the intensity of its effect. Effects of a drug are greatest when concentrations of the drug in body tissues are changing fastest, especially if they are increasing.

4. The person's *drug use history* may influence the effects of a drug. A given amount of alcohol, for example, will generally affect a habitual drinker less than an occasional drinker. Tolerance to some drugs, such as LSD, builds rapidly. To experience the same effect, a user has to abstain from the drug for a period of time before that dosage will again exert its original effects.

5. The *method of use* (or *route of administration*) has a direct effect on how strong a response a drug produces. Methods of use include ingestion, inhalation, injection, and absorption through the skin or tissue linings. Drugs are usually injected in one of three ways: intravenously (IV, or mainlining), intramuscularly (IM), or subcutaneously (SC, or skin popping).

User Factors

Certain physical and psychological characteristics also help determine how a person will respond to a drug. Body mass is one variable. The effects of a certain dose of a drug on a 100-pound person will be twice as great as on a 200-pound person. Other variables include general health and genetic factors. For example, some people have an inherited ability to rapidly metabolize a cough suppressant called dextromethorphan, which also has psychoactive properties. These people must take a higher-than-normal dose to get a given cough-suppressant effect.

If a person's biochemical state is already altered by another drug, this too can make a difference. Some drugs intensify the effects of other drugs, as is the case with alcohol and sedatives. Some drugs block the effects of other drugs, such as when a tranquilizer is used to relieve anxiety caused by cocaine. Interactions between drugs, including many prescription and OTC medications, can be unpredictable and dangerous.

One physical condition that requires special precautions is pregnancy. It can be risky for a woman to use any drugs at all during pregnancy, including alcohol and common OTC preparations like cough medicine. The risks are greatest during the first trimester, when the fetus's body is rapidly forming and even small biochemical alterations in the mother can have a devastating effect on fetal development. Even later, the fetus is more susceptible than the mother to the adverse effects of any drugs she takes. The fetus may even become physically dependent on a drug being taken by the mother and suffer withdrawal symptoms after birth.

Sometimes a person's response to a drug is strongly influenced by the user's expectations about how he or she will react (the psychological *set*). With large doses, the drug's chemical properties seem to have the strongest effect on the user's response. But with small doses, psychological (and social) factors are often more important. When people strongly believe that a given drug will affect them a certain way, they are likely to experience those effects regardless of the drug's pharmacological properties. In one study, regular users of marijuana reported a moderate level of intoxication (**high**) after using a cigarette that smelled and tasted like marijuana but contained no THC, the active ingredient in marijuana. This is an example of the **placebo effect**— when a person receives an inert substance yet responds as if it were an active drug. In other studies, subjects who smoked low doses of real marijuana that they believed to be a placebo experienced no effects from the drug. Clearly, the user's expectations had a greater effect on the smokers than the drug itself.

Social Factors

The *setting* is the physical and social environment surrounding the drug use. If a person uses marijuana at home with trusted friends and pleasant music, the effects are likely to be different from the effects if the same dose is taken in an austere experimental laboratory with an impassive research technician. Similarly, the dose of alcohol that produces mild euphoria and stimulation at a noisy, active cocktail party might induce sleepiness and slight depression when taken at home while alone.

REPRESENTATIVE PSYCHOACTIVE DRUGS

The following sections introduce six representative groups of psychoactive drugs (Figure 7.1): opioids, central nervous system (CNS) depressants, central nervous system stimulants, marijuana and other cannabis products, hallucinogens, and inhalants.

TERMS

time-action function   The relationship between the time elapsed since a drug was taken and the intensity of its effect.

high   The subjectively pleasing effects of a drug, usually felt quite soon after the drug is taken.

placebo effect   A response to an inert or innocuous medication given in place of an active drug.

Category	Representative drugs	Street names	Appearance	Methods of use	Short-term effects
Opioids 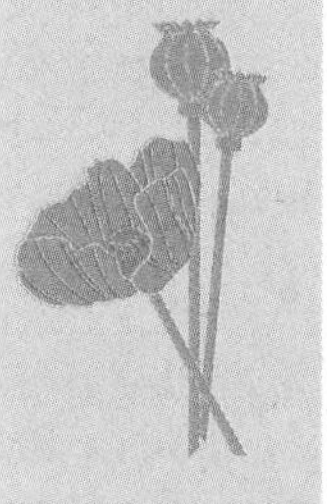	Heroin	Dope, H, junk, brown sugar, smack	White/dark brown powder; dark tar or coal-like substance	Injected, smoked, snorted	Relief of anxiety and pain; euphoria; lethargy, apathy, drowsiness, confusion, inability to concentrate; nausea, constipation, respiratory depression
	Opium	Big O, black stuff, hop	Dark brown or black chunks	Swallowed, smoked	
	Morphine	M, Miss Emma, monkey, white stuff	White crystals, liquid solution	Injected, swallowed, smoked	
	Oxycodone, codeine, hydrocodone	Oxy, O.C., killer, Captain Cody, schoolboy, vike	Tablets, powder made from crushing tablets	Swallowed, injected, snorted	
Central nervous system depressants 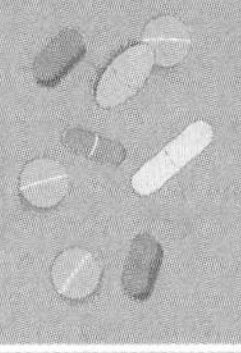	Barbiturates	Barbs, reds, red birds, yellows, yellow jackets	Colored capsules	Swallowed, injected	Reduced anxiety, mood changes, lowered inhibitions, impaired muscle coordination, reduced pulse rate, drowsiness, loss of consciousness, respiratory depression
	Benzodiazepines (e.g., Valium, Xanax, Rohypnol)	Candy, downers, tranks, roofies, forget-me pill	Tablets	Swallowed, injected	
	Methaqualone	Ludes, quad, quay	Tablets	Injected, swallowed	
	Gamma hydroxy butyrate (GHB)	G, Georgia home boy, grievous bodily harm	Clear liquid, white powder	Swallowed	
Central nervous system stimulants 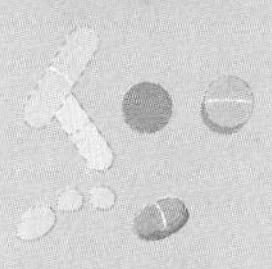	Amphetamine, methamphetamine	Bennies, speed, black beauties, uppers, chalk, crank, crystal, ice, meth	Tablets, capsules, white powder, white crystals	Injected, swallowed, smoked, snorted	Increased heart rate, blood pressure, metabolism; increased mental alertness and energy; nervousness, insomnia, impulsive behavior; reduced appetite
	Cocaine, crack cocaine	Blow, C, candy, coke, flake, rock, toot	White powder, beige pellets or rocks	Injected, smoked, snorted	
	Ritalin	JIF, MPH, R-ball, Skippy	Tablets	Injected, swallowed, snorted	
Marijuana and other cannabis products 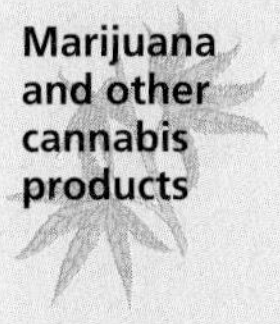	Marijuana	Dope, grass, joints, Mary Jane, reefer, skunk, weed	Dried leaves and stems	Smoked, swallowed	Euphoria, slowed thinking and reaction time, confusion, anxiety, impaired balance and coordination, increased heart rate
	Hashish	Hash, hemp, boom, gangster	Dark, resin-like compound formed into rocks or blocks	Smoked, swallowed	
Hallucinogens 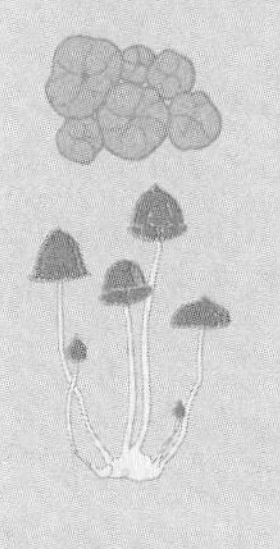	LSD	Acid, boomers, blotter, yellow sunshines	Blotter paper, liquid, gelatin tabs, pills	Swallowed, absorbed through mouth tissues	Altered states of perception and feeling; nausea; increased heart rate, blood pressure; delirium; impaired motor function; numbness, weakness
	Mescaline (peyote)	Buttons, cactus, mesc	Brown buttons, liquid	Swallowed, smoked	
	Psilocybin	Shrooms, magic mushrooms	Dried mushrooms	Swallowed	
	Ketamine	K, special K, cat valium, vitamin K	Clear liquid, white or beige powder	Injected, snorted, smoked	
	PCP	Angel dust, hog, love boat, peace pill	White to brown powder, tablets	Injected, swallowed, smoked, snorted	
	MDMA (ecstasy)	X, peace, clarity, Adam	Tablets	Swallowed	
Inhalants 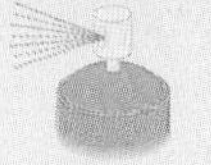	Solvents, aerosols, nitrites, anesthetics	Laughing gas, poppers, snappers, whippets	Household products, sprays, glues, paint thinner, petroleum products	Inhaled through nose or mouth	Stimulation, loss of inhibition, slurred speech, loss of motor coordination, loss of consciousness

FIGURE 7.1 Commonly abused drugs and their effects.

SOURCES: The Partnership for a Drug-Free America. 2006. *Drug Guide by Name* (http://www.drugfree.org/portal/drug_guide; retrieved August 7, 2006); U.S. Drug Enforcement Agency. 2006. *Photo Library* (http://www.usdoj.gov/dea/photo_library.html; retrieved August 7, 2006); U.S. Drug Enforcement Agency. 2005. *Drug Information* (http://www.usdoj.gov/dea/concern.concern.htm; retrieved August 7, 2006); National Institute on Drug Abuse. 2004. *Commonly Abused Drugs* (http://www.drugabuse.gov/DrugPages/DrugsofAbuse.html; retrieved August 7, 2006).

Opioids

Also called *narcotics,* **opioids** are natural or synthetic (laboratory-made) drugs, such as opium, morphine, heroin, methadone, codeine, hydrocodone, oxycodone, meperidine, and fentanyl. Opioids relieve pain, cause drowsiness, and induce **euphoria**. Especially in small doses, opioids have beneficial medical uses, including pain relief and cough suppression. Opioids tend to reduce anxiety and produce lethargy, apathy, and an inability to concentrate. Opioid users become less active and less responsive to frustration, hunger, and sexual stimulation. These ef-

fects are more pronounced in novice users; with repeated use, many effects diminish.

Opioids are typically injected or absorbed into the body from the stomach, intestines, nasal membranes (from snorting or sniffing), or lungs (from smoking). Effects depend on the method of administration. If brain levels of the drug change rapidly, more immediate effects will result. Although the euphoria associated with opioids is an important factor in their abuse, many people experience a feeling of uneasiness when they first use these drugs. Users also often feel nauseated and vomit, and they may have other unpleasant sensations. Even so, the abuse of opioids often results in dependence. Tolerance can develop rapidly and be pronounced. Withdrawal symptoms include cramps, chills, sweating, nausea, tremors, irritability, and feelings of panic.

Users who sniff or snort avoid the special disease risks of injection drug use, including HIV infection, dependence can readily result from sniffing and smoking heroin. In addition, the potentially high but variable purity of street heroin poses a risk of unintentional overdose. Symptoms of overdose include respiratory depression, coma, and constriction of the pupils; death can result.

Nonmedical use of prescription pain relievers that contain oxycodone and hydrocodone, including Oxycontin and Vicodin, has increased in recent years. When taken as prescribed in tablet form, these drugs treat moderate to severe chronic pain and do not typically lead to abuse. However, like other opioids, use of prescription painkillers can lead to abuse and dependence. Oxycodone and hydrocodone can be abused orally; the long-acting form of oxycodone is also sometimes crushed and snorted or dissolved and injected, providing a powerful heroin-like high. When taken in large doses or combined with other drugs, oxycodone and hydrocodone can cause fatal respiratory depression.

Central Nervous System Depressants

Central nervous system **depressants,** also known as **sedative-hypnotics,** slow down the overall activity of the **central nervous system (CNS).** The result can range from mild **sedation** to death. CNS depressants include alcohol, barbiturates, and other sedatives.

Types The various types of barbiturates (downers or downs) are similar in chemical composition and action, but they differ in how quickly and how long they act. Antianxiety agents, also called sedatives or **tranquilizers,** include the benzodiazepines such as Xanax, Valium, Librium, clonazepam (Klonopin), and flunitrazepam (Rohypnol, also called roofies). Other CNS depressants include methaqualone (Quaalude), ethchlorvynol (Placidyl), chloral hydrate ("mickey"), and gamma hydroxy butyrate (GHB, or "liquid ecstasy").

Effects CNS depressants reduce anxiety and cause mood changes, impaired muscular coordination, slurring

TERMS

opioid Any of several natural or synthetic drugs that relieve pain and cause drowsiness and/or euphoria; examples are opium, morphine, and heroin; also called a *narcotic.*

euphoria An exaggerated feeling of well-being.

depressant, or sedative-hypnotic A drug that decreases nervous or muscular activity, causing drowsiness or sleep.

central nervous system (CNS) The brain and spinal cord.

sedation The induction of a calm, relaxed, often sleepy state.

tranquilizer A CNS depressant that reduces tension and anxiety.

Club Drugs

Club drugs are part of popular dance culture. Some people refer to club drugs as soft drugs because they see them as recreational—for the casual, weekend user—rather than as addictive. But club drugs have many potential negative effects and are particularly potent and unpredictable when mixed with alcohol. Substitute drugs are often sold in place of club drugs, putting users at risk for taking dangerous combinations of unknown drugs.

MDMA *(ecstasy, E, X, XTC, Adam, hug drug, lover's speed):* Taken in pill form, MDMA (methylenedioxymethamphetamine) is a stimulant with mildly hallucinogenic and amphetamine-like effects. Users may experience euphoria, increased energy, and a heightened sense of belonging. Using MDMA can produce dangerously high body temperature and potentially fatal dehydration; some users experience confusion, depression, anxiety, paranoia, muscle tension, involuntary teeth clenching, blurred vision, nausea, and seizures. Even low doses can affect concentration, judgment, and driving ability. Tolerance can develop, leading users to take the drug more frequently, to use higher doses, or to combine MDMA with other drugs to enhance the drug's effects.

In addition to MDMA, many ecstasy tablets include other drugs such as methamphetamine, ephedrine, or cocaine. At high doses or mixed with other drugs, MDMA is extremely dangerous; most deaths linked to MDMA have occurred as a result of multidrug toxicity or traumatic injuries.

MDMA increases the activity of three neurotransmitters: serotonin, dopamine, and norepinephrine. Increases in serotonin are likely the cause of the drug's mood-elevating effects, but use of MDMA can deplete the brain of serotonin and may cause an emotional let-down (sadness, irritability, etc.) in the days following use.

MDMA users perform worse than nonusers on complex cognitive tasks of memory, attention, and general intelligence. Long-term effects may include physical symptoms and psychological problems such as confusion or paranoia. Research suggests that pregnant women who use MDMA are at increased risk for having a baby with congenital malformations and long-term impairment in memory and other cognitive functions.

LSD *(acid, boomers, yellow sunshines, red dragon):* A potent hallucinogen, LSD (lysergic acid diethylamide) is sold in tablets or capsules, in liquid form, or on small squares of paper called blotters. LSD increases heart rate and body temperature and may cause nausea, tremors, sweating, numbness, and weakness.

Ketamine *(special K, vitamin K, K, cat valium, jet):* A veterinary anesthetic that can be taken in powdered or liquid form, ketamine may cause hallucinations and impaired attention and memory. At higher doses, ketamine can cause delirium, amnesia, high blood pressure, and potentially fatal respiratory problems. Tolerance to ketamine develops rapidly.

GHB *(Georgia home boy, G, grievous bodily harm, liquid ecstasy):* GHB (gamma hydroxybutyrate) can be produced in clear liquid, white powder, tablet, and capsule form. GHB is a CNS depressant that in large doses or when taken in combination with alcohol or other depressants can cause sedation, loss of consciousness, respiratory arrest, and death. GHB may cause prolonged and potentially life-threatening withdrawal symptoms.

Some products sold as dietary supplements for bodybuilding, weight loss, or insomnia contain the chemically similar compounds GBL (gamma butyrolactone) or BD (butanediol). It is illegal to sell products containing GHB, GBL, or BD for human consumption. The FDA has issued several warnings to prevent such items from being sold to the public.

Rohypnol *(roofies, roche, forget-me pill):* Taken in tablet form, Rohypnol (flunitrazepam) is a sedative that is ten times more potent than Valium. Its effects, which are magnified by alcohol, include reduced blood pressure, dizziness, confusion, gastrointestinal disturbances, and loss of consciousness. Users of Rohypnol may develop physical and psychological dependence on the drug.

Several club drugs are used as "date rape drugs." Because they can be added to beverages surreptitiously, these drugs may be unknowingly consumed by intended rape victims. In addition to depressant effects, some drugs also cause *anterograde amnesia,* the loss of memory of things occurring while under the influence of the drug. Because of concern about such drugs, Congress passed the "Drug-Induced Rape Prevention and Punishment Act," which increased federal penalties for use of any controlled substance to aid in sexual assault.

---

of speech, and drowsiness or sleep. Mental functioning is also affected, but the degree varies from person to person and also depends on the kind of task the person is trying to do. Most people become drowsy with small doses, although a few become more active.

From Use to Abuse People are usually introduced to CNS depressants either through a medical prescription or through drug-using peers. The use of Rohypnol and GHB is often associated with dance clubs and raves. Most CNS depressants, including alcohol, can lead to classical physical dependence. Tolerance, sometimes for up to 15 times the usual dose, can develop with repeated use. Tranquilizers have been shown to produce physical dependence even at ordinary prescribed doses. Withdrawal symptoms can be more severe than those accompanying opioid dependence. They may begin as anxiety, shaking, and weakness but may turn into convulsions and possibly cardiovascular collapse and death.

While intoxicated, people on depressants cannot function well. They are confused and are frequently obstinate, irritable, and abusive. Even prescription use of benzodiazepines has been associated with an increased risk of automobile crashes. After long-term use, depressants like alcohol can lead to poor health and brain damage, with impaired ability to reason and make judgments.

Too much depression of the central nervous system slows respiration and may stop it entirely. CNS depressants are particularly dangerous in combination with another depressant, such as alcohol. Rohypnol is ten times more potent than Valium and can be fatal if combined with alcohol. GHB is often produced clandestinely, resulting in widely varying degrees of purity; it has been responsible for many poisonings and a number of deaths.

Central Nervous System Stimulants

CNS **stimulants** speed up the activity of the nervous or muscular system, causing the heart rate to accelerate, blood pressure to rise, blood vessels to constrict, the pupils of the eyes and the bronchial tubes to dilate, and gastric and adrenal secretions to increase. There is greater muscular tension and sometimes an increase in motor activity. Small doses usually make people feel more awake and alert, less fatigued and bored. The most common CNS stimulants are cocaine, amphetamines, nicotine, ephedrine, and caffeine.

Cocaine Usually derived from the leaves of coca shrubs that grow high in the Andes in South America, cocaine—also known as coke or snow—is a potent CNS stimulant. It is usually snorted and absorbed through the nasal mucosa or injected intravenously, providing rapid increases of the drug's concentration in the blood and therefore fast, intense effects. Another method of use involves processing cocaine with baking soda and water, yielding the ready-to-smoke form of cocaine known as crack. Crack is typically available as small beads or pellets smokable in glass pipes.

EFFECTS The effects of cocaine are usually intense but short-lived. The euphoria lasts from 5 to 20 minutes and ends abruptly, to be replaced by irritability, anxiety, or slight depression. When cocaine is absorbed via the lungs, by either smoking or inhalation, it reaches the brain in about 10 seconds, and the effects are particularly intense. This is part of the appeal of smoking crack. The effects

TERMS

stimulant A drug that increases nervous or muscular activity.

state dependence A situation in which information learned in a drug-induced state is difficult to recall when the effect of the drug wears off.

from IV injections occur almost as quickly—in about 20 seconds. Since the mucous membranes in the nose briefly slow absorption, the onset of effects from snorting takes 2–3 minutes. Heavy users may inject cocaine intravenously every 10–20 minutes to maintain the effects.

The larger the cocaine dose and the more rapidly it is absorbed into the bloodstream, the greater the immediate—and sometimes lethal—effects. Sudden death from cocaine is most commonly the result of excessive CNS stimulation that causes convulsions and respiratory collapse, irregular heartbeat, extremely high blood pressure, blood clots, and possibly heart attack or stroke. Although rare, fatalities can occur in healthy young people; among people age 18–59, cocaine users are seven times more likely than nonusers to have a heart attack. Chronic cocaine use produces inflammation of the nasal mucosa, which can lead to persistent bleeding and ulceration of the septum between the nostrils. The use of cocaine may also cause paranoia and/or aggressiveness.

COCAINE USE DURING PREGNANCY A woman who uses cocaine during pregnancy is at higher risk for miscarriage, premature labor, and stillbirth. She is more likely to deliver a low-birth-weight baby who has a small head circumference. Her infant may be at increased risk for defects of the genitourinary tract, cardiovascular system, central nervous system, and extremities. It is difficult to pinpoint the effects of cocaine because many women who use cocaine also use tobacco and/or alcohol. Infants whose mothers use cocaine may also be born intoxicated. Cocaine also passes into breast milk and can intoxicate a breastfeeding infant.

Amphetamines Amphetamines (uppers) are a group of synthetic chemicals that are potent CNS stimulants. Some common drugs in this family are amphetamine (Benzedrine), dextroamphetamine (Dexedrine), and methamphetamine (Methedrine). According to the CDC's 2007 Youth Risk Behavior Surveillance, 4.5% of American high school students reported using methamphetamine at least once during their lifetime (see the box "The Meth Epidemic").

EFFECTS Small doses of amphetamines usually make people feel more alert. Amphetamines generally increase motor activity but do not measurably alter a normal, rested person's ability to perform tasks calling for challenging motor skills or complex thinking. When amphetamines do improve performance, it is primarily by counteracting fatigue and boredom. Amphetamines in small doses also increase heart rate and blood pressure and change sleep patterns. They are sometimes used to curb appetite, but after a few weeks the user develops tolerance and needs higher doses. When people stop taking the drug, their appetite usually returns, and they gain back the weight they lost.

FROM USE TO ABUSE Much amphetamine abuse begins as an attempt to cope with a temporary situation. A student

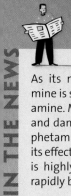
The Meth Epidemic

As its name suggests, methamphetamine is similar to the stimulant amphetamine. Meth, however, is more addictive and dangerous than most forms of amphetamine because it is more toxic and its effects last longer. Methamphetamine is highly addictive; many casual users rapidly become regular users.

What Are Meth's Effects?

By stimulating dopamine activity in the brain, meth increases the user's ability to stay awake and perform physical activity. Meth's other short-term effects can include euphoria, rapid breathing, increased body temperature (hyperthermia), insomnia, tremors, anxiety, and convulsions.

In the long term, meth's effects can be devastating. Severe weight loss, heart attack, stroke, hallucinations, violence, paranoia, and psychotic behavior have all been linked to meth addiction. Brain damage similar to that found in Parkinson's disease and Alzheimer's disease has been reported in long-term meth users. Meth use causes extensive tooth decay and tooth loss, a condition referred to as "meth mouth." The drug takes a severe toll on the user's heart, increasing heart rate and blood pressure, damaging blood vessels, and causing irregular heartbeat. Such damage can be fatal.

Who Uses Meth?

According to estimates from the Substance Abuse and Mental Health Services Administration, about 1.3 million Americans have used meth at least once in the past year. The highest rates of use are among young adults age 18–25.

Although methamphetamine is often called "poor man's cocaine," its users are not all poor or poorly educated; rather, they span the socioeconomic spectrum. The drug spread east from the West Coast and is now found in all 50 states, in rural, suburban, and urban areas. Meth producers are finding ways to attract younger users, such as by designing candy-flavored meth, which makes the drug easier to take and more appealing to children. Many drug enforcement and government officials say methampethamine is the number-one drug problem in the United States today.

Related Issues

Along with the physical problems suffered by meth users, the drug has led to a growing array of social and emotional problems. For example, because meth diminishes the user's judgment, many meth addicts engage in unsafe sex, increasing their risk of infection from a variety of transmittable diseases, especially HIV and hepatitis C. Meth use is also associated with domestic violence and family breakdown.

Another problem unique to meth is its do-it-yourself appeal to users and dealers. The drug is relatively easy to make, using commonly available chemicals, and clandestine meth labs in residential living rooms and basements have sprung up across the country. One of the chemicals used in making meth is pseudoephedrine, a drug found in products used to relieve nasal or sinus congestion, such as Sudafed and other cold and allergy medications. To limit access to this drug, Congress passed the Combat Methamphetamine Epidemic Act of 2005 as part of the Patriot Act, requiring behind-the-counter sale of products containing pseudoepinehprine and two other drugs used to make meth.

Methamphetamine production is also very dangerous. The use of caustic and highly explosive chemicals puts meth "cooks" at risk for injury and death from explosion and fire.

Treatment Options

Cognitive behavioral therapy is widely viewed as the best approach to treatment for meth addiction; therapy helps users identify the root causes of their addiction and teaches them skills needed to quit. In some cases, antidepressants or antianxiety medications are prescribed, but there currently is no single effective pharmacological treatment for methamphetamine addiction. In studies, the drug Prometa has been effective in helping meth addicts break their addiction. Further studies are under way.

---

cramming for an exam or an exhausted long-haul truck driver can go a little longer by taking amphetamines. Unfortunately, the likelihood of making bad judgments significantly increases. The stimulating effects may also wear off suddenly, and the user may precipitously feel exhausted or fall asleep ("crash").

Another problem is **state dependence,** the phenomenon whereby information learned in a certain drug-induced state is difficult to recall when the person is not in that same physiological state. Test performance may deteriorate when students use drugs to study and then take tests in their normal, nondrug state.

DEPENDENCE Repeated use of amphetamines, even in moderate doses, often leads to tolerance and the need for increasingly larger doses. Long-term use of amphetamines at high doses can cause paranoia, hallucinations, delusions, and incoherence. Methamphetamine users have signs of brain damage similar to those seen in Parkinson's disease patients that appear to persist even after drug use ceases, causing impaired memory and motor coordination. Withdrawal symptoms may include muscle aches and tremors, profound fatigue, deep depression, despair, and apathy. Chronic high-dose use is often associated with pronounced psychological cravings and obsessive drug-seeking behavior.

Women who use amphetamines during pregnancy risk premature birth, stillbirth, low birth weight, and early infant death. Babies born to amphetamine-using mothers have a higher incidence of cleft palate, cleft lip, and deformed limbs. They may also experience symptoms of withdrawal from amphetamines.

REPRESENTATIVE PSYCHOACTIVE DRUGS   **163**

Ritalin A stimulant with amphetamine-like effects, Ritalin (methylphenidate) is used to treat attention-deficit/hyperactivity disorder (ADHD). When taken orally at prescribed levels, it has little potential for abuse. When injected or snorted, however, dependence and tolerance can rapidly result.

Caffeine Caffeine is probably the most popular psychoactive drug and also one of the most ancient. It is found in coffee, tea, cocoa, soft drinks, headache remedies, and OTC preparations like NōDōz (Table 7.3). In ordinary doses, caffeine produces greater alertness and a sense of well-being. It also decreases feelings of fatigue or boredom; using caffeine may enable a person to keep at physically tiring or repetitive tasks longer. Such use is usually followed, however, by a sudden letdown. Caffeine does not noticeably influence a person's ability to perform complex mental tasks unless fatigue, boredom, or other factors have already affected normal performance.

Caffeine mildly stimulates the heart and respiratory system, increases muscular tremor, and enhances gastric secretion. Higher doses may cause nervousness, anxiety, irritability, headache, disturbed sleep, and gastric irritation or peptic ulcers. In people with high blood pressure, caffeine can cause blood pressure to rise even more; in people with type 2 diabetes, caffeine may cause glucose and insulin levels to rise after meals. Some people, especially children, are quite vulnerable to the adverse effects of caffeine. They become hyperactive and overly sensitive to any stimulation in their environment.

Drinks containing caffeine are rarely harmful for most people, but some tolerance develops, and withdrawal symptoms of irritability, headaches, and even mild depression do occur. People can usually avoid problems by simply decreasing their daily intake of caffeine.

Marijuana and Other Cannabis Products

Marijuana is the most widely used illegal drug in the United States (cocaine is second). More than 40% of Americans have tried marijuana at least once; among 21–25-year-olds, more than 54% have tried marijuana. In 2007, 12.6% of college students reported using marijuana at least once within the past month.

Marijuana is a crude preparation of various parts of the Indian hemp plant *Cannabis sativa,* which grows in most parts of the world. THC (tetrahydrocannabinol) is the main active ingredient in marijuana. Based on THC content, the

Table 7.3	Caffeine Content of Popular Beverages	
	Serving Size	Typical Caffeine Level (mg)*
Coffee		
Regular coffee, brewed	8 oz.	95
Regular coffee, instant	8 oz.	93
Espresso	1 oz.	64
Decaffeinated coffee, brewed	8 oz.	5
Decaffeinated coffee, instant	8 oz.	2
Tea		
Regular tea, brewed	8 oz.	47
Snapple Iced Tea	16 oz.	18
Nestea	12 oz.	17
SoBe Green Tea	8 oz.	14
Lipton Brisk Iced Tea, Lemon	12 oz.	10
Decaffeinated tea, brewed	8 oz.	2
Green tea, brewed	8 oz.	Varies
Soda		
Code Red Mountain Dew	12 oz.	54
Mello Yello	12 oz.	53
Diet Coke	12 oz.	47
Dr. Pepper, Diet Dr. Pepper	12 oz.	41
Sunkist Orange Soda	12 oz.	41
Pepsi	12 oz.	38
Coca-Cola Classic, Cherry Coca-Cola, Diet Cherry Coca-Cola, Diet Pepsi	12 oz.	35
A&W Crème Soda	12 oz.	29
Barq's Root Beer	12 oz.	23
Energy Drinks		
No Name	8.4 oz.	280
SoBe No Fear	16 oz.	174
Monster Energy, Rockstar	16 oz.	160
SoBe Adrenaline Rush	16 oz.	152
Full Throttle, Full Throttle Fury	16 oz.	144
AMP Energy Drink	16 oz.	143
Red Bull	8.3 oz.	76
Vault	8 oz.	47

*Caffeine levels vary greatly by brand of product, manner of preparation, and amount consumed. The amounts shown here are averages based on tests conducted by a variety of organizations. The U.S. Food and Drug Administration limits the amount of caffeine in cola and pepper soft drinks to 71 milligrams per 12-ounce serving. To find the exact amount of caffeine in any product, check that product's label.

SOURCES: Center for Science in the Public Interest. 2007. *Caffeine Content of Food & Drugs* (http://www.cspinet.org/new/cafchart.html; retrieved February 3, 2009); Mayo Clinic. 2007. *How Much Caffeine Is in Your Daily Habit?* (http://www.mayoclinic.com/health/caffeine/AN01211; retrieved February 3, 2009); U.S. Department of Agriculture, Agricultural Research Service. 2007. *USDA National Nutrient Database for Standard Reference, Release 20* (http://www.ars.usda.gov/ba/bhnrc/ndl; retrieved February 3, 2009).

potency of marijuana preparations varies widely. Marijuana plants that grow wild often have less than 1% THC in their leaves. When selected strains are cultivated by separation of male and female plants (*sinsemilla*), the bud leaves from the flowering tops may contain 7–8% THC. Marijuana is usually smoked, but it can also be ingested.

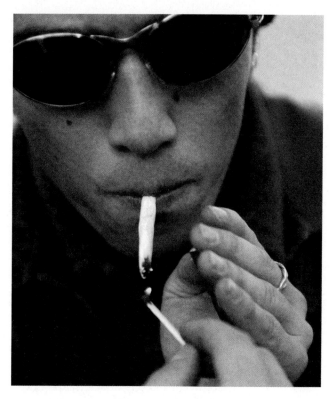

Marijuana is the most widely used illegal drug in the United States.

Short-Term Effects and Uses   The effects of a low dose of marijuana are strongly influenced by the user's expectations and past experiences. At low doses, users typically experience euphoria, a heightening of subjective sensory experiences, a slowing down of the perception of passing time, and a relaxed, laid-back attitude. With moderate doses, these effects become stronger, and the user may have impaired memory function, disturbed thought patterns, lapses of attention, and feelings of **depersonalization**, in which the mind seems to be separated from the body.

The effects of marijuana in higher doses are determined mostly by the drug itself rather than by the user's expectations and setting. Very high doses produce marked sensory distortion and changes in body image, causing some users to become anxious or panicky.

Physiologically, marijuana increases heart rate and dilates certain blood vessels in the eyes, which creates the characteristic bloodshot eyes. THC affects parts of the brain controlling balance, coordination, and reaction time; thus marijuana use impairs driving performance. The combination of alcohol and marijuana makes driving even riskier.

According to the Institute of Medicine some compounds in marijuana may have legitimate medical use, such as easing pain, reducing nausea, and increasing appetite. These benefits led several states to approve the use of "medical marijuana" by extremely ill patients, with physician monitoring. However, because growing, selling, or possessing marijuana is a federal crime, the Su-preme Court has held that state laws permitting medical marijuana use cannot supersede federal law, which means that anyone who uses marijuana for medical reasons—even in a state that approves such use—can still be prosecuted under federal drug laws.

Long-Term Effects   The most probable long-term effect of smoking marijuana is respiratory damage, including impaired lung function and chronic bronchial irritation. Although there is no evidence linking marijuana use to lung cancer, it may cause changes in lung tissue that promote cancer growth. Marijuana users may be at increased risk for emphysema and cancer of the head and neck; among people with chronic conditions like cancer and AIDS, marijuana use is associated with increased risk of fatal lung infections. Heavy users may experience learning problems, as well as subtle impairments of attention and memory that may or may not be reversible following long-term abstinence. Long-term use may also decrease testosterone levels and sperm counts and increase sperm abnormalities.

Heavy marijuana use during pregnancy may cause impaired fetal growth and development, low birth weight, and increased risk of ectopic pregnancy. Marijuana may act synergistically with alcohol to increase the damaging effects of alcohol on the fetus. THC rapidly enters breast milk and may impair an infant's early motor development.

Dependence   Regular users of marijuana can develop tolerance; some develop dependence, and researchers estimate that 1.5% of Americans meet the APA criteria for marijuana dependence. Withdrawal symptoms may occur in the majority of dependent or heavy users; common symptoms include anger or aggression, irritability, nervousness or restlessness, sleep difficulties, and decreased appetite or weight loss.

Hallucinogens

Hallucinogens are a group of drugs whose predominant pharmacological effect is to alter the user's perceptions, feelings, and thoughts. Hallucinogens include LSD (lysergic acid diethylamide), mescaline, psilocybin, STP

(4-methyl-2,5-dimethoxyamphetamine), DMT (dimethyltryptamine), MDMA (3,4-methylene-dioxymethamphetamine), ketamine, and PCP (phencyclidine). These drugs are most commonly ingested or smoked.

LSD LSD is one of the most powerful psychoactive drugs. Tiny doses will produce noticeable effects in most people, such as an altered sense of time, visual disturbances, an improved sense of hearing, mood changes, and distortions in how people perceive their bodies. Dilation of the pupils and slight dizziness, weakness, and nausea may also occur. With larger doses, users may experience a phenomenon known as **synesthesia**, feelings of depersonalization, and other alterations in the perceived relationship between the self and external reality.

Many hallucinogens induce tolerance so quickly that after only one or two doses their effects decrease substantially. The user must then stop taking the drug for several days before his or her system can be receptive to it again. These drugs cause little drug-seeking behavior and no physical dependence or withdrawal symptoms.

The immediate effects of low doses of hallucinogens are largely determined by expectations and setting. Many effects are hard to describe because they involve subjective and unusual dimensions of awareness—the **altered states of consciousness** for which these drugs are famous. For this reason, hallucinogens have acquired a certain aura not associated with other drugs. People have taken LSD in search of a religious or mystical experience or in the hope of exploring new worlds.

A severe panic reaction can result from taking any dose of LSD. Even after the drug's chemical effects have worn off, spontaneous flashbacks and other psychological disturbances can occur. **Flashbacks** are perceptual distortions and bizarre thoughts that occur after the drug has been entirely eliminated from the body.

Other Hallucinogens Most other hallucinogens have the same general effects as LSD, but there are some variations. For example, a DMT or ketamine high does not last as long as an LSD high; an STP high lasts longer. MDMA (ecstasy) has both hallucinogenic and amphetamine-like properties. Tolerance to MDMA develops quickly, and high doses can cause anxiety, delusions, and paranoia.

PCP reduces and distorts sensory input, especially proprioception, the sensation of body position and movement; it creates a state of sensory deprivation. Because it can be easily made, PCP is often available illegally and is sometimes used as an inexpensive replacement for other psychoactive drugs. The effects of ketamine are similar to those of PCP—confusion, agitation, aggression, and lack of coordination—but they tend to be less predictable. Tolerance to either drug can develop rapidly.

Mescaline, derived from the peyote cactus, is the ceremonial drug of the Native American Church. It causes effects similar to LSD, including altered perception and feeling; increased body temperature, heart rate, and blood pressure; weakness and trembling; and sleeplessness. Mescaline is expensive, so most street mescaline is diluted LSD or a mixture of other drugs. Hallucinogenic effects can be obtained from certain mushrooms (*Psilocybe mexicana,* or "magic mushrooms"), certain morning glory seeds, nutmeg, jimsonweed, and other botanical products, but unpleasant side effects, such as dizziness, have limited the popularity of these products.

Inhalants

Inhaling certain chemicals can produce effects ranging from heightened pleasure to delirium and death. Inhalants fall into several major groups: (1) volatile solvents, which are found in products such as paint thinner, glue, and gasoline; (2) aerosols, which are sprays that contain propellants and solvents; (3) nitrites, such as butyl nitrite and amyl nitrite; and (4) anesthetics, which include nitrous oxide, or laughing gas.

Inhalant use is difficult to control because inhalants are easy to obtain. They are present in a variety of seemingly harmless products, from dessert-topping sprays to underarm deodorants, that are both inexpensive and legal. Using the drugs also requires no illegal or suspicious paraphernalia. Inhalant users get high by sniffing, snorting, "bagging" (inhaling fumes from a plastic bag), or "huffing" (placing an inhalant-soaked rag in the mouth).

Although different in makeup, nearly all inhalants produce effects similar to those of anesthetics, which slow down body functions. Low doses may cause users to feel slightly stimulated; at higher doses, users may feel less inhibited and less in control. Sniffing high concentrations of the chemicals in solvents or aerosol sprays can cause a loss of consciousness, heart failure, and death. High concentrations of any inhalant can also cause death from suffocation by displacing the oxygen in the lungs and central nervous system. Deliberately inhaling from a bag or in a closed area greatly increases the chances of suffocation. Other possible effects of the excessive or long-term use of

TERMS

synesthesia A condition in which a stimulus evokes not only the sensation appropriate to it but also another sensation of a different character, such as when a color evokes a specific smell.

altered states of consciousness Profound changes in mood, thinking, and perception.

flashback A perceptual distortion or bizarre thought that recurs after the chemical effects of a drug have worn off.

inhalants include damage to the nervous system (impaired perception, reasoning, memory, and muscular coordination); hearing loss; increased risk of cancer; and damage to the liver, kidneys, and bone marrow.

DRUG USE: THE DECADES AHEAD

Drug research will undoubtedly provide new information, new treatments, and new chemical combinations in the decades ahead. Although the use of some drugs, both legal and illegal, has declined dramatically since the 1970s, the use of others has held steady or increased. Mounting public concern has led to great debate and a wide range of opinions about what should be done. Efforts to combat the problem include workplace drug testing, tougher law enforcement and prosecution, and treatment and education.

Drugs, Society, and Families

According to the National Institute on Drug Abuse, the cost to society of illicit drug abuse alone is $181 billion annually. That figure exceeds $500 billion when combined with the costs of alcohol and tobacco use, including health care, criminal justice, and lost productivity. But the costs are more than just financial; they are also paid in human pain and suffering.

The criminal justice system is inundated with people accused of crimes related to drug possession, sale, or use. The FBI reports that more than 1.8 million arrests are made annually for drug violations; at any given time, more than 100,000 people are in jail for violating drug laws. Many assaults and murders are committed when people try to acquire or protect drug territories, settle disputes about drugs, or steal from dealers. Violence and the use of guns are more common in neighborhoods where drug trafficking is prevalent. Addicts commit more robberies and burglaries than criminals not on drugs. People under the influence of drugs, especially alcohol, are more likely to commit violent crimes like rape and murder than people who do not use drugs (see the box "Drug Use and Ethnicity: Risk Factors and Protective Factors").

Drug use is also a health care issue for society. In the United States, illegal drug use leads to more than 800,000 emergency room admissions and nearly 20,000 deaths annually. Although it is in the best interest of society to treat addicts who want help, but there is not nearly enough space in treatment facilities to help the millions of Americans who need immediate treatment. Drug addicts who want to quit, especially those among the urban poor, often have to wait a year or more for acceptance into a residential care or other treatment program. Drug abuse also takes a toll on individuals and families. Children born to women who use drugs such as alcohol, tobacco, or cocaine may have long-term health problems. Drug use in families can become a vicious cycle. Observing adults around them using drugs, children assume it is an acceptable way to deal with problems. Problems such as abuse, neglect, lack of opportunity, and unemployment become contributing factors to drug use and serve to perpetuate the cycle.

Legalizing Drugs

Pointing out that many of the social problems associated with drugs are related to prohibition rather than to the effects of the drugs themselves, some people have argued for various forms of drug legalization or decriminalization. Proposals range from making drugs such as marijuana and heroin available by prescription to allowing licensed dealers to sell some of these drugs to adults. Proponents argue that legalizing some currently illicit drugs—but putting controls on them similar to those used for alcohol, tobacco, and prescription drugs—could eliminate many of the problems related to drug use.

Opponents of drug legalization argue that allowing easier access to drugs would expose many more people to possible abuse and dependence. Drugs would be cheaper and easier to obtain, and drug use would be more socially acceptable. Legalizing drugs could cause an increase in drug use among children and teenagers. Opponents point out that alcohol and tobacco are major causes of disease and death in our society and that they should not be used as models for other practices.

Drug Testing

According to data from recent surveys, the majority of substance users hold full-time jobs and constitute a significant public health problem in the workplace. Drug use in the workplace not only creates health problems for individual users, but it has a negative effect on productivity and on safety of coworkers. People who use drugs at work face

Drug Use and Ethnicity: Risk Factors and Protective Factors

connect™

Surveys of the U.S. population find a variety of trends in drug use and abuse among ethnic groups (see table). In addition to these general trends, there are also trends relating to the use of specific drugs among different groups.

However, as is true for many areas of health, ethnic trends are influenced by a complex interplay of other factors:

• *Educational status:* Adults with four or more years of college are more likely to have *tried* illicit drugs than are people of the same age who never finished high school, but *current* drug use is lower among college graduates than among people with less education. Among teens, poor school performance is associated with increased risk for illicit drug use.

• *Employment status:* Most adult drug users are employed, but rates of current drug use are much higher among people who are unemployed or who work part-time compared with those who are employed full-time.

• *Parental education and socioeconomic status:* Students from poor families have higher rates of *early* drug use compared with students from wealthier families, but by the twelfth grade, the differences disappear. Socioeconomic status and parental education are closely linked.

• *Geographic area:* Current drug use in the United States is highest in the West and South; drug use is also higher in metropolitan and urban areas compared with more rural areas. People living in communities with high rates of poverty, crime, and unemployment have higher than average rates of drug use and abuse. Specific drugs may also be more available—and their abuse more prevalent—in certain regions or communities.

Strong cultural identity is associated with reduced risk of drug use and abuse among all groups. Some factors believed to contribute to lower rates of drug use among these groups include the following:

• *Parental and community disapproval of drug and alcohol use:* Parents of Asian American children tend to have more restrictive drug and alcohol use norms than African American and white parents. Black parents tend to monitor their children's activities and friendships more closely than white parents. Parental disapproval of drug use is often tied to greater perceived risk of drug use—and lower rates of drug use—among teens.

• *Close family ties:* Asian American teens are the likeliest to come from intact homes. Respect for authority and family loyalty are strongly valued among many Asian American populations. Black teens, although least likely to come from intact homes, often come from single-parent households with close extended family ties. Teens from cohesive and stable families are less likely to use drugs.

• *Focus on schooling and education:* Teens from families who value education and where parents help with homework and limit weeknight time with friends have lower rates of drug use.

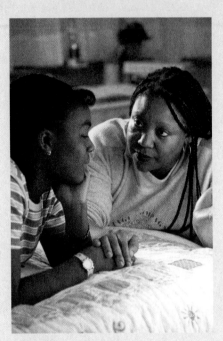

Asian Americans have twice the rate of college graduation compared with other groups.

SOURCES: Johnston, L. D., et al. 2008. *Monitoring the Future: National Results on Adolescent Drug Use: Overview of Key Findings, 2007.* Bethesda, Md.: National Institute on Drug Abuse; Office of Applied Studies, Substance Abuse and Mental Health Services Administration. 2008. *Results from the 2007 National Survey on Drug Use and Health: National Findings* (http://oas.samhsa.gov/nhsda.htm; retrieved May 1, 2008).

National Survey Results, 2007

	Lifetime Drug Use	Past Year Drug Use	Past Month Drug Use				Past Year Illicit Drug Dependence
			Age 12–17	Age 18–25	Age 26 and Older	All Ages	
White	50.3	14.9	10.2	21.9	5.9	8.2	2.7
Black or African American	43.1	16.0	9.4	18.7	7.5	9.5	3.7
Hispanic or Latino	34.2	12.2	8.1	14.6	4.3	6.6	2.5
Asian American	22.8	7.2	6.0	11.7	2.6	4.2	1.1
American Indian and Alaska Native	54.6	18.4	N/A	N/A	8.5	12.6	4.0
Native Hawaiian and Pacific Islander American	N/A	13.3	N/A	9.0	N/A	N/A	3.6
Two or more races	51.5	22.1	9.2	25.9	9.1	11.8	5.1

Note: Results shown in percentages of each population group.

N/A = Data not available for 2007.

higher rates of absenteeism, poor health, and a greater likelihood of harming themselves or others in the workplace.

Statistics from the federal government show that 8.2% of full-time workers used illicit drugs between 2002 and 2004. Illicit drug use is highest among workers in the food industry and construction sectors, while heavy alcohol use is greatest among construction, mining, and repair workers. Premature death, illness, and disability—factors associated with the economic and health burden of lost productivity—are estimated to run as high as $114 billion for drug use and $179 billion for heavy alcohol use.

The extent of the problem has given rise to the development of workplace policies to help workers regain their health and well-being such as drug testing and referral services. Despite controversial aspects of drug testing in the workplace, a growing number of U.S. workers recognize the need for such screening. Most drug testing involves a urine test; a test for alcohol involves a blood test or a breath test. If a person tests positive for drugs, the employer may provide drug counseling or treatment, suspend the employee until he or she tests negative, or fire the individual.

Treatment for Drug Dependence

Regardless of the therapeutic approach used for drug dependence, many individuals undergoing treatment will often slide back into their drug habits. Preventing relapse and maintaining long-term cessation of drug use are complex medical goals. Relapse prevention research is increasingly focusing on expanding the repertoire of behavioral skills to overcome dependence. Medications are also used in treating addiction.

Medication-Assisted Treatment   Medications can reduce the craving for the abused drug or block or oppose its effects. Perhaps the best-known medication for drug abuse is methadone, a synthetic drug used as a substitute for heroin. Use of methadone prevents withdrawal reactions and reduces the craving for heroin; it enables dependent people to function normally in social and vocational activities, although they remain dependent on methadone. The narcotic buprenorphine, approved in 2002 for treatment of opioid addiction, also reduces cravings.

Medication therapy is relatively simple and inexpensive and is therefore popular among patients, health care providers, and insurance companies. However, the relapse rate is high. Combining drug therapy with psychological and social services improves success rates, underscoring the importance of psychological factors in drug dependence.

Treatment Centers   Treatment centers offer a variety of short-term and long-term services, including hospitalization, detoxification, counseling, and other mental health services. The therapeutic community is a specific type of center, a residential program run in a completely drug-free atmosphere. Administered by ex-addicts, these programs use confrontation, strict discipline, and unrelenting peer pressure to attempt to resocialize the addict with a different set of values. Halfway houses, transitional settings between a 24-hour-a-day program and independent living, can be an important phase of treatment.

Self-Help Groups and Peer Counseling   Groups such as Alcoholics Anonymous (AA) and Narcotics Anonymous (NA) have helped many people. People treated in drug substitution programs or substance-abuse treatment centers are often urged or required to join a self-help group as part of their recovery. These groups follow a 12-step program. Group members' first step is to acknowledge that they have a problem over which they have no control. Peer support is a critical ingredient of these programs, and members usually meet at least once a week. Each member is paired with a sponsor to call on for advice and support if the temptation to relapse becomes overwhelming. Chapters of AA and NA meet on some college campuses; community-based chapters are listed in the phone book and in local newspapers.

Many colleges also have peer counseling programs, in which students are trained to help other students who have drug problems. A peer counselor's role may be as limited as referring a student to a professional with expertise in substance dependence for an evaluation or as involved as helping arrange a leave of absence from school for participation in a drug-treatment program.

Harm Reduction Strategies   Recognizing that many attempts at treatment are at first unsuccessful and that a drug-free society may be an unobtainable goal, some experts advocate the use of harm reduction strategies. The goal of harm reduction is to minimize the negative effects of drug use and abuse; a common example is the use of designated drivers to reduce alcohol-related motor vehicle crashes. In terms of illicit drugs, drug substitution programs such as methadone maintenance are one form of harm reduction; although participants remain drug dependent, the negative individual and social consequences of their drug use is reduced. Syringe exchange programs, designed to reduce transmission of HIV and hepatitis C, are another harm reduction approach. Some experts advocate free testing of street drugs for purity and potency to help users avoid unintentional toxicity or overdose.

Codependency   Drug abuse takes a toll on friends and family members, and counseling can help people work

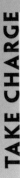
If Someone You Know Has a Drug Problem . . .

Changes in behavior and mood in someone you know may signal a growing dependence on drugs. Signs that a person's life is beginning to focus on drugs include the following:

- Sudden withdrawal or emotional distance

- Rebellious or unusually irritable behavior

- A loss of interest in usual activities or hobbies

- A decline in school performance

- A sudden change in the chosen group of friends

- Changes in sleeping or eating habits

- Frequent borrowing of money or stealing

- Secretive behavior about personal possessions, such as a backpack or the contents of a drawer

- Deterioration of physical appearance

If you believe a family member or friend has a drug problem, obtain information about resources for drug treatment available on your campus or in your community. Communicate your concern, provide him or her with information about treatment options, and offer your support during treatment. If the person continues to deny having a problem, you may want to talk with an experienced counselor about setting up an intervention—a formal, structured confrontation designed to end denial by having family, friends, and other caring individuals present their concerns to the drug user. And finally, examine your relationship with the abuser for signs of codependency. If necessary, get help for yourself; friends and family of drug users can often benefit from counseling.

---

through painful feelings of guilt and powerlessness. **Codependency,** in which a person close to the drug abuser is controlled by the abuser's behavior, sometimes develops. Codependent people may come to believe that love, approval, and security are contingent on their taking care of the abuser. People can become codependent because they want to help when someone they love becomes dependent on a drug. They may assume their good intentions will persuade the drug user to stop.

Codependent people often engage in behaviors that remove or soften the effects of drug use on the user—so-called *enabling* behaviors. However, the habit of enabling can inhibit a drug-dependent person's recovery because the person never has to experience the consequences of his or her behavior.

Have you ever been an enabler in a relationship? You may have, if you've ever done any of the following:

- Given someone one more chance to stop abusing drugs, then another, and another . . .

- Made excuses or lied for someone to his or her friends, teachers, or employer

- Joined someone in drug use and blamed others for your behavior

- Loaned money to someone to continue drug use

- Stayed up late waiting for or gone out searching for someone who uses drugs

- Felt embarrassed or angry about the actions of someone who uses drugs

- Ignored the drug use because the person got defensive when you brought it up

- Not confronted a friend or relative who was obviously intoxicated or high on a drug

If you come from a codependent family or see yourself developing codependency relationships or engaging in enabling behaviors, consider acting now to make changes in your patterns of interaction.

Preventing Drug Abuse

Obviously, the best solution to drug abuse is prevention. Government attempts at prevention tend to focus on controlling supply—stopping the production, importation, and distribution of illegal drugs. Other solutions are based on lowering demand—developing persuasive antidrug educational programs. Indirect approaches to prevention involve building young people's self-esteem, improving their academic skills, and increasing their recreational opportunities. Direct approaches involve giving information about the adverse effects of drugs and teaching tactics that help students resist peer pressure to use drugs in various situations.

Prevention efforts need to focus on the different motivations individuals have for using and abusing specific drugs at different ages. For example, adolescents in junior or senior high school are often more responsive to peer counselors. Many young adults tend to be influenced by efforts that focus on health education. For all ages, it is important to provide nondrug alternatives—such as recreational facilities, counseling, greater opportunities for

TERMS **codependency** A relationship in which a non–substance-abusing partner or family member is controlled by the abuser's behavior; codependent people frequently engage in enabling behaviors.

leisure activities, and places to socialize—that speak to the individual's or group's specific reasons for using drugs. Reminding young people that most people, no matter what age, do not use drugs is a critical part of preventing substance abuse.

The Role of Drugs in Your Life

Whatever your experience has been up to now, it's likely that you will encounter drugs at some point in your life. To make sure you'll have the inner resources to resist peer pressure and make your own decision, cultivate a variety of activities you enjoy doing, realize that you are entitled to have your own opinion, and don't neglect your self-esteem.

Before you try a psychoactive drug, consider the following questions:

- *What are the risks involved?* Many drugs carry an immediate risk of injury or death. Most involve the longer-term risk of abuse and dependence.

- *Is using the drug compatible with your goals?* Consider how drug use will affect your education and career objectives, your relationships, your future happiness, and the happiness of those who love you.

- *What are your ethical beliefs about drug use?* Consider whether using a drug would cause you to go against your personal ethics, religious beliefs, social values, or family responsibilities.

- *What are the financial costs?* Many drugs are expensive, especially if you become dependent on them.

- *Are you trying to solve a deeper problem?* Drugs will not make emotional pain go away; in the long run, they will only make it worse. If you are feeling depressed or anxious, seek help from a mental health professional instead of self-medicating with drugs.

Like all aspects of health-related behavior, making responsible decisions about drug use depends on information, knowledge, and insight into yourself. Many choices are possible; making the ones that are right for you is what counts.

QUESTIONS FOR CRITICAL THINKING AND REFLECTION

Do you know someone who may have a drug problem? What steps, if any, have you taken to help that person? If you were using drugs and felt that things had gone out of control, what would you want your friends to do for you?

TIPS FOR TODAY AND THE FUTURE
RIGHT NOW YOU CAN

- If you are a regular caffeine user, look for ways to cut back.
- Consider whether you or someone you know might benefit from drug counseling. Find out what types of services are available on campus or in your area.

IN THE FUTURE YOU CAN

- Investigate the drug-related attitudes of people you know. For example, talk to two older adults and two fellow students about their attitudes toward legalizing marijuana. What are the differences in their opinions, and how do they account for them?
- Analyze media portrayals of drug use. As you watch TV shows and movies, take note of the way they depict drug use among people of different ages and backgrounds. How realistic are the portrayals, in your view? Think about the influence they have on you and your peers.

SUMMARY

- Addictive behaviors are reinforcing. Addicts experience a strong compulsion for the behavior and a loss of control over it; an escalating pattern of abuse with serious negative consequences may result.

- The sources or causes of addiction include heredity, personality, lifestyle, and environmental factors. People may use an addictive behavior as a means of alleviating stress or painful emotions.

- Many common behaviors are potentially addictive, including gambling, shopping, sexual activity, Internet use, eating, and working.

- Drug abuse is a maladaptive pattern of drug use that persists despite adverse social, psychological, or medical consequences.

- Drug dependence involves taking a drug compulsively, which includes neglecting constructive activities because of it and continuing to use it despite experiencing adverse effects resulting from its use. Tolerance and withdrawal symptoms are often present.

- Reasons for using drugs include the lure of the illicit; curiosity; rebellion; peer pressure; and the desire to alter one's mood or escape boredom, anxiety, depression, or other psychological problems.

- Psychoactive drugs affect the mind and body by altering brain chemistry. The effect of a drug depends on the properties of the drug and how it's used (drug factors),

Changing Your Drug Habits

This behavior change strategy focuses on one of the most commonly used drugs—caffeine. If you are concerned about your use of a different drug or another type of addictive behavior, you can devise your own plan based on this one and on the steps outlined in Chapter 1.

Because caffeine supports certain behaviors that are characteristic of our culture, such as sedentary, stressful work, you may find yourself relying on coffee (or tea, chocolate, or cola) to get through a busy schedule. Such habits often begin in college. Fortunately, it's easier to break a habit before it becomes entrenched as a lifelong dependency.

Self-Monitoring

Keep a log of how much caffeine you eat or drink. Use a measuring cup to measure coffee or tea. Using Table 7.3, convert the amounts you drink into an estimate expressed in milligrams of caffeine. Be sure to include all forms, such as chocolate bars and OTC medications, as well as caffeine candy, colas, cocoa or hot chocolate, chocolate cake, tea, and coffee.

Self-Assessment

At the end of the week, add up your daily totals and divide by 7 to get your daily average in milligrams. How much is too much? At more than 250 mg per day, you may well be experiencing some adverse symptoms. If you are experiencing at least five of the following symptoms, you may want to cut down: restlessness, nervousness, excitement, insomnia, flushed face, excessive sweating, gastrointestinal problems, muscle twitching, rambling thoughts and speech, irregular heartbeat, periods of inexhaustibility, and excessive pacing or movement.

Set Limits

Can you restrict your caffeine intake to a daily total, and stick to this contract? If so, set a cutoff point, such as one cup of coffee. Pegging it to a specific time of day can be helpful, because then you won't confront a decision at any other point (and possibly fail). If you find you cannot stick to your limit, you may want to cut out caffeine altogether; abstinence can be easier than moderation for some people. If you experience caffeine withdrawal symptoms (headache, fatigue), you may want to cut your intake more gradually.

Find Other Ways to Keep Up Your Energy

If you are fatigued, it makes sense to get enough sleep or exercise more, rather than drowning the problem in coffee or tea. Different people need different amounts of sleep; you may also need more sleep at different times, such as during a personal crisis or an illness. Also, exercise raises your metabolic rate for hours afterward—a handy fact to exploit when you want to feel more awake and want to avoid an irritable caffeine jag. And if you've been compounding your fatigue by not eating properly, try filling up on complex carbohydrates such as whole-grain bread or crackers instead of candy bars.

Tips on Cutting Out Caffeine Here are some more ways to decrease your consumption of caffeine:

■ Keep some noncaffeinated drinks on hand, such as decaffeinated coffee, herbal teas, mineral water, bouillon, or hot water.

■ Alternate between hot and very cold liquids.

■ Fill your coffee cup only halfway.

■ Avoid the office or school lunchroom or cafeteria and the chocolate sections of the grocery store. (Often people drink coffee or tea and eat chocolate simply because they're available.)

■ Read labels of over-the-counter medications to check for hidden sources of caffeine.

---

the physical and psychological characteristics of the user (user factors), and the physical and social environment surrounding the drug use (social factors).

• Opioids relieve pain, cause drowsiness, and induce euphoria; they reduce anxiety and produce lethargy, apathy, and an inability to concentrate.

• CNS depressants slow down the overall activity of the nerves; they reduce anxiety and cause mood changes, impaired muscular coordination, slurring of speech, and drowsiness or sleep.

• CNS stimulants speed up the activity of the nerves, causing acceleration of the heart rate, a rise in blood pressure, dilation of the pupils and bronchial tubes, and an increase in gastric and adrenal secretions.

• Marijuana usually causes euphoria and a relaxed attitude at low doses; very high doses produce feelings of depersonalization and sensory distortion. The long-term effects may include chronic bronchitis and cancer; use during pregnancy may impair fetal growth.

• Hallucinogens alter perception, feelings, and thought and may cause an altered sense of time, visual disturbances, and mood changes.

• Inhalants are present in a variety of harmless products; they can cause delirium. Their use can lead to loss of consciousness, heart failure, suffocation, and death.

• Economic and social costs of drug abuse include the financial costs of law enforcement, treatment, and health care and the social costs of crime, violence, and family problems. Drug testing and drug legalization have been proposed to address some of the problems related to drug abuse.

• Approaches to treatment include medication, treatment centers, self-help groups, and peer counseling; many programs also offer counseling to family members.

FOR MORE INFORMATION

BOOKS

Aue, P. W. 2006. *Teen Drug Abuse: Opposing Viewpoints.* San Diego: Greenhaven Press. *Explores key issues relating to drug use and abuse by teenagers.*

Hanson, G. R., et al. 2008. *Drugs and Society,* 10th ed. Boston: Jones & Bartlett. *Discusses the impact of drug abuse on individuals' lives and on the broader society.*

Karch, S. B. 2006. *Drug Abuse Handbook,* 2nd ed. London: CRC Press. *Explores drug abuse from a variety of perspectives, including clinical and criminological.*

Ksir, C., C. L. Hart, and O. S. Ray. 2008. *Drugs, Society, and Human Behavior,* 12th ed. New York: McGraw-Hill. *Examines drugs and behavior from the behavioral, pharmacological, historical, social, legal, and clinical perspectives.*

Lessa, N. R., et al. 2006. *Wiley Concise Guides to Mental Health: Substance Use Disorders.* New York: Wiley. *A clearly written introduction to the diagnosis and treatment of various kinds of substance abuse.*

Murphy, P. J. M., and M. Shlafer. 2006. *Over-the-Counter Drugs of Abuse.* New York: Chelsea House Publications. *An up-to-date discussion of nonprescription medicines and their abuse.*

Rosen Publishing. 2006. *Drug Abuse and Society Series.* New York: Rosen Publishing. *A series of short books, each exploring a different type of drugs—from prescription medicine to club drugs—and their use and abuse.*

ORGANIZATIONS, HOTLINES, AND WEB SITES

Center for On-Line Addiction. Contains information about Internet and cybersex addiction.
  http://netaddiction.com
ClubDrugs.Org. Provides information on drugs commonly classified as "club drugs."
  http://www.clubdrugs.org
Do It Now Foundation. Provides youth-oriented information about drugs.
  http://www.doitnow.org
Drug Enforcement Administration: Drugs of Abuse. Provides basic facts about major drugs of abuse, including penalties for drug trafficking.
  http://www.dea.gov/concern/concern.htm
Gamblers Anonymous. Includes questions to help diagnose gambling problems and resources for getting help.
  http://www.gamblersanonymous.org
Higher Education Center for Alcohol and Other Drug Abuse and Violence Prevention. Gives information about alcohol and drug abuse on campus and links to related sites.
  http://www.edc.org/hec

Indiana Prevention Resource Center. A clearinghouse of information and links on substance-abuse topics, including specific psychoactive drugs and issues such as drug testing and drug legalization.
  http://www.drugs.indiana.edu
Narcotics Anonymous (NA). Similar to Alcoholics Anonymous, NA sponsors 12-step meetings and provides other support services for drug abusers.
  http://www.na.org
There are also 12-step programs that focus on specific drugs:
  Cocaine Anonymous
    http://www.ca.org
  Marijuana Anonymous
    http://www.marijuana-anonymous.org
National Center on Addiction and Substance Abuse (CASA) at Columbia University. Provides information about the costs of substance abuse to individuals and society.
  http://www.casacolumbia.org
National Clearinghouse for Alcohol and Drug Information. Provides statistics, information, and publications on substance abuse, including resources for people who want to help friends and family members overcome substance-abuse problems.
  http://ncadi.samhsa.gov
National Council on Problem Gambling. Provides information and help for people with gambling problems and their families, including a searchable directory of counselors.
  http://www.ncpgambling.org
National Drug Information, Treatment, and Referral Hotlines. Sponsored by the SAMHSA Center for Substance Abuse Treatment, these hotlines provide information on drug abuse and on HIV infection as it relates to substance abuse; referrals to support groups and treatment programs are available.
  800-662-HELP
  800-729-6686 (Spanish)
  800-487-4889 (TDD for hearing impaired)
National Institute on Drug Abuse. Develops and supports research on drug-abuse prevention programs; fact sheets on drugs of abuse are available on the Web site or via recorded phone messages, fax, or mail.
  http://www.drugabuse.gov
Substance Abuse and Mental Health Services Administration (SAMHSA). Provides statistics, information, and other resources related to substance-abuse prevention and treatment.
  http://www.samhsa.gov

See also the listings for Chapters 10 and 11.

SELECTED BIBLIOGRAPHY

American Psychiatric Association. 2000. *Diagnostic and Statistical Manual of Mental Disorders,* Fourth Edition, Text Revision. *(DSM-IV-TR).* Washington, D.C.: American Psychiatric Association.

Beers, M. H., et. al. 2006. *The Merck Manual of Diagnosis and Therapy,* 18th ed. New York: Wiley.

Braine, N. 2004. Long-term effects of syringe exchange on risk behavior and HIV prevention. *AIDS Education and Prevention* 16(3): 264–275.

Budney, A. J., et al. 2004. Review of the validity and significance of cannabis withdrawal syndrome. *American Journal of Psychiatry* 161(11): 1967–1977.

Centers for Disease Control and Prevention. 2006. Methamphetamine Use and HIV Risk Behaviors Among Heterosexual Men. *Morbidity and Mortality Weekly Report* (55)10: 273–277.

Colfax, G., et al. 2005. Longitudinal patterns of methamphetamine, popper (amyl nitrite), and cocaine use and high-risk sexual behavior among a cohort of San Francisco men who have sex with men. *Journal of Urban Health,* 28 February [epub].

Compton, W. M., et al. 2004. Prevalence of marijuana use disorder in the United States. *Journal of the American Medical Association* 291(17): 2114–2121.

Delaney-Black, V., et al. 2004. Prenatal cocaine: Quantity of exposure and gender moderation. *Journal of Developmental and Behavioral Pediatrics* 25(4): 254–263.

Grant, J. E., et al. 2006. Multicenter investigation of the opioid antagonist nalmefene in the treatment of pathological gambling. *American Journal of Psychiatry* 163(2): 303–312.

Hurd, Y. L., et al. 2005. Marijuana impairs growth in mid-gestation fetuses. *Neurotoxicology and Teratology* 27(2): 221–229.

Iannone, M., et al. 2006. Electrocortical effects of MDMA are potentiated by acoustic stimulation in rats. *BMC Neuroscience* 7: 13.

Jefferson, D. J. 2005. America's most dangerous drug. *Newsweek,* 8 August, 41–48.

Johnston, L. D., et al. 2008. *Monitoring the Future: National Results on Adolescent Drug Use: Overview of Key Findings, 2007.* Bethesda, Md.: National Institute on Drug Abuse.

Juliano, L. M., and R. R. Griffiths. 2004. A critical review of caffeine withdrawal: Empirical validation of symptoms and signs, incidence, severity, and associated features. *Psychopharmacology* 176(1): 1–29.

Kim, S. W., et al. 2006. Pathological gambling and mood disorders: Clinical associations and treatment implications. *Journal of Affective Disorders* 92(1): 109–116.

Lane, J. D., et al. 2004. Caffeine impairs glucose metabolism in type 2 diabetes. *Diabetes Care* 27(8): 2047–2048.

Lynch, W. J., P. K. Maciejewski, and M. N. Potenza. 2004. Psychiatric correlates of gambling in adolescents and young adults grouped by age at gambling onset. *Archives of General Psychiatry* 61(11): 1116–1122.

Mahowald, M. L., J. A. Singh, and P. Majeski. 2005. Opioid use by patients in an orthopedics spine clinic. *Arthritis and Rheumatology* 52(1): 312–321.

McBride, B. F., et al. 2004. Electrocardiographic and hemodynamic effects of a multicomponent dietary supplement containing ephedra and caffeine. *Journal of the American Medical Association* 291(4): 216–221.

McCusker, R. R., et al. 2006. Caffeine content of energy drinks, carbonated sodas, and other beverages. *Journal of Analytical Toxicology* 30(2): 112–114.

Messinis, L., et al. 2006. Neuropsychological deficits in long-term frequent cannabis users. *Neurology* 66(5): 737–739.

National Institute on Drug Abuse. 2008. *NIDA InfoFacts: Treatment Approaches for Drug Addiction* (http://www.drugabuse.gov/infofacts/treatmeth.html; retrieved February 3, 2009).

Office of Applied Studies, Substance Abuse and Mental Health Services Administration. 2008. *Results from the 2007 National Survey on Drug Use and Health: National Findings* (http://oas.samhsa.gov/nhsda.htm; retrieved February 3, 2009).

Opioid abuse. 2004. *Journal of the American Medical Association* 291(11): 1394.

Parrott, A. C. 2005. Chronic tolerance to recreational MDMA (3,4-methylenedioxymethamphetamine) or ecstasy. *Journal of Psychopharmacology* 19(1): 71–83.

Ramaekers, J. G., et al. 2004. Dose-related risk of motor vehicle crashes after cannabis use. *Drug and Alcohol Dependence* 73(2): 109–119.

Ren, S., et al. 2006. Effect of long-term cocaine use on regional left ventricular function as determined by magnetic resonance imaging. *American Journal of Cardiology* 97(7): 1085–1088.

Savoca, M. R., et al. 2005. Association of ambulatory blood pressure and dietary caffeine in adolescents. *American Journal of Hypertension* 18(1): 116–120.

Singer, L. T., et al. 2004. Cognitive outcomes of preschool children with prenatal cocaine exposure. *Journal of the American Medical Association* 291(20): 2448–2456.

Substance Abuse and Mental Health Services Administration. 2005 Nonmedical oxycodone users: A comparison with heroin users. *The NSDUH Report,* January.

Substance Abuse and Mental Health Services Administration, Office of Applied Studies. 2007. *Drug Abuse Warning Network, 2005: National Estimates of Drug-Related Emergency Department Visits.* Rockville, Md.: Substance Abuse and Mental Health Services Administration, DAWN Series D-29, DHHS Publication No. (SMA) 07-4256.

Wareing, M., et al. 2005. Visuo-spatial working memory deficits in current and former users of MDMA ("ecstasy"). *Human Psychopharmacology* 20(2): 115–23.

Waska, R. 2006. Addictions and the quest to control the object. *American Journal of Psychoanalysis* 66(1): 43–62.

Zakzanis, K. K., and Z. Campbell. 2006. Memory impairment in now abstinent MDMA users and continued users: A longitudinal follow-up. *Neurology* 66(5): 740–741.

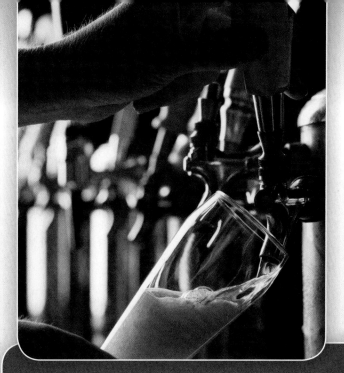

LOOKING   HEAD>>   >

AFTER READING   HAPTER
YOU   OULD B   TO:

- Explai   ow alcoh   d an   d by
  the b

- Descri   m
  drinki

- Descri
  their c

- List the
  they co

- Explain
  ated wi

- Describe
  prepare plans to stop using
  environmental tobacco smoke

ALCOHOL AND TOBACCO

8

W hen we think about drugs, most of us think of either the over-the-counter medications we get for colds and coughs or illicit drugs like marijuana and cocaine. The truth is that the most common and widely used drugs in the United States—and the ones responsible for the most illnesses, injuries, and deaths—are **alcohol** and **tobacco.** Alcohol use is associated with more than 75,000 deaths per year among Americans, and tobacco use is associated with more than 440,000 deaths per year.

Alcohol has a mixed role in human life. Used in moderation, alcohol can enhance social occasions by loosening inhibitions and creating a pleasant feeling of relaxation. But like other drugs, alcohol has physiological effects on the body that can impair functioning in the short term and cause devastating damage in the long term. For some people, alcohol becomes an addiction, leading to a lifetime of recovery or, for a few, to debilitation and death.

Tobacco use affects the health of people at all stages of life and from all walks of life. On average, a male smoker loses about 13 years from his life; a female smoker loses nearly 15 years. Nonsmokers also suffer, especially the children of parents who smoke. Exposure to environmental tobacco smoke (ETS) kills thousands of nonsmokers every year. Smoking is the leading cause of preventable death in the United States. This chapter examines the complexities of alcohol and tobacco use in the United States.

THE NATURE OF ALCOHOL

If you have ever been around people who are drinking, you probably noticed that alcohol seems to affect different people in different ways. One person may seem to get drunk after just a drink or two, while another appears to tolerate a great deal of alcohol without becoming intoxicated. These differences can be explained by looking at

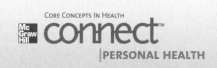

the chemistry of alcohol and how it is absorbed and metabolized by the body.

Alcoholic Beverages

There are several basic types of alcoholic beverages, but ethyl alcohol (or ethanol, often abbreviated as ETOH)is the psychoactive ingredient in each of them:

- Beer is a mild intoxicant brewed from a mixture of grains. By volume, beer usually contains 3–6% alcohol.

- Ales and malt liquors contain 6–8% alcohol by volume.

- Wines are made by fermenting the juices of grapes or other fruits. In table wines, the concentration of alcohol is about 9–14%. *Fortified wines,* so called because extra alcohol is added to them, include sherry, port, and Madeira. They contain about 20% alcohol.

- Hard liquor—such as gin, whiskey, rum, tequila, vodka, and liqueur—is made by *distilling* brewed or fermented grains or other plant products. Hard liquors usually contain 35–50% alcohol.

The concentration of alcohol in a beverage is indicated by its **proof value,** which is two times the percentage concentration. For example, if a beverage is 100 proof, it contains 50% alcohol. The proof value of hard liquor can usually be found on the bottle's label. When alcohol consumption is discussed, the term **one drink** (or *a standard drink*) means the amount of a beverage that typically contains about 0.6 ounce of alcohol.

Alcohol provides 7 calories per gram, and the alcohol in one drink (14–17 grams) supplies about 100–120 calories. Most alcoholic beverages also contain some carbohydrate, so, for example, one beer provides about 150 total calories. The "light" in light beer refers to calories; a light beer typically has close to the same alcohol content as a regular beer and about 100 calories. A 5-ounce glass of red wine has 100 calories; white wine has 96. A 3-ounce

margarita supplies 157 calories, a 6-ounce cosmopolitan has 143 calories, and a 6-ounce rum and Coke contains about 180 calories.

Absorption

When a person ingests alcohol, about 20% is rapidly absorbed from the stomach into the bloodstream. About 75% is absorbed through the upper part of the small intestine. Any remaining alcohol enters the bloodstream further along the gastrointestinal tract. Once in the bloodstream, alcohol produces feelings of intoxication. The rate of absorption is affected by a variety of factors. For example, the carbonation in a beverage like champagne increases the rate of alcohol absorption. Artificial sweeteners (commonly used in drink mixers) have been shown to have the same effect. Food in the stomach slows the rate of absorption, as does the drinking of highly concentrated alcoholic beverages such as hard liquor.

Metabolism and Excretion

Because alcohol easily moves through most biological membranes, it is rapidly distributed throughout most body tissues via the bloodstream. The main site of alcohol **metabolism** is the liver, though a small amount of alcohol is metabolized in the stomach (see the box "Metabolizing Alcohol: Our Bodies Work Differently"). About 2–10% of ingested alcohol is not metabolized in the liver or other tissues but is excreted unchanged by the lungs, kidneys, and sweat glands. Excreted alcohol causes the telltale smell on a drinker's breath and is the basis of breath and urine analyses for alcohol levels.

Alcohol readily enters the human brain, affecting neurotransmitters, the chemicals that carry messages between brain cells. With chronic heavy usage, however, alcohol's effects become permanent, resulting in permanent disruption of brain function and changes in brain structure.

Alcohol Intake and Blood Alcohol Concentration

Blood alcohol concentration (BAC), a measure of intoxication, is determined by the amount of alcohol consumed in a given amount of time and by individual factors:

- *Body weight:* In most cases, a smaller person develops a higher BAC than a larger person after drinking the same amount of alcohol (Figure 8.1). A smaller person has less overall body tissue into which alcohol can be distributed.

- *Percent body fat:* A person with a higher percentage of body fat will usually develop a higher BAC than a more muscular person of the same weight. Alcohol does not concentrate as much in fatty tissue as in muscle and most other tissues, in part because fat has fewer blood vessels.

TERMS

alcohol The intoxicating ingredient in fermented or distilled beverages; a colorless, pungent liquid.

tobacco The leaves of cultivated tobacco plants prepared for smoking, chewing, or use as snuff.

proof value Two times the percentage of alcohol by volume; a beverage that is 50% alcohol by volume is 100 proof.

one drink The amount of a beverage that typically contains about 0.6 ounce of alcohol; also called *a standard drink.*

metabolism The chemical transformation of food and other substances in the body into energy and wastes.

blood alcohol concentration (BAC) The amount of alcohol in the blood in terms of weight per unit volume; used as a measure of intoxication.

Metabolizing Alcohol: Our Bodies Work Differently

DIMENSIONS OF DIVERSITY

Do you notice that you react differently to alcohol than some of your friends? If so, you may be witnessing genetic differences in alcohol metabolism that are associated with ethnicity. Alcohol is metabolized mainly in the liver, where it is converted by an enzyme (alcohol dehydrogenase) to a toxic substance called acetaldehyde. Acetaldehyde is responsible for many of alcohol's noxious effects. Ideally, it is quickly broken down by another enzyme (acetaldehyde dehydrogenase).

But some people, primarily those of Asian descent, have inherited ineffective or inactive variations of the latter enzyme. Other people, including some of African descent and some Jewish population groups, have forms of alcohol dehydrogenase that metabolize alcohol to acetaldehyde unusually quickly. In either case, the result is a buildup of acetaldehyde when these people drink alcohol. They experience a reaction called *flushing syndrome*. Their skin feels hot, their heart and respiration rates increase, and they may get a headache, vomit, or break out in hives. The severity of their reaction is affected by the inherited form of their alcohol-metabolizing enzymes. Drinking makes some people so uncomfortable that it's unlikely they could ever become addicted to alcohol.

The body's response to acetaldehyde is the basis for treating alcohol abuse with the drug disulfiram (Antabuse), which inhibits the action of acetaldehyde dehydrogenase. When a person taking disulfiram ingests alcohol, acetaldehyde levels increase rapidly, and he or she develops an intense flushing reaction along with weakness, nausea, vomiting, and other disagreeable symptoms.

How people behave in relation to alcohol is influenced in complex ways by many factors, including social and cultural ones. But in this case at least, individual choices and behavior are strongly influenced by a specific genetic characteristic.

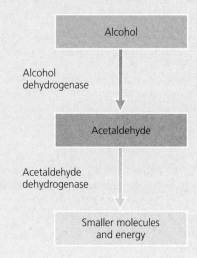

- *Sex:* Women metabolize less alcohol in the stomach than men do because the stomach enzyme that breaks down alcohol before it enters the bloodstream is four times more active in men than in women. This means that more unmetabolized alcohol is released into the bloodstream in women. Because women are also generally smaller than men and have a higher percentage of body fat, women will have a higher BAC than men after consuming the same amount of alcohol. Hormonal fluctuations may also affect the rate of alcohol metabolism, making a woman more susceptible to high BACs at certain times during her menstrual cycle (usually just prior to the onset of menstruation).

BAC also depends on the balance between the rate of alcohol absorption and the rate of alcohol metabolism. A man who weighs 150 pounds and has normal liver function metabolizes about 0.3 ounce of alcohol per hour, the equivalent of about half a 12-ounce bottle of beer or a 5-ounce glass of wine. The rate of alcohol metabolism varies among individuals and is largely determined by genetic factors and drinking behavior. Although the rate of alcohol absorption can be slowed by factors like food, the metabolic rate *cannot* be influenced by exercise, breathing deeply, eating, drinking coffee, or taking other drugs. The rate of alcohol metabolism is the same whether a person is asleep or awake.

If a person absorbs slightly less alcohol each hour than he or she can metabolize in an hour, the BAC remains low.

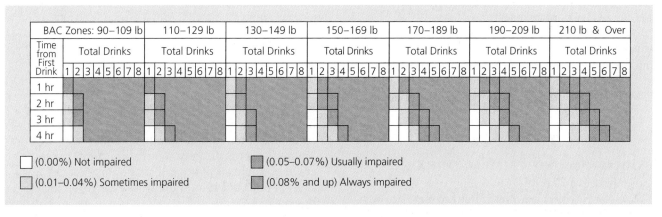

FIGURE 8.1 Approximate blood alcohol concentration and body weight. This chart illustrates the BAC an average person of a given weight would reach after drinking the specified number of drinks in the time shown. The legal limit for BAC in all states is 0.08%; for drivers under 21 years of age, many states have zero-tolerance laws that set BAC limits of 0.01% or 0.02%.

Table 8.1	The Effects of Alcohol	
BAC (%)	Common Behavioral Effects	Hours Required to Metabolize Alcohol
0.00–0.05	Slight change in feelings, usually relaxation and euphoria. Decreased alertness.	2–3
0.05–0.10	Emotional instability, with exaggerated feelings and behavior. Reduced social inhibitions. Impairment of reaction time and fine motor coordination. Increasingly impaired during driving. Legally drunk at 0.08%.	3–6
0.10–0.15	Unsteadiness in standing and walking. Loss of peripheral vision. Driving is extremely dangerous.	6–10
0.15–0.30	Staggering gait. Slurred speech. Pain and other sensory perceptions greatly impaired.	10–24
More than 0.30	Stupor or unconsciousness. Anesthesia. Death possible at 0.35% and above. Can result from rapid or binge drinking with few earlier effects.	More than 24

People can drink large amounts of alcohol this way over a long period of time without becoming noticeably intoxicated; however, they do run the risk of significant long-term health hazards. If a person drinks alcohol more quickly than it can be metabolized, the BAC will steadily increase, and he or she will become more and more drunk (Table 8.1).

ALCOHOL AND HEALTH

The effects of alcohol consumption on health depend on the individual, the circumstances, and the amount of alcohol consumed.

The Immediate Effects of Alcohol

Alcohol is a CNS depressant, and its effects vary because body systems are affected to different degrees at different BACs. At any given BAC, the effects of alcohol are more pronounced when the BAC is rapidly increasing than when it is slowly increasing, steady, or decreasing. The effects of alcohol are more pronounced if a person drinks on an empty stomach, because alcohol is absorbed more quickly and the BAC rises more quickly.

Low Concentrations of Alcohol   The effects of alcohol can first be felt at a BAC of about 0.03–0.05% and may include light-headedness, relaxation, and a release of inhibitions. Most drinkers experience mild euphoria and become more sociable. When people drink in social settings, alcohol often seems to act as a stimulant, enhancing conviviality or assertiveness. This apparent stimulation occurs because alcohol depresses inhibitory centers in the brain.

Higher Concentrations of Alcohol   At higher concentrations, the pleasant effects tend to be replaced by more negative ones: interference with motor coordination, verbal performance, and intellectual functions. The drinker often becomes irritable or emotional. When the BAC reaches 0.1%, most sensory and motor functioning is reduced, and many people become sleepy. Vision, smell, taste, and hearing become less acute. At 0.2%, most drinkers are completely unable to function, either physically or psychologically, because of the pronounced depression of the central nervous system, muscles, and other body systems. Coma usually occurs at a BAC of 0.35%, and any higher level can be fatal. Small doses of alcohol may improve sexual functioning for individuals who are especially anxious or self-conscious, but higher doses often have negative effects, such as reduced erectile response. (Chronic effects of heavy drinking include reduction of testosterone levels and impairment of sperm production.)

Alcohol Hangover   Alcohol's effects wear off slowly. The symptoms of a hangover include headache, shakiness, nausea, diarrhea, fatigue, and impaired mental functioning. During a hangover, heart rate and blood pressure increase, making some individuals more vulnerable to heart attacks. Electroencephalography (brain wave measurement) shows diffuse slowing of brain waves for up to 16 hours after BAC drops to zero. Studies of pilots, drivers, and skiers all indicate that coordination and cognition are impaired in a person with a hangover, increasing the risk of injury.

Alcohol Poisoning   Drinking large amounts of alcohol over a short period of time can rapidly raise the BAC into

QUESTIONS FOR CRITICAL THINKING AND REFLECTION
Have you ever had a hangover or watched someone else suffer through one? Did the experience affect your attitude about drinking? In what way?

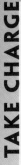

TAKE CHARGE

Dealing with an Alcohol Emergency

Remember: Being very drunk is potentially life-threatening. Helping a drunken friend could save a life.

• Be firm but calm. Don't engage the person in an argument or discuss her drinking behavior while she is intoxicated.

• Get the person out of harm's way—don't let her drive or wander outside. Don't let her drink any more alcohol.

• If the person is unconscious, don't assume she is just "sleeping it off." Place her on her side with her knees up. This position will help prevent choking if the person should vomit.

• Stay with the person—you need to be ready to help if she vomits or stops breathing.

• Don't try to give the person anything to eat or drink, including coffee or other drugs. Don't give cold showers or try to make her walk around. None of these things help anyone to sober up, and they can be dangerous.

Call 911 immediately in any of the following instances:

• You can't wake the person even with shouting or shaking.

• The person is taking fewer than 8 breaths per minute or her breathing seems shallow or irregular.

• You think the person took other drugs in addition to alcohol.

• The person has had an injury, especially a blow to the head.

• The person drank a large amount of alcohol within a short period of time and then became unconscious. Death caused by alcohol poisoning most often occurs when the blood alcohol level rises very quickly due to rapid ingestion of alcohol.

If you aren't sure what to do, call 911. You may save a life.

---

the lethal range. Death from alcohol poisoning may be caused either by central nervous system and respiratory depression or by inhaling fluid or vomit into the lungs. The amount of alcohol it takes to make a person unconscious is dangerously close to a fatal dose. Although passing out may prevent someone from drinking more, BAC can keep rising during unconsciousness, because the body continues absorbing ingested alcohol into the bloodstream. Special care should be taken to ensure the safety of anyone who has been drinking heavily, especially if the person becomes unconscious (see the box "Dealing with an Alcohol Emergency").

Using Alcohol with Other Drugs Alcohol-drug combinations are a leading cause of drug-related deaths. Using alcohol while taking a medication that can cause CNS depression increases the effects of both drugs, potentially leading to coma, respiratory depression, and death. Such drugs include barbiturates, Valium-like drugs, narcotics such as codeine, and OTC antihistamines such as Benadryl. For people who consume three or more drinks per day, use of OTC pain relievers like aspirin, ibuprofen, or acetaminophen increases the risk of stomach bleeding or liver damage. Some antibiotics and diabetes medications can also interact dangerously with alcohol. Many illegal drugs are especially dangerous when combined with alcohol. Life-threatening overdoses occur at much lower doses when heroin and other narcotics are combined with alcohol.

Alcohol-Related Injuries and Violence The combination of impaired judgment, weakened sensory perception, reduced inhibitions, impaired motor coordination, and increased aggressiveness and hostility that characterizes alcohol intoxication can be dangerous. Through ho-micide, suicide, automobile crashes, and other traumatic incidents, alcohol use is linked to more than 75,000 American deaths each year. Among successful suicides, alcohol use is common, as well. Alcohol use more than triples the chances of fatal injuries during leisure activities such as swimming and boating, and more than half of all fatal falls and serious burns happen to people who have been drinking.

> **QUICK STATS**
>
> **Nearly 500,000** emergency room visits resulted from using alcohol or alcohol/drug combinations in 2005.
>
> —Drug Abuse Warning Network, 2007

Alcohol and Aggression Alcohol use contributes to over 50% of all murders, assaults, and rapes. Alcohol is frequently found in the bloodstream of victims as well as perpetrators. In 2007, more than 2,600,000 arrests were made for alcohol-related offenses. However, only some people become violent under alcohol's influence. These people are often predisposed to aggressive behavior and are highly impulsive. Some may have an underlying psychiatric condition called *antisocial personality disorder*. Alcohol is an important component of gang life, affirming masculinity and male togetherness and contributing to gang violence.

Alcohol abuse can wreak havoc on home life. Marital discord and domestic violence often occur in the presence of excess alcohol. Heavy drinking by parents is associated with child abuse, typically emotional or psychological abuse.

Alcohol and Sexual Decision Making Alcohol seriously affects a person's ability to make wise decisions about sex. Heavy drinkers are more likely to have multiple sex partners and to engage in other forms of high-risk sexual behavior. For all these reasons, rates of sexually transmitted infections (including HIV) and unwanted pregnancy are higher among people who drink heavily than among people who drink moderately or not at all. Women who binge-drink are at increased risk for rape and other forms of nonconsensual sex.

Drinking and Driving

In 2007, about 32% of more than 41,000 crash fatalities involved drivers with a BAC of 0.08% or higher. Each year, more than 275,000 people are injured in alcohol-related (BAC of 0.01% or higher) car crashes—an average of one person injured every 2 minutes. In the 2007 National Survey on Drug Use and Health, 13.7% of Americans age 18 and older admitted to using alcohol before driving.

People who drink and drive are unable to drive safely because their judgment is impaired, their reaction time is slower, and their coordination is reduced. Some driving skills are affected at BACs of 0.02% and lower. The *dose-response function* is the relationship between the amount of alcohol or drug consumed and the type and intensity of the resulting effect. Higher doses of alcohol are associated with a much greater probability of automobile crashes (Figure 8.2). A person driving with a BAC of 0.14% is more than 40 times more likely to be involved in a crash than someone with no alcohol in his or her blood. For those with a BAC above 0.14%, the risk of a fatal crash is estimated to be 380 times higher.

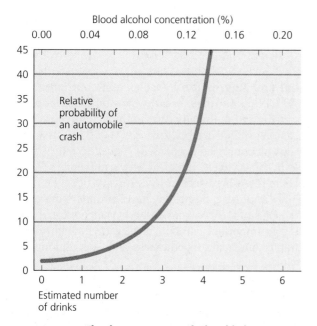

FIGURE 8.2 The dose-response relationship between BAC and automobile crashes.

In addition to an increased risk of injury and death, driving while intoxicated can have serious legal consequences. Since 2003, the legal limit for BAC has been 0.08% in all states and the District of Columbia. There are stiff penalties for drunk driving, including fines, loss of license, confiscation of vehicle, and jail time. Under current zero-tolerance laws in many states, drivers under age 21 who have consumed *any* alcohol may have their license suspended. If you are out of your home and drinking, find alternative transportation or have a *designated driver* who doesn't drink and can provide safe transportation home.

It's more difficult to protect yourself against someone else who drinks and drives. Learn to be alert to the erratic driving that signals an impaired driver. Warning signs include wide, abrupt, and illegal turns; straddling the center line or lane marker; driving against traffic; driving on the shoulder; weaving, swerving, or nearly striking an object or another vehicle; following too closely; erratic speed; driving with headlights off at night; and driving with the window down in very cold weather. If you see any of these signs, try the following strategies:

- If the driver is ahead of you, maintain a safe following distance. Don't try to pass.
- If the driver is behind you, turn right at the nearest intersection, and let the driver pass.
- If the driver is approaching your car, move to the shoulder and stop. Avoid a head-on collision by sounding your horn or flashing your lights.
- When approaching an intersection, slow down and stay alert for vehicles that don't appear to be slowing.
- Make sure your safety belt is fastened and children are in approved safety seats.
- Report suspected impaired drivers to the nearest police station by phone.

The Effects of Chronic Use

Because alcohol is distributed throughout most of the body, it can affect many different organs and tissues (Figure 8.3).

The Digestive System Even in the short term, alcohol can alter the functioning of the liver. Within just a few days of heavy alcohol consumption, fat begins to accumulate in liver cells, resulting in the development of "fatty liver." If drinking continues, inflammation of the

> Chronic liver disease is the **12th** leading cause of death in the United States.
>
> —National Center for Health Statistics, 2008

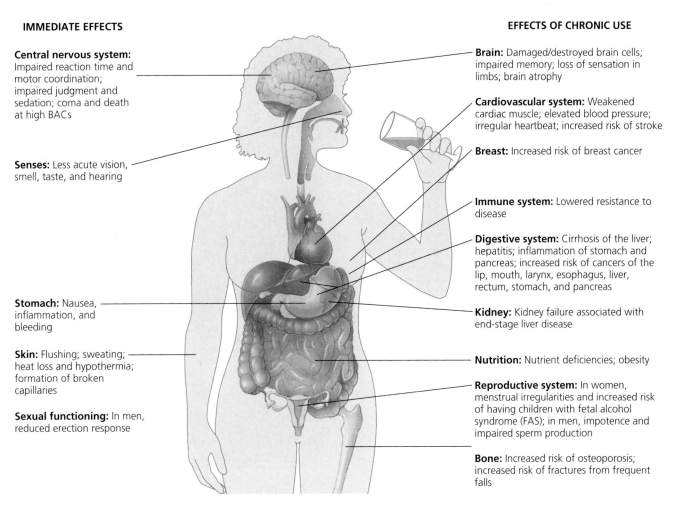

Central nervous system: Impaired reaction time and motor coordination; impaired judgment and sedation; coma and death at high BACs

Senses: Less acute vision, smell, taste, and hearing

Stomach: Nausea, inflammation, and bleeding

Skin: Flushing; sweating; heat loss and hypothermia; formation of broken capillaries

Sexual functioning: In men, reduced erection response

Brain: Damaged/destroyed brain cells; impaired memory; loss of sensation in limbs; brain atrophy

Cardiovascular system: Weakened cardiac muscle; elevated blood pressure; irregular heartbeat; increased risk of stroke

Breast: Increased risk of breast cancer

Immune system: Lowered resistance to disease

Digestive system: Cirrhosis of the liver; hepatitis; inflammation of stomach and pancreas; increased risk of cancers of the lip, mouth, larynx, esophagus, liver, rectum, stomach, and pancreas

Kidney: Kidney failure associated with end-stage liver disease

Nutrition: Nutrient deficiencies; obesity

Reproductive system: In women, menstrual irregularities and increased risk of having children with fetal alcohol syndrome (FAS); in men, impotence and impaired sperm production

Bone: Increased risk of osteoporosis; increased risk of fractures from frequent falls

FIGURE 8.3 The immediate and long-term effects of alcohol abuse.

liver can occur, resulting in alcoholic hepatitis, a frequent cause of hospitalization and death in alcoholics. With continued alcohol use, liver cells are progressively damaged and then permanently destroyed. The destroyed cells are replaced by fibrous scar tissue, a condition known as **cirrhosis.** People with cirrhosis who continue to drink have only a 50% chance of surviving 5 or more years.

Alcohol can inflame the pancreas, causing nausea, vomiting, abnormal digestion, and severe pain. Unlike cirrhosis, which usually occurs after years of fairly heavy alcohol use, pancreatitis can occur after just one or two severe binge-drinking episodes. Acute pancreatitis is often fatal; in survivors it can develop into a chronic condition.

The Cardiovascular System   The effects of alcohol on the cardiovascular system depend on the amount of alcohol consumed. Moderate doses of alcohol—one drink or less a day for women and one to two drinks a day for men—may reduce the risk of heart disease and heart attack in some people. However, higher doses of alcohol have harmful effects on the cardiovascular system. In

some people, more than two drinks a day will elevate blood pressure, making stroke and heart attack more likely. Some alcoholics show a weakening of the heart muscle, a condition known as **cardiac myopathy.** Binge drinking can cause "holiday heart," a syndrome characterized by serious abnormal heart rhythms, which usually appear within 24 hours of a binge episode.

Cancer   The U.S. Department of Health and Human Services lists alcoholic beverages as human carcinogens. Chronic alcohol consumption is a clear risk factor for cancers of the mouth, throat, larynx, and esophagus. Five or six daily drinks, especially combined with smoking, increase risk of these cancers by a factor of 50 or more.

cirrhosis   A disease in which the liver is severely damaged by alcohol, other toxins, or infection.

cardiac myopathy   Weakening of the heart muscle through disease.

TERMS

Alcohol also is largely responsible for the most common form of liver cancer. Recent studies show that breast cancer risk, although still small, begins to increase at two to three drinks per day, and continues to rise with increasing numbers of daily drinks.

Brain Damage   Imaging studies document that many alcoholics experience brain shrinkage with loss of both grey and white matter, reduced blood flow, and slowed metabolic rates in some brain regions. About half of the alcoholics in the United States have cognitive impairments, ranging from mild to severe. These include memory loss, dementia, and compromised problem-solving and reasoning abilities. Malnutrition, particularly thiamine deficiency, contributes to severe brain damage and the disabling condition known as Wernicke-Korsakoff syndrome.

Mortality   Excessive alcohol consumption is a factor in several of the leading causes of death for Americans. Average life expectancy among alcoholics is about 15 years less than among nonalcoholics. About half the deaths caused by alcohol are due to chronic conditions such as cirrhosis and cancer; the other half are due to acute conditions or events such as car crashes, falls, and suicide.

The Effects of Alcohol Use During Pregnancy

During pregnancy, alcohol and its metabolic product acetaldehyde readily cross the placenta, potentially harming the developing fetus. Damage to the fetus depends on the amount of alcohol consumed and the stage of the pregnancy. Early in pregnancy, heavy drinking can cause spontaneous abortion or miscarriage. Alcohol in early pregnancy can also cause a collection of birth defects known as **fetal alcohol syndrome (FAS)**. Children with FAS have a characteristic mixture of deformities, and their physical and mental growth is slower than normal.

FAS is a permanent, incurable condition that causes lifelong disability; it is among the most common preventable causes of mental retardation in the Western world. Full-blown FAS occurs in up to 15 out of every 10,000 live births in the United States. About three times as many babies are born with **alcohol-related neurodevelopmental disorder (ARND)**. Children with ARND appear physically normal but often have significant learning and behavioral disorders. The

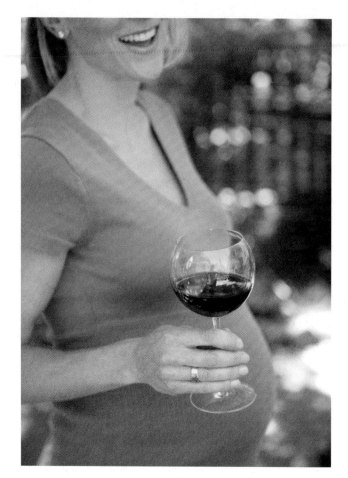
Experts warn that there is no safe level of alcohol consumption during pregnancy.

whole range of FAS and ARND is commonly called *fetal alcohol spectrum disorder (FASD)*.

No one is sure exactly how much alcohol causes FASD or ARND, but a recent study found that children born to mothers who drank as little as one and a half drinks per week during their pregnancy weighed less and were shorter at age 14 than children of mothers who drank nothing during pregnancy. Such evidence has led experts to assert that no amount of alcohol during pregnancy is safe.

Women who are trying to conceive, or who are sexually active without using effective contraception, are also advised to abstain from alcohol to avoid inadvertently harming their baby in the first few days or weeks of pregnancy. And because alcohol quickly enters breast milk, many physicians advise mothers to abstain from drinking alcohol if they are breastfeeding.

Possible Health Benefits of Alcohol

Numerous studies have shown that, on average, light to moderate drinkers live longer than either abstainers or heavy drinkers. Alcohol consumption appears to confer health benefits primarily to middle-aged or older individuals.

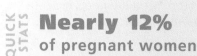

Nearly 12%
of pregnant women consume alcohol, and almost 4% are binge drinkers.

—SAMHSA, 2008

If you are 35 or younger, your odds of dying *increase* in direct proportion to the amount of alcohol you drink. Among people under age 35, even light drinkers have slightly higher mortality rates than nondrinkers. In other words, young adults who drink *any* amount of alcohol are more likely to die than nondrinkers of the same age.

Alcohol's benefits relate to heart health. The lowest rates of coronary heart disease (CHD) deaths occur with moderate alcohol use, which in studies had a positive effect on both healthy people and individuals at risk for CHD. In a 2006 study of men age 50 and over, those who drank moderately each day reduced their risk of CHD by about 40%, compared to men who never drank. The difference was not as great in women. Moderate drinking may improve heart health by raising blood levels of HDL (the beneficial form of cholesterol), by thinning the blood, and by reducing inflammation and the risk of dangerous blood clots, all of which can contribute to the risk of a heart attack. Some evidence also suggests that moderate drinkers may be less likely to develop or better able to manage a variety of other conditions, including diabetes, high blood pressure, strokes, arterial blockages in the legs, cognitive decline (including Alzheimer's disease), and benign prostate enlargement.

ALCOHOL ABUSE AND DEPENDENCE

The CDC estimates that about 60% of Americans age 18 and older drink alcohol routinely or infrequently. Approximately 15% of Americans are former drinkers, and 25% are lifetime abstainers. According to the National Survey on Drug Abuse and Health for 2007, almost 7% of Americans were classified as heavy alcohol users. Heavy drinkers account for over half of all the alcohol consumed, as well as a disproportionate amount of the social, economic, and medical costs of alcohol abuse (estimated at over $180 billion per year). Excessive alcohol use is the third leading lifestyle-related cause of death.

Abuse Versus Dependence

The American Psychiatric Association's *Diagnostic and Statistical Manual of Mental Disorders* makes a distinction between substance abuse and substance dependence. Al-

cohol abuse is recurrent alcohol use that has negative consequences, such as drinking in dangerous situations (before driving, for instance), or drinking patterns that result in academic, professional, interpersonal, or legal difficulties. **Alcohol dependence,** or **alcoholism,** involves more extensive problems with alcohol use, usually involving physical tolerance and withdrawal. Alcoholism is discussed in greater detail later in the chapter.

How can you tell if you or someone you know is becoming alcohol-dependent? Look for the following warning signs:

- Drinking alone or secretively
- Using alcohol deliberately and repeatedly to perform or get through difficult situations
- Feeling uncomfortable on certain occasions when alcohol is not available
- Escalating alcohol consumption beyond an already established drinking pattern
- Consuming alcohol heavily in risky situations, such as before driving
- Getting drunk regularly or more frequently than in the past
- Drinking in the morning or at other unusual times

Binge Drinking

The National Institute on Alcohol Abuse and Alcoholism defines **binge drinking** as a pattern of alcohol use that brings a person's BAC up to 0.08% or above (typically four drinks for men or three drinks for women), consumed within about 2 hours. The National Survey on Drug Use and Health defines binge drinking as having five or more drinks within about 2 hours, at least once within 30 days; the 2007 survey estimated that 23% of people over the age of 12 were binge drinkers. Almost 7% were heavy drinkers, defined as having five or more drinks on the same occasion on each of 5 or more days in the past 30 days.

Among Americans under 21 years old, most drinking is in the form of a binge. However, a sizeable number of those 25 years or older are binge drinkers, and about 75% of the alcohol consumed by adults in the United States meets the definition of binge drinking.

Binge drinking has a profound effect on students' lives (see the box "College Binge Drinking"). Frequent binge drinkers were found to be three to seven times more likely than non–binge drinkers to engage in unplanned or unprotected sex, to drive after drinking, and to get hurt or injured (Table 8.2). Binge drinkers were also more likely to miss classes, get behind in schoolwork, and argue with friends. The more frequent the binges, the more problems the students encountered. Despite their experiences, fewer than 1% of the binge drinkers identified themselves as problem drinkers.

Alcoholism

As mentioned earlier, alcoholism, or alcohol dependence, is usually characterized by tolerance to alcohol and withdrawal symptoms.

Patterns and Prevalence   Alcoholism occurs among people of all ethnic groups and at all socioeconomic levels. There are different patterns of alcohol dependence, including these four common ones: (1) regular daily intake of large amounts, (2) regular heavy drinking limited to weekends, (3) long periods of sobriety interspersed with binges of daily heavy drinking lasting for weeks or months, and (4) heavy drinking limited to periods of stress.

Once established, alcoholism often exhibits a pattern of exacerbations and remissions. Alcoholism is not hopeless, however; many alcoholics do achieve permanent abstinence.

TERMS

hallucination   A false perception that does not correspond to external reality, such as seeing visions or hearing voices that are not there.

delirium tremens (the DTs)   A state of confusion brought on by the reduction of alcohol intake in an alcohol-dependent person; other symptoms are sweating, trembling, anxiety, hallucinations, and seizures.

VITAL STATISTICS		
Table 8.2	The Effects of Binge Drinking on College Students	

	Percentage of Students Experiencing Problems	
Alcohol-Related Problem	**Non–Binge Drinkers**	**Frequent Binge Drinkers**
Drove after drinking alcohol	18	58
Did something they regretted	17	62
Argued with friends	10	43
Engaged in unplanned sex	9	41
Missed a class	9	60
Got behind in schoolwork	9	42
Had unprotected sex	4	21
Got hurt or injured	4	28
Got into trouble with police	2	14
Had five or more of these problems since school year began	4	48

SOURCE: Wechsler, H., and B. Wuethrich. 2003. *Dying to Drink: Confronting Binge Drinking on College Campuses*, reprint ed. Emmaus, Pa.: Rodale.

Health Effects   *Tolerance* means that a drinker needs more alcohol to achieve intoxication or the desired effect, that the effects of continued use of the same amount of alcohol are diminished, or that the drinker can function adequately at doses or a BAC that would produce significant impairment in a casual user. Heavy users of alcohol may need to consume about 50% more than they originally needed in order to experience the same degree of intoxication.

Withdrawal symptoms include trembling hands (shakes, or jitters), a rapid pulse and accelerated breathing rate, insomnia, nightmares, anxiety, and gastrointestinal upset. More severe withdrawal symptoms occur in about 5% of alcoholics. These include seizures (sometimes called rum fits), confusion, and **hallucinations.** Still less common is **delirium tremens (the DTs),** a medical emergency characterized by severe disorientation, confusion, epileptic-like seizures, and vivid hallucinations, often of vermin and small animals. The mortality rate from DTs can be as high as 15%.

Alcoholics face all the physical health risks associated with intoxication and chronic drinking described earlier. Some of the damage is compounded by nutritional deficiencies that often accompany alcoholism. A mental problem associated with alcohol use is profound memory gaps (commonly known as blackouts).

Social and Psychological Effects   Alcohol use causes more serious social and psychological problems than all other forms of drug abuse combined. For every person

College Binge Drinking

College binge drinking, a serious problem for decades, has recently come under a harsh spotlight due largely to highly publicized alcohol-related tragedies on campus. Deaths from alcohol overdose, alcohol-related injuries (including motor vehicle crashes), violent crimes, student riots, and serious vandalism have all drawn attention to the epidemic of heavy drinking on college campuses.

To many people, heavy drinking is considered a normal and integral part of college life. But research has shown that heavy drinking has had a devastating impact on far too many students—drinkers and nondrinkers alike—as well as on their families and communities.

Drinking on campus is pervasive. Approximately 80% of college students drink alcohol; that's more than use cigarettes, marijuana, or cocaine combined. Research on college students across the United States shows that nearly half (44%) of students binge-drink. Other sources estimate that about 40% binge-drink, and about 20% binge three or more times over a two-week period.

Every year, an estimated 1700 college students age 18–24 die from overdoses and alcohol-related injuries. Another 600,000 sustain unintentional alcohol-related injuries, 700,000 are assaulted by other students who have been drinking, and 100,000 are victims of alcohol-related date rape or sexual assault.

These statistics have shocked many students, administrators, and parents into demanding changes in college attitudes and policies regarding alcohol. In response, the Task Force of the National Advisory Council on Alcohol Abuse and Alcoholism was formed. Its report documents the extent of the alcohol problem and is a call to action for colleges and their surrounding communities to re-examine their alcohol policies and overhaul the campus drinking culture. These efforts, according to the Task Force, must focus on three levels:

1. Ultimately, *individual students* must take responsibility for their own behavior, but programs that encourage and support development of healthy attitudes toward alcohol are often needed. These programs should target students at increased risk of developing alcohol problems.

2. The *student body as a whole* must work to discourage alcohol abuse. This effort might include promoting alcohol-free activities, reducing the availability of alcohol, and avoiding social and commercial promotion of alcohol on campus. Fraternities, sororities, eating clubs, and other campus organizations should be held accountable if underage or otherwise inappropriate alcohol use takes place on their premises.

3. *Colleges and surrounding communities* must cooperate to discourage excessive drinking. Those who enable students to drink irresponsibly must be held accountable.

The U.S. Surgeon General, in his 2007 Call to Action to Prevent and Reduce Underage Drinking, suggests eliminating alcohol sponsorship of athletic events and other social activities. Working together, students, faculty, administrators, parents, and the community have begun to put an end to the destructive culture of heavy drinking on college campuses. At some schools, there is an effort to shift classes to Fridays and even Saturdays, after it was found that binge drinking increases when students don't have Friday classes. Increasingly, incoming students are required to take a 3-hour online class about alcohol. And there is stricter punishment for underage drinking and public drunkenness on some campuses, with the likelihood of suspension for repeat offenders.

who is an alcoholic, another three or four people are directly affected.

Alcoholics frequently suffer from mental disorders in addition to their substance dependence. Alcoholics are much more likely than nonalcoholics to suffer from clinical depression, panic disorder, schizophrenia, and antisocial personality disorders. People with anxiety or panic attacks may try to use alcohol to lessen their anxiety, even though alcohol often makes these disorders worse.

Causes of Alcoholism The precise causes of alcoholism are unknown, but many factors are probably involved. Some studies suggest that as much as 50–60% of a person's risk for alcoholism is determined by genetic factors but not all children of alcoholics become alcoholic, and it is clear that other factors are involved. A person's risk of developing alcoholism may be increased by certain personality disorders, having grown up in a violent or otherwise troubled household, and imitating the alcohol abuse of peers and other role models. People who begin drinking excessively in their teens are especially prone to binge drinking and alcoholism later in life. Certain social factors have also been linked with alcoholism, including urbanization, disappearance of the extended family, a general loosening of kinship ties, increased mobility, and changing values.

Treatment Some alcoholics recover without professional help. How often this occurs is unknown, but possibly as many as one-third stop drinking on their own or reduce their drinking enough to eliminate problems. Often these spontaneous recoveries are linked to an alcohol-related crisis, such as a blackout or alcohol-related automobile crash, a health problem, or the threat of being fired. Most alcoholics, however, require a treatment program of some kind in order to stop drinking. Many different kinds of programs exist. No single treatment works for everyone, so a person may have to try different programs before finding the right one.

One of the oldest and best-known recovery programs is Alcoholics Anonymous (AA). AA consists of self-help groups that meet several times each week in many communities and follow a 12-step program. Important steps for people in these programs include recognizing that they are "powerless over alcohol" and must seek help from a "higher power" in order to regain control of their lives. By verbalizing these steps, the alcoholic directly addresses the denial that is often prominent in alcoholism and other addictions. Many AA members have a sponsor of their choosing who is available by phone 24 hours a day for individual support and crisis intervention.

Other recovery approaches are available. Some, like Rational Recovery and Women for Sobriety, deliberately avoid any emphasis on higher spiritual powers. A more controversial approach to problem drinking is offered by the group Moderation Management, which encourages people to manage their drinking behavior by limiting intake or abstaining.

Al-Anon is a companion program to AA for families and friends of alcoholics. In Al-Anon, spouses and others explore how they enabled the alcoholic to drink by denying, rationalizing, or covering up his or her drinking and how they can change this codependent behavior.

Employee assistance programs and school-based programs represent another approach to alcoholism treatment. Inpatient hospital rehabilitation is useful for some alcoholics, especially if they have serious medical or mental problems or if life stressors threaten to overwhelm them.

There are also several medical treatments for alcoholism:

- *Disulfiram* (Antabuse) inhibits the metabolic breakdown of acetaldehyde and causes patients to flush and feel ill when they drink, thus theoretically inhibiting impulse drinking.
- *Naltrexone* reduces the craving for alcohol and decreases its pleasant, reinforcing effects without making the user feel ill.
- *Injectable naltrexone* is a single monthly shot administered by a health professional.
- *Acamprosate* (Campral) helps people maintain abstinence after they have stopped drinking by acting on brain pathways related to alcohol abuse.

18 million Americans who needed treatment for alcohol abuse did not receive any treatment in 2007.

—SAMHSA, 2008

Table 8.3 Users and Abusers of Alcohol in the U.S., by Demographic Characteristics: 2007

	Past Year Prevalence (Percentage)	
	Alcohol Use	Alcohol Abuse or Dependence
Gender		
Men	69.5	10.6
Women	62.2	4.6
Ethnicity		
White	70.4	8.0
Black or African American	54.5	6.3
American Indian and Alaska Native	59.3	10.9
Native Hawaiian and other Pacific Islander	72.3	7.3
Asian American	49.6	4.3
Hispanic or Latino	57.2	7.0
Two or more races	64.3	8.6
Total Population	**65.7**	**7.5**

SOURCE: Office of Applied Studies, Substance Abuse and Mental Health Services Administration. 2008. *Results from the 2007 National Survey on Drug Use and Health: National Findings* (http://oas.samhsa.gov/nsduh; retrieved February 4, 2009).

In people who abuse alcohol and have significant depression or anxiety, the use of antidepressant or anti-anxiety medication can improve both mental health and drinking behavior. In addition, drugs such as diazepam (Valium) are sometimes prescribed to replace alcohol during initial stages of withdrawal. Such chemical substitutes are usually useful for only a week or so, because alcoholics are at particularly high risk for developing dependence on other drugs.

Gender and Ethnic Differences

Alcohol abusers come from all socioeconomic levels and cultural groups, but there are notable differences in patterns of drinking between men and women and among different ethnic groups (Table 8.3).

QUESTIONS FOR CRITICAL THINKING AND REFLECTION

Do you know anyone with a serious alcohol problem? From what you have read in this chapter, would you say that person abuses alcohol or is dependent on it? What effects, if any, has this person's problem had on your life? Have you thought about getting support or help?

Drinking Behavior and Responsibility

Examine Your Attitudes and Behavior

Think about how you really feel about drinking: Is it of little consequence to you or perhaps even an intrusion into your college experience? Or is alcohol the key ingredient for any and all fun activities? How do you perceive nondrinkers at a party where others are drinking?

Also consider the sources of your ideas about alcohol. How was alcohol used in your family when you were growing up? How is it used—or how do you think it's used—by students at your school? And how is alcohol use portrayed in advertisements you're exposed to? What effect do they have on you and your attitudes about drinking?

Finally, carefully examine your drinking behavior. If you drink alcohol, what are your reasons for doing so? Is your drinking behavior moderate and responsible? Or do you frequently overindulge and suffer negative consequences? Try tracking your alcohol use in your health journal for a week or two to help evaluate your drinking behavior.

Drinking Moderately and Responsibly

• *Drink slowly and space your drinks.* Sip your drinks, and alternate them with nonalcoholic choices. Don't drink alcoholic beverages to quench your thirst, and avoid drinks made with carbonated mixers.

• *Eat before and while drinking.* Don't drink on an empty stomach. Food in your stomach will slow the rate at which alcohol is absorbed.

• *Know your limits and your drinks.* Learn how different BACs affect you and how to keep your BAC and behavior under control.

• *Be aware of the setting.* In dangerous situations, abstinence is the only appropriate choice.

• *Use designated drivers.* Arrange carpools to and from parties or events where alcohol will be served. Rotate the responsibility for acting as a designated driver.

• *Learn to enjoy activities without alcohol.* If you can't have fun without drinking, you may have a problem with alcohol.

Encourage Responsible Drinking in Others

• *Encourage responsible attitudes.* Learn to express disapproval about someone who has drunk too much. Don't treat the choice to abstain as strange. The majority of American adults drink moderately or not at all.

• *Be a responsible host.* Serve only enough alcohol for each guest to have a moderate number of drinks, and serve lots of nonalcoholic choices. Always serve food along with alcohol, and stop serving alcohol an hour or more before people will leave. Insist that a guest who drinks too much take a taxi, ride with someone else, or stay overnight rather than drive.

• *Hold drinkers fully responsible for their behavior.* Pardoning unacceptable behavior fosters the attitude that the behavior is due to the drug rather than the person.

• *Take community action.* Find out about prevention programs on your campus or in your community. Consider joining an action group such as Students Against Destructive Decisions (SADD) or Mothers Against Drunk Driving (MADD); visit www.sadd.org and www.madd.org.

Men Among white American men, excessive drinking often begins in the teens or twenties and progresses gradually through the thirties until the individual is clearly identifiable as an alcoholic by the time he is in his late thirties or early forties (see the box "Drinking Behavior and Responsibility.") Other men remain controlled drinkers until later in life, sometimes becoming alcoholic in association with retirement, the loss of friends and loved ones, boredom, illness, or psychological disorders.

Women Women tend to become alcoholic at a later age and with fewer years of heavy drinking. It is not unusual for women in their forties or fifties to become alcoholic after years of controlled drinking. Women alcoholics develop cirrhosis and other medical complications somewhat more often than men. Women alcoholics may have more medical problems because they are less likely to seek early treatment. In addition, there may be an inherently greater biological risk for women who drink.

African Americans Although as a group African Americans use less alcohol than most other groups (includ-

ing whites), they face disproportionately high levels of alcohol-related birth defects, cirrhosis, cancer, hypertension, and other medical problems. In addition, blacks are more likely than members of other ethnic groups to be victims of alcohol-related homicides, criminal assaults, and injuries. AA groups of predominantly African Americans are effective, perhaps because essential elements of AA—sharing common experiences, mutual acceptance of one another as human beings, and trusting a higher power—are already a part of African American culture.

Latinos Drinking patterns among Latinos vary significantly, depending on their specific cultural background and how long they and their families have lived in the United States. Drunk driving and cirrhosis are the most common causes of alcohol-related death and injury among Hispanic men. Hispanic women are more likely to abstain from alcohol than white or black women, but those who do drink are at special risk for problems. Treating the entire family as a unit is an important part of treatment because family pride, solidarity, and support are important aspects of Latino culture. Some Hispanics may do better if treatment efforts are integrated with the techniques of folk healers and spiritists.

Asian Americans   As a group, Asian Americans have lower-than-average rates of alcohol abuse. However, acculturation may somewhat weaken the generally strong Asian taboos and community sanctions against alcohol misuse. For many Asian Americans, though, the genetically based physiological aversion to alcohol remains a deterrent to abuse. Ethnic agencies, health care professionals, and ministers seem to be the most effective sources of treatment, when needed.

American Indians and Alaska Natives   Alcohol abuse is one of the most widespread and severe health problems among American Indians and Alaska Natives, especially for adolescents and young adults. The rate of alcoholism among American Indians is twice that of the general population, and the death rate from alcohol-related causes is about eight times higher. Treatment may be more effective if it reflects tribal values.

Helping Someone with an Alcohol Problem

Helping a friend or relative with an alcohol problem requires skill and tact. Start by making sure you are not enabling someone to continue excessively using alcohol. Enabling takes many forms, such as making excuses for the alcohol abuser—for example, saying "he has the flu" when it is really a hangover. Another important step is open, honest labeling—"I think you have a problem with alcohol." Such explicit statements usually elicit emotional rebuttals and may endanger a relationship. However, you are not helping your friends by allowing them to deny their problems with alcohol or other drugs. Taking action shows that you care. Even when problems are acknowledged, there is usually reluctance to get help. Your best role might be to obtain information about the available resources and persistently encourage their use.

QUESTIONS FOR CRITICAL THINKING AND REFLECTION

Are you aware of the campus and community resources that can help someone overcome an alcohol problem? For example, does your school offer alternatives to keg parties or other events where alcohol is traditionally provided? Are there dorms, Greek organizations, or clubs whose members agree to abstain from alcohol? Are counseling services readily available to students?

WHO USES TOBACCO?

In spite of the known health hazards—and despite increasing public and private efforts to restrict smoking—nearly 71 million Americans are smokers, with thousands more joining their ranks every day. In 2006, nearly 24% of men and 18% of women smoked cigarettes. Rates of smoking varied, based on gender, age, ethnicity, and education level (Table 8.4).

Although all states ban the sale of tobacco to anyone under 18 years of age, at least 500 million packs of cigarettes and 26 million containers of chewing tobacco are consumed by minors each year. Each day, roughly 1300 teenagers become regular smokers; at least one-third of them will die prematurely because of tobacco. In 2007, about 3.5% of 13-year-old Americans said they had used tobacco products in the last month. Among high school students, about 20% smoke cigarettes at least occasionally and 14% smoke cigars. An estimated 8%, including 10% of white male students, use spit tobacco. Male college athletes and professional baseball players report even higher rates of spit tobacco use.

Men and women with other drug-abuse problems frequently use tobacco. Smoking also is more prevalent among people with mental disorders than among the rest of the population: 40% of people with major depression, social phobias, and generalized anxiety disorder are smokers, as are 80% of people with schizophrenia. Such findings suggest that underlying psychological or phy-

Table 8.4	Who Smokes?		
	Percentage of Smokers		
	Men	**Women**	**Total**
Ethnic Group (age ≥ 18)			
White	24.3	19.7	21.9
Black	27.6	19.2	23.0
Asian	16.8	4.6	10.4
American Indian/ Alaskan Native	35.6	29.0	32.4
Latino	20.1	10.1	15.2
Education (age ≥ 25)			
≤ 8 years	22.3	12.3	17.4
9–11 years	40.1	36.4	35.4
12 years (no diploma)	27.9	23.3	25.6
GED	51.3	40.2	46.0
12 years (diploma)	27.6	20.4	23.8
Associate degree	25.4	17.8	21.2
Undergraduate degree	10.8	8.4	9.6
Graduate degree	7.3	5.8	6.6
Total	**23.9**	**18.0**	**20.8**

SOURCE: Centers for Disease Control and Prevention. 2007. Cigarette smoking among adults—United States, 2006. *Morbidity and Mortality Weekly Report* 56(44): 1157–1161.

siological traits may predispose people to drug use, including tobacco.

WHY PEOPLE USE TOBACCO

Although people start smoking for a variety of reasons, they usually become long-term smokers after becoming addicted to nicotine—the key psychoactive ingredient in tobacco smoke.

Nicotine Addiction

The primary reason people continue to use tobacco is that they have become addicted to a powerful psychoactive drug: **nicotine.** Many researchers consider nicotine to be the most physically addictive of all the psychoactive drugs.

Some neurological studies indicate that nicotine acts on the brain in much the same way as cocaine and heroin. Nicotine reaches the brain via the bloodstream seconds after it is inhaled or, in the case of spit tobacco, absorbed through membranes of the mouth or nose. It triggers the release of powerful chemical messengers in the brain, including epinephrine, norepinephrine, and dopamine. But unlike street drugs, most of which are used to achieve a high, nicotine's primary attraction seems to lie in its ability to modulate everyday emotions.

At low doses, nicotine acts as a stimulant. It increases heart rate and blood pressure. In adults, nicotine can enhance alertness, concentration, rapid information processing, memory, and learning. In some circumstances, nicotine acts as a mild sedative. Most commonly, nicotine relieves symptoms such as anxiety, irritability, and mild depression in tobacco users who are experiencing withdrawal. Nicotine addiction fulfills the criteria for substance dependence, including loss of control, tolerance, and withdrawal.

Loss of Control Three out of four smokers want to quit but find they cannot. Regular tobacco users live according to a rigid cycle of need and gratification. On average, they can go no more than 40 minutes between doses of nicotine; otherwise, they begin feeling edgy and irritable and have trouble concentrating. If ignored, nicotine cravings build until getting tobacco becomes a paramount concern, crowding out other thoughts. Tobacco users become

adept at keeping a steady amount of nicotine circulating in the blood and going to the brain. They may plan their daily schedule around opportunities to satisfy their nicotine cravings; this loss of control and personal freedom can affect all the dimensions of wellness (see the box "Tobacco Use and Religion: Global Views" on p. 190).

Tolerance and Withdrawal Using tobacco builds up tolerance. Where one cigarette may make a beginning smoker nauseated and dizzy, a long-term smoker may have to chain-smoke a pack or more to experience the same effects. For most regular tobacco users, sudden abstinence from nicotine produces predictable withdrawal symptoms, which come on several hours after the last dose of nicotine and can include severe cravings, insomnia, confusion, tremors, difficulty concentrating, fatigue, muscle pains, headache, nausea, irritability, anger, and depression. Although most of these symptoms of physical dependence pass in 2 or 3 days, many ex-smokers report intermittent urges to smoke for years after quitting.

Social and Psychological Factors

Social and psychological forces combine with physiological addiction to maintain the tobacco habit. Many people, for example, have established habits of smoking while doing something else—while talking, working, drinking, and so on. The spit tobacco habit is also associated with certain situations, such as studying or playing sports. It is difficult for these people to break their habits because the activities they associate with tobacco use continue to trigger their urge.

About 2.4 million Americans started smoking in 2006; 61.2% were younger than 18.

—SAMHSA, 2007

QUICK STATS

Why Start in the First Place?

Children and teenagers constitute 90% of all new smokers in this country. Every day, 1300 teenagers and many younger children start smoking, while hundreds of others take up snuff or chewing tobacco. The average age for starting smokers is 13; for spit tobacco users, 10. Children—especially girls—are beginning to experiment with tobacco at ever-younger ages. The earlier people begin smoking,

nicotine A poisonous, addictive substance found in tobacco and responsible for many of the effects of tobacco.

TERMS

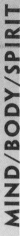
Religious traditions can best assist adult smokers by reminding them of two principles: one, the value of liberation from any form of slavery, and two, respect for life and the body.

Tobacco Use as a Violation of Religious Principles

All religions condemn tobacco use for its damaging effects on the body. Most religions regard the human body as the dwelling place of the spirit; as such, it deserves care and respect.

The Baha'i faith, for example, strongly discourages smoking as unclean and unhealthy. Some Protestant churches consider tobacco use a violation of the body. For Hindus, smoking goes against one of the primary spiritual practices, the care of the body. The Roman Catholic Church endorses the age-old adage "a sound mind in a sound body." For Muslims, one of the five essential principles on which religious law is based is protection of the integrity of the individual. In Judaism, people are urged to "choose life" and to choose whatever strengthens the capacity to live. Buddhists believe that the body doesn't belong to the person at all—even suicide is considered murder—and one must do nothing to harm it.

Most religions also contend that dependence and addiction run counter to ideas of freedom, choice, and human dignity. Buddhism teaches a path of freedom—a way of life without dependence on anything. Hindus regard tobacco use as a dependence that is not necessary for the preservation of health. Protestant churches caution that any form of dependence is contrary to the notion of Christian freedom.

Another argument against tobacco use is the immorality of imposing secondhand smoke on nonsmokers, which is seen as inflicting harm on others.

The Role of Individual Responsibility

Most religions focus on the role of individual responsibility in overcoming dependence on tobacco. In Buddhism, for example, people must assume responsibility for their habits; they practice introspection to understand the cause of problems within themselves and the effects of their actions on others. The principles of Islam are based on notions of responsibility and protection; you are responsible for your body and health.

Religion and Tobacco Control

Different religions share common views on how the problem of tobacco use should be approached. The Islamic view is that the campaign to control tobacco use must be based on awareness, responsibility, and justice. According to the Geneva Interreligious Platform (a project involving Hindus, Buddhists, Jews, Christians, Muslims, and Baha'is), the best approach is prevention. Here, the rights of nonsmokers clearly prevail over the freedom of smokers. In support of this position, the common religious exhortation not to do unto others what you would not have them do unto you can be invoked.

---

the more likely they are to become heavy smokers—and to die of tobacco-related disease.

Young people start using tobacco for a variety of reasons. Many young, white, male athletes, for example, begin using spit tobacco to emulate their favorite professional athletes. Young women often take up smoking because they think it will help them lose weight or stay thin. Most often, however, young people start smoking simply because their peers are already doing it.

Rationalizing the Dangers Making the decision to smoke requires minimizing or denying both the health risks of tobacco use and the tremendous pain, disability, emotional trauma, family stress, and financial expense involved in tobacco-related diseases such as cancer and emphysema. A sense of invincibility, characteristic of many adolescents and young adults, also contributes to the decision to use tobacco.

Many teenagers believe they will be able to stop smoking when they want. In fact, adolescents are more vulnerable to nicotine than are older tobacco users. Compared with older smokers, adolescents become heavy smokers and develop dependence after fewer cigarettes.

Emulating Smoking in the Media In the top-grossing films in 2002–2003, smoking was portrayed in more than 73% of the films, including 82% of PG-13 films; smoking was often shown positively as a means to relieve tension or as something to do while socializing. Negative consequences resulting from tobacco use were depicted for only 3% of the major characters who used tobacco. By showing smoking in an unrealistically positive light, films may be acting as advertisement.

Studies of adolescents have consistently found a strong association between seeing tobacco use in films and trying cigarettes. Teens may be particularly sensitive to on-screen portrayals of smoking because they are in the process of developing adult identities; during this period, they may try out different personas, including those of their favorite movie stars. Some groups suggest an automatic R rating for any film that shows tobacco use, equating smoking with violence, strong language, sexuality, and nudity in determining a film's rating.

HEALTH HAZARDS

Tobacco adversely affects nearly every part of the body, including the brain, stomach, mouth, and reproductive organs.

Tobacco Smoke: A Toxic Mix

Tobacco smoke contains hundreds of damaging chemical substances, including acetone (nail polish remover), ammonia, hexamine (lighter fluid), and toluene (industrial solvent). Smoke from a typical unfiltered cigarette contains about 5 billion particles per cubic millimeter—50,000 times as many as are found in an equal volume of smoggy urban air. These particles, when condensed, form a brown, sticky mass called **cigarette tar.**

Carcinogens and Poisons At least 43 chemicals in tobacco smoke are linked to the development of cancer. Some, such as benzo(a)pyrene and urethane, are **carcinogens;** that is, they directly cause cancer. Other chemicals, such as formaldehyde, are **cocarcinogens;** they do not themselves cause cancer but combine with other chemicals to stimulate the growth of certain cancers, at least in laboratory animals. Tobacco also contains poisonous substances, including arsenic and hydrogen cyanide. In addition to being an addictive psychoactive drug, nicotine is also a poison and can be fatal in high doses. Many cases of nicotine poisoning occur each year in toddlers and infants who pick up and eat cigarette butts they find at home or on the playground.

Cigarette smoke contains carbon monoxide, the deadly gas in automobile exhaust, in concentrations 400 times greater than is considered safe in industrial workplaces.

Carbon monoxide displaces oxygen in red blood cells, depleting the body's supply of oxygen needed for extra work. Carbon monoxide also impairs visual acuity, especially at night.

Additives Tobacco manufacturers use additives to manipulate the taste and effect of cigarettes and other tobacco products.

Additives include sugars as flavor enhancers to mask the harsh, bitter taste of tobacco, so smokers can inhale more smoke and absorb more nicotine. Other flavor components, such as theobromine and glycyrrhizin, act as bronchodilators, opening the lungs' airways and making it easier for nicotine to get into the bloodstream.

Ammonia boosts the amount of addictive nicotine delivered by cigarettes. Some additives are intended to make **sidestream smoke** (the uninhaled smoke from a burning cigarette) less obvious and objectionable.

Nearly 600 chemicals, approved as safe when used as food additives, are used in manufacturing cigarettes, but some form cancer-causing agents when heated or burned.

"Light" and Low-Tar Cigarettes Some smokers switch to low-tar, low-nicotine, or filtered cigarettes because they believe them to be healthier alternatives. But there is no such thing as a safe cigarette, and smoking behavior is a more important factor in tar and nicotine intake than the type of cigarette smoked. Smokers who switch to a low-nicotine brand often compensate by smoking more cigarettes, inhaling more deeply, taking larger or more frequent puffs, or blocking ventilation holes with lips or fingers to offset the effects of filters.

Studies have found that people who smoke "light" cigarettes inhale up to eight times as much tar and nicotine as printed on the label. Studies also show that smokers of light cigarettes are less likely to quit than smokers of regular cigarettes, probably due to the misperception that light cigarettes are safer.

Menthol Cigarettes About 70% of African American smokers smoke menthol cigarettes, as compared to 30%

TERMS

cigarette tar A brown, sticky mass created when the chemical particles in tobacco smoke condense.

carcinogen Any substance that causes cancer.

cocarcinogen A substance that works with a carcinogen to cause cancer.

sidestream smoke The uninhaled smoke from a burning cigarette.

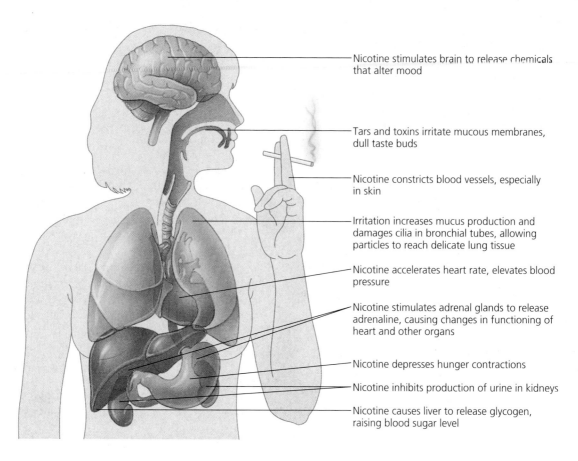

Nicotine stimulates brain to release chemicals that alter mood

Tars and toxins irritate mucous membranes, dull taste buds

Nicotine constricts blood vessels, especially in skin

Irritation increases mucus production and damages cilia in bronchial tubes, allowing particles to reach delicate lung tissue

Nicotine accelerates heart rate, elevates blood pressure

Nicotine stimulates adrenal glands to release adrenaline, causing changes in functioning of heart and other organs

Nicotine depresses hunger contractions

Nicotine inhibits production of urine in kidneys

Nicotine causes liver to release glycogen, raising blood sugar level

FIGURE 8.4   The short-term effects of smoking a cigarette.

of whites. Studies have found that blacks absorb more nicotine than other groups and metabolize it more slowly; they also have lower rates of successful quitting. The anesthetizing effect of menthol, which may allow smokers to inhale more deeply and hold smoke in their lungs for a longer period, may be partly responsible for these differences.

The Immediate Effects of Smoking

The beginning smoker often has symptoms of mild nicotine poisoning: dizziness; faintness; rapid pulse; cold, clammy skin; and sometimes nausea, vomiting, and diarrhea. The effects of nicotine on smokers vary, depending greatly on the size of the nicotine dose and how much tolerance previous smoking has built up. Nicotine can either excite or tranquilize the nervous system, depending on dosage.

Nicotine has many other immediate effects (Figure 8.4). It stimulates the part of the brain called the **cerebral cortex.** It also stimulates the adrenal glands to discharge adrenaline. Nicotine inhibits the formation of urine; constricts the blood vessels, especially in the skin; accelerates the heart rate; and elevates blood pressure. Higher blood pressure, faster heart rate, and constricted blood vessels require the heart to pump more blood.

Smoking depresses hunger contractions and dulls the taste buds; smokers who quit often notice that food tastes much better.

The Long-Term Effects of Smoking

Smoking is linked to many deadly and disabling diseases. Total amount of tobacco smoke inhaled is a key factor contributing to disease. People who smoke more cigarettes per day, inhale deeply, puff frequently, smoke cigarettes down to the butts, or begin smoking at an early age run a greater risk of disease than do those who smoke more moderately or who do not smoke at all.

Cardiovascular Disease   Although lung cancer tends to receive the most publicity, **coronary heart disease (CHD),** is actually the most widespread single cause of death for cigarette smokers. CHD often results from **atherosclerosis,** a condition in which fatty deposits called **plaques** form on the inner walls of heart arteries, causing them to narrow and stiffen. Smoking and exposure to environmental tobacco smoke (ETS) permanently accelerate the rate of plaque accumulation in the coronary arteries—50% for smokers, 25% for ex-smokers, and 20% for people regularly exposed to ETS. If the plaque completely blocks the flow of blood to a portion of the heart, a heart attack (**myocardial infarction**) occurs. CHD can also interfere with the heart's electrical activity, resulting in disturbances of the normal heartbeat rhythm.

Smokers have a death rate from CHD that is 70% higher than that of nonsmokers. The risks of CHD decrease rapidly when a person stops smoking; this is particularly true for younger smokers, whose coronary arteries have not yet been extensively damaged. Cigarette smoking has also been linked to other cardiovascular diseases, including the following:

- *Stroke,* a sudden interference with the circulation of blood in a part of the brain, resulting in the destruction of brain cells
- *Aortic aneurysm,* a bulge in the aorta caused by a weakening in its walls
- *Pulmonary heart disease,* a disorder of the right side of the heart, caused by changes in the blood vessels of the lungs

Lung Cancer and Other Cancers Cigarette smoking is the primary cause of lung cancer. Those who smoke two or more packs of cigarettes a day have lung cancer death rates 12–25 times greater than those of nonsmokers. The dramatic rise in lung cancer rates among women in the past 40 years clearly parallels the increase of smoking in this group; lung cancer now exceeds breast cancer as the leading cause of cancer deaths among women. The risk of developing lung cancer increases with the number of cigarettes smoked each day, the number of years of smoking, and the age at which the person started smoking. Evidence suggests that after 1 year without smoking, the risk of lung cancer decreases substantially. After 10 years, the risk of lung cancer among ex-smokers is 50% lower than that of continuing smokers.

Research has also linked smoking to cancers of the trachea, mouth, pharynx, esophagus, larynx, pancreas, bladder, kidney, breast, cervix, stomach, liver, colon, and skin.

Chronic Obstructive Pulmonary Disease The lungs of a smoker are constantly exposed to dangerous chemicals and irritants, and they must work harder to function adequately. The stresses placed on the lungs by smoking can permanently damage lung function and lead to *chronic obstructive pulmonary disease (COPD),* also known as chronic obstructive lung disease (COLD), or chronic lower respiratory disease. COPD is the fourth leading cause of death in the United States. This progressive and disabling disorder consists of several different but related diseases; emphysema and chronic bronchitis are two of the most common.

Emphysema is a disabling condition in which the walls of the lungs' air sacs lose their elasticity and are gradually destroyed. The lungs' ability to obtain oxygen and remove carbon dioxide is impaired. A person with emphysema is breathless, is constantly gasping for air, and has the feeling of drowning. The heart must pump harder and may become enlarged. People with emphysema often die from a damaged heart. There is no known way to reverse this disease. In its advanced stage, the victim is bedridden and severely disabled.

Chronic bronchitis is a persistent, recurrent inflammation of the bronchial tubes. When the cell lining of the bronchial tubes is irritated, it secretes excess mucus. Bronchial congestion is followed by a chronic cough, which makes breathing more and more difficult. If smokers have chronic bronchitis, they face a greater risk of lung cancer, no matter how old they are or how many cigarettes they smoke. Chronic bronchitis seems to be a shortcut to lung cancer.

Even when a smoker shows no signs of lung impairment or disease, cigarette smoking causes other respiratory damage. Normally the cells lining the bronchial tubes secrete mucus, a sticky fluid that collects particles of soot, dust, and other substances in inhaled air. Mucus is carried up to the mouth by the continuous motion of the cilia, hairlike structures that protrude from the inner surface of the bronchial tubes. If the cilia are destroyed or impaired, or if the pollution of inhaled air is more than the system can remove, the protection provided by cilia is lost.

Cigarette smoke first slows and then stops the action of the cilia. Eventually it destroys them, leaving delicate membranes exposed to injury from substances inhaled in cigarette smoke or from the polluted air. This interfer-

cerebral cortex The outer layer of the brain, which controls complex behavior and mental activity.

coronary heart disease (CHD) Cardiovascular disease caused by hardening of the arteries that supply oxygen to the heart muscle; also called *coronary artery disease.*

atherosclerosis Cardiovascular disease caused by the deposit of fatty substances (called *plaque*) in the walls of the arteries.

plaque A deposit on the inner wall of blood vessels; blood can coagulate around plaque and form a clot.

myocardial infarction A heart attack caused by the complete blockage of a main coronary artery.

emphysema A disease characterized by a loss of lung tissue elasticity and breakup of the air sacs, impairing the lungs' ability to obtain oxygen and remove carbon dioxide.

chronic bronchitis Recurrent, persistent inflammation of the bronchial tubes.

TERMS

ence with the functioning of the respiratory system often leads rapidly to the conditions known as smoker's throat and smoker's cough, as well as to shortness of breath. Other respiratory effects of smoking include a worsening of allergy and asthma symptoms and an increase in the smoker's susceptibility to colds.

Additional Health, Cosmetic, and Economic Concerns   People who smoke are more likely to develop peptic ulcers and heartburn, raising the risk of esophageal cancer. Smokers are twice as likely as nonsmokers to experience erectile dysfunction (impotence), and smoking is linked to reduced fertility in both men and women. Smokers are at increased risk for tooth decay and gum and periodontal diseases, with symptoms appearing by the mid-20s. Smoking dulls the senses of taste and smell and increases the risk for hearing loss and blindness. Smokers have higher rates of motor vehicle crashes, fire-related injuries, and back pain. Smoking can cause premature skin wrinkling, premature baldness, stained teeth, discolored fingers, and a persistent tobacco odor in clothes and hair. In 2008, the average per-pack price of cigarettes was $4.32. A pack-a-day habit costs nearly $1600 each year for cigarettes alone. In addition, smoking contributes to osteoporosis, increases the risk of complications from diabetes, and accelerates the course of multiple sclerosis.

Cumulative Effects   The cumulative effects of tobacco use fall into two general categories. The first category is reduced life expectancy. A male who takes up smoking before age 15 and continues to smoke is only half as likely to live to age 75 as a male who never smokes. Females who have similar smoking habits also have a reduced life expectancy.

The second category involves quality of life. A national health survey begun in 1964 shows that smokers spend one-third more time away from their jobs because of illness than nonsmokers. Both men and women smokers show a greater rate of acute and chronic disease than people who have never smoked (see the box "Gender and Tobacco Use"). Smokers become disabled at younger ages than nonsmokers and have more years of unhealthy life as well as a shorter life span.

Other Forms of Tobacco Use

Many smokers have switched from cigarettes to other forms of tobacco, such as spit (smokeless) tobacco, cigars

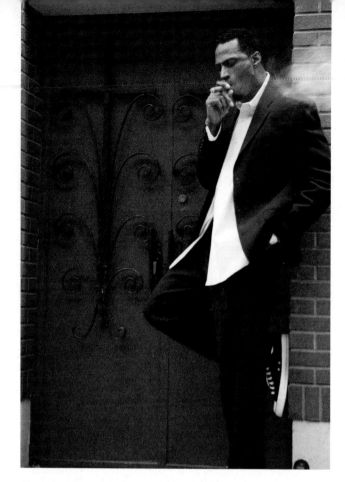

Cigars contain more tobacco than cigarettes and so produce more tar when smoked. Cigar smokers face an increased risk of cancer even if they don't inhale the smoke.

and pipes, and clove cigarettes and bidis. These alternatives, however, are far from safe.

Spit (Smokeless) Tobacco   More than 6.6 million adults and about 8% of all high school students are current spit tobacco users. Spit tobacco comes in two major forms: snuff and chewing tobacco (chew). In snuff, the tobacco leaf is processed into a coarse, moist powder and mixed with flavorings. Snuff is usually sold in small tins. Users place a "pinch," "dip," or "quid" between the lower lip or cheek and gum and suck on it. In chewing tobacco, the tobacco leaf may be shredded ("leaf"), pressed into bricks or cakes ("plugs"), or dried and twisted into ropelike strands ("twists"). Chew is usually sold in pouches. Users place a wad of tobacco in their mouth and then chew or suck it to release the nicotine. All types of smokeless tobacco cause an increase in saliva production, and the resulting tobacco juice is spit out or swallowed.

The nicotine in spit tobacco—along with flavorings and additives—is absorbed through the gums and lining of the mouth. Holding an average-size dip in the mouth for 30 minutes delivers about the same amount of nicotine as two or three cigarettes. Because of its nicotine content, spit tobacco is highly addictive. Some users keep it in their mouth even while sleeping.

Gender and Tobacco Use

American men are currently more likely than women to smoke, but women younger than age 23 are becoming smokers at a faster rate than any other population segment. As the rate of smoking among women approaches that of men, so do rates of tobacco-related illness and death. More American women now die each year from lung cancer than from breast cancer.

Although overall risks of tobacco-related illness are similar for women and men, sex appears to make a difference in some diseases. Women, for example, are more at risk for smoking-related blood clots and strokes than are men, and the risk is even greater for women using oral contraceptives. Among men and women with the same smoking history, the odds for developing three major types of cancer, including lung cancer, is 1.2–1.7 times higher in women.

For both men and women, tobacco use is associated with increased incidence of sex-specific health problems. Men who smoke increase their risk of erectile dysfunction and infertility due to reduced sperm density and motility. Women who smoke have higher rates of osteoporosis, thyroid-related diseases, and depression.

Women who smoke also have risks associated with reproduction and the reproductive organs. Smoking is associated with greater menstrual bleeding, greater duration of painful menstrual cramps, and more variability in menstrual cycle length. Smokers have a more difficult time becoming pregnant, and they reach menopause on average a year or two earlier than nonsmokers. They face increased chances of miscarriage or placental disorders that lead to bleeding and premature delivery; rates of ectopic

pregnancy, preeclampsia, and stillbirth are also higher among women who smoke. Smoking is a risk factor for cervical cancer.

When women decide to try to stop smoking, they are more likely than men to join a support group. Overall, though, women are less successful than men in quitting. Women report more severe withdrawal symptoms and are more likely than men to report cravings in response to social and behavioral cues associated with smoking.

For men, relapse to smoking is often associated with work or social pressure; women are more likely to relapse when sad or depressed or concerned about weight gain. Nicotine replacement therapy appears to work better for men, whereas the non-nicotine medication bupropion appears to work better for women.

Although not as dangerous as smoking cigarettes, the use of spit tobacco carries many health risks. Changes can occur in the mouth after only a few weeks of use. Gums and lips become dried and irritated and may bleed. White or red patches may appear inside the mouth; this condition, known as *leukoplakia*, can lead to oral cancer. About 25% of regular spit tobacco users have *gingivitis* (inflammation) and recession of the gums and bone loss around the teeth, especially where the tobacco is usually placed. The senses of taste and smell are usually dulled.

One of the most serious effects of spit tobacco is an increased risk of oral cancer—cancers of the lip, tongue, cheek, throat, gums, roof and floor of the mouth, and larynx. Spit tobacco contains at least 28 chemicals known to cause cancer, and long-term snuff use may increase the risk of oral cancer by as much as 50 times. Surgery to treat oral cancer is often disfiguring and may involve removing parts of the face, tongue, cheek, or lip.

Cigars and Pipes The popularity of cigars is highest among white males age 18–44 with higher-than-average income and education, but women are also smoking cigars in record numbers. Cigar use is also growing among young people: In government surveys, 12% of American high school students reported having smoked at least one cigar in the previous month. Less than 1% of Americans, mostly males who also smoke cigarettes, are pipe smokers.

Cigars are made from rolled whole tobacco leaves; pipe tobacco is made from shredded leaves and often flavored. Users absorb nicotine through the gums and lining of the mouth. Cigars contain more tobacco than cigarettes and

so contain more nicotine and produce more tar when smoked. Large cigars may contain as much tobacco as a whole pack of cigarettes and take 1–2 hours to smoke.

The smoke from cigars contains many of the same toxins and carcinogens as the smoke from cigarettes, some in much higher quantities. The health risks of cigars depend on the number of cigars smoked and whether the smoker inhales. Because most cigar and pipe users do not inhale, they have a lower risk of cancer and cardiovascular and respiratory diseases than cigarette smokers. However, their risks are substantially higher than those of nonsmokers.

Nicotine addiction is another concern. Most adults who smoke cigars do so only occasionally, and there is little evidence that use of cigars by adults leads to addiction. The recent rise in cigar use among teens has raised concerns, however, because nicotine addiction almost always develops in the teen or young adult years.

Clove Cigarettes and Bidis Clove cigarettes, also called "kreteks" or "chicartas," are made of tobacco mixed with chopped cloves; they are imported primarily from Indonesia and Pakistan. Clove cigarettes contain almost twice as much tar, nicotine, and carbon monoxide as conventional cigarettes and so have all the same health hazards. Some chemical constituents of cloves may also be dangerous. For example, eugenol, an anesthetic compound found in cloves, may impair the respiratory system's ability to detect and defend against foreign particles. There have been a number of serious respiratory injuries and deaths from the use of clove cigarettes.

QUESTIONS FOR CRITICAL THINKING AND REFLECTION

Do you know anyone who has suffered from an illness related to tobacco use? If so, what problems did that person face? What was the outcome? Did the experience have any effect on your views about using tobacco?

Bidis, or "beadies," are small cigarettes imported from India that contain species of tobacco different from those used by U.S. cigarette manufacturers. The tobacco in bidis is hand-rolled in Indian ebony leaves (tendu) and then often flavored; clove, mint, chocolate, and fruit varieties are available. Bidis contain up to four times more nicotine than U.S. cigarettes and twice as much tar.

THE EFFECTS OF SMOKING ON THE NONSMOKER

Tens of thousands of nonsmokers die each year because of exposure to secondhand smoke. Further, the medical and societal costs of tobacco use are enormous.

Environmental Tobacco Smoke

The U.S. Environmental Protection Agency (EPA) has designated **environmental tobacco smoke (ETS)**—more commonly called *secondhand smoke*—a Class A carcinogen. In 2006, the Surgeon General issued a report concluding that there is no safe level of exposure to ETS.

Environmental tobacco smoke consists of mainstream smoke and sidestream smoke. Smoke exhaled by smokers is referred to as **mainstream smoke.** Sidestream smoke enters the atmosphere from the burning end of a cigarette, cigar, or pipe. Nearly 85% of the smoke in a room where someone is smoking comes from sidestream smoke. Undiluted sidestream smoke, because it is not filtered through either a cigarette filter or a smoker's lungs, has twice as much tar and nicotine, three times as much benzo(a)pyrene, almost three times as much carbon monoxide, and three times as much ammonia.

In rooms where people are smoking, levels of carbon monoxide can exceed those permitted by Federal Air Quality Standards for outside air. The carcinogens in the secondhand smoke from a single cigar exceeds that of

three cigarettes, and cigar smoke contains up to 30 times more carbon monoxide.

ETS Effects   Nonsmokers subjected to ETS frequently develop coughs, headaches, nasal discomfort, and eye irritation. Other symptoms range from breathlessness to sinus problems. People with allergies tend to suffer the most.

ETS causes 3000 lung cancer deaths and about 35,000 deaths from heart disease each year in people who do not smoke. ETS also aggravates asthma and increases the risk for breast and cervical cancers. Scientists have been able to measure changes that contribute to lung tissue damage and potential tumor promotion in the bloodstreams of healthy young test subjects who spend just 3 hours in a smoke-filled room. After just 30 minutes of exposure to ETS, the function in the coronary arteries of healthy nonsmokers is reduced to the same level as that of smokers. And nonsmokers can still be affected by the harmful effects of ETS hours after they have left a smoky environment. Carbon monoxide, for example, lingers in the bloodstream 5 hours later.

Infants, Children, and ETS   Infants exposed to smoke are more likely to die of sudden infant death syndrome (SIDS) than babies not exposed to ETS. ETS causes up to 18,600 cases of low birth weight each year. Children under 5 whose primary caregiver smokes ten or more cigarettes per day have measurable blood levels of nicotine and tobacco carcinogens. Chemicals in tobacco smoke also show up in breast milk, and breastfeeding may pass more chemicals to the infant of a smoking mother than does direct exposure. ETS triggers 150,000– 300,000 cases of bronchitis, pneumonia, and other respiratory infections in infants and toddlers up to age 18 months each year.

Older children suffer, too. ETS is a risk factor for asthma in children who have not previously displayed symptoms of the disease, and it aggravates the symptoms of children who already have asthma. ETS is also linked to reduced lung function and fluid buildup in the middle ear, a contributing factor in middle-ear infections, a leading reason for childhood surgery. Later in life, people exposed to ETS as children are at increased risk for lung cancer, emphysema, and chronic bronchitis.

Smoking and Pregnancy

Smoking almost doubles a pregnant woman's chance of having a miscarriage, and it significantly increases her risk of ectopic pregnancy. Maternal smoking causes an

environmental tobacco smoke (ETS)   Smoke that enters the atmosphere from the burning end of a cigarette, cigar, or pipe, as well as smoke that is exhaled by smokers; also called *secondhand smoke.*

mainstream smoke   Smoke that is inhaled by a smoker and then exhaled into the atmosphere.

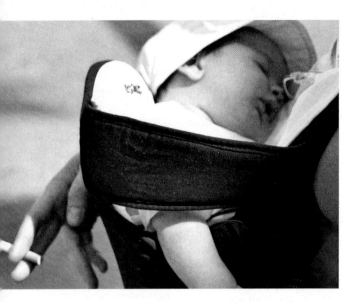
Millions of American infants and children are regularly exposed to environmental tobacco smoke.

estimated 4600 infant deaths in the United States each year, primarily due to premature delivery and smoking-related problems with the placenta. Maternal smoking is a major factor in low birth weight, which puts newborns at high risk for infections and other serious problems. If a nonsmoking mother is regularly exposed to ETS, her infant is also at greater risk for low birth weight.

THINKING ABOUT THE ENVIRONMENT

The buildings in which you live, work, and learn are important parts of your environment, as are the skies and oceans. The health and safety of indoor air are threatened by secondhand smoke, just as the outside air is threatened by other forms of pollution.

The U.S. Surgeon General reported in 2006 that more than 40% of all nonsmokers are routinely exposed to tobacco smoke, typically indoors. Roughly 30% of indoor workers are not protected by smoke-free workplace rules. The Surgeon General also reported the following:

- Children exposed to secondhand smoke are more likely to die of sudden infant death syndrome and to develop severe infections.

- Adults exposed to secondhand smoke experience immediate harmful effects on the cardiovascular system and increased risk of coronary heart disease and lung cancer.

- There is no safe level of exposure to secondhand smoke.

- Completely eliminating indoor smoking is the only way to fully protect nonsmokers from exposure to secondhand smoke. Ventilating buildings or separating smokers from nonsmokers is not sufficient.

Babies born to mothers who smoke more than two packs a day perform poorly on developmental tests in the first hours after birth, compared to babies of nonsmoking mothers. Later in life, obesity, hyperactivity, short attention span, and lower scores on spelling and reading tests all occur more frequently in children whose mothers smoked during pregnancy than in those born to nonsmoking mothers. Prenatal tobacco exposure has also been associated with behavioral problems in children.

The Cost of Tobacco Use to Society

The annual health-related costs of smoking exceed $167 billion. These costs far exceed the tax revenues that states collect on the sale of tobacco products.

In order to recoup public health care expenditures, 43 states filed suit against tobacco companies, and in 1998 the Master Settlement Agreement (MSA) was signed. The MSA required the tobacco companies to pay states $206 billion over 25 years; it also limits or bans certain types of advertising, promotions, and lobbying. Many of the provisions of the deal are designed to limit youth exposure and access to tobacco. In exchange, the tobacco industry settled the state lawsuits and is protected from future suits by states, counties, towns, and other public entities.

The MSA, however, did not prevent individuals from suing the tobacco industry, and a number of lawsuits moved forward, some resulting in huge fines against tobacco companies. The industry was dealt another potential blow in August 2006, when a U.S. District Court judge ordered tobacco companies to stop marketing cigarettes with labels like "light" and "low-tar." The judge found that tobacco companies had violated racketeering laws by conspiring for years to deceive the public about the health risks of smoking. As court battles continue, tobacco companies seek new markets in developing countries, and tobacco use is poised to become the leading cause of death worldwide.

WHAT CAN BE DONE?

There are many ways to act against this public health threat.

Action at Many Levels

Thousands of local ordinances across the nation restrict or ban smoking in restaurants, stores, workplaces, and even public outdoor areas. An assessment made in 2006 found that 42% of Americans live in municipalities with smoke-free restaurants and 30% live in locations with smoke-free workplaces. At least 260 colleges and universities now have totally smoke-free campuses or prohibit smoking in residential buildings. As local nonsmoking laws proliferate, evidence mounts that environmental restrictions are effective in encouraging smokers to quit.

QUESTIONS FOR CRITICAL THINKING AND REFLECTION

What are your views on the government's role in regulating tobacco products? Is there currently enough regulation, or should the government go further in controlling the production and marketing of these products? What events or experiences have shaped your views on this issue?

At the state level, many tough anti-tobacco laws have been passed. As of January 2008, comprehensive smoke-free air laws were in effect in 21 states, the District of Columbia, and Puerto Rico. California has one of the most aggressive—and successful—tobacco control programs, combining taxes on cigarettes, graphic advertisements, and bans on smoking in bars and restaurants. At the federal level, smoking has been banned on virtually all domestic airplane flights, and the U.S. Defense Department has banned smoking at all military work sites.

Smoking is also banned on many international air flights, as well as in many restaurants and hotels and on public transportation in some countries. The World Health Organization has taken the lead in international anti-tobacco efforts by sponsoring the Framework Convention on Tobacco Control. Another international activity is the annual commemoration of World No Tobacco Day (May 31), on which smokers are encouraged to stop smoking for 1 day.

Such local, state, national, and international efforts represent progress, but health activists warn that tobacco industry influence remains strong. The tobacco industry contributes heavily to sympathetic legislative officeholders and candidates. Since 1999, tobacco interests have spent more than $115 million on federal lobbying activities.

Individual Action

Nonsmokers have the right not only to breathe clean air but also to take action to help solve one of society's most serious public health threats. Here are a few actions you can take: When a smoker violates a no-smoking designation, complain. If your favorite restaurant or shop doesn't have a nonsmoking policy, ask the manager to adopt one. If you see children buying tobacco, report this illegal activity to the facility manager or the police. Learn more about addiction and tobacco cessation so you can better

support the tobacco users you know. Vote for candidates who support anti-tobacco measures; contact local, state, and national representatives to express your views.

You can also cancel your subscriptions to magazines that carry tobacco advertising and send a letter to the publisher explaining your decision. Voice your opinion about other positive representations of tobacco use. (A recent study found that more than two-thirds of children's animated feature films have featured tobacco or alcohol use with no clear message that such practices were unhealthy.) Volunteer with the American Lung Association, the American Cancer Society, or the American Heart Association.

HOW A TOBACCO USER CAN QUIT

Giving up tobacco is a long-term process. Research shows that tobacco users move through predictable stages—from being uninterested in stopping, to thinking about change, to making a concerted effort to stop, to finally maintaining abstinence. But most attempt to quit several times before they finally succeed. Relapse is a normal part of the process.

The Benefits of Quitting

Giving up tobacco provides immediate health benefits to men and women of all ages (Table 8.5). The younger people are when they stop smoking, the more pronounced the health improvements. And these improvements gradually but invariably increase as the period of nonsmoking lengthens. It's never too late to quit, though. According to a U.S. Surgeon General's report, people who quit smoking, regardless of age, live longer than people who continue to smoke.

Options for Quitting

Most tobacco users—76% in a recent survey—want to quit, and half of those who want to quit will make an attempt this year. What are their options? No single method works for everyone, but each does work for some people some of the time. Choosing to quit requires developing a strategy for success. Some people quit cold turkey, whereas others taper off slowly. There are over-the-counter and prescription products that help many people (see the box "Smoking Cessation Products" for more on these options). Behavioral factors that have been shown to increase the chances of a smoker's permanent smoking cessation are support from others and regular exercise. Support can come from friends and family and/or formal group programs sponsored by organizations such as the American Cancer Society and the American Lung Association or by your college health center or community hospital.

Free telephone quitlines are emerging as a popular and effective strategy to help stop smoking. Quitlines are staffed by trained counselors who help each caller plan a personal quitting strategy, usually including a combination of nicotine replacement therapy, changes in daily habits, and emotional support. In 2004, the Department of Health and Human Services established a national toll-free number, 1-800-QUITNOW (1-800-784-8669), to serve as a single access point for smokers seeking information and assistance in quitting.

Most smokers in the process of quitting experience both physical and psychological effects of nicotine withdrawal, and exercise can help with both. For many smokers, their tobacco use is associated with certain times and places—following a meal, for example. Resolving to walk after dinner instead of lighting up provides a distraction from cravings and eliminates the cues that trigger a desire to smoke. In addition, many people worry about weight gain associated with quitting. Although most ex-smokers do gain a few pounds, at least temporarily, incorporating exercise into a new tobacco-free routine lays the foundation for healthy weight management. The health risks of adding a few pounds are far outweighed by the risks of continued smoking; it's estimated that a smoker would have to gain 75–100 pounds to equal the health risks of smoking a pack a day.

Table 8.5	Benefits of Quitting Smoking

Within 20 minutes of your last cigarette:
- You stop polluting the air
- Blood pressure drops to normal
- Pulse rate drops to normal
- Temperature of hands and feet increases to normal

8 hours:
- Carbon monoxide level in blood drops to normal
- Oxygen level in blood increases to normal

24 hours:
- Chance of heart attack decreases

48 hours:
- Nerve endings start regrowing
- Ability to smell and taste is enhanced

2–3 months:
- Circulation improves
- Walking becomes easier
- Lung function increases up to 30%

1–9 months:
- Coughing, sinus congestion, fatigue, and shortness of breath all decrease

1 year:
- Heart disease death rate is half that of a smoker

5 years:
- Stroke risk drops nearly to the risk for nonsmokers

10 years:
- Lung cancer death rate drops to 50% of that of continuing smokers
- Incidence of other cancers (mouth, throat, larynx, esophagus, bladder, kidney, and pancreas) decreases
- Risk of ulcer decreases

15 years:
- Risk of lung cancer is about 25% of that of continuing smokers
- Risks of heart disease and death are close to those for nonsmokers

SOURCES: American Lung Association. 2002. *Benefits of Quitting* (http://www.lungusa.org/tobacco/quit_ben.html; retrieved August 18, 2006); American Cancer Society. 2000. *Quitting Smoking* (http://www.cancer.org/tobacco/quitting.html; retrieved August 18, 2006).

QUESTIONS FOR CRITICAL THINKING AND REFLECTION

What anti-smoking ordinances are in effect in your community? Does your school prohibit smoking on campus? Do you think these rules have been effective in reducing smoking or exposure to ETS? Do you support such regulations? Why or why not?

TIPS FOR TODAY AND THE FUTURE

The responsible use of alcohol means drinking in moderation or not at all. The best approach to tobacco use is never to start.

RIGHT NOW YOU CAN

- Consider whether there is a history of alcohol abuse or dependence in your family.
- Take stock of the number of alcoholic beverages in your home. Does there always seem to be a lot on hand? Do you find yourself purchasing alcohol frequently? What do your purchasing habits say about your drinking?
- If you smoke, think about the next time you'll want a cigarette. Visualize yourself enjoying this activity without smoking.

IN THE FUTURE YOU CAN

- Think about the next party you plan to attend. Decide how much you will drink at the party, and how you will get home afterward.
- If you have a family member who smokes, resolve to talk to that person, offering support if he or she is interested in quitting.
- If you smoke, resolve to quit. Research options for quitting and choose one you think will work best for you.

Smoking Cessation Products

connect™

Each year, millions of Americans visit their doctors in the hope of finding a drug that can help them stop smoking. Although pharmacological options are limited, the few available drugs have proved successful.

Chantix (Varinicline)

The newest smoking cessation drug, marketed under the name Chantix, works in two ways: It reduces nicotine cravings, easing the withdrawal process, and it blocks the pleasant effects of nicotine. The drug acts on neurotransmitter receptors in the brain.

Unlike most smoking cessation products currently on the market, Chantix is not a nicotine replacement. For this reason, smokers may be advised to continue smoking for the first few days of treatment, to avoid withdrawal and to allow the drug to build up in their system. The approved course of treatment is 12 weeks, but the duration and recommended dosage depend on several factors, including the smoker's general health and the length and severity of his or her nicotine addiction.

Side effects reported with Chantix include nausea, headache, vomiting, sleep disruptions, and change in taste perception. Chantix is not recommended for women who are pregnant or nursing.

Zyban (Bupropion)

Bupropion is an antidepressant (prescribed under the name Wellbutrin) as well as a smoking cessation aid (prescribed under the name Zyban). As a smoking cessation aid, bupropion eases the symptoms of nicotine withdrawal and reduces the urge to smoke. Like Chantix, it acts on neurotransmitter receptors in the brain.

Bupropion users have reported an array of side effects, but they are rare. Side effects may be reduced by changing the dosage, taking the medicine at a different time of day, or taking it with or without food. Zyban and Wellbutrin should not be taken together.

Nicotine Replacement Products

The most widely used smoking cessation products replace the nicotine that the user would normally get from tobacco, reducing withdrawal symptoms and cravings. Although still harmful, nicotine replacement products provide a cleaner form of nicotine, without the thousands of poisons and tars produced by burning tobacco. Less of the product is used over time, as the need for nicotine decreases.

Nicotine replacement products come in several forms, including patches, gum, lozenges, nasal sprays, and inhalers. They are available in a variety of strengths and can be worked into many different smoking cessation strategies. Most are available without a prescription.

The nicotine patch is popular because it can be applied and forgotten until it needs to be removed or changed, usually every 16 or 24 hours. Placed on the upper arm or torso, it releases a steady stream of nicotine, which is absorbed through the skin. The main side effects are skin irritation and redness. Nicotine gum and nicotine lozenges have the advantage of allowing the smoker to use them whenever he or she craves nicotine. Side effects of nicotine gum include mouth sores and headaches; nicotine lozenges can cause nausea and heartburn. Nicotine nasal sprays and inhalers are available only by prescription.

Although all these products have proved to be effective in helping users stop smoking, experts recommend them only as one part of a complete smoking cessation program. Such a program should include regular professional counseling and physician monitoring.

As with any significant change in health-related behavior, giving up tobacco requires planning, sustained effort, and support. It is an ongoing process, not a one-time event. The Behavior Change Strategy describes the steps that successful quitters follow.

SUMMARY

• After being absorbed into the bloodstream in the stomach and small intestine, alcohol is transported throughout the body. The liver metabolizes alcohol as blood circulates through it.

• Alcohol is a CNS depressant. At low doses, it tends to make people feel relaxed.

• Alcohol use increases the risk of injury and violence; drinking before driving is particularly dangerous, even at low doses.

• Continued alcohol use has negative effects on the digestive and cardiovascular systems and increases cancer risk and overall mortality.

• Pregnant women who drink risk giving birth to children with a cluster of birth defects known as fetal alcohol syndrome (FAS). Even occasional drinking during pregnancy can cause brain injury in the fetus.

• Alcohol abuse involves drinking in dangerous situations or drinking to a degree that causes academic, professional, interpersonal, or legal difficulties.

• Alcohol dependence, or alcoholism, is characterized by more extensive problems with alcohol, usually involving tolerance and withdrawal.

• Binge drinking is a common form of alcohol abuse on college campuses that has negative effects on both drinking and nondrinking students.

- Physical consequences of alcoholism include the direct effects of tolerance and withdrawal, as well as all the problems associated with chronic drinking. Psychological problems include memory loss and additional mental disorders such as depression.

- Treatment approaches include mutual support groups like AA, job- and school-based programs, inpatient hospital programs, and pharmacological treatments.

- Smoking is the largest preventable cause of ill health and death in the United States. Nevertheless, millions of Americans continue to use tobacco.

- People who begin smoking are usually imitating others or responding to seductive advertising. Smoking is associated with low education level and the use of other drugs.

- Tobacco smoke is made up of hundreds of different chemicals, including some that are carcinogenic or poisonous or that damage the respiratory system.

- Nicotine acts on the nervous system as a stimulant or a depressant. It can cause blood pressure and heart rate to increase, straining the heart.

- Cardiovascular disease is the most widespread cause of death for cigarette smokers. Cigarette smoking is the primary cause of lung cancer and is linked to many other cancers and respiratory diseases.

- The use of spit tobacco leads to nicotine addiction and is linked to oral cancers.

- Cigars, pipes, clove cigarettes, and bidis are not safe alternatives to cigarettes.

- Environmental tobacco smoke (ETS) contains high concentrations of toxic chemicals and can cause headaches, eye and nasal irritation, and sinus problems. Children whose parents smoke are especially susceptible to respiratory diseases.

- Smoking during pregnancy increases the risk of miscarriage, stillbirth, congenital abnormalities, premature birth, and low birth weight. SIDS, behavior problems, and long-term impairments in development are also risks.

- Giving up smoking is a difficult and long-term process. Although most ex-smokers quit on their own, some smokers benefit from stop-smoking programs, OTC and prescription medications, and support groups.

FOR MORE INFORMATION

BOOKS

Dean, Michael. 2007. *Empty Cribs: The Impact of Smoking on Child Health.* New York: Arts & Sciences Publishing. *Examines the effects of smoking on children, before and after birth.*

Gilman, S. L., ed. 2004. *Smoke: A Global History of Smoking.* London: Reaktion Books. *A look at smoking and its effects, including history and issues related to culture, art, and gender.*

Herrick, C. 2007. *100 Questions & Answers About Alcoholism & Drug Addiction.* Boston: Jones and Bartlett. *Answers a range of specific questions about alcohol abuse, dependence, and treatment options.*

How to Quit Smoking Without Gaining Weight. 2004. New York: American Lung Association.

Kinney, J. 2009. *Loosening the Grip: A Handbook of Alcohol Information,* 9th ed. New York: McGraw-Hill. *A fascinating book about alcohol, including information on physical effects, abuse, alcoholism, and cultural aspects of alcohol use.*

Seaman, B. 2006. *Binge: Campus Life in an Age of Disconnection and Excess.* New York: Wiley. *An exploration of campus life at 12 residential colleges and universities, with discussions on the effects of student isolation, peer pressure, and drinking on today's students.*

Wholey, D. 2007. *Why Do I Keep Doing That?* Deerfield Beach, Fla.: Health Communications. *An optimistic approach to breaking self-destructive habits.*

ORGANIZATIONS, HOTLINES, AND WEB SITES

Action on Smoking and Health (ASH). An advocacy group that provides statistics, news briefs, and other information.
   http://ash.org

Al-Anon Family Group Headquarters. Provides information and referrals to local Al-Anon and Alateen groups. The Web site includes a self-quiz to determine if you are affected by someone's drinking.
   888-4AL-ANON
   http://www.al-anon.alateen.org

Alcoholics Anonymous (AA) World Services. Provides general information on AA, literature on alcoholism, and information about AA meetings and related 12-step organizations.
   212-870-3400
   http://www.aa.org

Alcohol Treatment Referral Hotline. Provides referrals to local intervention and treatment providers.
   800-ALCOHOL

American Cancer Society (ACS). Sponsor of the annual Great American Smokeout; provides information on the dangers of tobacco, as well as tools for prevention and cessation for both smokers and users of spit tobacco.
   http://www.cancer.org

American Lung Association. Provides information on lung diseases, tobacco control, and environmental health.
   http://www.lungusa.org

Bacchus and Gamma Peer Education Network. An association of college- and university-based peer education programs that focus on prevention of alcohol abuse.
   http://www.bacchusgamma.org

CDC's Tobacco Information and Prevention Source (TIPS). Provides research results, educational materials, and tips on how to quit smoking; Web site includes special sections for kids and teens.
   http://www.cdc.gov/tobacco

The College Alcohol Study. Harvard School of Public Health. Provides information about and results from the recent studies of binge drinking on college campuses.
   http://www.hsph.harvard.edu/cas

College Drinking Prevention. Includes information about alcohol, including myths about alcohol use and an interactive look at how alcohol affects the body.
   http://www.collegedrinkingprevention.gov

Kicking the Tobacco Habit

You can look forward to a longer and healthier life if you join the 47 million Americans who have quit using tobacco. The steps for quitting described below are discussed in terms of the most popular tobacco product in the United States—cigarettes—but they can be adapted for all forms of tobacco.

Gather Information

Collect personal smoking information in a detailed journal about your smoking behavior. Write down the time you smoke each cigarette of the day, the situation you are in, how you feel, where you smoke, and how strong your craving for the cigarette is, plus any other information that seems relevant. Part of the job is to identify patterns of smoking that are connected with routine situations (for example, the coffee break smoke, the after-dinner cigarette, the tension-reduction cigarette). Use this information to discover the behavior patterns involved in your smoking habit.

Make the Decision to Quit

Choose a date in the near future when you expect to be relatively stress-free and can give quitting the energy and attention it will require. Don't choose a date right before or during finals week, for instance. Consider making quitting a gift: Choose your birthday as your quit date, for example, or make quitting a Father's Day or Mother's Day present. You might also want to coordinate your quit date with a buddy—a fellow tobacco user who wants to quit or a nonsmoker who wants to give up another bad habit or begin an exercise program. Tell your friends and family when you plan to quit. Ask them to offer encouragement and help hold you to your goal.

Decide what approach to quitting will work best for you. Will you go cold turkey, or will you taper off? Will you use nicotine patches or gum? Will you join a support group or enlist the help of a buddy? Prepare a contract for quitting, as discussed in Chapter 1. Set firm dates and rewards, and sign the contract. Post it in a prominent place.

Prepare to Quit

One of the most important things you can do to prepare to quit is to develop and practice nonsmoking relaxation techniques. Many smokers find that they use cigarettes to help them unwind in tense situations or to relax at other times. If this is true for you, you'll need to find and develop effective substitutes. It takes time to become proficient at relaxation techniques, so begin practicing before your quit date. Refer to the detailed discussion of relaxation techniques in Chapter 2.

Other things you can do to help prepare for quitting include the following:

- Make an appointment to see your physician. Ask about OTC and prescription aids for tobacco cessation and whether one or more might be appropriate for you.

- Make a dentist's appointment to have your teeth cleaned the day after your target quit date.

- Start an easy exercise program, if you're not exercising regularly already.

- Buy some sugarless gum. Stock your kitchen with low-calorie snacks.

- Clean out your car, and air out your house. Send your clothes out for dry cleaning.

- Throw away all your cigarette-related paraphernalia (ashtrays, lighters, etc.).

- The night before your quit day, get rid of all your cigarettes. Have fun with this—get your friends or family to help you tear them up.

- Make your last few days of smoking inconvenient: Smoke only outdoors and when alone. Don't do anything else while you smoke.

Quitting

Your first few days without cigarettes will probably be the most difficult. It's hard to give up such a strongly ingrained habit, but remember that millions of Americans have done it—and you can, too. Plan and rehearse the steps you will take when you experience a powerful craving. Avoid or control situations that you know from your journal are powerfully associated with your smoking (see the table). If your hands feel empty without a cigarette, try holding or fiddling with a small object such as a paper clip or pencil.

Social support can also be a big help. Arrange with a buddy to help you with your weak moments, and call him or her whenever you feel overwhelmed by an urge to smoke. Tell people you've just quit. You may discover many inspiring former smokers who can encourage you and reassure you that it's possible to quit and lead a happier, healthier life. Find a formal support group to join if you think it will help.

Maintaining Nonsmoking

The lingering smoking urges that remain once you've quit should be carefully tracked and controlled because they can cause relapses if left unattended. Keep track of these urges in your journal to help you deal with them. If certain situations still trigger the urge for a cigarette, change something about

Environmental Protection Agency Indoor Air Quality/ETS. Provides information and links about secondhand smoke.

http://www.epa.gov/smokefree

Moderation Management Network. Controversial self-help program designed to help early problem drinkers limit their drinking; not intended for serious alcohol abusers or alcoholics.

http://www.moderation.org

Mothers Against Drunk Driving (MADD). Supports efforts to develop solutions to the problems of drunk driving and underage drinking;

provides news, information, and brochures about many topics, including a guide for giving a safe party.

http://www.madd.org

National Association for Children of Alcoholics (NACoA). Provides information and support for children of alcoholics.

888-554-COAS

http://www.nacoa.net

National Clearinghouse for Alcohol and Drug Information/Prevention Online. Provides statistics and information on alcohol abuse, in-the situation to break past associations. If stress or boredom causes strong smoking urges, use a relaxation technique, take a brisk walk, have a stick of gum, or substitute some other activity for smoking.

Don't set yourself up for a relapse. If you allow yourself to get overwhelmed at school or work or to gain weight, it will be easier to convince yourself that now isn't the right time to quit. This *is* the right time. Continue to practice time-management and relaxation techniques. Exercise regularly, eat sensibly, and get enough sleep. These habits will not only ensure your success at remaining tobacco-free but also serve you well in stressful times throughout your life. In fact, former smokers who have quit for at least 3 months report reduced stress levels, probably because quitting smoking lowers overall arousal.

Watch out for patterns of thinking that can make nonsmoking more difficult. Focus on the positive aspects of not smoking, and give yourself lots of praise—you deserve it. Stick with the schedule of rewards you developed for your contract.

Keep track of the emerging benefits that come from having quit. Items that might appear on your list include improved stamina, an increased sense of pride at having kicked a strong addiction, a sharper sense of taste and smell, no more smoker's cough, and so on. Keep track of the money you're saving by not smoking, and spend it on things you really enjoy. And if you do lapse, be gentle with yourself. Lapses are a normal part of quitting. Forgive yourself, and pick up where you left off.

Strategies for Dealing with High-Risk Smoking Situations

Cues and High-Risk Situations	Suggested Strategies
Awakening in morning	Brush your teeth as soon as you wake up. Take a shower or bath.
Drinking coffee	Do something else with your hands. Drink tea or another beverage instead.
Eating meals	Sit in nonsmoking sections of restaurants. Get up from the table right after eating, and start another activity. Brush your teeth right after eating.
Driving a car	Have the car cleaned when you quit smoking. Chew sugarless gum or eat a low-calorie snack. Take public transportation or ride your bike. Turn on the radio and sing along.
Socializing with friends who smoke	Suggest nonsmoking events (movies, theater, shopping). Tell friends you've quit and ask them not to smoke around you, offer you cigarettes, or give you cigarettes if you ask for them.
Drinking at a bar, restaurant, or party	Try to take a nonsmoker with you, or associate with nonsmokers. Let friends know you've just quit. Moderate your intake of alcohol (it can weaken your resolve).
Encountering stressful situations	Practice relaxation techniques. Take some deep breaths. Get out of your room or house. Go somewhere that doesn't allow smoking. Take a shower, chew gum, call a friend, or exercise.

SOURCES: Strategies adapted with permission from *Postgraduate Medicine* 90(1), July 1991.

cluding resources for people who want to help friends and family members overcome alcohol-abuse problems.
    http://ncadi.samhsa.gov
National Council on Alcoholism and Drug Dependence (NCADD). Provides information and counseling referrals.
    212-269-7797; 800-NCA-CALL (24-hour Hope Line)
    http://www.ncadd.org
National Institute on Alcohol Abuse and Alcoholism (NIAAA). Provides booklets and other publications on a variety of alcohol-related top-ics, including fetal alcohol syndrome, alcoholism treatment, and alcohol use and minorities.
    http://www.niaaa.nih.gov
Nicotine Anonymous. A 12-step program for tobacco users.
    http://www.nicotine-anonymous.org
Rational Recovery. A free self-help program that offers an alternative to 12-step programs; the emphasis is on learning the skill of abstinence.
    http://www.rational.org

Smokefree.Gov. Provides step-by-step strategies for quitting as well as expert support via telephone or instant messaging.

http://www.smokefree.gov

World Health Organization Tobacco Free Initiative. Promotes the goal of a tobacco-free world.

http://www.who.int/tobacco/en

SELECTED BIBLIOGRAPHY

American Cancer Society. 2008. *Cancer Facts and Figures, 2008.* Atlanta, Ga.: American Cancer Society.

American Lung Association. 2008. *State Legislated Actions on Tobacco Issues (SLATI), 19th Edition* (http://slati.lungusa.org/reports/SLATI_07.pdf; retrieved February 6, 2009).

American Lung Association. 2008. *State of Tobacco Control 2007.* New York: American Lung Association.

American Nonsmokers' Rights Foundation. 2009. *Colleges and Universities with Smokefree Air Policies: January 4, 2009.* (http://www.no-smoke.org/pdf/ smokefreecollegesuniversities.pdf; retrieved February 6, 2009).

Anton, R. F., et al. 2006. Combined pharmacotherapies and behavioral interventions for alcohol dependence: The COMBINE study: A randomized controlled trial. *Journal of the American Medical Association* 295(17): 2003–2017.

Campaign for Tobacco-Free Kids. 2008. *State Cigarette Tax Rates and Rank, Date of Last Increase, Annual Pack Sales and Revenues, and Related Data, August 2008* (http://tobaccofreekids.org/research/factsheets/pdf/0099. pdf; retrieved February 6, 2009).

Centers for Disease Control and Prevention. 2007. Cigarette smoking among adults—United States, 2006. *Morbidity and Mortality Weekly Report* 56(44): 1157–1161.

Centers for Disease Control and Prevention. 2008. *Behavioral Risk Factor Surveillance System Survey Data, 2007.* Atlanta, Georgia: U.S. Department of Health and Human Services, Centers for Disease Control and Prevention.

Centers for Disease Control and Prevention. 2008. *Early Release of Selected Estimates Based on Data from the January–March 2008 National Health Interview Survey* (http://www.cdc.gov/nchs/data/nhis/earlyrelease/ earlyrelease200809.pdf; retrieved September 29, 2008).

Centers for Disease Control and Prevention. 2008. Surveillance for cancers associated with tobacco use—United States, 1999–2004. *Morbidity and Mortality Weekly Report* 57(SS-08): 1–33.

Centers for Disease Control and Prevention. 2008. Youth risk behavior surveillance—United States, 2007. *Morbidity and Mortality Weekly Report* 57(SS-04): 1–131.

Centers for Disease Control and Prevention. 2004. Alcohol-attributable deaths and years of potential life lost, United States, 2001. *Morbidity and Mortality Weekly Report* 53(37): 866–870.

College Drinking Prevention. 2007. *A Snapshot of Annual High-Risk College Drinking Consequences* (http://www.collegedrinkingprevention.gov/ StatsSummaries/snapshot.aspx; retrieved February 4, 2009).

Collins, G. B., et al. 2006. Drug adjuncts for treating alcohol dependence. *Cleveland Clinic Journal of Medicine* 73(7): 641–644.

Costello, R. M. 2006. Long-term mortality from alcoholism: A descriptive analysis. *Journal of Studies on Alcohol* 67(5): 694–699.

Department of Health and Human Services. 2007. *The Surgeon General's Call to Action to Prevent and Reduce Underage Drinking.* Washington, D.C.: Department of Health and Human Services, Office of the Surgeon General.

Fiore, M. C., et al. 2008. *Treating Tobacco Use and Dependence: 2008 Update. Clinical Practice Guideline.* Rockville, Md.: U.S. Department of Health and Human Services, Public Health Service.

Food and Drug Administration. 2008. *Consumer Update: New Safety Warnings for Chantix* (http://www.fds.gov/consumer/updates/chantix020508 .html; retrieved September 27, 2008).

Gades, N. M., et al. 2005. Association between smoking and erectile dysfunction: A population-based study. *American Journal of Epidemiology* 161(4): 346–351.

Heilig, M., and M. Egli. 2006. Pharmacological treatment of alcohol dependence: Target symptoms and target mechanisms. *Pharmacology and Therapeutics* 111(3): 855–876.

Hingson, R., et al. 2005. Magnitude of alcohol-related mortality and morbidity among U.S. college students ages 18–24. *Annual Review of Public Health* 26: 259–279.

Hingson, R. W., et al. 2006. Age at drinking onset and alcohol dependence: Age at onset, duration, and severity. *Archives of Pediatrics and Adolescent Medicine* 160(7): 739–746.

Mannino, D. M., and A. S. Buist. 2007. Global burden of COPD: Risk factors, prevalence, and future trends. *Lancet* 370(9589): 765–773.

National Institute on Alcohol Abuse and Alcoholism. 2006. *Young Adult Drinking.* Alcohol Alert No. 68. Bethesda, Md.: National Institute on Alcohol Abuse and Alcoholism.

Office of Applied Studies, Substance Abuse and Mental Health Services Administration. 2008. *Results from the 2007 National Survey on Drug Use and Health: National Findings* (http://www.drugabusestatistics.samhsa .gov; retrieved February 6, 2009).

Perreira, K. M., and K. E. Cortes. 2006. Explaining Race/Ethnicity and Nativity Differences in Alcohol and Tobacco Use During Pregnancy. *American Journal of Public Health,* 27 July [epub].

Titus-Ernstoff, L., et al. 2008. Longitudinal study of viewing smoking in movies and initiation of smoking by children. *Pediatrics* 121(1): 15–21.

U.S. Surgeon General. 2006. *The Health Consequences of Involuntary Exposure to Tobacco Smoke* (http://www.surgeongeneral.gov/library/ secondhandsmoke/ report/; retrieved May 6, 2008).

Vineis, P., et al. 2005. Environmental tobacco smoke and risk of respiratory cancer and chronic obstructive pulmonary disease in former smokers and never smokers in the EPIC prospective study. *British Medical Journal* 330(7486): 277.

World Health Organization. 2008. *The Global Tobacco Crisis* (http://www .who.int/tobacco/mpower/mpower_report_tobacco_crisis_2008.pdf; retrieved September 27, 2008).

Yolton, K., et al. 2005. Exposure to environmental tobacco smoke and cognitive abilities among U.S. children and adolescents. *Environmental Health Perspectives* 113(1): 98–103.

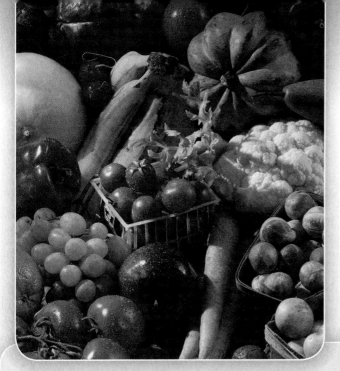

LOOKING AHEAD>>>>>

**AFTER READING THIS CHAPTER,
YOU SHOULD BE ABLE TO:**

- List the essential nutrients, and describe the functions they perform in the body

- Describe the guidelines that have been developed to help people choose a healthy diet, avoid nutritional deficiencies, and reduce their risk of diet-related chronic diseases

- Discuss nutritional guidelines for vegetarians and for special population groups

- Explain how to use food labels and other consumer tools to make informed choices about foods

- Put together a personal nutrition plan based on affordable foods that you enjoy and that will promote wellness, today as well as in the future

NUTRITION BASICS

9

In your lifetime, you'll spend about 6 years eating—about 70,000 meals and 60 tons of food. What you eat can have profound effects on your health and well-being. Your nutritional habits help determine your risk of major chronic diseases, including heart disease, cancer, stroke, and diabetes. Choosing foods that provide the nutrients you need while limiting the substances linked to disease should be an important part of your daily life.

Choosing a healthy diet is a two-part process. First, you have to know which nutrients you need and in what amounts. Second, you have to translate those requirements into a diet consisting of foods you like that are both available and affordable. Once you know what constitutes a healthy diet for you, you can adjust your current diet to bring it into line with your goals.

This chapter explains the basic principles of **nutrition.** It introduces the six classes of essential nutrients, explaining their roles in the functioning of the body. It also provides guidelines that you can use to design a healthy diet plan.

NUTRITIONAL REQUIREMENTS: COMPONENTS OF A HEALTHY DIET

You probably think about your diet in terms of the foods you like to eat. What's important for your health, though, are the nutrients contained in those foods. Your body requires proteins, fats, carbohydrates, vitamins, minerals, and water—about 45 **essential nutrients.** In this context, the word *essential* means that you must get these substances from food because your body is unable to manufacture them, or at least not fast enough to meet your physiological needs.

The body needs some essential nutrients in relatively large amounts; these *macronutrients* include protein, fat, and carbohydrate. *Micronutrients,* such as vitamins and minerals, are required in much smaller amounts. Your body obtains these nutrients through the process of **digestion,** in which the foods you eat are broken down into compounds your gastrointestinal tract can absorb and your body can use (Figure 9.1).

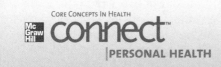

CORE CONCEPTS IN HEALTH

Mc Graw Hill **connect**™

|PERSONAL HEALTH

http://www.mcgrawhillconnect.com/personalhealth

The energy in foods is expressed as **kilocalories.** One kilocalorie represents the amount of heat it takes to raise the temperature of 1 liter of water 1°C. A person needs about 2000 kilocalories per day to meet his or her energy needs. In common usage, people usually refer to kilocalories as *calories,* which is technically a much smaller energy unit: (1 kilocalorie contains 1000 calories). This text uses the familiar word *calorie* to stand for the larger energy unit; you'll also find the word *calorie* used on food labels.

Of the six classes of essential nutrients, three supply energy:

- Fat = 9 calories per gram
- Protein = 4 calories per gram
- Carbohydrate = 4 calories per gram

Alcohol, though not an essential nutrient, also supplies energy, providing 7 calories per gram. The high caloric content of fat is one reason experts often advise against high fat consumption; most of us do not need the extra calories to meet energy needs. Regardless of their source, calories consumed in excess of energy needs are converted to fat and stored in the body. But just meeting energy needs is not enough; our bodies need enough of the essential nutrients to grow and function properly.

Proteins—The Basis of Body Structure

Proteins form important parts of the body's main structural components: muscles and bones. Proteins also form important parts of blood, enzymes, some hormones, and

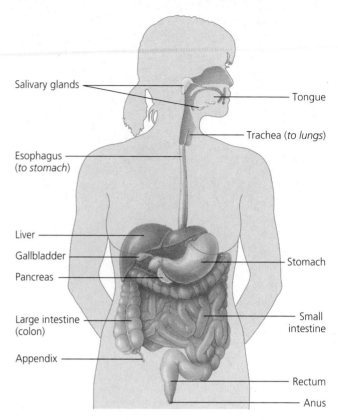

FIGURE 9.1   The digestive system.   Food is partially broken down by being chewed and mixed with saliva in the mouth. After traveling to the stomach via the esophagus, food is broken down further by stomach acids and other secretions. As food moves through the digestive tract, it is mixed by muscular contractions and broken down by chemicals. Most absorption of nutrients occurs in the small intestine, aided by secretions from the pancreas, gallbladder, and intestinal lining. The large intestine reabsorbs excess water; the remaining solid wastes are collected in the rectum and excreted through the anus.

cell membranes. As mentioned earlier, proteins also provide energy (4 calories per gram) for the body.

Amino Acids   The building blocks of proteins are called **amino acids.** Twenty common amino acids are found in food; nine of these are essential: histidine, isoleucine, leucine, lysine, methionine, phenylalanine, threonine, tryptophan, and valine. The other eleven amino acids can be produced by the body, given the presence of the needed components supplied by foods.

Complete and Incomplete Proteins   Individual protein sources are considered *complete* if they supply all the essential amino acids in adequate amounts and *incomplete* if they do not. Meat, fish, poultry, eggs, milk, cheese, and soy provide complete proteins. Incomplete proteins, which come from other plant sources such as **legumes** and nuts, are good sources of most essential amino acids but are usually low in one or two.

Certain combinations of vegetable proteins, such as wheat and peanuts in a peanut butter sandwich, allow each vegetable protein to make up for the amino acids missing in the other protein. The combination yields a complete protein. Many traditional food pairings, such as beans and rice or corn and beans, emerged as dietary staples because they are complementary proteins. Vegetarians should include a variety of vegetable protein sources in their diets to make sure they get all the essential amino acids in adequate amounts. About two-thirds of the protein in the American diet comes from animal sources (meat and dairy products); therefore, the American diet is rich in essential amino acids.

Recommended Protein Intake Adequate daily intake of protein for adults is 0.8 gram per kilogram (0.36 gram per pound) of body weight, corresponding to 50 grams of protein per day for someone who weighs 140 pounds and 65 grams of protein for someone who weighs 180 pounds. Most Americans meet or exceed the protein intake needed for adequate nutrition. If you consume more protein than your body needs, the extra protein is synthesized into fat for energy storage or burned for energy requirements. A little extra protein is not harmful, but it can contribute fat to the diet because protein-rich foods are often fat-rich as well. A very high protein intake can also strain the kidneys.

A fairly broad range of protein intakes is associated with good health, and the Food and Nutrition Board recommends that the amount of protein adults eat should fall within the range of 10–35% of total daily calorie intake, depending on the individual's age. The average American diet includes about 15–16% of total daily calories as protein.

Fats—Essential in Small Amounts

Fats, also known as *lipids*, are the most concentrated source of energy, at 9 calories per gram. The fats stored in your body represent usable energy, they help insulate your body, and they support and cushion your organs. Fats in the diet help your body absorb fat-soluble vitamins, and add important flavor and texture to foods. Fats are the major fuel for the body during rest and light activity. Two fats, linoleic acid and alpha-linolenic acid, are essential components of the diet.

Types and Sources of Fats Most of the fats in foods are fairly similar in composition, generally including a molecule of glycerol (an alcohol) with three fatty acid chains attached to it. The resulting structure is called a *triglyceride*. Animal fat, for example, is primarily made of triglycerides. Within a triglyceride, differences in the fatty

acid structure result in different types of fats. Depending on this structure, a fat may be unsaturated, monounsaturated, polyunsaturated, or saturated. (The essential fatty acids—linoleic and alpha-linolenic acids—are both polyunsaturated.) The different types of fatty acids have different characteristics and different effects on your health.

Food fats are usually composed of both saturated and unsaturated fatty acids; the dominant type of fatty acid determines the fat's characteristics. Food fats containing large amounts of saturated fatty acids are usually solid at room temperature; they are generally found naturally in animal products. The leading sources of saturated fat in the American diet are red meats (hamburger, steak, roasts), whole milk, cheese, hot dogs, and lunch meats. Food fats containing large amounts of monounsaturated and polyunsaturated fatty acids usually come from plant sources and are liquid at room temperature. Olive, canola, safflower, and peanut oils contain mostly monounsaturated fatty acids. Soybean, corn, and cottonseed oils contain mostly polyunsaturated fatty acids.

Hydrogenation There are notable exceptions to these generalizations. When unsaturated vegetable oils undergo the process of **hydrogenation**, a mixture of saturated and unsaturated fatty acids is produced. Hydrogenation also changes some unsaturated fatty acids to **trans fatty acids**, unsaturated fatty acids with an atypical shape that affects their behavior in the body. Food manufacturers use hydrogenation to increase the stability of an oil so it can be reused for deep frying, to improve the texture of certain foods, and to extend the shelf life of foods made with oil. Hydrogenation also transforms a liquid oil into margarine or vegetable shortening.

Leading sources of trans fats in the American diet are deep-fried fast foods such as french fries and fried chicken (typically fried in vegetable shortening rather than oil); baked and snack foods such as pot pies, cakes, cookies, pastries, doughnuts, and chips; and stick margarine. In general, the more solid a hydrogenated oil is, the more saturated and trans fats it contains; for example, stick margarines typically contain more saturated and trans fats than do tub or squeeze margarines. Small amounts of trans fatty acids are found naturally in meat and milk.

Hydrogenated vegetable oils are not the only plant fats that contain saturated fats. Palm and coconut oils, although derived from plants, are also highly saturated. However, fish oils, derived from an animal source, are rich in polyunsaturated fats.

Fats and Health   Different types of fats have very different effects on health. Many studies have examined the effects of dietary fat intake on blood **cholesterol** levels and the risk of heart disease. Saturated and trans fatty acids raise blood levels of **low-density lipoprotein (LDL),** or "bad" cholesterol, thereby increasing a person's risk of heart disease. Unsaturated fatty acids lower LDL. Monounsaturated fatty acids, such as those found in olive and canola oils, may also increase levels of **high-density lipoproteins (HDL),** or "good" cholesterol, providing even greater benefits for heart health. In large amounts, trans fatty acids may lower HDL. Saturated fats have been found to impair the ability of HDLs to prevent inflammation of the blood vessels, one of the key factors in vascular disease; they have also been found to reduce the ability of the blood vessels to react normally to stress. Thus, to reduce the risk of heart disease, it is important to choose unsaturated fats instead of saturated and trans fats.

Most Americans consume more saturated fat than trans fat (11% versus 2–4% of total daily calories). However, health experts are particularly concerned about trans fats because of their double negative effect on heart health—they both raise LDL and lower HDL—and because there is less public awareness of trans fats. Since January 2006, food labels have included trans fat content. Consumers can also check for the presence of trans fats by examining the ingredient list of a food for partially hydrogenated oil or vegetable shortening.

Although saturated and trans fats pose health hazards, other fats can be beneficial. When used in place of saturated fats, monounsaturated fatty acids, as found in avocados, most nuts, and olive, canola, peanut, and safflower oils, improve cholesterol levels and may help protect against some cancers. **Omega-3 fatty acids,** a form of polyunsaturated fat found primarily in fish, may be even

more healthful. Omega-3s and the compounds the body makes from them have a number of heart-healthy effects; nutritionists recommend that Americans increase the proportion of omega-3s in their diet by eating fish two or more times a week. Salmon, tuna, trout, mackerel, herring, sardines, and anchovies are all good sources of omega-3s; lesser amounts are found in plant foods, including dark-green leafy vegetables; walnuts; flaxseeds; and canola, walnut, and flaxseed oils.

Most of the polyunsaturated fats currently consumed by Americans are omega-6 fatty acids, primarily from corn oil and soybean oil. However, some nutritionists recommend that people reduce the proportion of omega-6s they consume in favor of omega-3s. To make this adjustment, use canola oil rather than corn oil in cooking, and check for corn, soybean, or cottonseed oil in products such as mayonnaise, margarine, and salad dressing.

In addition to its effects on heart disease risk, dietary fat can affect health in other ways. Diets high in fatty red meat are associated with an increased risk of certain forms of cancer, especially colon cancer. A high-fat diet can also make weight management more difficult. Because fat is a concentrated source of calories, a high-fat diet is often a high-calorie diet that can lead to weight gain. In addition, there is some evidence that calories from fat are more easily converted to body fat than calories from protein or carbohydrate. The types of fatty acids and their effects on health are summarized in Figure 9.2.

Recommended Fat Intake   To meet the body's demand for essential fats, adult men need about 17 grams per day of linoleic acid and 1.6 grams per day of alpha-linolenic acid; adult women need 12 grams of linoleic acid and 1.1 grams of alpha-linolenic acid. It takes only 3–4 teaspoons (15–20 grams) of vegetable oil per day incorporated into your diet to supply the essential fats. Most Americans consume sufficient amounts of the essential fats; limiting unhealthy fats is a much greater health concern.

Limits for total fat, saturated fat, and trans fat intake have been set by a number of government and research organizations. In 2002, the Food and Nutrition Board of the Institute of Medicine released recommendations for the balance of energy sources in a healthful diet. These new recommendations, called Acceptable Macronutrient Distribution Ranges (AMDRs), are based on ensuring adequate intake of essential nutrients while also reducing the risk of chronic diseases such as heart disease and cancer. As with protein, a range of levels of fat consumption is associated with good health; the AMDR for total fat is

TERMS

cholesterol   A waxy substance found in the blood and cells and needed for synthesis of cell membranes, vitamin D, and hormones.

low-density lipoprotein (LDL)   Blood fat that transports cholesterol to organs and tissues; excess amounts result in the accumulation of deposits on artery walls.

high-density lipoprotein (HDL)   Blood fat that helps transport cholesterol out of the arteries, thereby protecting against heart disease.

omega-3 fatty acids   Polyunsaturated fatty acids commonly found in fish oils that are beneficial to cardiovascular health.

carbohydrate   An essential nutrient; sugars, starches, and dietary fiber are all carbohydrates.

	Type of Fatty Acid	Found In[a]	Possible Effects on Health
Keep Intake Low	SATURATED 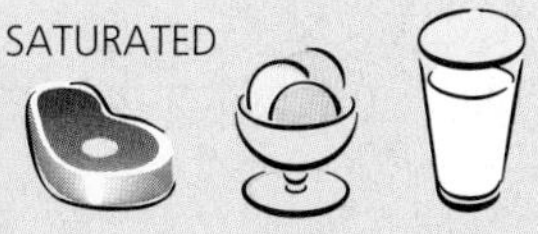	Animal fats (especially fatty meats and poultry fat and skin) Butter, cheese, and other high-fat dairy products Palm and coconut oils	Raises total cholesterol and LDL cholesterol levels Increases risk of heart disease May increase risk of colon and prostate cancers
	TRANS 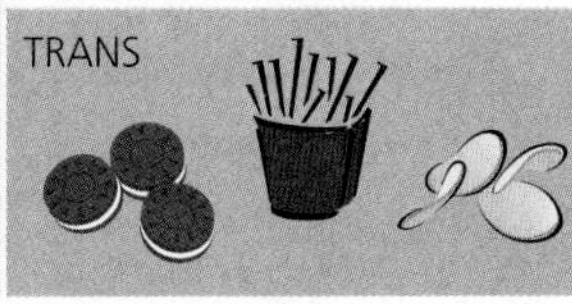	French fries and other deep-fried fast foods Stick margarines, shortening Packaged cookies and crackers Processed snacks and sweets	Raises total cholesterol and LDL cholesterol levels Lowers HDL cholesterol levels May increase risk of heart disease and breast cancer
Choose Moderate Amounts	MONOUNSATURATED 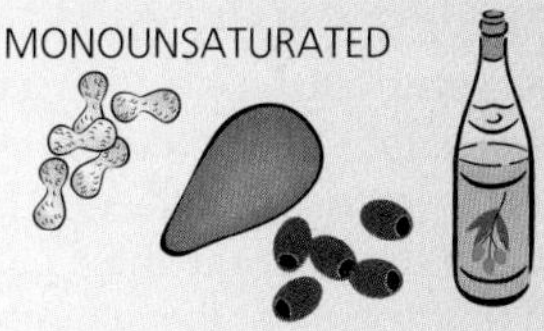	Olive, canola, and safflower oils Avocados, olives Peanut butter (without added fat) Many nuts, including almonds, cashews, pecans, and pistachios	Lowers total cholesterol and LDL cholesterol levels May reduce blood pressure and lower triglyceride levels (a risk factor for CVD) May reduce risk of heart disease, stroke, and some cancers
	POLYUNSATURATED (two groups)[b]		
	Omega-3 fatty acids 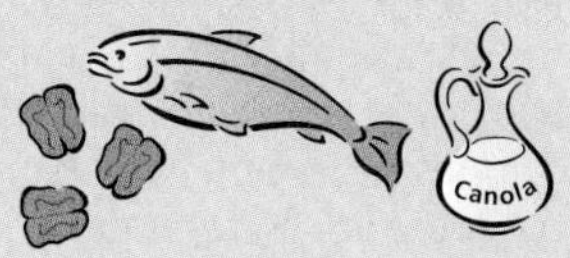	Fatty fish, including salmon, white albacore tuna, mackerel, anchovies, and sardines Lesser amounts in walnut, flaxseed, canola, and soybean oils; tofu; walnuts; flaxseeds; and dark green leafy vegetables	Reduces blood clotting and inflammation and inhibits abnormal heart rhythms Lowers triglyceride levels (a risk factor for CVD) May lower blood pressure in some people May reduce risk of fatal heart attack, stroke, and some cancers
	Omega-6 fatty acids 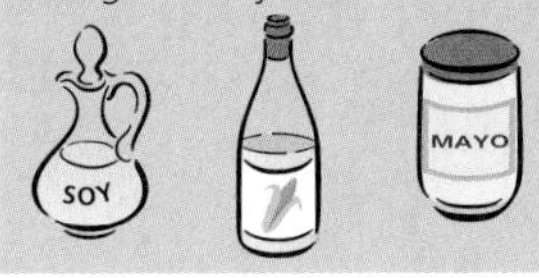	Corn, soybean, and cottonseed oils (often used in margarine, mayonnaise, and salad dressing)	Lowers total cholesterol and LDL cholesterol levels May lower HDL cholesterol levels May reduce risk of heart disease May slightly increase risk of cancer if omega-6 intake is high and omega-3 intake is low

[a] Food fats contain a combination of types of fatty acids in various proportions; for example, canola oil is composed mainly of monounsaturated fatty acids (62%) but also contains polyunsaturated (32%) and saturated (6%) fatty acids. Food fats are categorized here according to their predominant fatty acid.

[b] The essential fatty acids are polyunsaturated: Linoleic acid is an omega-6 fatty acid and alpha-linolenic acid is an omega-3 fatty acid.

FIGURE 9.2   Types of fatty acids and their possible effects on health.

20–35% of total calories. Although more difficult for consumers to monitor, AMDRs have also been set for omega-6 fatty acids (5–10%) and omega-3 fatty acids (0.6–1.2%) as part of total fat intake. Because any amount of saturated and trans fats increases the risk of heart disease, the Food and Nutrition Board recommends that saturated fat and trans fat intake be kept as low as possible; most fat in a healthy diet should be unsaturated.

For advice on setting individual intake goals, see the box "Setting Intake Goals for Protein, Fat, and Carbohydrate." To determine how close you are to meeting your personal intake goals for fat, keep a running total over the course of the day. For prepared foods, food labels list the number of grams of fat, protein, and carbohydrate; the breakdown for popular fast-food items can be found in the appendix. Nutrition information is also available in many grocery stores, in inexpensive published nutrition guides, and online. By checking these resources, you can keep track of the total grams of fat, protein, and carbohydrate you eat and assess your current diet. You can still eat high-fat foods, but it makes sense to limit the size of your portions and to balance your intake with low-fat foods.

Carbohydrates—An Ideal Source of Energy

Carbohydrates are needed in the diet primarily to supply energy for body cells. Some cells, such as those found in the brain and other parts of the nervous system and in blood, use only carbohydrates for fuel. During high-intensity exercise, muscles also use primarily carbohydrates for fuel.

Simple and Complex Carbohydrates   Carbohydrates are classified into two groups: simple and complex. Simple carbohydrates include sucrose (table sugar), fructose (fruit sugar, honey), maltose (malt sugar), and lactose (milk sugar). Simple carbohydrates provide much of the sweetness in foods and are found naturally in fruits and milk and are added to soft drinks, fruit drinks, candy, and sweet desserts. There is no evidence that any type of simple carbohydrate is more nutritious than others.

Complex carbohydrates include starches and most types of dietary fiber. Starches are found in a variety of plants, especially grains (wheat, rye, rice, oats, barley, millet), legumes (dry beans, peas, and lentils), and tubers (potatoes

Setting Intake Goals for Protein, Fat, and Carbohydrate

Goals have been established by the Food and Nutrition Board to help ensure adequate intake of the essential amino acids, fatty acids, and carbohydrate. The daily goals for adequate intake for adults are as follow:

	Men	Women
Protein	56 grams	46 grams
Fat: Linoleic acid	17 grams	12 grams
Alpha-linolenic acid	1.6 grams	1.1 grams
Carbohydrate	130 grams	130 grams

Protein intake goals can be calculated more specifically by multiplying your body weight in kilograms by 0.8 or your body weight in pounds by 0.36. (Refer to the Nutrition Resources section at the end of the chapter for information for specific age groups and life stages.)

To meet your daily energy needs, you need to consume more than the minimally adequate amounts of the energy-providing nutrients listed above, which alone supply only about 800–900 calories. The Food and Nutrition Board provides additional guidance in the form of Acceptable Macronutrient Distribution Ranges (AMDRs). The ranges can help you balance your intake of the energy-providing nutrients in ways that ensure adequate intake while reducing the risk of chronic disease. The AMDRs for protein, total fat, and carbohydrate are as follow:

Protein	10–35% of total daily calories
Total fat	20–35% of total daily calories
Carbohydrate	45–65% of total daily calories

To set individual goals, begin by estimating your total daily energy (calorie) needs; if your weight is stable, your current energy intake is the number of calories you need to maintain your weight at your current activity level. Next, select percentage goals for protein, fat, and carbohydrate. You can allocate your total daily calories among the three classes of macronutrients to suit your preferences; just make sure that the three percentages you select total 100% and that you meet the minimum intake goals listed. Two samples reflecting different total energy intake and nutrient intake goals are shown in the table below.

To translate your own percentage goals into daily intake goals expressed in calories and grams, multiply the appropriate percentages by total calorie intake and then divide the results by the corresponding calories per gram. For example, a fat limit of 35% applied to a 2200-calorie diet would be calculated as follows: 0.35 × 2200 = 770 calories of total fat; 770 ÷ 9 calories per gram = 86 grams of total fat. (Remember that fat has 9 calories per gram and that protein and carbohydrate have 4 calories per gram.)

Two Sample Macronutrient Distributions

		Sample 1		Sample 2	
Nutrient	AMDR	Individual Goals	Amounts for a 1600-Calorie Diet	Individual Goals	Amounts for a 2800-Calorie Diet
Protein	10–35%	15%	240 calories = 60 grams	30%	840 calories = 210 grams
Fat	20–35%	30%	480 calories = 53 grams	25%	700 calories = 78 grams
Carbohydrate	45–65%	55%	880 calories = 220 grams	45%	1260 calories = 315 grams

SOURCE: Food and Nutrition Board, Institute of Medicine, National Academies. 2002. *Dietary Reference Intakes: Applications in Dietary Planning,* Washington, D.C.: National Academies Press. Reprinted with permission from the National Academies Press, Washington, D.C.

and yams). Most other vegetables contain a mixture of complex and simple carbohydrates.

During digestion in the mouth and small intestine, your body breaks down carbohydrates into simple sugar molecules, such as **glucose,** for absorption. Once glucose is in the bloodstream, the pancreas releases the hormone insulin, which allows cells to take up glucose and use it for energy. The liver and muscles also take up glucose to provide carbohydrate storage in the form of **glycogen.** Some people have problems controlling blood glucose levels, a disorder called *diabetes mellitus.*

→ Refined Carbohydrates Versus Whole Grains Complex carbohydrates can be further divided between refined, or processed, carbohydrates and unrefined carbohydrates, or **whole grains.** Before they are processed, all grains are whole grains, consisting of an inner layer, germ; a middle layer, the endosperm; and an outer layer, bran. During processing, the germ and bran are often removed, leaving just the starchy endosperm. The refinement of whole grains transforms whole-wheat flour to white flour, brown rice to white rice, and so on.

Refined carbohydrates usually retain all the calories of their unrefined counterparts, but they tend to be much

Choosing More Whole-Grain Foods

Whole-grain foods are good weapons against heart disease, diabetes, high blood pressure, stroke, and certain cancers. They are also low in fat and so can be a good choice for managing weight.

What Are Whole Grains?

The first step in increasing your intake of whole grains is to correctly identify them. The following are whole grains:

whole wheat	whole-grain corn
whole rye	popcorn
whole oats	brown rice
oatmeal	whole-grain barley

More unusual choices include bulgur (cracked wheat), millet, kasha (roasted buckwheat kernels), quinoa, wheat and rye berries, amaranth, wild rice, graham flour, whole-grain kamut, whole-grain spelt, and whole-grain triticale.

Wheat flour, unbleached flour, enriched flour, and de-germinated corn meal are not whole grains. Wheat germ and wheat bran are also not whole grains, but they are the constituents of wheat typically left out when wheat is processed and so are healthier choices than regular wheat flour, which typically contains just the endosperm.

Reading Food Packages to Find Whole Grains

To find packaged foods rich in whole grains, read the list of ingredients and check for special health claims related to whole grains. The *first* item on the list of ingredients should be one of the whole grains listed above. In addition, the FDA allows manufacturers to include special health claims for foods that contain 51% or more whole-grain ingredients. Such products may contain a statement such as the following on their packaging: "Rich in whole grain," "Made with 100% whole grain," or "Diets rich in whole-grain foods may help reduce the risk of heart disease and certain cancers." However, many whole-grain products will not carry such claims.

Incorporating Whole Grains into Your Daily Diet

• *Bread:* Look for sandwich breads, bagels, English muffins, buns, and pita breads with a whole grain listed as the first ingredient.

• *Breakfast cereals:* Check the ingredient list for whole grains. Whole-grain choices include oatmeal, muesli, shredded wheat, and some types of raisin bran, bran flakes, wheat flakes, toasted oats, and granola.

• *Rice:* Choose brown rice or rice blends that include brown rice.

• *Pasta:* Look for whole-wheat, whole-grain kamut, or whole-grain spelt pasta.

• *Tortillas:* Choose whole-wheat or whole-corn tortillas.

• *Crackers and snacks:* Some varieties of crackers are made from whole grains, including some flatbreads or crispbreads, woven wheat crackers, and rye crackers. Other whole-grain snack possibilities include popcorn, popcorn cakes, brown rice cakes, whole-corn tortilla chips, and whole-wheat fig cookies. Be sure to check food labels for fat content, as many popular snacks are high in fat.

• *Mixed-grain dishes:* Combine whole grains with other foods to create healthy mixed dishes. Possibilities include tabouli; soups made with hulled barley or wheat berries; and pilafs, casseroles, and salads made with brown rice, whole-wheat couscous, kasha, millet, wheat bulgur, or quinoa.

If your grocery store doesn't carry all of these items, try your local health food store.

---

lower in fiber, vitamins, minerals, and other beneficial compounds. Unrefined carbohydrates tend to take longer to chew and digest than refined ones; they also enter the bloodstream more slowly. This slower digestive pace tends to make people feel full sooner and for a longer period. Also, a slower rise in blood glucose levels following consumption of complex carbohydrates may help in the management of diabetes. Whole grains are also high in dietary fiber and so have all the benefits of fiber (discussed later). Consumption of whole grains has been linked to a reduced risk of heart disease, diabetes, high blood pressure, stroke, and certain forms of cancer. For all these reasons, whole grains are recommended over those that have been refined (see the box "Choosing More Whole-Grain Foods").

Glycemic Index and Glycemic Response Insulin and glucose levels rise and fall following a meal or snack containing any type of carbohydrate. Some foods cause a quick and dramatic rise in glucose and insulin levels; others have a slower, more moderate effect. A food that has a rapid effect on blood glucose levels is said to have a high **glycemic index.** Research findings have been mixed, but some studies have found that a meal containing high glycemic index foods may increase appetite, and that over the long term,

glucose   A simple sugar that is the body's basic fuel.

glycogen   An animal starch stored in the liver and muscles.

whole grain   The entire edible portion of a grain such as wheat, rice, or oats, consisting of the germ, endosperm, and bran. During milling or processing, parts of the grain are removed, often leaving just the endosperm.

glycemic index   A measure of how the ingestion of a particular food affects blood glucose levels.

diets rich in these foods may increase risk of diabetes and heart disease for some people. High glycemic index foods do not, as some popular diets claim, directly cause weight gain beyond the calories they contain.

Attempting to base food choices on glycemic index is a difficult task, however. Although unrefined complex carbohydrates and high-fiber foods generally tend to have a low glycemic index, patterns are less clear for other types of foods and do not follow an easy distinction such as that of simple versus complex carbohydrates. For example, some fruits with fairly high levels of simple carbohydrates have only a moderate effect on blood glucose levels, whereas white rice, potatoes, and white bread, which are rich in complex carbohydrates, have a high glycemic index. The body's response to carbohydrates also depends on many other factors, such as how foods are combined and prepared and the fitness status of the individual.

This complexity is one reason major health organizations have not issued specific guidelines for glycemic index. For people with particular health concerns, glycemic index may be an important consideration; however, it should not be the sole criterion for food choices. Remember that most unrefined grains, fruits, vegetables, and legumes are rich in nutrients, have a relatively low energy density, and have a low to moderate glycemic index. Choose a variety of vegetables daily, and avoid heavy consumption of white potatoes. Limit foods that are high in added sugars but provide few other nutrients. Some studies have singled out regular soda, with its large dose of rapidly absorbable sugar, as specifically linked to increased diabetes risk.

Recommended Carbohydrate Intake On average, Americans consume 200–300 grams of carbohydrate per day, well above the 130 grams needed to meet the body's requirement for essential carbohydrate. A range of intakes is associated with good health, and experts recommend that adults consume 45–65% of total daily calories as carbohydrate, about 225–325 grams of carbohydrate for someone consuming 2000 calories per day. The focus should be on consuming a variety of foods rich in complex carbohydrates, especially whole grains.

Although the Food and Nutrition Board set an AMDR for added sugars of 25% or less of total daily calories, many health experts recommend an even lower intake. World Health Organization guidelines suggested a limit of 10% of total daily calories from added sugars; limits set by the USDA in 2005 are even lower, with a maximum of about 8 teaspoons (32 grams) suggested for someone consuming 2000 calories per day. Foods high in added sugar are generally high in calories and low in nutrients and fiber, thus providing empty calories. The simple carbohydrates in your diet should come mainly from fruits, which are excellent sources of vitamins and minerals, and from low-fat or fat-free milk and other dairy products, which are high in protein and calcium.

Fiber—A Closer Look

Fiber is the term given to nondigestible carbohydrates provided by plants. Instead of being digested, like starch, fiber passes through the intestinal tract and provides bulk for feces in the large intestine, which in turn facilitates elimination. In the large intestine, some types of fiber are broken down by bacteria into acids and gases, which explains why consuming too much fiber can lead to intestinal gas. Because humans cannot digest fiber, it is not a source of carbohydrate in the diet; however, the consumption of fiber is necessary for good health.

Types of Fiber The Food and Nutrition Board has defined two types of fiber: dietary fiber and functional fiber. **Dietary fiber** refers to the nondigestible carbohydrates (and the noncarbohydrate substance lignin) that are present naturally in plants such as grains, legumes, and vegetables. **Functional fiber** refers to nondigestible carbohydrates that have been either isolated from natural sources or synthesized in a lab and then added to a food product or dietary supplement. **Total fiber** is the sum of dietary and functional fiber.

Fibers have different properties that lead to different physiological effects in the body. For example, **soluble (viscous) fiber** such as that found in oat bran or legumes can delay stomach emptying, slow the movement of glucose into the blood after eating, and reduce absorption of cholesterol. **Insoluble fiber,** such as that found in wheat bran or psyllium seed, increases fecal bulk and helps prevent constipation, hemorrhoids, and other digestive disorders. A diet high in fiber can help reduce the risk of type 2 diabetes and heart disease as well as improve gastrointestinal health. Some studies have linked high-fiber diets with reduced risk of colon and rectal cancer; other studies have suggested that other characteristics of diets rich in fruits, vegetables, and whole grains may be responsible for this reduction in risk.

Sources of Fiber   All plant foods contain some dietary fiber. Fruits, legumes, oats (especially oat bran), and barley all contain the viscous types of fiber that help lower blood glucose and cholesterol levels. Wheat (especially wheat bran), other grains and cereals, and vegetables are good sources of cellulose and other fibers that help prevent constipation. Psyllium, which is often added to cereals or used in fiber supplements and laxatives, improves intestinal health and also helps control glucose and cholesterol levels. The processing of packaged foods can remove fiber, so it is important to rely on fresh fruits and vegetables and foods made from whole grains as your main sources of fiber.

Recommended Fiber Intake   To reduce the risk of chronic disease and maintain intestinal health, the Food and Nutrition Board recommends a daily fiber intake of 38 grams for adult men and 25 grams for adult women. Americans currently consume about half this amount. Fiber should come from foods, not supplements, which should be used only under medical supervision.

Vitamins—Organic Micronutrients

Vitamins are organic (carbon-containing) substances required in small amounts to regulate various processes within living cells (Table 9.1). Humans need 13 vitamins; 4 are fat-soluble (A, D, E, and K), and 9 are water-soluble (C, and the 8 B-complex vitamins: thiamin, riboflavin, niacin, vitamin B-6, folate, vitamin B-12, biotin, and pantothenic acid).

Functions of Vitamins   Many vitamins help chemical reactions take place. They provide no energy to the body directly but help unleash the energy stored in carbohydrates, proteins, and fats. Vitamins are critical in the production of red blood cells and the maintenance of the nervous, skeletal, and immune systems. Some vitamins act as **antioxidants,** which help preserve healthy cells in the body. Key vitamin antioxidants include vitamin E, vitamin C, and the vitamin A precursor beta-carotene.

Sources of Vitamins   The human body does not manufacture most of the vitamins it requires and must obtain them from foods. Vitamins are abundant in fruits, vegetables, and grains. In addition, many processed foods, such as flour and breakfast cereals, contain added vitamins. A few vitamins are made in certain parts of the body: The skin makes vitamin D when it is exposed to sunlight, and intestinal bacteria make vitamin K.

Vitamin Deficiencies   If your diet lacks a particular vitamin, characteristic symptoms of deficiency can develop. (Table 9.1 lists the signs of certain vitamin deficiencies.) For example, *scurvy* is a potentially fatal illness caused by a long-term lack of vitamin C. Children who do not get enough vitamin D can develop *rickets,* which leads to potentially disabling bone deformations. Vitamin A deficiency may cause blindness, and seizures can develop in people whose diet lacks vitamin B-6. Low intake of folate and vitamins B-6 and B-12 has been linked to an increased risk of heart disease.

New research is tying vitamin deficiencies with other health risks, as well. For example, two recent studies showed that a lack of vitamin K may contribute to bone brittleness and contribute to bone fractures. Several studies have associated vitamin D deficiency with an increased risk of cardiovascular disease in adults, and show that the vitamin plays an important role in arterial health and blood clotting. A 2008 study also raised the possibility that women with certain types of breast cancer may be more likely to die from their cancer if they do not get enough vitamin D.

Vitamin deficiency diseases are most often seen in developing countries; they are relatively rare in the United States because vitamins are readily available from our food supply. Still, many Americans consume less-than-recommended amounts of several vitamins. Even in the face of new findings, however, experts warn that there is not yet enough evidence to prove that everyone should begin taking vitamin supplements.

Extra vitamins in the diet can also be harmful, especially when taken as supplements. Megadoses of fat-soluble vitamins are particularly dangerous because the excess is stored in the body rather than excreted, increasing the risk of toxicity. Even when vitamins are not taken in excess, relying on supplements for an adequate intake of vitamins can be a problem. There are many substances in foods other than vitamins and minerals, and some of these compounds may have important health effects.

Minerals—Inorganic Micronutrients

Minerals are inorganic (non–carbon-containing) elements you need in relatively small amounts to help regulate

	Table 9.1	**Facts About Vitamins**		
Vitamin	**Important Dietary Sources**	**Major Functions**	**Signs of Prolonged Deficiency**	**Toxic Effects of Megadoses**
Fat-Soluble				
Vitamin A	Liver, milk, butter, cheese, and fortified margarine; carrots, spinach, and other orange and deep-green vegetables and fruits	Maintenance of vision, skin, linings of the nose, mouth, digestive and urinary tracts, immune function	Night blindness; dry, scaling skin; increased susceptibility to infection; loss of appetite; anemia; kidney stones	Liver damage, miscarriage and birth defects, headache, vomiting and diarrhea, vertigo, double vision, bone abnormalities
Vitamin D	Fortified milk and margarine, fish oils, butter, egg yolks (sunlight on skin also produces vitamin D)	Development and maintenance of bones and teeth, promotion of calcium absorption	Rickets (bone deformities) in children; bone softening, loss, and fractures in adults	Kidney damage, calcium deposits in soft tissues, depression, death
Vitamin E	Vegetable oils, whole grains, nuts and seeds, green leafy vegetables, asparagus, peaches	Protection and maintenance of cellular membranes	Red blood cell breakage and anemia, weakness, neurological problems, muscle cramps	Relatively nontoxic, but may cause excess bleeding or formation of blood clots
Vitamin K	Green leafy vegetables; smaller amounts widespread in other foods	Production of factors essential for blood clotting and bone metabolism	Hemorrhaging	None reported
Water-Soluble				
Bitoin	Cereals, yeast, egg yolks, soy flour, liver; widespread in foods	Synthesis of fat, glycogen, and amino acids	Rash, nausea, vomiting, weight loss, depression, fatigue, hair loss	None reported
Folate	Green leafy vegetables, yeast, oranges, whole grains, legumes, liver	Amino acid metabolism, synthesis of RNA and DNA, new cell synthesis	Anemia, weakness, fatigue, irritability, shortness of breath, swollen tongue	Masking of vitamin B-12 deficiency
Niacin	Eggs, poultry, fish, milk, whole grains, nuts, enriched breads and cereals, meats, legumes	Conversion of carbohydrates, fats, and protein into usable forms of energy	Pellagra (symptoms include diarrhea, dermatitis, inflammation of mucous membranes, dementia)	Flushing of the skin, nausea, vomiting, diarrhea, liver dysfunction, glucose intolerance
Pantothenic acid	Animal foods, whole grains, broccoli, potatoes; widespread in foods	Metabolism of fats, carbohydrates, and proteins	Fatigue, numbness and tingling of hands and feet, gastrointestinal disturbances	None reported
Riboflavin	Dairy products, enriched breads and cereals, lean meats, poultry, fish, green vegetables	Energy metabolism; maintenance of skin, mucous membranes, and nervous system structures	Cracks at corners of mouth, sore throat, skin rash, hypersensitivity to light, purple tongue	None reported
Thiamin	Whole-grain and enriched breads and cereals, organ meats, lean pork, nuts, legumes	Conversion of carbohydrates into usable forms of energy, maintenance of appetite and nervous system function	Beriberi (symptoms include muscle wasting, mental confusion, anorexia, enlarged heart, nerve changes)	None reported
Vitamin B-6	Eggs, poultry, fish, whole grains, nuts, soybeans, liver, kidney, pork	Metabolism of amino acids and glycogen	Anemia, convulsions, cracks at corners of mouth, dermatitis, nausea, confusion	Neurological abnormalities and damage
Vitamin B-12	Meat, fish, poultry, fortified cereals	Synthesis of blood cells; other metabolic reactions	Anemia, fatigue, nervous system damage, sore tongue	None reported
Vitamin C	Peppers, broccoli, spinach, brussels sprouts, citrus fruits, strawberries, tomatoes, potatoes, cabbage, other fruits and vegetables	Maintenance and repair of connective tissue, bones, teeth, and cartilage; promotion of healing; aid in iron absorption	Scurvy, anemia, reduced resistance to infection, loosened teeth, joint pain, poor wound healing, hair loss, poor iron absorption	Urinary stones in some people, acid stomach from ingesting supplements in pill form, nausea, diarrhea, headache, fatigue

SOURCES: Food and Nutrition Board, Institute of Medicine. 2006. *Dietary Reference Intakes: The Essential Guide to Nutrient Requirements.* Washington, D.C.: The National Academies Press. The complete Dietary Reference Intake reports are available from the National Academy Press (http://www.nap.edu); Shils, M. E., et al., eds. 2005. *Modern Nutrition in Health and Disease,* 10th ed. Baltimore: Lippincott Williams & Wilkins.

Table 9.2   Facts About Selected Minerals

Mineral	Important Dietary Sources	Major Functions	Signs of Prolonged Deficiency	Toxic Effects of Megadoses
Calcium	Milk and milk products, tofu, fortified orange juice and bread, green leafy vegetables, bones in fish	Formation of bones and teeth, control of nerve impulses, muscle contraction, blood clotting	Stunted growth in children, bone mineral loss in adults; urinary stones	Kidney stones, calcium deposits in soft tissues, inhibition of mineral absorption, constipation
Fluoride	Fluoridated water, tea, marine fish eaten with bones	Maintenance of tooth and bone structure	Higher frequency of tooth decay	Increased bone density, mottling of teeth, impaired kidney function
Iodine	Iodized salt, seafood, processed foods	Essential part of thyroid hormones, regulation of body metabolism	Goiter (enlarged thyroid), cretinism (birth defect)	Depression of thyroid activity, hyperthyroidism in susceptible people
Iron	Meat and poultry, fortified grain products, dark green vegetables, dried fruit	Component of hemoglobin, myoglobin, and enzymes	Iron-deficiency anemia, weakness, impaired immune function, gastrointestinal distress	Nausea, diarrhea, liver and kidney damage, joint pains, sterility, disruption of cardiac function, death
Magnesium	Widespread in foods and water (except soft water); especially found in grains, legumes, nuts, seeds, green vegetables, milk	Transmission of nerve impulses, energy transfer, activation of many enzymes	Neurological disturbances, cardiovascular problems, kidney disorders, nausea, growth failure in children	Nausea, vomiting, diarrhea, central nervous system depression, coma; death in people with impaired kidney function
Phosphorus	Present in nearly all foods, especially milk, cereal, peas, eggs, meat	Bone growth and maintenance, energy transfer in cells	Impaired growth, weakness, kidney disorders, cardio-respiratory and nervous system dysfunction	Drop in blood calcium levels, calcium deposits in soft tissues, bone loss
Potassium	Meats, milk, fruits, vegetables, grains, legumes	Nerve function and body water balance	Muscular weakness, nausea, drowsiness, paralysis, confusion, disruption of cardiac rhythm	Cardiac arrest
Selenium	Seafood, meat, eggs, whole grains	Defense against oxidative stress, regulation of thyroid hormone action	Muscle pain and weakness, heart disorders	Hair and nail loss, nausea and vomiting, weakness, irritability
Sodium	Salt, soy sauce, salted foods, tomato juice	Body water balance, acid-base balance, nerve function	Muscle weakness, loss of appetite, nausea, vomiting; deficiency is rarely seen	Edema, hypertension in sensitive people
Zinc	Whole grains, meat, eggs, liver, seafood (especially oysters)	Synthesis of proteins, RNA, and DNA; wound healing; immune response; ability to taste	Growth failure, loss of appetite, impaired taste acuity, skin rash, impaired immune function, poor wound healing	Vomiting, impaired immune function, decline in blood HDL levels, impaired copper absorption

SOURCES: Food and Nutrition Board, Institute of Medicine. 2006. *Dietary Reference Intakes: The Essential Guide to Nutrient Requirements.* Washington, D.C.: The National Academies Press. The complete Dietary Reference Intake reports are available from the National Academy Press (http://www.nap.edu); Shils, M. E., et al., eds. 2005. *Modern Nutrition in Health and Disease,* 10th ed. Baltimore: Lippincott Williams & Wilkins.

body functions, aid in the growth and maintenance of body tissues, and help release energy (Table 9.2). There are about 17 essential minerals. The major minerals, those that the body needs in amounts exceeding 100 milligrams per day, include calcium, phosphorus, magnesium, sodium, potassium, and chloride. The essential trace minerals, those that you need in minute amounts, include copper, fluoride, iodide, iron, selenium, and zinc.

Characteristic symptoms develop if an essential mineral is consumed in a quantity too small or too large for good health. The minerals commonly lacking in the American diet are iron, calcium, potassium, and magnesium. Iron-deficiency **anemia** is a problem in many age groups, and researchers fear poor calcium intakes in childhood are sowing the seeds for future **osteoporosis,** especially in women (see the box "Eating for Healthy Bones").

anemia   A deficiency in the oxygen-carrying material in the red blood cells.

osteoporosis   A condition in which the bones become extremely thin and brittle and break easily.

TERMS

Eating for Healthy Bones

Osteoporosis is a condition in which the bones become dangerously thin and fragile over time. An estimated 10 million Americans over age 50 have osteoporosis, and another 34 million are at risk. Women account for about 80% of osteoporosis cases. Most bone mass is built by age 18. After bone density peaks between ages 25 and 35, bone mass is lost over time. To prevent osteoporosis, the best strategy is to build as much bone as possible during your youth and do everything you can to maintain it as you age. Up to 50% of bone loss is determined by controllable lifestyle factors. Key nutrients for bone health include the following:

- **Calcium.** Consuming an adequate amount of calcium is important throughout life to build and maintain bone mass. Milk, yogurt, and calcium-fortified orange juice, bread, and cereals are all good sources.

- **Vitamin D.** Vitamin D is necessary for bones to absorb calcium; a daily intake of 5 micrograms is recommended for adults age 19–50. Vitamin D can be obtained from foods and is manufactured by the skin when exposed to sunlight. Candidates for vitamin D supplements include people who don't eat many foods rich in vitamin D; those who don't expose their face, arms, and hands to the sun (without sunscreen) for 5–15 minutes a few times each week; and people who live north of an imaginary line roughly between Boston and the Oregon–California border (the sun is weaker in northern latitudes).

- **Vitamin K.** Vitamin K promotes the synthesis of proteins that help keep bones strong. Broccoli and leafy green vegetables are rich in vitamin K.

- **Other nutrients.** Other nutrients that may play an important role in bone health include vitamin C, magnesium, potassium, manganese, zinc, copper, and boron.

On the flip side, there are several dietary substances that may have a *negative* effect on bone health, especially if consumed in excess: alcohol, sodium, caffeine, and retinol (a form of vitamin A).

In addition, weight-bearing aerobic exercise helps maintain bone mass throughout life, and strength training improves bone density, muscle mass, strength, and balance.

Water—Vital but Often Ignored

Water is the major component in both foods and the human body: You are composed of about 50–60% water. Your need for other nutrients, in terms of weight, is much less than your need for water. You can live up to 50 days without food, but only a few days without water.

Water is distributed all over the body, among lean and other tissues and in blood and other body fluids. Water is used in the digestion and absorption of food and is the medium in which most of the chemical reactions take place within the body. Some water-based fluids, like blood, transport substances around the body, whereas other fluids serve as lubricants or cushions. Water also helps regulate body temperature.

Water is contained in almost all foods, particularly in liquids, fruits, and vegetables. The foods and fluids you consume provide 80–90% of your daily water intake; the remainder is generated through metabolism. You lose water each day in urine, feces, and sweat and through evaporation from your lungs.

Most people can maintain a healthy water balance by consuming beverages at meals and drinking fluids in response to thirst. The Food and Nutrition Board has set levels of adequate water intake to maintain hydration; all fluids, including those containing caffeine, can count toward your total daily fluid intake. Under these guidelines, men need to consume about 3.7 total liters of water, with 3.0 liters (about 13 cups) coming from beverages; women need 2.7 total liters, with 2.2 liters (about 9 cups) coming from beverages. (See Table 1 in the Nutrition Resources section at the end of the chapter for information on specific age groups.) If you exercise vigorously or live in a hot climate, you need to consume additional fluids to maintain a balance between water consumed and water lost.

Other Substances in Food

Many substances in food are not essential nutrients but may influence health.

Antioxidants When the body uses oxygen or breaks down certain fats or proteins as a normal part of metabolism, it gives rise to substances called **free radicals.** Environmental factors such as cigarette smoke, exhaust fumes, radiation, excessive sunlight, certain drugs, and stress can increase free radical production. A free radical is a chemically unstable molecule that reacts with fats, proteins, and DNA, damaging cell membranes and mutating genes. Free radicals have been implicated in aging, cancer, cardiovascular disease, and other degenerative diseases like arthritis.

Antioxidants found in foods can help protect the body from damage by free radicals in several ways. Some prevent or reduce the formation of free radicals; others remove free radicals from the body; still others repair some types of free radical damage after it occurs. Some antioxidants, such as vitamin C, vitamin E, and selenium, are also essential nutrients. Others—such as the carotenoids found in yellow, orange, and deep-green vegetables—are not. Researchers recently identified the top antioxidant-containing foods and beverages as blackberries, walnuts, strawberries, artichokes, cranberries, brewed coffee, raspberries, pecans, blueberries, cloves, grape juice, unsweetened baking choc-

QUESTIONS FOR CRITICAL THINKING AND REFLECTION

Experts say that two of the most important factors in a healthy diet are eating the "right" kinds of carbohydrates and the "right" kinds of fats. Based on what you've read so far in this chapter, which are the "right" carbohydrates and fats? How would you say your own diet stacks up when it comes to carbs and fats?

olate, sour cherries, and red wine. Also high in antioxidants are brussels sprouts, kale, cauliflower, and pomegranates.

Phytochemicals   Antioxidants fall into the broader category of **phytochemicals,** substances found in plant foods that may help prevent chronic disease. Researchers have just begun to identify and study all the different compounds found in foods, and many preliminary findings are promising. For example, certain substances found in soy foods may help lower cholesterol levels. Sulforaphane, a compound isolated from broccoli and other **cruciferous vegetables,** may render some carcinogenic compounds harmless. Allyl sulfides, a group of chemicals found in garlic and onions, appear to boost the activity of cancer-fighting immune cells.

If you want to increase your intake of phytochemicals, it is best to eat a variety of fruits, vegetables, and grains rather than relying on supplements. Like many vitamins and minerals, isolated phytochemicals may be harmful if taken in high doses. In addition, it is likely that their health benefits are the result of chemical substances working in combination.

NUTRITIONAL GUIDELINES: PLANNING YOUR DIET

Various tools have been created by scientific and government groups to help people design healthy diets. The **Dietary Reference Intakes (DRIs)** are standards for nutrient intake designed to prevent nutritional deficiencies and reduce the risk of chronic disease. **Dietary Guidelines for Americans** have been established to promote health and reduce the risk for major chronic diseases through diet and physical activity. Further guidance symbolized by **MyPyramid** provides daily food intake patterns that meet the DRIs and are consistent with the Dietary Guidelines for Americans.

Dietary Reference Intakes (DRIs)

The Food and Nutrition Board establishes dietary standards, or recommended intake levels, for Americans of all ages. The current set of standards, called Dietary Refer-

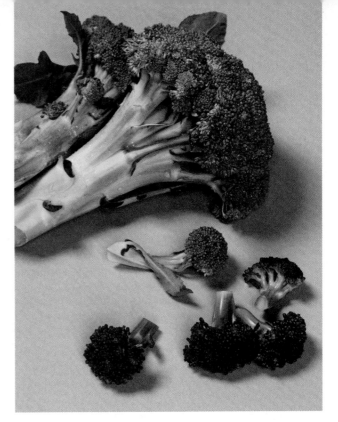

Cruciferous vegetables like broccoli are rich in phytochemicals and essential vitamins and minerals.

ence Intakes (DRIs), is relatively new, having been introduced in 1997. The DRIs are frequently reviewed and are updated as new nutrition-related information becomes available. The DRIs present different categories of nutrients in easy-to-read table format. An earlier set of standards, called the Recommended Dietary Allowances (RDAs), focused on preventing nutritional deficiency diseases such as anemia. The DRIs have a broader focus because of

TERMS

free radical   An electron-seeking compound that can react with fats, proteins, and DNA, damaging cell membranes and mutating genes in its search for electrons.

phytochemical   A naturally occurring substance found in plant foods that may help prevent and treat chronic diseases like cancer and heart disease; *phyto* means plant.

cruciferous vegetables   Vegetables of the cabbage family, including cabbage, broccoli, brussels sprouts, kale, and cauliflower; the flower petals of these plants form the shape of a cross, hence the name.

Dietary Reference Intakes (DRIs)   An umbrella term for four types of nutrient standards: Estimated Average Requirement (EAR), Adequate Intake (AI), Recommended Dietary Allowance (RDA), Tolerable Upper Intake Level (UL).

Dietary Guidelines for Americans   General principles of good nutrition intended to help prevent certain diet-related diseases.

MyPyramid   A food-group plan that provides practical advice to ensure a balanced intake of the essential nutrients.

research that looked not just at the prevention of nutrient deficiencies but also at the role of nutrients in promoting health and preventing chronic diseases.

The DRIs include standards for both recommended intakes and maximum safe intakes. The recommended intake of each nutrient is expressed as either a *Recommended Dietary Allowance (RDA)* or *Adequate Intake (AI)*. An AI is set when there is not enough information available to set an RDA value; regardless of the type of standard used, however, the DRI represents the best available estimate of intake for optimal health. The *Tolerable Upper Intake Level (UL)* is the maximum daily intake that is unlikely to cause health problems in a healthy person.

Because of lack of data, ULs have not been set for all nutrients. This does not mean that people can tolerate chronic intakes of these vitamins and minerals above recommended levels. Like all chemical agents, nutrients can produce adverse effects if intakes are excessive. There is no established benefit from consuming nutrients at levels above the RDA or AI. The DRIs can be found in the Nutrition Resources section at the end of the chapter.

Because the DRIs are too cumbersome to use as a basis for food labels, the U.S. Food and Drug Administration (FDA) uses another set of dietary standards, the **Daily Values.** The Daily Values are based on several different sets of guidelines and include standards for fat, cholesterol, carbohydrate, dietary fiber, and selected vitamins and minerals. The Daily Values represent appropriate intake levels for a 2000-calorie diet. The percent Daily Value shown on a food label shows how well that food contributes to your recommended daily intake.

Dietary Guidelines for Americans

To provide general guidance for choosing a healthy diet, the U.S. Department of Agriculture (USDA) and the U.S. Department of Health and Human Services (DHHS) have jointly issued Dietary Guidelines for Americans, most recently in 2005. These guidelines are intended for healthy children age 2 and older and adults of all ages. Key recommendations include the following:

- Consume a variety of nutrient-dense foods within and among the basic food groups, while staying within energy needs.

- Control calorie intake to manage body weight.

- Be physically active every day.

- Increase daily intake of foods from certain groups: fruits and vegetables, whole grains, and fat-free or low-fat milk and milk products.

- Choose fats wisely for good health, limiting intake of saturated and trans fats.

- Choose carbohydrates wisely for good health, limiting intake of added sugars.

- Choose and prepare foods with little salt, and consume potassium-rich foods.

- If you drink alcoholic beverages, do so in moderation.

- Keep foods safe to eat.

Following these guidelines promotes health and reduces risk for chronic diseases.

Adequate Nutrients Within Calorie Needs Many people consume more calories than they need while failing to meet recommended intakes for all nutrients. The DRIs provide a foundation not only for current health but also for reducing chronic disease risk.

Two eating plans that translate nutrient recommendations into food choices are the USDA's MyPyramid and the DASH eating plan. You can obtain all the nutrients you need by choosing the recommended number of daily servings from basic food groups and following the advice about selecting nutrient-dense foods within the groups.

Weight Management Overweight and obesity are a major public health problem in the United States. Calorie intake and physical activity work together to influence body weight. Most Americans need to reduce the amount of calories they consume, increase their level of physical activity, and make wiser food choices. Many adults gain weight slowly over time, but even small changes in behavior can help avoid weight gain.

Physical Activity Regular physical activity improves fitness, helps manage weight, promotes psychological well-being, and reduces risk of heart disease, high blood pressure, cancer, and diabetes. Become active if you are inactive, and maintain or increase physical activity if you are already active. The amount of daily physical activity recommended for you depends on your current health status and goals.

Food Groups to Encourage The Dietary Guidelines for Americans and MyPyramid both emphasize eating a wide range of foods. Central to these plans are fruits, vegetables, whole grains, and low-fat and fat-free dairy products. Each of these food groups offers a nearly endless array of choices. The discussion of MyPyramid, which comes later in this chapter, provides detailed information on choices and serving sizes.

Fats The type and amount of fats consumed can make a difference for health. A diet low in saturated fat, trans

Environmental issues—including booming populations and changing weather patterns—have coupled with fuel shortages to create a potential global food crisis. In 2008, evidence of such a crisis began to mount, even as worldwide production of many food staples reached all-time highs.

- The growing demand for corn to create ethanol (an alternative to gasoline) has driven up corn prices and greatly reduced the amount of grain used for human and animal consumption.

- Driven by fears of future shortages, the price of rice rose by more than 75% between December 2007 and April 2008. Some rice-producing countries began restricting rice exports to meet their own needs for the staple.

- Riots erupted in Haiti, Egypt, Bangladesh, and other countries in the spring of 2008, as residents protested food shortages and high prices. Many experts warned that at current rates, the world's poorest people soon would not be able to feed themselves.

For more information on the environment and health, see Chapter 14.

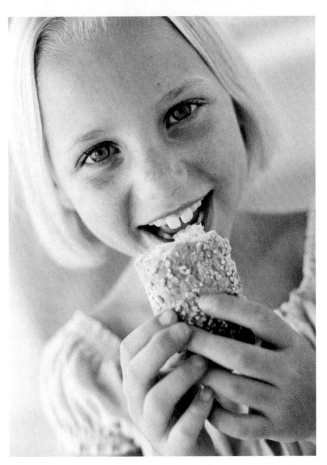

Half of your daily grain servings should come from whole grains. To check if a food contains whole grains, read the ingredient list on the food label.

fat, and cholesterol helps keep blood cholesterol low and reduces the risk for heart disease. Goals for fat intake for most adults are as follows:

Total fat: 20–35% of total daily calories

Saturated fat: Less than 10% of total daily calories

Trans fat: As little as possible

Cholesterol: Less than 300 mg per day

Most fats in the diet should come from sources of unsaturated fats, such as fish, nuts, and vegetable oils (see the box "Going Trans Fat–Free").

Cholesterol is found only in animal foods. If you need to reduce your cholesterol intake, limit your intake of foods that are particularly high in cholesterol, including egg yolks, dairy fats, certain shellfish, and liver and other organ meats; watch your serving sizes of animal foods. Food labels list the fat and cholesterol content of foods.

Two servings per week of fish rich in heart-healthy omega-3 fatty acids are also recommended for people at high risk for heart disease. However, for certain groups, intake limits are set for varieties of fish that may contain mercury. Fish rich in omega-3 fatty acids include salmon, mackerel, and trout.

Carbohydrates Fruits, vegetables, whole grains, and fat-free or low-fat milk can provide the recommended amount of carbohydrate. Choose fiber-rich foods often—for example, whole fruits, whole grains, and legumes.

People who consume foods and beverages high in added sugars tend to consume more calories but smaller amounts of vitamins and minerals than those who limit their intake of added sugars. A food is likely high in sugar if one of the following appears first or second in the list of ingredients or if several are listed: sugar (any type, including beet, brown, invert, raw, and cane), corn syrup or sweetener, fruit juice concentrate, honey, malt syrup, molasses, syrup, cane juice, dextrose, fructose, glucose, lactose, maltose, or sucrose.

To reduce added sugar consumption, cut back on soft drinks, candies, sweet desserts, fruit drinks, and other foods high in added sugars. Watch out for specialty drinks like café mochas, chai tea, smoothies, and sports drinks, which can contain hundreds of extra calories from sugar. Drink water rather than sweetened drinks, and don't let sodas and other sweets crowd out more nutritious foods, such as low-fat milk. Regular soda is the leading source of

Daily Values A simplified version of the RDAs used on food labels; also included are values for nutrients with no RDA per se.

TERMS

Going Trans Fat–Free

What do the cities of New York, Philadelphia, and Tiburon, California, have in common? They were the first three cities in the United States to be trans fat–free. In 2004, restaurants in Tiburon, a suburb of San Francisco, voluntarily stopped using cooking oils containing trans fat. The grassroots effort in Tiburon served as a model for regulations passed in 2006 and 2007 to limit the amount of trans fat served in New York and Philadelphia restaurants. Since then, nine other American cities have enacted similar regulations. In 2008, California enacted legislation banning the use of trans fats statewide; the law, which will be in full effect in 2011, restricts the use of trans fats in restaurants and in the preparation of food for retail sale.

What Are Trans Fats?

Trans fats are unsaturated fatty acids that have a physical structure more like saturated fatty acids. Although trans fats are found in small amounts naturally in milk, beef, and lamb, most trans fats are formed through the process of hydrogenation. Many popular food items contain trans fat (see table).

Hydrogenation makes liquid oils into solid or semisolid fats. These partially hydrogenated oils have a longer shelf life and ideal physical properties for use in baked goods such as pastries, pie crusts, pizza dough, biscuits, cookies, and crackers. Partially hydrogenated oils are used for deep-fat frying because they have a long fry life.

The use of partially hydrogenated oils in restaurant and commercially prepared foods grew throughout the 1960s, 1970s, and 1980s in response to public health recommendations to reduce saturated fat intake from animal fats and tropical oils (such as palm and coconut oil).

Why Worry About Trans Fats?

In the 1990s, studies began to show that trans fats had similar effects in the body as saturated fat. Research found that trans fats were actually worse for heart health because they not only raise LDL cholesterol but also lower HDL cholesterol. A recent study found that a 2% increase in dietary intake from trans fat was associated with a 23% increase in heart disease. Studies also suggest that trans fats may promote obesity and diabetes.

Can Trans Fats Be Eliminated?

Health organizations recommend that trans fat intake be as low as possible. More and more products in the grocery store are available trans fat–free, and as consumer interest in trans fat–free restaurants grows, it will be easier for consumers to limit trans fats when eating out.

Denmark has made it illegal for any food to contain more than 2% trans fat, and Canada is considering a nationwide ban on trans fats in restaurants. In 2004, the U.S. Center for Science in the Public Interest petitioned the FDA to ban trans fat as a food ingredient.

Reducing Your Trans Fat Intake

Start by reading food labels; trans fat content is required to be listed. A serving of a food can contain up to 0.5 gram of trans fat and still show zero grams on the Nutrition Fact label and the words "trans fat-free" on the label. So check the ingredient list. If partially hydrogenated oil is included in the list, then the product contains trans fat.

Next, check the product's calorie and saturated fat content. Trans fat–free foods are not healthier if they contain more saturated fat or more calories from added sugars. Ask at restaurants whether trans fat–free oils are used in cooking. Proposals being considered in some states could require national chain restaurants to include information about calorie content of their foods, which could also help consumers make smart choices.

Trans Fat Content of Common Food Items			
Product	**Common Serving Size**	**Total Fat (g)**	**Trans Fat (g)**
French fries	Medium pkg (147 g)	27	8
Stick margarine	1 tbsp	11	3
Tub margarine	1 tbsp	7	0.5
Shortening	1 tbsp	13	4
Potato chips	Small bag (42.5 g)	11	3
Doughnut	1	18	5
Candy bar	1 (40 g)	10	3
Pound cake	1 slice (80 g)	16	4.5

SOURCES: Mozaffarian, D., et al. 2006. Trans fatty acids and cardiovascular disease. *New England Journal of Medicine* 354(15): 1601–1613; Eckel, R. H., et al. 2006. Understanding the complexity of trans fatty acid reduction in the American diet. American Heart Association Trans Fat Conference 2006. Report of the *Trans Fat Conference Planning Group. Circulation* 115(16): 2231–2246; American Heart Association. 2009. *Trans Fats* (http://www.americanheart.org/presenter.jhtml?identifier=3045792; retrieved February 9, 2009); Center for Science in the Public Interest. 2009. *Trans Fat* (http://www.cspinet.org/transfat; retrieved February 9, 2009); U.S. Food and Drug Administration, Center for Food Safety and Applied Nutrition. 2006 Update. *Questions and Answers about Trans Fat Nutrition Labeling* (http://vm.cfsan.fda.gov/~dms/qatrans2.html; retrieved February 9, 2009); U.S. Food and Drug Administration. 2003. *Revealing Trans Fats* (http://www.fda.gov/FDAC/features/2003/503_fats.html; retrieved February 9, 2009).

both added sugars and calories in the American diet, but it provides little in the way of nutrients except sugar. The 10 teaspoons of sugar in a 12-ounce soda can exceed the recommended daily limit for added sugars for someone consuming 2000 calories per day.

Sodium and Potassium Many people can reduce their chance of developing high blood pressure or lower already elevated blood pressure by consuming less salt; reducing blood pressure lowers the risk for stroke, heart disease, and kidney disease. We need only small amounts

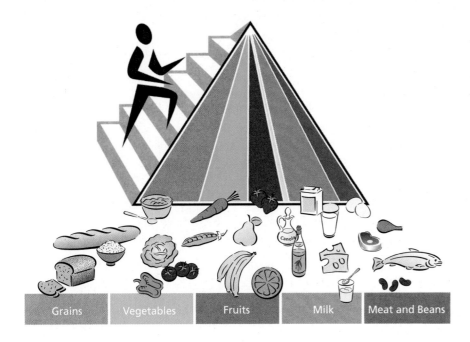

FIGURE 9.3 USDA's MyPyramid.
The USDA food guidance system, called MyPyramid, can be personalized based on an individual's sex, age, and activity level; visit MyPyramid.gov to obtain a food plan appropriate for you. MyPyramid contains five main food groups plus oils (yellow band). Key consumer messages include the following:

- Grains: Make half your grains whole

- Vegetables: Vary your veggies

- Fruits: Focus on fruits

- Milk: Get your calcium-rich foods

- Meat and Beans: Go lean with protein

SOURCE: U.S. Department of Agriculture. 2005. *MyPyramid* (http://www.mypyramid.gov; retrieved February 9, 2009).

| Grains | Vegetables | Fruits | Milk | Meat and Beans |

of salt (1500 mg per day for adults); most Americans consume much more salt than they need. The goal is to reduce sodium intake to less than 2300 milligrams per day, the equivalent of about 1 teaspoon of salt. Certain groups, including people with hypertension, African Americans, and older adults, benefit from an even lower sodium intake (no more than 1500 mg per day).

Salt is found mainly in processed and prepared foods; smaller amounts may also be added during cooking or at the table. To lower your intake of salt, choose fresh or plain frozen meat, poultry, seafood, and vegetables most often; these are lower in salt than processed forms are. Check and compare the sodium content in processed foods, including frozen dinners, cheeses, soups, salad dressings, sauces, and canned mixed dishes. Add less salt during cooking and at the table, and limit your use of high-sodium condiments like soy sauce, ketchup, mustard, pickles, and olives. Use lemon juice, herbs, and spices instead of salt to enhance the flavor of foods.

Along with lowering salt intake, increasing potassium intake helps lower blood pressure. Fruits, vegetables, and most milk products are available in forms that contain no salt, and many of these are sources of potassium. Potassium-rich foods include leafy green vegetables, sweet and white potatoes, winter squash, soybeans, tomato sauce, bananas, peaches, apricots, cantaloupes, and orange juice.

Alcoholic Beverages Alcoholic beverages supply calories but few nutrients. Drinking in moderation—that is, no more than one drink per day for women and no more than two drinks per day for men—is associated with mortality reduction among some groups, primarily males age 45 and older and women age 55 and older. Among younger people, alcohol use provides little if any health benefit, and heavy drinking is associated with motor vehicle injuries and deaths, liver disease, stroke, violence, and other health problems.

USDA's MyPyramid

Many Americans are familiar with the USDA Food Guide Pyramid, the food guidance system that was first released in 1992. Since the initial release of the Pyramid, scientists have updated both nutrient recommendations (the DRIs) and the Dietary Guidelines for Americans. So, as the 2005 Dietary Guidelines were prepared, the USDA reassessed its overall food guidance system and released MyPyramid in April 2005 (Figure 9.3).

A variety of experts have proposed other food-group plans. Some of these address perceived shortcomings in the USDA plans, and some adapt the basic 1992 Pyramid to special populations. The USDA Center for Nutrition Policy and Promotion (www.usda.gov/cnpp) has more on alternative food plans for special populations such as young children, older adults, and people choosing particular ethnic diets. MyPyramid is available in Spanish, and there are special adaptations of MyPyramid for children age 6–11 and for pregnant or breastfeeding women (www.MyPyramid.gov).

Another food plan that has received attention in recent years is the Mediterranean diet, which emphasizes vegetables, fruits, and whole grains; daily servings of beans, legumes, and nuts; moderate consumption of fish, poultry,

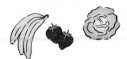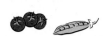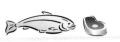

Daily Amount of Food from Each Group

Food group amounts shown in cups (c) or ounce-equivalents (oz-eq), with number of daily servings (srv) shown in parentheses; vegetable subgroup amounts are per week

Calorie level	1600	1800	2000	2200	2400	2600	2800	3000
Grains	5 oz-eq	6 oz-eq	6 oz-eq	7 oz-eq	8 oz-eq	9 oz-eq	10 oz-eq	10 oz-eq
Whole grains	3 oz-eq	3 oz-eq	3 oz-eq	3.5 oz-eq	4 oz-eq	4.5 oz-eq	5 oz-eq	5 oz-eq
Other grains	2 oz-eq	3 oz-eq	3 oz-eq	3.5 oz-eq	4 oz-eq	4.5 oz-eq	5 oz-eq	5 oz-eq
Vegetables	2 c (4 srv)	2.5 c (5 srv)	2.5 c (5 srv)	3c (6 srv)	3 c (6 srv)	3.5 c (7 srv)	3.5 c (7 srv)	4 c (8 srv)
Dark green	2 c/wk	3 c/wk	3 c/wk	3 c/wk	3 c/wk	3 c/wk	3 c/wk	3 c/wk
Orange	1.5 c/wk	2 c/wk	2 c/wk	2 c/wk	2 c/wk	2.5 c/wk	2.5 c/wk	2.5 c/wk
Legumes	2.5 c/wk	3 c/wk	3 c/wk	3 c/wk	3 c/wk	3.5 c/wk	3.5 c/wk	3.5 c/wk
Starchy	2.5 c/wk	3 c/wk	3 c/wk	6 c/wk	6 c/wk	7 c/wk	7 c/wk	9 c/wk
Other	5.5 c/wk	6.5 c/wk	6.5 c/wk	7 c/wk	7 c/wk	8.5 c/wk	8.5 c/wk	10 c/wk
Fruits	1.5 c (3 srv)	1.5 c (3 srv)	2 c (4 srv)	2 c (4 srv)	2 c (4 srv)	2 c (4 srv)	2.5 c (5 srv)	2.5 c (5 srv)
Milk	3 c	3 c	3 c	3 c	3 c	3 c	3 c	3 c
Lean meat and beans	5 oz-eq	5 oz-eq	5.5 oz-eq	6 oz-eq	6.5 oz-eq	6.5 oz-eq	7 oz-eq	7 oz-eq
Oils	5 tsp	5 tsp	6 tsp	6 tsp	7 tsp	8 tsp	8 tsp	10 tsp

The discretionary calorie allowances shown below are the calories remaining at each level after nutrient-dense foods in each food group are selected. Those trying to lose weight may choose not to use discretionary calories. For those wanting to maintain weight, discretionary calories may be used to increase the amount of food from each food group; to consume foods that are not in the lowest fat form or that contain added sugars; to add oil, fat, or sugars to foods; or to consume alcohol. The amounts below show how discretionary calories may be divided between solid fats and added sugars.

Discretionary calories	132	195	267	290	362	410	426	512
Solid fats	11 g	15 g	18 g	19 g	22 g	24 g	24 g	29 g
Added sugars	12 g (3 tsp)	20 g (5 tsp)	32 g (8 tsp)	38 g (9 tsp)	48 g (12 tsp)	56 g (14 tsp)	60 g (15 tsp)	72 g (18 tsp)

FIGURE 9.4 MyPyramid food intake patterns. To determine an appropriate amount of food from each group, find the column with your approximate daily energy intake. That column lists the daily recommended intake from each food group. Visit MyPyramid.gov for a personalized intake plan and for intakes for other calorie levels.

SOURCE: U.S. Department of Health and Human Services and U.S. Department of Agriculture. 2005. *Dietary Guidelines for Americans, 2005, Appendix A. Eating Patterns* (http://www.health.gov/dietaryguidelines/dga2005/document/html/appendixA.htm; retrieved February 9, 2009).

and dairy products; and the use of olive oil over other types of fat, especially saturated fat. The Mediterranean diet has been associated with lower rates of heart disease and cancer, and recent studies have found a link between the diet and a greatly reduced risk of Alzheimer's disease.

Key Messages of MyPyramid The new MyPyramid symbol has been developed to remind consumers to make

healthy food choices and to be active every day. Key messages include the following:

- *Personalization* is represented by the person on the steps and the MyPyramid.gov site, which includes individualized recommendations, interactive assessments of food intake and physical activity, and tips.

- *Daily physical activity,* represented by the person climbing the steps, is important for maintaining a healthy weight and reducing the risk of chronic disease.

- *Moderation* of food intake is represented by the narrowing of each food group from bottom to top.

- *Proportionality* is represented by the different widths of the food group bands.

- *Variety* is represented by the six color bands; foods from all groups are needed daily for good health.

- *Gradual improvement* is a good strategy; people can benefit from taking small steps each day.

The MyPyramid chart in Figure 9.4 shows the food intake patterns recommended for different levels of calorie intake; Table 9.3) provides guidance for determining an appropriate calorie intake for weight maintenance. Use the table to identify an energy intake that is about right for you; then refer to the appropriate column in Figure 9.4. A personalized version of MyPyramid recommendations can also be found at www.MyPyramid.gov. Each food group is described briefly below. Past experiences have shown that many Americans have trouble identifying serving sizes, so recommended daily intakes from each group are now given in terms of cups and ounces (see the box "Judging Portion Sizes" on p. 224).

Grains Foods from this group are usually low in fat and rich in complex carbohydrates, dietary fiber (if grains are unrefined), and many vitamins and minerals, including thiamin, riboflavin, iron, niacin, folic acid (if enriched or fortified), and zinc. Someone eating 2000 calories a day should include 6 ounce-equivalents each day, with half of those servings from whole grains such as whole-grain bread. The following count as 1 ounce-equivalent:

- 1 slice of bread
- 1 small (2½-inch diameter) muffin
- 1 cup ready-to-eat cereal flakes
- ½ cup cooked cereal, rice, grains, or pasta
- 1 6-inch tortilla

Choose foods that are typically made with little fat or sugar (bread, rice, pasta) over those that are high in fat and sugar (croissants, chips, cookies, doughnuts).

Vegetables Vegetables contain carbohydrates, dietary fiber, vitamin A, vitamin C, folate, potassium, and other nutrients. They are also naturally low in fat. In a 2000-calorie diet, 2½ cups (5 servings) of vegetables should be included daily. Each of the following counts as 1 serving (½ cup or equivalent) of vegetables:

- ½ cup raw or cooked vegetables
- 1 cup raw leafy salad greens
- ½ cup vegetable juice

Table 9.3	MyPyramid Daily Calorie Intake Levels		
Age (years)	Sedentary[a]	Moderately Active[b]	Active[c]
Child			
2–3	1000	1000–1400	1000–1400
Female			
4–8	1200–1400	1400–1600	1400–1800
9–13	1400–1600	1600–2000	1800–2200
14–18	1800	2000	2400
19–30	1800–2000	2000–2200	2400
31–50	1800	2000	2200
51+	1600	1800	2000–2200
Male			
4–8	1200–1400	1400–1600	1600–2000
9–13	1600–2000	1800–2200	2000–2600
14–18	2000–2400	2400–2800	2800–3200
19–30	2400–2600	2600–2800	3000
31–50	2200–2400	2400–2600	2800–3000
51+	2000–2200	2200–2400	2400–2800

[a]A lifestyle that includes only the light physical activity associated with typical day-to-day life.
[b]A lifestyle that includes physical activity equivalent to walking about 1.5 to 3 miles per day at 3 to 4 miles per hour (30–60 minutes a day of moderate physical activity), in addition to the light physical activity associated with typical day-to-day life.
[c]A lifestyle that includes physical activity equivalent to walking more than 3 miles per day at 3 to 4 miles per hour (60 or more minutes a day of moderate physical activity), in addition to the light physical activity associated with typical day-to-day life.

SOURCE: U.S. Department of Agriculture. 2005. *MyPyramid Food Intake Pattern Calorie Levels* (http://www.mypyramid.gov/downloads/ MyPyramid _Calorie_Levels.pdf; retrieved February 9, 2009).

Because vegetables vary in the nutrients they provide, it is important to consume a variety of types of vegetables to obtain maximum nutrition. Many Americans consume only a few types of vegetables, with white potatoes (baked or served as french fries) being the most popular. To help boost variety, MyPyramid recommends servings from five different subgroups within the vegetables group; try to consume vegetables from several subgroups each day. (For clarity, Figure 9.4 shows servings from the subgroups in terms of weekly consumption.)

Only 24% of Americans eat five or more servings of fruits and vegetables daily.

—Behavioral Risk Factor Surveillance System, 2007

QUICK STATS

- Dark green vegetables like spinach, chard, collards, bok choy, broccoli, kale, romaine, and turnip and mustard greens

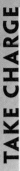

Judging Portion Sizes

Studies have shown that most people underestimate the size of their food portions, in many cases by as much as 50%. If you need to retrain your eye, try using measuring cups and spoons and an inexpensive kitchen scale when you eat at home. For quick estimates, use the following equivalents:

- 1 teaspoon of margarine = the tip of your thumb
- 1 ounce of cheese = your thumb, four dice stacked together, or an ice cube
- 3 ounces of chicken or meat = a deck of cards or an audio-cassette tape
- 1 cup of pasta = a small fist or a tennis ball

- ½ cup of rice or cooked vegetables = an ice cream scoop or one-third of a can of soda
- 2 tablespoons of peanut butter = a ping-pong ball or large marshmallow
- 1 medium potato = a computer mouse
- 1–2-ounce muffin or roll = plum or large egg
- 2-ounce bagel = hockey puck or yo-yo
- 1 medium fruit (apple or orange) = baseball
- ¼ cup nuts = golf ball
- Small cookie or cracker = poker chip

- Orange and deep yellow vegetables like carrots, winter squash, sweet potatoes, and pumpkin
- Legumes like pinto beans, kidney beans, black beans, lentils, chickpeas, soybeans, split peas, and tofu; legumes can be counted as servings of vegetables *or* as alternatives to meat
- Starchy vegetables like corn, green peas, and white potatoes
- Other vegetables; tomatoes, bell peppers (red, orange, yellow, or green), green beans, and cruciferous vegetables like cauliflower are good choices

Fruits Fruits are rich in carbohydrates, dietary fiber, and many vitamins, especially vitamin C. For someone eating a 2000-calorie diet, 2 cups (4 servings) of fruits are recommended daily. The following each count as 1 serving (½ cup or equivalent) of fruit:

- ½ cup fresh, canned, or frozen fruit
- ½ cup fruit juice (100% juice)
- 1 small whole fruit
- ¼ cup dried fruit

Good choices from this group are citrus fruits and juices, melons, pears, apples, bananas, and berries. Choose whole fruits often—they are higher in fiber and often lower in calories than fruit juices. Fruit *juices* typically contain

more nutrients and less added sugar than fruit *drinks*. For canned fruits, choose those packed in 100% fruit juice or water rather than in syrup.

Milk This group includes all milk and milk products, such as yogurt, cheeses (except cream cheese), and dairy desserts, as well as lactose-free and lactose-reduced products. Foods from this group are high in protein, carbohydrate, calcium, riboflavin, and vitamin D (if fortified). Those consuming 2000 calories per day should include 3 cups of milk or the equivalent daily. Each of the following counts as the equivalent of 1 cup:

- 1 cup milk or yogurt
- ½ cup ricotta cheese
- 1½ ounces natural cheese
- 2 ounces processed cheese

Cottage cheese is lower in calcium than most other cheeses; ½ cup is equivalent to ¼ cup milk. Ice cream is also lower in calcium and higher in sugar and fat than many other dairy products; one scoop counts as ⅓ cup milk. To limit calories and saturated fat in your diet, it is best to choose servings of low-fat and fat-free items from this group.

Meat and Beans This group includes meat, poultry, fish, dry beans and peas, eggs, nuts, and seeds. These foods provide protein, niacin, iron, vitamin B-6, zinc, and thiamin; the animal foods in the group also provide vitamin B-12. For someone consuming a 2000-calorie diet, 5½ ounce-equivalents is recommended. Each of the following counts as equivalent to 1 ounce:

- 1 ounce cooked lean meat, poultry, or fish
- ¼ cup cooked dry beans (legumes) or tofu
- 1 egg
- 1 tablespoon peanut butter
- ½ ounce nuts or seeds

vegan A vegetarian who eats no animal products at all.

lacto-vegetarian A vegetarian who includes milk and cheese products in the diet.

lacto-ovo-vegetarian A vegetarian who eats no meat, poultry, or fish but does eat eggs and milk products.

partial vegetarian, semivegetarian, or pescovegetarian A vegetarian who includes eggs, dairy products, and/or small amounts of poultry and seafood in the diet.

One egg at breakfast, ½ cup of pinto beans at lunch, and a 3-ounce (cooked weight) hamburger at dinner would add up to the equivalent of 6 ounces of lean meat for the day. To limit your intake of fat and saturated fat, choose lean cuts of meat and skinless poultry, and watch your serving sizes carefully. Choose at least one serving of plant proteins, such as black beans, lentils, or tofu, every day.

Oils The Oils group represents the oils that are added to foods during processing, cooking, or at the table; oils and soft margarines include vegetable oils and soft vegetable oil table spreads that have no trans fats. These are major sources of vitamin E and unsaturated fatty acids, including the essential fatty acids. For a 2000-calorie diet, 6 teaspoons of oils per day are recommended. One teaspoon is the equivalent of the following:

- 1 teaspoon vegetable oil or soft margarine
- 1 tablespoon salad dressing or light mayonnaise

Foods that are mostly oils include nuts, olives, avocados, and some fish. The following portions include about 1 teaspoon of oil: 8 large olives, ⅙ medium avocado, ½ tablespoon peanut butter, and ⅓ ounce roasted nuts. Food labels can help consumers identify the type and amount of fat in various foods.

Discretionary Calories, Solid Fats, and Added Sugars The suggested intakes from the basic food groups in MyPyramid assume that nutrient-dense forms are selected from each group; nutrient-dense forms are those that are fat-free or low-fat and that contain no added sugars. If this pattern is followed, then a small amount of additional calories can be consumed—the *discretionary calorie allowance*. Figure 9.4 on page 222 shows the discretionary calorie allowance at each calorie level in MyPyramid.

People who are trying to lose weight may choose not to use discretionary calories. For those wanting to maintain weight, discretionary calories may be used to increase the amount of food from a food group; to consume foods that are not in the lowest fat form or that contain added sugars; to add oil, fat, or sugars to foods; or to consume alcohol. The amounts shown in Figure 9.4 show how discretionary calories may be divided between solid fats and added sugars. The values for additional fat target no more than 30% of total calories from fat and less than 10% of calories from saturated fat. Examples of discretionary solid fat calories include choosing higher-fat meats such as sausages, or chicken with skin, or whole milk instead of fat-free milk and topping foods with butter. For example, a cup of whole milk has 60 calories more than a cup of fat-free milk; these 60 calories would be counted as discretionary calories.

The suggested amounts of added sugars may be helpful limits for including some sweetened foods or beverages in the daily diet without exceeding energy needs or under-consuming other nutrients. For example, in a 2000-calorie diet, MyPyramid lists 32 grams (8 teaspoons) for discretionary intake of added sugars. In the American diet, added sugars are often found in sweetened beverages (regular soda, sweetened teas, fruit drinks), dairy products (ice cream, some yogurts), and grain products (bakery goods). For example, a 20-ounce regular soda has 260 calories from added sugars that would be counted as discretionary calories. The current American diet includes higher-than-recommended levels of sugar intake.

The Vegetarian Alternative

Some people choose a diet in which foods of animal origin (meat, poultry, fish, eggs, milk) are eliminated or restricted. Many do so for health reasons; vegetarian diets tend to be lower in saturated fat, cholesterol, and animal protein and higher in complex carbohydrates, dietary fiber, folate, vitamins C and E, carotenoids, and phytochemicals. Some people adopt a vegetarian diet out of concern for the environment, for financial considerations, or for reasons related to ethics or religion.

Types of Vegetarian Diets There are various vegetarian styles; the wider the variety of the diet eaten, the easier it is to meet nutritional needs. **Vegans** eat only plant foods. **Lacto-vegetarians** eat plant foods and dairy products. **Lacto-ovo-vegetarians** eat plant foods, dairy products, and eggs. Others can be categorized as **partial vegetarians**, **semivegetarians**, or **pescovegetarians**; these individuals eat plant foods, dairy products, eggs, and usually a small selection of poultry, fish, and other seafood.

A Food Plan for Vegetarians MyPyramid can be adapted for use by vegetarians with only a few key modifications. For the meat and beans group, vegetarians can focus on the nonmeat choices of dry beans (legumes), nuts, seeds, eggs, and soy foods like tofu (soybean curd) and tempeh (a cultured soy product). Vegans and other vegetarians who do not consume any dairy products must find other rich sources of calcium. Fruits, vegetables, and whole grains are healthy choices for people following all types of vegetarian diets.

A healthy vegetarian diet emphasizes a wide variety of plant foods. Although plant proteins are generally of lower quality than animal proteins, choosing a variety of plant foods will supply all of the essential amino acids. Choosing minimally processed and unrefined foods will maximize nutrient value and provide ample dietary fiber. Daily consumption of a variety of plant foods in amounts that meet total energy needs can provide all

4% of Americans describe their typical diet as vegetarian.

—Harris Interactive, 2006

How Different Are the Nutritional Needs of Women and Men?

connect™

When it comes to nutrition, men and women have a lot in common. Both sexes need the same essential nutrients, and the Dietary Guidelines for Americans apply equally to both. But beyond the basics, men and women need different amounts of essential nutrients and have different nutritional concerns.

Women tend to be smaller and weigh less than men, and thus have lower energy requirements and need to consume fewer calories than men to maintain a healthy weight. For most nutrients, women need the same or slightly lower amounts than men. But because women consume fewer calories, they may have more difficulty getting adequate amounts of all essential nutrients and need to focus on nutrient-dense foods.

Two nutrients of special concern to women are calcium and iron. Low calcium intake may be linked to the development of osteoporosis in later life. The *Healthy People 2010* report sets a goal of increasing from 40% to 75% the proportion of women age 20–49 who meet the dietary recommendation for calcium. Fat-free and low-fat dairy products and fortified cereal, bread, and orange juice are good choices for calcium-rich foods.

Menstruating women also have higher iron needs than other groups, and low iron intake can lead to iron-deficiency anemia. Lean red meat, green leafy vegetables, and fortified breakfast cereals are good sources of iron. As discussed earlier, all women capable of becoming pregnant should consume adequate folic acid from fortified foods and/or supplements.

Men are seldom thought of as having nutritional deficiencies because they generally have high-calorie diets. However, many men have a diet that does not follow recommended food intake patterns and includes more red meat and fewer fruits, vegetables, and whole grains than recommended. This dietary pattern is linked to heart disease and some types of cancer. A high intake of calories can lead to weight gain over time if a man's activity level decreases as he ages. To reduce chronic disease risk, men should focus on increasing their consumption of fruits, vegetables, and whole grains to obtain vitamins, minerals, fiber, and phytochemicals.

The "Fruits and Veggies—More Matters" initiative is the result of a partnership of health organizations led by the Centers for Disease Control and Prevention and the Produce for Better Health Foundation. The goal is to increase consumption of fruits and vegetables. Information found in stores, online, and on packaging will help both men and women make healthful choices.

---

needed nutrients, except vitamin B-12 and possibly vitamin D.

Dietary Challenges for Special Population Groups

The Dietary Guidelines for Americans and MyPyramid provide a basis that everyone can use to create a healthy diet. However, some population groups face special dietary challenges (see the box "How Different Are the Nutritional Needs of Women and Men?").

Children and Teenagers Perhaps the best thing a parent can do for younger children is to provide them with a variety of foods. Add vegetables to casseroles and fruit to cereal; offer fruit and vegetable juices or homemade yogurt or fruit shakes instead of sugary drinks. Allowing children to help prepare meals is another good way to increase overall food consumption and variety. Many children and teenagers enjoy eating at fast-food restaurants; they should be encouraged to select the healthiest choices from fast-food menus (see the appendix) and to complete the day's diet with low-fat, nutrient-rich foods.

College Students Foods that are convenient for college students are not always the healthiest choices. It is easy for students who eat in buffet-style dining halls or food courts to overeat, and the foods offered are not necessarily high in essential nutrients and low in fat. The same is true of meals at fast-food restaurants, another convenient source of quick and inexpensive meals for busy students. Although no food is entirely bad, consuming a wide variety of foods is critical for a healthy diet (see the box "Eating Strategies for College Students").

Older Adults Nutrient needs do not change much as people age, but because older adults tend to become less active, they require fewer calories to maintain body weight. At the same time, the absorption of nutrients tends to be lower in older adults because of age-related changes in the digestive tract. Thus, they must consume nutrient-dense foods in order to meet their nutritional requirements. As discussed earlier, foods fortified with vitamin B-12 and/or B-12 supplements are recommended for people over age 50. Because constipation is a common problem, consuming foods high in fiber and getting adequate fluids are important goals.

Athletes Key dietary concerns for athletes are meeting their increased energy requirements and drinking enough fluids during practice and throughout the day to remain fully hydrated. Endurance athletes may also benefit from increasing the amount of carbohydrate in the diet to 60–70% of total daily calories; this increase should come in the form of complex, rather than simple, carbohydrates. Athletes for whom maintaining low body weight and body fat is important—such as skaters, gymnasts, and wrestlers—should consume adequate nutrients and avoid falling into unhealthy patterns of eating.

People with Special Health Concerns Many Americans have special health concerns that affect their dietary

Eating Strategies for College Students

General Guidelines

• Eat slowly, and enjoy your food. Set aside a separate time to eat, and don't eat while you study.

• Eat a colorful, varied diet. The more colorful your diet is, the more varied and rich in fruits and vegetables it will be. Many Americans eat few fruits and vegetables, despite the fact that these foods are typically inexpensive, delicious, rich in nutrients, and low in fat and calories.

• Eat breakfast. You'll have more energy in the morning and be less likely to grab an unhealthy snack later on.

• Choose healthy snacks—fruits, vegetables, grains, and cereals—as often as you can.

• Drink water more often than soft drinks or other sweetened beverages. Rent a mini-refrigerator for your dorm room and stock up on healthy beverages.

• Pay attention to portion sizes.

• Combine physical activity with healthy eating. You'll feel better and have a much lower risk of many chronic diseases. Even a little exercise is better than none.

Eating in the Dining Hall

• Choose a meal plan that includes breakfast, and don't skip it.

• If menus are posted or distributed, decide what you want to eat before you get in line, and stick to your choices. Consider what you plan to do and eat for the rest of the day before making your choices.

• Ask for large servings of vegetables and small servings of meat and other high-fat main dishes. Build your meals around grains and vegetables.

• Try whole grains like brown rice, whole-wheat bread, and whole-grain cereals.

• Choose leaner poultry, fish, or bean dishes rather than high-fat meats and fried entrees.

• Ask that gravies and sauces be served on the side.

• Choose broth-based or vegetable soups rather than cream soups.

• At the salad bar, load up on leafy greens, beans, and fresh vegetables. Avoid mayonnaise-coated salads, bacon, croutons, and high-fat dressings. Put dressing on the side, and dip your fork into it rather than pouring it over the salad.

• Drink nonfat milk, water, or 100% fruit juice rather than heavily sweetened fruit drinks, whole milk, or soft drinks.

• Choose fruit for dessert rather than pastries or cookies.

Eating in Fast-Food Restaurants

• Most fast-food chains can provide a brochure with a nutritional breakdown of the foods on the menu. Ask for it.

• Order small single burgers with no cheese instead of double burgers with many toppings.

• Ask for items to be prepared without mayonnaise, tartar sauce, sour cream, or other high-fat sauces. Ketchup, mustard, and fat-free mayonnaise or sour cream are better choices and are available at many fast-food restaurants.

• Choose whole-grain buns or bread for burgers and sandwiches.

• Choose chicken items made from chicken breast, not processed chicken.

• Order vegetable pizzas without extra cheese.

• If you order french fries or onion rings, get the smallest size, and/or share them with a friend. Better yet, get a salad or fruit cup instead.

Eating on the Run

Are you chronically short of time? Pack these items for a quick snack or meal: fresh or dried fruit, fruit juices, raw fresh vegetables like carrots, plain bagels, bread sticks, whole-wheat fig bars, low-fat cheese sticks or cubes, low-fat crackers or granola bars, fat-free or low-fat yogurt, snack-size cereal boxes, pretzels, rice or corn cakes, plain popcorn, soup (if you have access to a microwave), or water.

QUESTIONS FOR CRITICAL THINKING AND REFLECTION

What factors influence your food choices—convenience, cost, availability, habit? Do you ever consider nutritional content or nutritional recommendations like those found in MyPyramid? If not, how big a change would it be for you to think of nutritional content first when choosing food? Is it something you could do easily?

needs. For example, women who are pregnant or breast-feeding require extra calories, vitamins, and minerals. People with diabetes benefit from a well-balanced diet that is low in simple sugars, high in complex carbohydrates, and relatively rich in monounsaturated fats. People with high blood pressure need to control their weight and limit their sodium consumption. If you have a health problem or concern that may require a special diet, discuss your situation with a physician or registered dietitian.

A PERSONAL PLAN: MAKING INFORMED CHOICES ABOUT FOOD

Now that you understand the basis of good nutrition and a healthy diet, you can put together a diet that works for you. Focus on the likely causes of any health problems in your life, and make specific dietary changes to address them. You may also have some specific areas of concern, such as interpreting food labels and dietary supplement labels, avoiding foodborne illnesses and environmental contaminants, and understanding food additives. We turn to these and other topics next.

Reading Food Labels

All processed foods regulated by either the FDA or the USDA include standardized nutrition information on their labels. Every food label shows serving sizes and the amount of fat, saturated fat, trans fat, cholesterol, sodium, total carbohydrate, dietary fiber, sugars, and protein in each serving. To make intelligent choices about food, learn to read and *understand* food labels (see the box "Using Food Labels").

Reading Dietary Supplement Labels

Dietary supplements include vitamins, minerals, amino acids, herbs, glandular extracts, enzymes, and other compounds. They may come in the form of tablets, capsules, liquids, or powders. Although dietary supplements are often thought to be safe and "natural," they contain powerful bioactive chemicals that have the potential for harm. About one-quarter of all pharmaceutical drugs are derived from botanical sources, and even essential vitamins and minerals can have toxic effects if consumed in excess.

In the United States, supplements are not legally considered drugs and are not regulated the same way drugs are. Before they are approved by the FDA and put on the market, drugs undergo clinical studies to determine safety, effectiveness, side effects and risks, possible interactions with other substances, and appropriate dosages. The FDA does not authorize or test dietary supplements, and supplements are not required to demonstrate either safety or effectiveness prior to marketing. Although dosage guidelines exist for some of the compounds in dietary supplements, dosages for many are not well established.

There are also key differences in how drugs and supplements are manufactured. FDA-approved medications are standardized for potency, and quality control and proof of purity are required. Dietary supplement manufacture is not as closely regulated, and there is no guarantee that a product even contains a given ingredient, let alone in the appropriate amount. The potency of herbal supplements tends to vary widely due to differences in growing and harvesting conditions, preparation methods, and storage. In addition, herbs can be contaminated or misidentified at any stage from harvest to packaging. To provide consumers with more reliable and consistent information about supplements, the FDA requires supplements to have labels similar to those found on foods (see the box "Using Dietary Supplement Labels" on page 230).

Protecting Yourself Against Foodborne Illness

Many people worry about additives or pesticide residues in their food, but a greater threat comes from microorganisms that cause foodborne illnesses. Raw or undercooked animal products, such as chicken, hamburger, and oysters, pose the greatest threat, although in recent years contaminated fruits and vegetables have been catching up.

Symptoms of foodborne illness include diarrhea, vomiting, fever, and weakness. Although the effects of foodborne illnesses are usually not serious, some groups, such as children, pregnant women, and the elderly, are more at risk for severe complications.

Most cases of foodborne illness are caused by pathogens, disease-causing microorganisms. The most common contaminants are *Campylobacter jejuni* (found in contaminated water, raw milk, and raw or undercooked poultry, meat, or shellfish), *Salmonella* bacteria (found in raw or undercooked eggs, poultry, and meat; milk and dairy products; seafood; fruits and vegetables, including sprouts; and inadequately refrigerated and reheated leftovers), *Shigella* bacteria (found in the human intestinal tract and usually transmitted via fecal contamination of food and water), *Escherichia coli* bacteria (found in the intestinal tracts of humans and animals, most commonly contaminate water, raw milk, raw to rare ground beef, unpasteurized juices, and fruits and vegetables), *Listeria monocytogenes* (found in soft cheeses, raw milk, improperly processed ice cream, raw leafy vegetables, hot dogs and lunch meats, and other meat, poultry, and processed foods), *Clostridium botulinum* (found in improperly canned foods, garlic in oil, sausages and other meat products, and vacuum-packed and tightly wrapped foods), and *Norovirus* (found in contaminated water, raw or

> **Americans spent $21.4 billion on dietary supplements in 2005.**
> —Council for Responsible Nutrition, 2007

> **About 40,000 cases of *Salmonella* infection occur annually in the United States.**
> —CDC, 2008

Using Food Labels

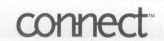

Food labels are designed to help consumers make food choices based on the nutrients that are most important to good health. In addition to listing nutrient content by weight, the label puts the information in the context of a daily diet of 2000 calories that includes no more than 65 grams of fat (approximately 30% of total calories). For example, if a serving of a particular product has 13 grams of fat, the label will show that the serving represents 20% of the daily fat allowance. If your daily diet contains fewer or more than 2000 calories, you need to adjust these calculations accordingly.

Food labels contain uniform serving sizes. This means that if you look at different brands of salad dressing, for example, you can compare calories and fat content based on the serving amount. (Food label serving sizes may be larger or smaller than MyPyramid serving size equivalents, however.) Regulations also require that foods meet strict definitions if their packaging includes the terms *light, low-fat,* or *high-fiber* (see below). Health claims such as "good source of dietary fiber" or "low in saturated fat" on packages are signals that those products can wisely be included in your diet. Overall, the food label is an important tool to help you choose a diet that conforms to My-Pyramid and the Dietary Guidelines.

Selected Nutrient Claims and What They Mean

Healthy A food that is low in fat, is low in saturated fat, has no more than 360–480 mg of sodium and 60 mg of cholesterol, *and* provides 10% or more of the Daily Value for vitamin A, vitamin C, protein, calcium, iron, or dietary fiber.

Light or lite One-third fewer calories or 50% less fat than a similar product.

Reduced or fewer At least 25% less of a nutrient than a similar product; can be ap-plied to fat ("reduced fat"), saturated fat, cholesterol, sodium, and calories.

Extra or added 10% or more of the Daily Value per serving when compared to what a similar product has.

Good source 10–19% of the Daily Value for a particular nutrient per serving.

High, rich in, or excellent source of 20% or more of the Daily Value for a particular nutrient per serving.

Low calorie 40 calories or less per serving.

High fiber 5 g or more of fiber per serving.

Good source of fiber 2.5–4.9 g of fiber per serving.

Fat-free Less than 0.5 g of fat per serving.

Low-fat 3 g of fat or less per serving.

Saturated fat-free Less than 0.5 g of saturated fat and 0.5 g of trans fatty acids per serving.

Low saturated fat 1 g or less of saturated fat per serving and no more than 15% of total calories.

Cholesterol-free Less than 2 mg of cholesterol and 2 g or less of saturated fat per serving.

Low cholesterol 20 mg or less of cholesterol and 2 g or less of saturated fat per serving.

Low sodium 140 mg or less of sodium per serving.

Very low sodium 35 mg or less of sodium per serving.

Lean Cooked seafood, meat, or poultry with less than 10 g of fat, 4.5 g or less of saturated fat, and less than 95 mg of cholesterol per serving.

Extra lean Cooked seafood, meat, or poultry with less than 5 g of fat, 2 g of saturated fat, and 95 mg of cholesterol per serving.

Note: The FDA has not yet defined nutrient claims relating to carbohydrate, so foods labeled low- or reduced-carbohydrate do not conform to any approved standard.

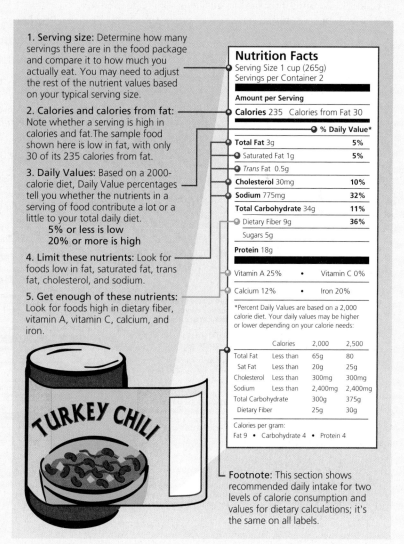

1. Serving size: Determine how many servings there are in the food package and compare it to how much you actually eat. You may need to adjust the rest of the nutrient values based on your typical serving size.

2. Calories and calories from fat: Note whether a serving is high in calories and fat. The sample food shown here is low in fat, with only 30 of its 235 calories from fat.

3. Daily Values: Based on a 2000-calorie diet, Daily Value percentages tell you whether the nutrients in a serving of food contribute a lot or a little to your total daily diet.
   5% or less is low
   20% or more is high

4. Limit these nutrients: Look for foods low in fat, saturated fat, trans fat, cholesterol, and sodium.

5. Get enough of these nutrients: Look for foods high in dietary fiber, vitamin A, vitamin C, calcium, and iron.

Nutrition Facts

Serving Size 1 cup (265g)
Servings per Container 2

Amount per Serving

Calories 235   Calories from Fat 30

	% Daily Value*
Total Fat 3g	5%
Saturated Fat 1g	5%
Trans Fat 0.5g	
Cholesterol 30mg	10%
Sodium 775mg	32%
Total Carbohydrate 34g	11%
Dietary Fiber 9g	36%
Sugars 5g	
Protein 18g	

Vitamin A 25%	•	Vitamin C 0%
Calcium 12%	•	Iron 20%

*Percent Daily Values are based on a 2,000 calorie diet. Your daily values may be higher or lower depending on your calorie needs:

		Calories	2,000	2,500
Total Fat	Less than		65g	80
Sat Fat	Less than		20g	25g
Cholesterol	Less than		300mg	300mg
Sodium	Less than		2,400mg	2,400mg
Total Carbohydrate			300g	375g
Dietary Fiber			25g	30g

Calories per gram:
Fat 9 • Carbohydrate 4 • Protein 4

Footnote: This section shows recommended daily intake for two levels of calorie consumption and values for dietary calculations; it's the same on all labels.

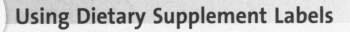

CRITICAL CONSUMER

Using Dietary Supplement Labels

Since 1999, specific types of information have been required on the labels of dietary supplements. In addition to basic information about the product, labels include a "Supplement Facts" panel, modeled after the "Nutrition Facts" panel used on food labels (see the label below). Under the Dietary Supplement Health and Education Act (DSHEA) and food labeling laws, supplement labels can make three types of health-related claims.

• *Nutrient-content claims,* such as "high in calcium," "excellent source of vitamin C," or "high potency." The claims "high in" and "excellent source of" mean the same as they do on food labels. A "high potency" single-ingredient supplement must contain 100% of its Daily Value; a "high potency" multi-ingredient product must contain 100% or more of the Daily Value of at least two-thirds of the nutrients present for which Daily Values have been established.

• *Health claims,* if they have been authorized by the FDA or another authoritative scientific body. The association between adequate calcium intake and lower risk of osteoporosis is an example of an approved health claim. Since 2003, the FDA has also allowed so-called *qualified* health claims for situations in which there is emerging but as yet inconclusive evidence for a particular claim. Such claims must include qualifying language such as "scientific evidence suggests but does not prove" the claim.

• *Structure-function claims,* such as "antioxidants maintain cellular integrity" or "this product enhances energy levels." Because these claims are not reviewed by the FDA, they must carry a disclaimer (see the sample label).

Tips for Choosing and Using Dietary Supplements

• Check with your physician before taking a supplement. Many are not meant for children, elderly people, women who are pregnant or breast-feeding, people with chronic illnesses, or people taking prescription or OTC medications.

• Choose brands made by nationally known food and drug manufacturers or house brands from large retail chains. Due to their size and visibility, such sources are likely to have high manufacturing standards.

• Look for the USP verification mark on the label, indicating that the product meets minimum safety and purity standards developed under the Dietary Supplement Verification Program by the United States Pharmacopeia (USP). The USP mark means that the product (1) contains the ingredients stated on the label, (2) has the declared amount and strength of ingredients, (3) will dissolve effectively, (4) has been screened for harmful contaminants, and (5) has been manufactured using safe, sanitary, and well-controlled procedures. The National Nutritional Foods Association (NNFA) has a self-regulatory testing program for its members; other, smaller associations and labs, including ConsumerLab.Com, also test and rate dietary supplements.

• Follow the cautions, instructions for use, and dosage given on the label.

• If you experience side effects, discontinue use of the product and contact your physician. Report any serious reactions to the FDA's MedWatch monitoring program (800-FDA-1088; http://www.fda.gov/medwatch).

For More Information About Dietary Supplements

ConsumerLab.Com: http://www.consumerlab.com

Food and Drug Administration: http://vm.cfsan.fda.gov/~dms/supplmnt.html

National Institutes of Health, Office of Dietary Supplements: http://dietary-supplements.info.nih.gov

Natural Products Association: http://www.naturalproductsassoc.org

U.S. Department of Agriculture: http://www.nal.usda.gov/fnic/etext/000015.html

U.S. Pharmacopeia: http://www.usp.org/uspverified/dietarysupplements

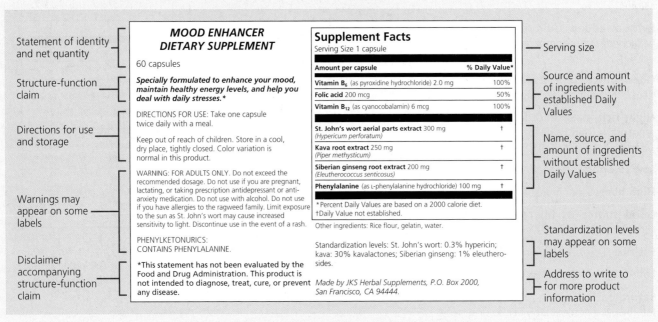

Safe Food Handling

- Don't buy food in containers that leak, bulge, or are severely dented. Refrigerated foods should be cold, and frozen foods should be solid.

- Refrigerate perishable items as soon as possible after purchase. Use or freeze fresh meats within 3–5 days and fresh poultry, fish, and ground meat within 1–2 days.

- Thaw frozen food in the refrigerator or in the microwave oven, not on the kitchen counter. Cook foods immediately after thawing.

- Thoroughly wash your hands with warm soapy water for 20 seconds before and after handling food, especially raw meat, fish, shellfish, poultry, or eggs.

- Make sure counters, cutting boards, dishes, utensils, and other equipment are thoroughly cleaned before and after use using hot soapy water. Wash dishcloths and kitchen towels frequently.

- If possible, use separate cutting boards for meat, poultry, and seafood and for foods that will be eaten raw, such as fruits and vegetables. Replace cutting boards once they become worn or develop hard-to-clean grooves.

- Thoroughly rinse and scrub fruits and vegetables with a brush, if possible, or peel off the skin.

- Cook foods thoroughly, especially beef, poultry, fish, pork, and eggs; cooking kills most microorganisms. Use a food thermometer to ensure that foods are cooked to a safe temperature. Hamburgers should be cooked to 160°F. Turn or stir microwaved food to make sure it is heated evenly throughout.

- Cook stuffing separately from poultry; or wash poultry thoroughly, stuff immediately before cooking, and transfer the stuffing to a clean bowl immediately after cooking. The temperature of cooked stuffing should reach 165°F.

- Keep hot foods hot (140°F or above) and cold foods cold (40°F or below); harmful bacteria can grow rapidly between these two temperatures. Refrigerate foods within 2 hours of purchase or preparation, and within 1 hour if the air temperature is above 90°F. Refrigerate foods at or below 40°F and freeze at or below 0°F. Use refrigerated leftovers within 3–4 days.

- Don't eat raw animal products, including raw eggs in homemade hollandaise sauce or eggnog. Use only pasteurized milk and juice.

- Cook eggs until they're firm, and fully cook foods containing eggs. Store eggs in the coldest part of the refrigerator, not in the door, and use them within 3–5 weeks.

- Because of possible contamination with *E. coli* O157:H7 and *Salmonella*, avoid raw sprouts. Even sprouts grown under clean conditions in the home can be risky because bacteria may be present in the seeds. Cook sprouts before eating them.

- According to the USDA, "When in doubt, throw it out." Even if a food looks and smells fine, it may not be safe. If you aren't sure that a food has been prepared, served, and stored safely, don't eat it.

Additional precautions are recommended for people at particularly high risk for foodborne illness—pregnant women, young children, older persons, and people with weakened immune systems or certain chronic illnesses. If you are a member of one of these groups, don't eat or drink any of the following products: unpasteurized juices; raw sprouts; unpasteurized (raw) milk and products made from unpasteurized milk; raw or undercooked meat, poultry, eggs, fish, and shellfish; and soft cheeses such as feta, Brie, Camembert, or blue-veined cheeses. To protect against *Listeria*, it's also important to avoid ready-to-eat foods such as hot dogs, luncheon meats, and cold cuts unless they are reheated until they are steaming hot.

insufficiently cooked shellfish, and salads contaminated by food handlers).

A potential new threat from food is bovine spongiform encephalopathy (BSE), or "mad cow disease," a fatal degenerative neurological disease caused by an abnormal protein that forms deposits in the brain. Visit the USDA Web site for more information (www.usda.gov).

Foodborne illness outbreaks associated with food-processing plants make headlines, but most cases of illness trace back to poor food handling in the home or in food-service establishments. To decrease your risk of foodborne illness, follow the guidelines in the box "Safe Food Handling."

Organic Foods

Some people who are concerned about pesticides and other environmental contaminants choose to buy foods that are **organic.** To be certified as organic by the USDA,

foods must meet strict production, processing, handling, and labeling criteria. Organic crops must meet limits on pesticide residues; for meat, milk, eggs, and other animal products to be certified organic, animals must be given organic feed and access to the outdoors and may not be given antibiotics or growth hormones. The use of genetic engineering, ionizing radiation, and sewage sludge is prohibited. Products can be labeled "100% organic" if they contain all organic ingredients and "organic" if they contain at least 95% organic ingredients; all such products may carry the USDA organic seal. A product with at

organic A designation applied to foods grown and produced according to strict guidelines limiting the use of pesticides, nonorganic ingredients, hormones, antibiotics, irradiation, genetic engineering, and other practices.

least 70% organic ingredients can be labeled "made with organic ingredients" but cannot use the USDA seal.

Some experts recommend that consumers who want to buy organic fruits and vegetables spend their money on those that carry lower pesticide residues than their conventional counterparts (the "dirty dozen"): apples, bell peppers, celery, cherries, imported grapes, nectarines, peaches, pears, potatoes, red raspberries, spinach, and strawberries. Experts also recommend buying organic beef, poultry, eggs, dairy products, and baby food. Fruits and vegetables that carry little pesticide residue whether grown conventionally or organically include asparagus, avocadoes, bananas, broccoli, cauliflower, corn, kiwi, mangoes, onions, papaya, pineapples, and peas. All foods are subject to strict pesticide limits; the debate about the health effects of small amounts of residue is ongoing.

Whether organic foods are better for your health or not, organic farming is better for the environment. It helps maintain biodiversity of crops and replenish the earth's resources; it is less likely to degrade soil, contaminate water, or expose farm workers to toxic chemicals. As multinational food companies get into the organic food business, however, consumers who want to support environmentally friendly farming methods should look for foods that are not only organic but locally grown.

Additives in Food

Today, some 2800 substances are intentionally added to foods to maintain or improve nutritional quality, to maintain freshness, to help in processing or preparation, or to alter taste or appearance. Additives make up less than 1% of our food. The most widely used are sugar, salt, and corn syrup; these three plus citric acid, baking soda, vegetable colors, mustard, and pepper account for 98% by weight of all food additives used in the United States.

Some additives may be of concern for certain people, either because they are consumed in large quantities or because they cause some type of reaction.

To avoid potential problems, eat a variety of foods in moderation. If you are sensitive to an additive, check

food labels when you shop, and ask questions when you eat out.

Food Irradiation

Food irradiation is the treatment of foods with gamma rays, X rays, or high-voltage electrons to kill potentially harmful pathogens, including bacteria, parasites, insects, and fungi that cause foodborne illness. It also reduces spoilage and extends shelf life. Few irradiated foods are currently on the market due to consumer resistance and skepticism. All primary irradiated foods (meat, vegetables, and so on) are labeled with the flowerlike radura symbol and a brief information label. Although irradiation kills most pathogens, proper handling of irradiated foods is still critical for preventing foodborne illness.

Genetically Modified Foods

Genetic engineering involves altering the characteristics of a plant, animal, or microorganism by adding, rearranging, or replacing genes in its DNA; the result is a **genetically modified (GM) organism.** New DNA may come from related species or from entirely different types of organisms. Many GM crops are already grown in the United States: About 75% of the current U.S. soybean crop has been genetically modified to be resistant to an herbicide used to kill weeds, and about 34% of the U.S. corn crop carries genes for herbicide resistance or pest resistance. Products made with GM organisms include juice, soda, nuts, tuna, frozen pizza, spaghetti sauce, canola oil, chips, salad dressings, and soup.

The potential benefits of GM foods cited by supporters include improved yields overall and in difficult growing conditions, increased disease resistance, improved nutritional content, lower prices, and less pesticide use. Critics of biotechnology argue that unexpected effects may occur: Gene manipulation could elevate levels of naturally occurring toxins or allergens, permanently change the gene pool and reduce biodiversity, and produce pesticide-resistant insects. Experience has shown that GM products are difficult to keep separate from non-GM products; animal escapes, cross-pollination, and contamination during processing are just a few ways GM organisms could potentially appear unexpectedly in the food supply or the environment.

According to the National Academy of Sciences, there is currently no proof that the GM food already on the market is unsafe. However, experts have recommended regulatory changes and further study of key issues, particularly the environmental effects of the escape of GM animals.

The FDA does not require special labeling for foods from genetically modified sources. Under current rules, the FDA requires special labeling only when a food's composition is changed significantly or when a known allergen such as a peanut gene is introduced into a food. The only foods guaranteed not to contain GM ingredients are those certified as organic.

Food Allergies and Food Intolerances

For some people, consuming a particular food causes symptoms such as itchiness, swollen lips, or abdominal pain. Adverse reactions like these may be due to a food allergy or a food intolerance, and symptoms may range from annoying to life-threatening.

A true **food allergy** is a reaction of the body's immune system to a food or food ingredient, usually a protein. This immune reaction can occur within minutes of ingesting the food, resulting in symptoms that affect the skin (hives), gastrointestinal tract (cramps or diarrhea), respiratory tract (asthma), or mouth (swelling of the lips or tongue). The most severe response is a systemic reaction called *anaphylaxis,* which involves a potentially life-threatening drop in blood pressure.

Although numerous food allergens have been identified, just eight foods account for more than 90% of the food allergies in the United States: cow's milk, eggs, peanuts, tree nuts (walnuts, cashews, and so on), soy, wheat, fish, and shellfish. Food labels are now required to state the presence of these eight allergens in plain language in the ingredient list. Individuals with food allergies, especially those prone to anaphylaxis, must diligently avoid trigger foods.

A food intolerance is a much more common source of adverse food reactions. In this case, the problem usually lies with metabolism rather than with the immune system. Lactose intolerance is a fairly common food intolerance. A more serious condition is intolerance of gluten, a protein component of some grains; in affected individuals, consumption of gluten damages the lining of the small intestine. Sulfite, a common food additive, can produce severe asthmatic reactions in sensitive individuals.

Many people with food intolerances can consume small amounts of the food that affects them; exceptions are gluten and sulfite, which must be avoided by sensitive individuals. Through trial and error, most people with food intolerances can adjust their intake of the trigger food to an appropriate level.

STATS

6 million Americans are allergic to shellfish, **1.8 million** are allergic to peanuts, and nearly **1 million** are truly allergic to dairy products.

—*Newsweek, 2007*

QUESTIONS FOR CRITICAL THINKING AND REFLECTION

What is the least healthy food you eat every day (either during meals or as a snack)? Identify at least one substitute that would be healthier but just as satisfying.

TIPS FOR TODAY AND THE FUTURE

Opportunities to improve your diet present themselves every day, and small changes add up.

RIGHT NOW YOU CAN

- Substitute a healthy snack for an unhealthy one.
- Drink a glass of water and put a bottle of water in your backpack for tomorrow.
- Plan to make healthy selections when you eat out, such as steamed vegetables instead of french fries or salmon instead of steak.

IN THE FUTURE, YOU CAN

- Visit the MyPyramid Web site at www.mypyramid.gov and use the online tools to create a personalized nutrition plan and begin tracking your eating habits.
- Learn to cook healthier meals. There are hundreds of free Web sites and low-cost cookbooks that provide recipes for healthy dishes.

SUMMARY

- To function at its best, the human body requires about 45 essential nutrients in specific proportions. People get the nutrients needed to fuel their bodies and maintain tissues and organ systems from foods; the body cannot synthesize most of them.

- Proteins, made up of amino acids, form muscles and bones and help make up blood, enzymes, hormones, and cell membranes. Foods from animal sources provide complete proteins; plants provide incomplete proteins.

- Fats, a concentrated source of energy, also help insulate the body and cushion the organs; 1 tablespoon of vegetable oil per day supplies the essential fats. Dietary fat intake should be 20–35% of total daily calories. Unsaturated fats should be favored over saturated and trans fats.

- Carbohydrates supply energy to the brain and other parts of the nervous system as well as to red blood cells. The body needs about 130 grams of carbohydrates a day, but more is recommended.

- Fiber includes nondigestible carbohydrates provided mainly by plants. Adequate intake of fiber (38 grams per

Improving Your Diet by Choosing Healthy Beverages

This Behavior Change Strategy focuses on choosing healthy beverages to increase intake of nutrients and decrease intake of empty calories from added sugars and fat. However, this model of dietary change can be applied to any modification you'd like to make to your diet.

Gather Data and Establish a Baseline

Begin by tracking your beverage consumption in your health journal. Write down the types and amounts of beverages you drink, including water. Also note where you were at the time and whether you obtained the beverage there or brought it with you. At the same time, investigate your options. Find out what other beverages you can easily obtain over the course of your daily routine. For example, what drinks are available in the dining hall where you eat lunch or at the food court where you often grab snacks? How many drinking fountains do you walk by over the course of the day? This information will help you put together a successful plan for change.

Analyze Your Data and Set Goals

Evaluate your beverage consumption by dividing your typical daily consumption between healthy and less healthy choices. Use the following guide as a basis, and add other beverages to the lists as needed.

Choose less often:

- Regular soda
- Sweetened bottled iced tea

- Fruit beverages made with little fruit juice (usually labeled fruit drinks, punches, beverages, blends, or ades)
- Whole milk

Choose more often:

- Water—plain, mineral, or sparkling
- Low-fat or fat-free milk
- Fruit juice (100% juice)
- Unsweetened herbal tea

How many beverages do you consume daily from each category? What would be a healthy and realistic goal for change? For example, if your beverage consumption is currently evenly divided between the "choose more often" and "choose less often" categories (four from each list), you might set a final goal for your behavior change program of increasing your healthy choices by two (to six from the "more often" list and two from the "less often" list).

Develop a Plan for Change

Once you've set your goal, you need to develop strategies that will help you choose healthy beverages more often. Consider the following possibilities:

- Keep healthy beverages on hand; if you live in a student dorm, rent a small refrigerator or keep bottled water, juice, fat-free milk, and other healthy choices in the dorm kitchen's refrigerator.
- Plan ahead, and put a bottle of water or 100% juice in your backpack every day.
- Check food labels on beverages for serving sizes, calories, and nutrients; compari-

son shop to find the healthiest choices, and watch your serving sizes. Use this information to make your "choose more often" list longer and more specific.

- If you eat out frequently, examine all the beverages available at the places you typically eat your meals. You'll probably find that healthy choices are available; if not, bring along your own drink or find somewhere else to eat.

- For a snack, try water and a piece of fruit rather than a heavily sweetened beverage.

- Create healthy beverages that appeal to you; for example, try adding slices of citrus fruit to water or mixing 100% fruit juice with sparkling water.

You may also need to make some changes in your routine to decrease the likelihood that you'll make unhealthy choices. For example, you might discover from your health journal that you always buy a soda after class when you pass a particular vending machine. If this is the case, try another route that allows you to avoid the machine. And try to guard against impulse buying by carrying water or a healthy snack with you every day.

To complete your plan, try some of the other behavior change strategies described in Chapter 1: Develop and sign a contract, set up a system of rewards, involve other people in your program, and develop strategies for challenging situations. Once your plan is complete, take action. Keep track of your progress in your health journal by continuing to monitor and evaluate your beverage consumption.

---

day for men and 25 grams per day for women) can help people manage diabetes and high cholesterol levels and improve intestinal health.

- The 13 vitamins needed in the diet are organic substances that promote specific chemical and cell processes within living tissue. Deficiencies or excesses can cause serious illnesses and even death.

- The approximately 17 minerals needed in the diet are inorganic substances that regulate body functions, aid in the growth and maintenance of body tissues, and help in the release of energy from foods.

- Water is used to digest and absorb food, transport substances around the body, lubricate joints and organs, and regulate body temperature.

- Foods contain other substances such as phytochemicals, which may not be essential nutrients but which reduce chronic disease risk.

- Dietary Reference Intakes (DRIs) are recommended intakes for essential nutrients that meet the needs of healthy people.

- The Dietary Guidelines for Americans address the prevention of diet-related diseases such as CVD, cancer, and diabetes. The guidelines advise us to consume a variety of foods while staying within calorie needs; manage body weight through calorie control and regular physical activity; eat more fruits, vegetables, whole grains, and reduced-fat dairy products; choose fats and carbohydrates wisely; eat less salt and more potassium; be moderate with alcohol intake; and handle foods safely.

• Choosing foods from each group in MyPyramid every day helps ensure the appropriate amounts of necessary nutrients.

• A vegetarian diet can meet human nutritional needs.

• Almost all foods have labels that show how much fat, cholesterol, protein, fiber, and sodium they contain. Dietary supplements also have uniform labels.

• Foodborne illnesses are a greater threat to health than additives and environmental contaminants. Other dietary issues of concern to some people include organic foods, food irradiation, genetic modification of foods, and food allergies and intolerances.

FOR MORE INFORMATION

BOOKS

Byrd-Bredbenner, C., et al. 2009. *Wardlaw's Perspectives in Nutrition,* 8th ed. New York: McGraw-Hill. *An easy-to-understand review of major concepts in nutrition.*

Duyff, R. L. 2006. *ADA Complete Food and Nutrition Guide,* 3rd ed. Hoboken, N.J.: Wiley. *An excellent review of current nutrition information.*

Insel, P. 2009. *Discovering Nutrition,* 4th ed. Sudbury, Mass.: Jones & Bartlett. *An introductory nutrition textbook covering a variety of key topics.*

Selkowitz, A. 2005. *The College Student's Guide to Eating Well on Campus,* revised ed. Bethesda, Md.: Tulip Hill Press. *Provides practical advice for students, including how to make healthy choices when eating in a dorm or restaurant and how to stock a first pantry.*

Warshaw, H. 2006. *What to Eat When You're Eating Out.* Alexandria, VA.: American Diabetes Association. *A registered dietician explains how to eat well when dining in restaurants; designed especially for those trying to manage their weight or a chronic condition such as diabetes.*

NEWSLETTERS

Environmental Nutrition (800-424-7887; http://www.environmental nutrition.com)

Nutrition Action Health Letter (202-332-9110; http://www.cspinet .org/nah)

Tufts University Health & Nutrition Letter (800-274-7581; http:// www.tuftshealthletter.com)

ORGANIZATIONS, HOTLINES, AND WEB SITES

American Dietetic Association. Provides a wide variety of nutrition-related educational materials.
    http://www.eatright.org

American Heart Association: Delicious Decisions. Provides basic information about nutrition, tips for shopping and eating out, and heart-healthy recipes.
    http://www.deliciousdecisions.org

FDA Center for Food Safety and Applied Nutrition. Offers information about topics such as food labeling, food additives, dietary supplements, and foodborne illness.
    http://vm.cfsan.fda.gov

Food Safety Hotlines. Provide information on safe purchase, handling, cooking, and storage of food.
    888-SAFEFOOD (FDA)
    800-535-4555 (USDA)

Gateways to Government Nutrition Information. Provide access to government resources relating to food safety and nutrition.
    http://www.foodsafety.gov
    http://www.nutrition.gov

Harvard School of Public Health Nutrition Source. Provides recent key research findings, including advice on interpreting news on nutrition; an overview of the Healthy Eating Pyramid, an alternative to the basic USDA pyramid; and suggestions for building a healthy diet.
    http://www.hsph.harvard.edu/nutritionsource

MyPyramid.gov. Provides personalized dietary plans and interactive food and activity tracking tools.
    http://www.mypyramid.gov

National Academies' Food and Nutrition Board. Provides information about the Dietary Reference Intakes and related guidelines.
    http://www.iom.edu/CMS/3788.aspx

National Cancer Institute: Eat 5 to 9 a Day for Better Health. Provides tips and recipes to help consumers increase their intake of fruits and vegetables.
    http://5aday.nci.nih.gov

Tufts University Nutrition Navigator. Provides descriptions and ratings for many nutrition-related Web pages.
    http://navigator.tufts.edu

USDA Center for Nutrition Policy and Promotion. Includes information on the Dietary Guidelines and MyPyramid.
    http://www.usda.gov/cnpp

USDA Food and Nutrition Information Center. Provides a variety of materials and extensive links relating to the Dietary Guidelines, food labels, MyPyramid, and many other topics.
    http://www.nal.usda.gov/fnic

Vegetarian Resource Group. Information and links for vegetarians and people interested in learning more about vegetarian diets.
    http://www.vrg.org

You can obtain nutrient breakdowns of individual food items from the following sites:

Nutrition Analysis Tool, University of Illinois, Urbana/Champaign
    http:/www.nat.uiuc.edu

USDA Nutrient Data Laboratory
    http://www.ars.usda.gov/ba/bhnrc/ndl

SELECTED BIBLIOGRAPHY

Aldana, S. G., et al. 2005. Effects of an intensive diet and physical activity modification program on the health risks of adults. *Journal of the American Dietetic Association* 105(3): 371–381.

American Heart Association. 2008. *Diet and Lifestyle Recommendations* (http://www.americanheart.org/presenter.jhtml?identifier=851; retrieved February 9, 2009).

American Heart Association. 2008. *Fish, Levels of Mercury and Omega-3 Fatty Acids* (http://www.americanheart.org/presenter.jhtml?identifier=3013797; retrieved February 9, 2009).

Centers for Disease Control and Prevention. 2005. *Foodborne Illness* (http://www.cdc.gov/ncidod/dbmd/diseaseinfo/files/foodborne_illness_FAQ.pdf; retrieved February 9, 2009).

Centers for Disease Control and Prevention. 2008. *Listeriosis* (http://www.cdc.gov/nczved/dfbmd/disease_listing/listeriosis_gi.html; retrieved February 9, 2009).

Cotton, P. A., et al. 2004. Dietary sources of nutrients among U.S. adults, 1994 to 1996. *Journal of the American Dietetic Association* 104: 921–930.

Council for Responsible Nutrition. 2005. *Dietary Supplements: Safe, Regulated and Beneficial* (http://www.crnusa.org/pdfs/CRN_FACT_DSSafeRegulatedBeneficial_07.pdf; retrieved February 9, 2009).

Food and Nutrition Board, Institute of Medicine. 2005. *Dietary Reference Intakes for Energy, Carbohydrate, Fiber, Fat, Fatty Acids, Cholesterol, Protein, and Amino Acids.* Washington, D.C.: National Academy Press.

Food and Nutrition Board, Institute of Medicine. 2005. *Dietary Reference Intakes for Water, Potassium, Sodium, Chloride, and Sulfate.* Washington, D.C.: National Academy Press.

A guide to the best and worst drinks. 2006. *Consumer Reports on Health,* July, 8–9.

Hanley, D. A., and K. S. Davison. 2005. Vitamin D insufficiency in North America. *Journal of Nutrition* 135(2): 332–337.

Harvard School of Public Health, Department of Nutrition. 2009. *The Nutrition Source: Knowledge for Healthy Eating* (http://www.hsph.harvard.edu/nutritionsource/index.html; retrieved February 9, 2009).

He, K., et al. 2004. Accumulated evidence on fish consumption and coronary heart disease mortality: A meta-analysis of cohort studies. *Circulation* 109: 2705–2711.

Lichtenstein, A. H., et al. 2006. Diet and Lifestyle Recommendations, Revision 2006. A Scientific Statement from the American Heart Association Nutrition Committee. *Circulation* 114(1): 82–96.

Liebman, B. 2006. Whole grains: The inside story. *Nutrition Action Health Letter* 33(4): 1–5.

Ma, Y., et al. 2005. Association between dietary carbohydrates and body weight. *American Journal of Epidemiology* 161(4): 359–367.

Mayo Clinic. 2008. *Food Pyramid: An Option for Better Eating* (http://www.mayoclinic.com/health/healthy-diet/NU00190; retrieved February 9, 2009).

Moreira N. 2005. *Soft Drinks as Top Calorie Culprit.* (http://www.sciencenews.org/articles/20050618/food.asp; retrieved May 12, 2008).

Mosaffarian, D., et al. 2006. Trans fatty acids and cardiovascular disease. *New England Journal of Medicine* 354(15): 1601–1613.

National Academy of Sciences, Institute of Medicine, Food and Nutrition Board. 2005. *Dietary Reference Intakes: Recommended Intakes for Individuals* (http://www.iom.edu/Object.File/Master/7/300/Webtablemacro.pdf; retrieved February 9, 2009).

Nicholls, S. J., et al. 2006. Consumption of saturated fat impairs the antiinflammatory properties of high-density lipoproteins and endothelial function. *Journal of the American College of Cardiology* 48(4): 715–720.

Pereira, M. A., et al. 2004. Dietary fiber and risk of coronary heart disease: A pooled analysis of cohort studies. *Archives of Internal Medicine* 164(4): 370–376.

U.S. Department of Agriculture and Centers for Disease Control and Prevention. 2007. *What We Eat in America, NHANES 2003–2004 Data: Nutrient Intakes: Mean Amounts and Percentages of Calories from Protein, Carbohydrate, Fat and Alcohol* (http://www.ars.usda.gov/Services/docs.htm?docid=14958; retrieved February 9, 2009).

U.S. Department of Health and Human Services and U.S. Department of Agriculture. 2005. *Dietary Guidelines for Americans 2005* (http://www.healthierus.gov/dietaryguidelines/index.html; retrieved February 9, 2009).

U.S. Department of Health and Human Services and U.S. Department of Agriculture. 2005. *Finding your way to a healthier you: Based on the Dietary Guidelines for Americans.* Home and Garden Bulletin No. 232-CP.

Vieth, R. 2006. What is the optimal vitamin D status for health? *Progress in Biophysics and Molecular Biology* 92(1): 26–32.

Nutrition Resources

Table 1 — Dietary Reference Intakes (DRIs): Recommended Levels for Individual Intake

Life Stage	Group	Biotin (µg/day)	Choline (mg/day)[a]	Folate (µg/day)[b]	Niacin (mg/day)[c]	Pantothenic Acid (mg/day)	Riboflavin (mg/day)
Infants	0–6 months	5	125	65	2	1.7	0.3
	7–12 months	6	150	80	4	1.8	0.4
Children	1–3 years	8	200	**150**	**6**	2	**0.5**
	4–8 years	12	250	**200**	**8**	3	**0.6**
Males	9–13 years	20	375	**300**	**12**	4	**0.9**
	14–18 years	25	550	**400**	**16**	5	**1.3**
	19–30 years	30	550	**400**	**16**	5	**1.3**
	31–50 years	30	550	**400**	**16**	5	**1.3**
	51–70 years	30	550	**400**	**16**	5	**1.3**
	>70 years	30	550	**400**	**16**	5	**1.3**
Females	9–13 years	20	375	**300**	**12**	4	**0.9**
	14–18 years	25	400	**400**[i]	**14**	5	**1.0**
	19–30 years	30	425	**400**[i]	**14**	5	**1.1**
	31–50 years	30	425	**400**[i]	**14**	5	**1.1**
	51–70 years	30	425	**400**[i]	**14**	5	**1.1**
	>70 years	30	425	**400**	**14**	5	**1.1**
Pregnancy	≤18 years	30	450	**600**[i]	**18**	6	**1.4**
	19–30 years	30	450	**600**[j]	**18**	6	**1.4**
	31–50 years	30	450	**600**[j]	**18**	6	**1.4**
Lactation	≤18 years	35	550	**500**	**17**	7	**1.6**
	19–30 years	35	550	**500**	**17**	7	**1.6**
	31–50 years	35	550	**500**	**17**	7	**1.6**
Tolerable Upper Intake Levels for Adults (19–70)			3500	1000[k]	35[h]		

Life Stage	Group	Thiamin (mg/day)	Vitamin A (µg/day)[d]	Vitamin B-6 (mg/day)	Vitamin B-12 (µg/day)	Vitamin C (mg/day)[e]	Vitamin D (µg/day)[f]	Vitamin E (mg/day)[g]
Infants	0–6 months	0.2	400	0.1	0.4	40	5	4
	7–12 months	0.3	500	0.3	0.5	50	5	5
Children	1–3 years	**0.5**	**300**	**0.5**	**0.9**	**15**	5	**6**
	4–8 years	**0.6**	**400**	**0.6**	**1.2**	**25**	5	**7**
Males	9–13 years	**0.9**	**600**	**1.0**	**1.8**	**45**	5	**11**
	14–18 years	**1.2**	**900**	**1.3**	**2.4**	**75**	5	**15**
	19–30 years	**1.2**	**900**	**1.3**	**2.4**	**90**	5	**15**
	31–50 years	**1.2**	**900**	**1.3**	**2.4**	**90**	5	**15**
	51–70 years	**1.2**	**900**	**1.7**	**2.4**[h]	**90**	10	**15**
	>70 years	**1.2**	**900**	**1.7**	**2.4**[h]	**90**	15	**15**
Females	9–13 years	**0.9**	**600**	**1.0**	**1.8**	**45**	5	**11**
	14–18 years	**1.0**	**700**	**1.2**	**2.4**	**65**	5	**15**
	19–30 years	**1.1**	**700**	**1.3**	**2.4**	**75**	5	**15**
	31–50 years	**1.1**	**700**	**1.3**	**2.4**	**75**	5	**15**
	51–70 years	**1.1**	**700**	**1.5**	**2.4**[h]	**75**	10	**15**
	>70 years	**1.1**	**700**	**1.5**	**2.4**[h]	**75**	15	**15**
Pregnancy	≤18 years	**1.4**	**750**	**1.9**	**2.6**	**80**	5	**15**
	19–30 years	**1.4**	**770**	**1.9**	**2.6**	**85**	5	**15**
	31–50 years	**1.4**	**770**	**1.9**	**2.6**	**85**	5	**15**
Lactation	≤18 years	**1.4**	**1200**	**2.0**	**2.8**	**115**	5	**19**
	19–30 years	**1.4**	**1300**	**2.0**	**2.8**	**120**	5	**19**
	31–50 years	**1.4**	**1300**	**2.0**	**2.8**	**120**	5	**19**
Tolerable Upper Intake Levels for Adults (19–70)			3000	100		2000	50	1000[k]

NOTE: The table includes values for the type of DRI standard—Adequate Intake (AI) or Recommended Dietary Allowance (RDA)—that has been established for that particular nutrient and life stage; RDAs are shown in **bold type.** The final row of the table shows the Tolerable Upper Intake Levels (ULs) for adults; refer to the full DRI report for information on other ages and life stages. A UL is the maximum level of daily nutrient intake that is likely to pose no risk of adverse effects. There is insufficient data to set ULs for all nutrients, but this does not mean that there is no potential for adverse effects; source of intake should be from food only to prevent high levels of intake of nutrients without established ULs. In healthy individuals, there is no established benefit from nutrient intakes above the RDA or AI.

[a] Although AIs have been set for choline, there are few data to assess whether a dietary supply of choline is needed at all stages of the life cycle, and it may be that the choline requirement can be met by endogenous synthesis at some of these stages.

[b] As dietary folate equivalents (DFE): 1 DFE 5 1 µg food folate 5 0.6 µg folate from fortified food or as a supplement consumed with food 5 0.5 µg of a supplement taken on an empty stomach.

[c] As niacin equivalents (NE): 1 mg niacin 5 60 mg tryptophan.

[d] As retinol activity equivalents (RAEs): 1 RAE 5 1 µg retinol, 12 µg β-carotene, or 24 µg α-carotene or β-cryptoxanthin. Preformed vitamin A (retinol) is abundant in animal-derived foods; provitamin A carotenoids are abundant in some dark yellow, orange, red, and deep-green fruits and vegetables. For preformed vitamin A and for provitamin A carotenoids in supplements, 1RE 5 1 RAE; for provitamin A carotenoids in foods, divide the REs by 2 to obtain RAEs. The UL applies only to preformed vitamin A.

Life Stage	Group	Vitamin K (μg/day)	Calcium (mg/day)	Chromium (μg/day)	Copper (μg/day)	Fluoride (mg/day)	Iodine (μg/day)
Infants	0–6 months	2.0	210	0.2	200	0.01	110
	7–12 months	2.5	270	5.5	220	0.5	130
Children	1–3 years	30	500	11	340	0.7	90
	4–8 years	55	800	15	440	1	90
Males	9–13 years	60	1300	25	700	2	120
	14–18 years	75	1300	35	890	3	150
	19–30 years	120	1000	35	900	4	150
	31–50 years	120	1000	35	900	4	150
	51–70 years	120	1200	30	900	4	150
	>70 years	120	1200	30	900	4	150
Females	9–13 years	60	1300	21	700	2	120
	14–18 years	75	1300	24	890	3	150
	19–30 years	90	1000	25	900	3	150
	31–50 years	90	1000	25	900	3	150
	51–70 years	90	1200	20	900	3	150
	>70 years	90	1200	20	900	3	150
Pregnancy	≤8 years	75	1300	29	1000	3	220
	19–30 years	90	1000	30	1000	3	220
	31–50 years	90	1000	30	1000	3	220
Lactation	≤18 years	75	1300	44	1300	3	290
	19–30 years	90	1000	45	1300	3	290
	31–50 years	90	1000	45	1300	3	290
Tolerable Upper Intake Levels for Adults (19–70)			2500		10,000	10	1100

Life Stage	Group	Iron (mg/day)[l]	Magnesium (mg/day)	Manganese (mg/day)	Molybdenum (μg/day)	Phosphorus (mg/day)	Selenium (μg/day)	Zinc (mg/day)[m]
Infants	0–6 months	0.27	30	0.003	2	100	15	2
	7–12 months	11	75	0.6	3	275	20	3
Children	1–3 years	7	80	1.2	17	460	20	3
	4–8 years	10	130	1.5	22	500	30	5
Males	9–13 years	8	240	1.9	34	1250	40	8
	14–18 years	11	410	2.2	43	1250	55	11
	19–30 years	8	400	2.3	45	700	55	11
	31–50 years	8	420	2.3	45	700	55	11
	51–70 years	8	420	2.3	45	700	55	11
	>70 years	8	420	2.3	45	700	55	11
Females	9–13 years	8	240	1.6	34	1250	40	8
	14–18 years	15	360	1.6	43	1250	55	9
	19–30 years	18	310	1.8	45	700	55	8
	31–50 years	18	320	1.8	45	700	55	8
	51–70 years	8	320	1.8	45	700	55	8
	>70 years	8	320	1.8	45	700	55	8
Pregnancy	≤8 years	27	400	2.0	50	1250	60	13
	19–30 years	27	350	2.0	50	700	60	11
	31–50 years	27	360	2.0	50	700	60	11
Lactation	≤18 years	10	360	2.6	50	1250	70	14
	19–30 years	9	310	2.6	50	700	70	12
	31–50 years	9	320	2.6	50	700	70	12
Tolerable Upper Intake Levels for Adults (19–70)		45	350[k]	11	2000	4000	400	40

[e]Individuals who smoke require an additional 35 mg/day of vitamin C over that needed by nonsmokers; nonsmokers regularly exposed to tobacco smoke should ensure they meet the RDA for vitamin C.

[f]As cholecalciferol: 1 μg cholecalciferol 5 40 IU vitamin D. DRI values are based on the absence of adequate exposure to sunlight.

[g]As α-tocopherol. Includes naturally occurring RRR-α-tocopherol and the 2R-stereoisomeric forms from supplements; does not include the 2S-stereoisomeric forms from supplements.

[h]Because 10–30% of older people may malabsorb food-bound B-12, those over age 50 should meet their RDA mainly with supplements or foods fortified with B-12.

[i]In view of evidence linking folate intake with neural tube defects in the fetus. It is recommended that all women capable of becoming pregnant consume 400 μg from supplements or fortified foods in addition to consuming folate from a varied diet.

[j]It is assumed that women will continue consuming 400 μg from supplements or fortified food until their pregnancy is confirmed and they enter prenatal care, which ordinarily occurs after the end of the periconceptional period-the critical time for formation of the neural tube.

[k]The UL applies only to intake from supplements, fortified foods, and/or pharmacological agents and not to intake from foods.

[l]Because the absorption of iron from plant foods is low compared to that from animal foods, the RDA for strict vegetarians is approximately 1.8 times higher than the values established for omnivores (14 mg/day for adult male vegetarians; 33 mg/day for premenopausal female vegetarians). Oral contraceptives (OCs) reduce menstrual blood losses, so women taking them need less daily iron; the RDA for premenopausal women taking OCs is 10.9 mg/day. For more on iron requirements for other special situations, refer to *Dietary Reference Intakes for Vitamin A, Vitamin K, Arsenic, Boron, Chromium, Copper, Iodine, Iron, Manganese, Molybdenum, Nickel, Silicon, Vanadium, and Zinc* (visit http://www.nap.edu for the complete report).

[m]Zinc absorption is lower for those consuming vegetarian diets so the zinc requirement for vegetarians is approximately twofold greater than for those consuming a nonvegetarian diet.

Life Stage	Group	Potassium (g/day)	Sodium (g/day)	Chloride (g/day)	Carbohydrate RDA/AI (g/day)	Carbohydrate AMDR[o] (%)	Total Fiber RDA/AI (g/day)	Total Fat AMDR[o] (%)
Infants	0–6 months	0.4	0.12	0.18	60	ND[q]	ND	[r]
	7–12 months	0.7	0.37	0.57	95	ND[q]	ND	[r]
Children	1–3 years	3.0	1.0	1.5	130	45–65	19	30–40
	4–8 years	3.8	1.2	1.9	130	45–65	25	25–35
Males	9–13 years	4.5	1.5	2.3	130	45–65	31	25–35
	14–18 years	4.7	1.5	2.3	130	45–65	38	25–35
	19–30 years	4.7	1.5	2.3	130	45–65	38	20–35
	31–50 years	4.7	1.5	2.3	130	45–65	38	20–35
	51–70 years	4.7	1.3	2.0	130	45–65	30	20–35
	>70 years	4.7	1.2	1.8	130	45–65	30	20–35
Females	9–13 years	4.5	1.5	2.3	130	45–65	26	25–35
	14–18 years	4.7	1.5	2.3	130	45–65	26	25–35
	19–30 years	4.7	1.5	2.3	130	45–65	25	20–35
	31–50 years	4.7	1.5	2.3	130	45–65	25	20–35
	51–70 years	4.7	1.3	2.0	130	45–65	21	20–35
	>70 years	4.7	1.2	1.8	130	45–65	21	20–35
Pregnancy	≤18 years	4.7	1.5	2.3	175	45–65	28	20–35
	19–30 years	4.7	1.5	2.3	175	45–65	28	20–35
	31–50 years	4.7	1.5	2.3	175	45–65	28	20–35
Lactation	≤18 years	5.1	1.5	2.3	210	45–65	29	20–35
	19–30 years	5.1	1.5	2.3	210	45–65	29	20–35
	31–50 years	5.1	1.5	2.3	210	45–65	29	20–35
Tolerable Upper Intake Levels for Adults (19–70)			2.3	3.6				

Life Stage	Group	Linoleic Acid RDA/AI (g/day)	Linoleic Acid AMDR[o] (%)	Alpha-linolenic Acid RDA/AI (g/day)	Alpha-linolenic Acid AMDR[o] (%)	Protein[n] RDA/AI (g/day)	Protein[n] AMDR[o] (%)	Water[p] (L/day)
Infants	0–6 months	4.4	ND[q]	0.5	ND[q]	9.1	ND[q]	0.7
	7–12 months	4.6	ND[q]	0.5	ND[q]	13.5	ND[q]	0.8
Children	1–3 years	7	5–10	0.7	0.6–1.2	13	5–20	1.3
	4–8 years	10	5–10	0.9	0.6–1.2	19	10–30	1.7
Males	9–13 years	12	5–10	1.2	0.6–1.2	34	10–30	2.4
	14–18 years	16	5–10	1.6	0.6–1.2	52	10–30	3.3
	19–30 years	17	5–10	1.6	0.6–1.2	56	10–35	3.7
	31–50 years	17	5–10	1.6	0.6–1.2	56	10–35	3.7
	51–70 years	14	5–10	1.6	0.6–1.2	56	10–35	3.7
	>70 years	14	5–10	1.6	0.6–1.2	56	10–35	3.7
Females	9–13 years	10	5–10	1.0	0.6–1.2	34	10–30	2.1
	14–18 years	11	5–10	1.1	0.6–1.2	46	10–30	2.3
	19–30 years	12	5–10	1.1	0.6–1.2	46	10–35	2.7
	31–50 years	12	5–10	1.1	0.6–1.2	46	10–35	2.7
	51–70 years	11	5–10	1.1	0.6–1.2	46	10–35	2.7
	>70 years	11	5–10	1.1	0.6–1.2	46	10–35	2.7
Pregnancy	≤18 years	13	5–10	1.4	0.6–1.2	71	10–35	3.0
	19–30 years	13	5–10	1.4	0.6–1.2	71	10–35	3.0
	31–50 years	13	5–10	1.4	0.6–1.2	71	10–35	3.0
Lactation	≤18 years	13	5–10	1.3	0.6–1.2	71	10–35	3.8
	19–30 years	13	5–10	1.3	0.6–1.2	71	10–35	3.8
	31–50 years	13	5–10	1.3	0.6–1.2	71	10–35	3.8

[n]Daily protein recommendations are based on body weight for reference body weights. To calculate for a specific body weight, use the following values: 1.5 g/kg for infants, 1.1 g/kg for 1–3 years, 0.95 g/kg for 4–13 years, 0.85 g/kg for 14–18 years, 0.8 g/kg for adults, and 1.1 g/kg for pregnant (using prepregnancy weight) and lactating women.

[o]Acceptable Macronutrient Distribution Range (AMDR), expressed as a percent of total daily calories, is the range of intake for a particular energy source that is associated with reduced risk of chronic disease while providing intakes of essential nutrients. If an individual consumes in excess of the AMDR, there is a potential for increasing the risk of chronic diseases and/or insufficient intakes of essential nutrients.

[p]Total water intake from fluids and food.

[q]Not determinable due to lack of data of adverse effects in this age group and concern with regard to lack of ability to handle excess amounts. Source of intake should be from food only to prevent high levels of intake.

[r]For infants, Adequate Intake of total fat is 31 grams/day (0–6 months) and 30 grams per day (7–12 months) from breast milk and, for infants 7–12 months, complementary food and beverages.

SOURCE: Reprinted with permission from *Dietary Reference Intakes: Applications in Dietary Planning,* copyright © 2003 by the National Academy of Sciences. Reprinted with permission from the National Academies Press, Washington, D.C.

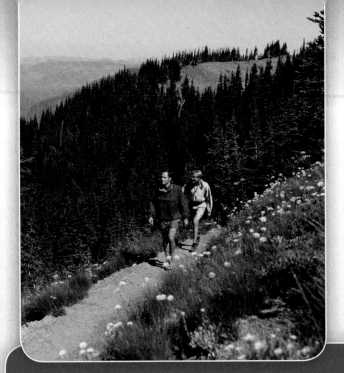

LOOKING AHEAD>>>>>

AFTER READING THIS CHAPTER, YOU SHOULD BE ABLE TO:

- Define physical fitness, and list the health-related components of fitness

- Explain the wellness benefits of physical activity and exercise

- Describe how to develop each of the health-related components of fitness

- Discuss how to choose appropriate exercise equipment, how to eat and drink for exercise, how to assess fitness, and how to prevent and manage injuries

- Put together a personalized exercise program that you enjoy and that will enable you to achieve your fitness goals

EXERCISE FOR HEALTH AND FITNESS

10

Your body is a wonderful moving machine made to work best when it is physically active. It readily adapts to practically any level of activity and exercise: The more you ask of your body—your muscles, bones, heart, lungs—the stronger and more fit it becomes. The opposite is also true. Left unchallenged, bones lose their density, joints stiffen, muscles become weak, and cellular energy systems begin to degenerate. To be truly healthy, human beings must be active. If approached correctly, physical activity and exercise can contribute immeasurably to overall wellness, add fun and joy to life, and provide the foundation for a lifetime of fitness.

WHAT IS PHYSICAL FITNESS?

Physical fitness is the body's ability to respond or adapt to the demands and stress of physical effort—that is, to perform moderate to vigorous levels of physical activity without becoming overly tired. Some components of fitness are related to specific activities or sports; others relate to general health. **Health-related fitness** includes cardiorespiratory endurance, muscular strength, muscular endurance, flexibility, and body composition. Health-related fitness helps you withstand physical challenges and protects you from diseases.

Cardiorespiratory Endurance

Cardiorespiratory endurance is the ability to perform prolonged, large-muscle, dynamic exercise at moderate to high intensity. When cardiorespiratory fitness is low, the heart has to work hard during normal daily activities and may not be able to work hard enough to sustain high-intensity physical activity in an emergency. Poor cardiorespiratory fitness is linked with heart disease, diabetes, colon cancer, stroke, depression, and anxiety. Regular cardiorespiratory **endurance training,** however, makes the heart stronger and improves the function of the entire cardiorespiratory system. As cardiorespiratory fitness improves, related physical functions also improve. The heart

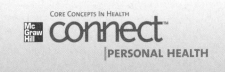

http://www.mcgrawhillconnect.com/personalhealth

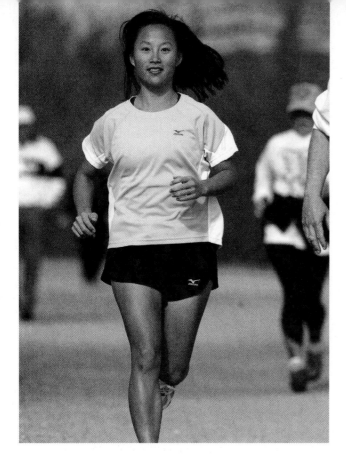
Cardiorespiratory endurance is a critical component of health-related fitness.

pumps more blood per heartbeat, resting heart rate slows and resting blood pressure decreases, blood volume increases, blood supply to tissues improves, and the body can cool itself better. A healthy heart can better withstand the strains of daily life, the stress of occasional emergencies, and the wear and tear of time. You can develop cardiorespiratory endurance through activities that involve continuous, rhythmic movements of large-muscle groups, such as the legs. Such activities include walking, jogging, cycling, and aerobic dancing.

Muscular Strength

Muscular strength is the amount of force a muscle can produce with a single maximum effort. It depends on such factors as the size of muscle cells and the ability of nerves to activate muscle cells. Strong muscles are important for everyday activities, such as climbing stairs, as well as for emergencies. They help keep the skeleton in proper alignment, preventing back and leg pain and providing the support necessary for good posture. Muscular strength has obvious importance in recreational activities. Strong people can hit a tennis ball harder, kick a soccer ball farther, and ride a bicycle uphill more easily.

Muscle tissue is an important element of overall body composition. Greater muscle mass makes possible a higher rate of metabolism and faster energy use, which help to maintain a healthy body weight. Strength training helps maintain muscle mass, function, and balance in older people, which greatly enhances their quality of life and prevents life-threatening injuries. Strength training has also been shown to benefit cardiovascular health and reduce the risk of osteoporosis (bone loss). Muscular strength can be developed by training with weights or by using the weight of the body for resistance during calisthenic exercises such as push-ups and curl-ups.

Muscular Endurance

Muscular endurance is the ability to resist fatigue and sustain a given level of muscle tension—that is, to hold a muscle contraction for a long time or to contract a muscle over and over again. It depends on such factors as the size of muscle cells, the ability of muscles to store fuel, and the blood supply to muscles. Muscular endurance is important for good posture and for injury prevention. Muscular endurance helps people cope with the physical demands of everyday life and enhances performance in sports and work. Like muscular strength, muscular endurance is developed by stressing the muscles with a greater load (weight) than they are used to. The degree to which strength or endurance develops depends on the type and amount of stress that is applied.

TERMS

physical fitness   The body's ability to respond or adapt to the demands and stress of physical effort.

health-related fitness   Physical capabilities that contribute to health, including cardiorespiratory endurance, muscular strength, muscular endurance, flexibility, and body composition.

cardiorespiratory endurance   The ability of the body to perform prolonged, large-muscle, dynamic exercise at moderate to high levels of intensity.

endurance training   Exercise intended specifically to improve cardiorespiratory endurance; usually involves prolonged, large-muscle, dynamic exercises.

muscular strength   The amount of force a muscle can produce with a single maximum effort.

muscular endurance   The ability of a muscle or group of muscles to remain contracted or to contract repeatedly for a long period of time.

Flexibility

Flexibility is the ability to move joints through their full range of motion. Flexible, pain-free joints are important for good health and well-being. Inactivity causes the joints to become stiffer with age. Stiffness, in turn, often causes older people to assume unnatural body postures that can stress joints and muscles. Stretching exercises can help ensure a healthy range of motion for all major joints.

Body Composition

Body composition refers to the proportion of fat and **fat-free mass** (muscle, bone, and water) in the body. Healthy body composition involves a high proportion of fat-free mass and an acceptably low level of body fat, adjusted for age and sex. A person with excessive body fat is more likely to experience health problems, including heart disease, high blood pressure, stroke, joint problems, diabetes, gallbladder disease, cancer, and back pain. The best way to lose fat is through a lifestyle that includes a sensible diet and exercise. The best way to add muscle mass is through resistance training such as weight training.

Skill-Related Components of Fitness

In addition to the five health-related components of physical fitness, the ability to perform a particular sport or activity may depend on **skill-related fitness** components such as speed, power, agility, balance, coordination, and reaction time. Skill-related fitness tends to be sport-specific and is best developed through practice. Some fitness experts contend that certain sports don't contribute to all the health-related components of physical fitness. Nevertheless, playing a sport can be fun, can help you build fitness, and may contribute to other areas of wellness.

PHYSICAL ACTIVITY AND EXERCISE FOR HEALTH AND FITNESS

Physical activity is any body movement carried out by the skeletal muscles and requiring energy. Quick, easy movements such as standing up or walking down a hallway require little energy or effort; more intense, sustained activities such as cycling 5 miles or running in a race require considerably more. **Exercise** refers to a subset of physical activity—planned, structured, repetitive movement of the body intended specifically to improve or maintain physical fitness. To develop fitness, a person must perform enough physical activity to stress the body and cause long-term physiological changes. Physical activity is essential to health and confers wide-ranging health benefits, but exercise is necessary to significantly improve physical fitness.

The Centers for Disease Control and Prevention (CDC) recently reported the following statistics about the physical activity levels of adult Americans:

- About 48% participate in some leisure-time physical activity, including 50% of men and 47% of women.
- Between 2001 and 2005, physical activity levels increased slightly among all age and ethnic groups, with the exception of Hispanic males.

The study also shows that education is an important factor in activity levels. For example, 54% of college graduates report doing some type of physical activity compared to 37% of high school dropouts. Other studies show that only about 12% of Americans exercise intensively at least five times per week, and 25% do some leisure-time strength training. Evidence is growing that for most Americans, becoming more physically active may be the single most important lifestyle change for promoting health and well-being (see the box "Exercise and Total Wellness.")

In 1996, the U.S. Surgeon General issued *Physical Activity and Health,* a landmark report designed to encourage Americans to become more active. One of its findings was that people can enjoy significant health benefits by including a moderate amount of physical activity on most, if not all, days of the week. This finding was echoed in the 2005 Dietary Guidelines for Americans, which recommended that all adults engage in at least 30 minutes of moderate-intensity physical activity, beyond usual activity, on most days of the week.

The recommendation was further refined in the publication *Physical Activity and Public Health: Updated Recommendations for Adults,* published jointly by the American College of Sports Medicine (ACSM) and the American Heart Association (AHA) in 2007. This report stated that adults need a minimum of 30 minutes of moderate-intensity aerobic (endurance) physical activity 5 days per week or 20 minutes of vigorous-intensity aerobic physical activity 3 days per week. Research shows that these levels of physical activity promote health and wellness in specific ways: by lowering the risk of high blood pressure, stroke,

QUESTIONS FOR CRITICAL THINKING AND REFLECTION

When you think about exercise, do you think of only one or two of the five components of health-related fitness, such as muscular strength or body composition? If so, where do you think your ideas come from? What role do the media play in shaping your ideas about fitness?

Exercise and Total Wellness

An active lifestyle provides a multitude of benefits. For example, physically active adults live from 2 to 4 years longer, on average, than do sedentary adults. The benefits of regular physical activity impact quality of life across multiple dimensions of wellness.

Physical Wellness In terms of general health, exercise increases your physical capacity so that you can meet the challenges of daily life with energy and vigor. Physical activity can help you generate more energy, increase your stamina, control your weight, manage stress, and boost your immune system.

Over the long term, even moderate physical activity can help you avoid illnesses such as heart disease, diabetes, high blood pressure, depression, osteoporosis, and some cancers. Evidence shows that exercise can even prevent premature death from several causes.

Emotional Wellness Exercise provides psychological and emotional benefits, contributing to your sense of competence and well-being. People who focus on staying active can also en-

joy an improved self-image and a higher level of self-confidence. Such healthy self-esteem can positively affect other aspects of your life, as well. For example, a good self-image can be helpful when dealing with others or when competing.

Intellectual Wellness Recent studies indicate that regular exercise is good for the brain—literally. One study shows that brain volume actually increases in adults who exercise regularly. Such gains in brain mass can improve cognitive functions and the overall health of the nervous system. Additionally, the process of mastering physical challenges—such as learning a proper golf swing—can boost intellectual fitness in the same manner as solving puzzles or engaging in other learning experiences.

Interpersonal Wellness Joining in physical activity with a friend or a group can be a boon to your interpersonal or social wellness, too. By sharing physical challenges with others, you can make new friends, deepen your existing relationships, and build a stronger overall network of support.

heart disease, type 2 diabetes, colon cancer, and osteoporosis and by reducing feelings of mild-to-moderate depression and anxiety.

The 2007 ACSM/AHA report defines moderate-intensity physical activity as activity that causes a noticeable increase in heart rate, such as a brisk walk. The report defines vigorous-intensity physical activity as activity that causes rapid breathing and a substantial increase in heart rate, as exemplified by jogging.

The daily total of physical activity can be accumulated in multiple bouts of 10 or more minutes—for example, two 10-minute bike rides to and from class and a brisk 10-minute walk to the store. More vigorous activity, as in a structured, systematic exercise program, is also needed to improve physical fitness; moderate physical activity alone is not enough. Physical fitness requires more intense movement that poses a substantially greater challenge to the body.

QUESTIONS FOR CRITICAL THINKING AND REFLECTION

Does your current lifestyle include enough physical activity—30 minutes of moderate-intensity activity 5 or more days a week—to support health and wellness? Does your lifestyle go beyond this level to include enough vigorous physical activity and exercise to build physical fitness? What changes could you make in your lifestyle to start developing physical fitness?

THE BENEFITS OF EXERCISE

The greater the demands made on the human body, the more it adjusts to meet the demands—it becomes fit. Over time, immediate, short-term adjustments translate into long-term changes and improvements (Figure 10.1). The goal of regular physical activity is to bring about these kinds of long-term changes and improvements in the body's functioning.

Improved Cardiorespiratory Functioning

During exercise, the cardiorespiratory system (heart, lungs, and circulatory system) must work harder to meet the

TERMS

flexibility The ability to move joints through their full range of motion.

body composition The proportion of fat and fat-free mass (muscle, bone, and water) in the body.

fat-free mass The nonfat component of the human body, consisting of skeletal muscle, bone, and water.

skill-related fitness Physical abilities that contribute to performance in a sport or activity, including speed, power, agility, balance, coordination, and reaction time.

physical activity Any body movement carried out by the skeletal muscles and requiring energy.

exercise Planned, structured, repetitive movement of the body intended to improve or maintain physical fitness.

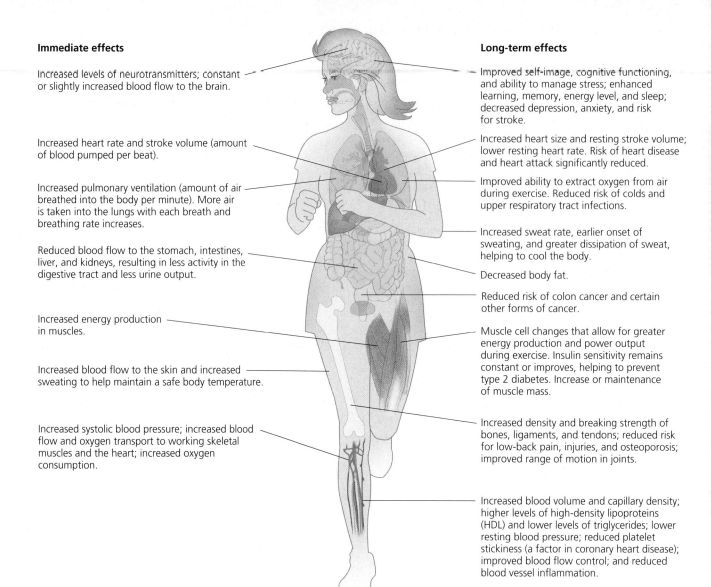

Immediate effects

Increased levels of neurotransmitters; constant or slightly increased blood flow to the brain.

Increased heart rate and stroke volume (amount of blood pumped per beat).

Increased pulmonary ventilation (amount of air breathed into the body per minute). More air is taken into the lungs with each breath and breathing rate increases.

Reduced blood flow to the stomach, intestines, liver, and kidneys, resulting in less activity in the digestive tract and less urine output.

Increased energy production in muscles.

Increased blood flow to the skin and increased sweating to help maintain a safe body temperature.

Increased systolic blood pressure; increased blood flow and oxygen transport to working skeletal muscles and the heart; increased oxygen consumption.

Long-term effects

Improved self-image, cognitive functioning, and ability to manage stress; enhanced learning, memory, energy level, and sleep; decreased depression, anxiety, and risk for stroke.

Increased heart size and resting stroke volume; lower resting heart rate. Risk of heart disease and heart attack significantly reduced.

Improved ability to extract oxygen from air during exercise. Reduced risk of colds and upper respiratory tract infections.

Increased sweat rate, earlier onset of sweating, and greater dissipation of sweat, helping to cool the body.

Decreased body fat.

Reduced risk of colon cancer and certain other forms of cancer.

Muscle cell changes that allow for greater energy production and power output during exercise. Insulin sensitivity remains constant or improves, helping to prevent type 2 diabetes. Increase or maintenance of muscle mass.

Increased density and breaking strength of bones, ligaments, and tendons; reduced risk for low-back pain, injuries, and osteoporosis; improved range of motion in joints.

Increased blood volume and capillary density; higher levels of high-density lipoproteins (HDL) and lower levels of triglycerides; lower resting blood pressure; reduced platelet stickiness (a factor in coronary heart disease); improved blood flow control; and reduced blood vessel inflammation.

FIGURE 10.1   Immediate and long-term effects of regular exercise.

body's increased demand for oxygen. Regular endurance exercise improves the functioning of the heart and the ability of the cardiorespiratory system to carry oxygen to body tissues. Exercise directly affects the health of your arteries, keeping them from stiffening or clogging with plaque and reducing the risk of cardiovascular disease. Exercise also improves sexual function and general vitality.

More Efficient Metabolism

Endurance exercise improves metabolism, the process that converts food to energy and builds tissue. A physically fit person is better able to generate energy, to use carbohydrates and fats for energy, and to regulate hormones. Exercise may also protect cells from damage from free radicals, destructive chemicals produced during normal metabolism, and from inflammation caused by high blood pres-

sure or cholesterol, nicotine, and overeating. Training activates antioxidant enzymes that prevent free radical damage and maintain the health of the body's cells.

Improved Body Composition

Exercise can improve body composition in several ways. Endurance exercise significantly increases daily calorie expenditure; it can also slightly raise *metabolic rate*, the rate at which the body burns calories, for several hours after an exercise session. Strength training increases muscle mass, thereby tip-

32% of Americans are at a weight considered to be healthy.

—*The Healthy People 2010 Database,* **2008**

STATS

Making Time for Physical Activity

"Too little time" is a common excuse for not being physically active. Learning to manage your time successfully is crucial if you are to maintain a wellness lifestyle. You can begin by keeping a record of how you are currently spending your time; in your health journal, use a grid broken into blocks of 15, 20, or 30 minutes to track your daily activities. Then analyze your record: List each type of activity and the total time you engaged in it on a given day—for example, sleeping, 7 hours; eating, 1.5 hours; studying, 3 hours; and so on. Take a close look at your list of activities, and prioritize them according to how important they are to you, from essential to somewhat important to not important at all.

Based on the priorities you set, make changes in your daily schedule by subtracting time from some activities in order to make time for physical activity. Look particularly carefully at your leisure-time activities and your methods of transportation; these are areas where it is easy to build in physical activity. Make changes using a system of trade-offs. For example, you may choose to reduce the total amount of time you spend playing computer games, listening to the radio, and chatting on the phone in order to make time for an after-dinner bike ride or a walk with a friend. You may decide to watch 10 fewer minutes of television in the morning in order to change your 5-minute drive to class into a 15-minute walk. The following are just a few ways to become more active:

- Take the stairs instead of the elevator or escalator.

- Walk to the post office, store, bank, or library when possible.

- Park your car a mile or even just a few blocks from your destination, and walk briskly.

- Do at least one chore every day that requires physical activity: Wash the windows or your car, clean your room or house, mow the lawn, or rake the leaves.

- Take study or work breaks to avoid sitting for more than 30 minutes at a time. Get up and walk around the library, office, or your home; go up and down a flight of stairs.

- Stretch when you stand in line or watch TV.

- When you take public transportation, get off one stop early and walk to your destination.

- Go dancing instead of to a movie.

- Put your remote controls in storage; when you want to change TV or radio stations, get up and do it by hand.

- Take the dog for a walk (or an extra walk) every day.

- If weather or neighborhood safety rule out walking outside, look for alternate locations—an indoor track, an enclosed shopping mall, or even a long hallway.

- Seize every opportunity to get up and walk around. Move more and sit less.

Visit the U.S. Department of Health and Human Services Small Step Web site (www.smallstep.gov) for more ideas.

---

ping the body composition ratio toward fat-free mass and away from fat. It can also help with losing fat because metabolic rate is directly proportional to fat-free mass: The more muscle mass, the higher the metabolic rate.

Disease Prevention and Management

Regular physical activity lowers your risk of many chronic, disabling diseases.

Cardiovascular Disease   A sedentary lifestyle is one of the six major risk factors for cardiovascular disease (CVD). Sedentary people have CVD death rates significantly higher than those of fit individuals. Physical inactivity increases the risk of CVD by 50–240%. The benefit of physical activity occurs at moderate levels of activity and rises with increasing levels of activity. Exercise positively affects the risk factors for CVD, including cholesterol levels and high blood pressure. Exercise also directly interferes with the disease process itself, directly lowering risk of heart disease and stroke.

Cancer   Studies have shown a relationship between increased physical activity and a reduced risk of cancer, but these findings are not conclusive. There is evidence that exercise reduces the risk of colon cancer and promising data that it reduces the risk of cancer of the breast and reproductive organs in women and prostate cancer in men.

Osteoporosis   A special benefit of exercise, especially for women, is protection against osteoporosis, a disease that results in loss of bone density and poor bone strength. Weight-bearing exercise, which includes almost everything except swimming, helps build bone during childhood and the teens and twenties. Strength training and impact exercises such as jumping rope can increase bone density throughout life. With stronger bones and muscles and better balance, fit people are less likely to experience debilitating falls and bone fractures.

Type 2 Diabetes   People with diabetes are prone to heart disease,

> **Nearly 73,000** Americans died of diabetes in 2006, making it the 7th leading cause of death that year.
>
> —National Center for Health Statistics, 2008

QUICK STATS

Exercise for People with Special Health Concerns

Regular, appropriate exercise is safe and beneficial for many people with chronic conditions or other special health concerns. For many people with special health concerns, in fact, the risks associated with *not* exercising are far greater than those associated with a moderate program of regular exercise.

If you have a special health concern and have hesitated becoming more active, one helpful strategy is to take a class or join an exercise group specifically designed for your condition. If you prefer to exercise at home, exercise videos are available for people with a variety of conditions.

The fitness recommendations for the general population presented in this chapter can serve as general guidelines for any exercise program. However, for people with special health concerns, certain precautions and monitoring may be required. *Anyone with special health concerns should consult a physician before beginning an exercise program.* Guidelines and cautions for some common conditions are described below:

Asthma

• Carry medication during workouts and avoid exercising alone. Use your inhaler before exercise, if recommended by your physician.

• Exercise regularly, and warm up and cool down slowly.

• When starting a fitness program, choose self-paced endurance activities, especially those involving interval training (short bouts of exercise followed by rest periods).

• When possible, avoid circumstances that may trigger an asthma attack, including cold, dry air or pollen or dust. Drink water to keep your airways moist, and in cold weather, cover your mouth with a mask or scarf to warm and humidify the air you breathe. Swimming is a good activity choice for people with asthma.

Diabetes

• Don't exercise alone; wear a bracelet identifying yourself as having diabetes.

• If you are taking insulin or another medication, you may need to adjust the timing and amount of each dose as you learn to balance your energy intake and output and your medication dosage.

• To prevent abnormally rapid absorption of injected insulin, inject it over a muscle that won't be exercised and wait at least an hour before exercising.

• Check blood sugar levels before, during, and after exercise, and adjust your diet or insulin dosage if needed. Avoid exercise if your blood sugar level is above 250 mg/dl, and ingest carbohydrates prior to exercise if your blood sugar level is below 100 mg/dl. Have high-carbohydrate foods available during a workout.

• Check your skin regularly for blisters and abrasions, especially on your feet.

Obesity

• For maximum benefit and minimum risk, begin with low- to moderate-intensity activities and increase intensity slowly as your fitness improves.

• To lose weight or maintain lost weight, exercise moderately 60 minutes or more every day.

• At first choose non- or low-weight-bearing activities like swimming, water exercises, cycling, or walking.

• Stay alert for symptoms of heat-related problems during exercise.

• Try to include as much lifestyle physical activity in your daily routine as possible.

• Include strength training in your program to build muscle mass.

Heart Disease and Hypertension

• Warm-up and cool-down sessions should be gradual and last at least 10 minutes.

• Exercise at a moderate rather than a high intensity; monitor your heart rate during exercise, and stop if you experience dizziness or chest pain.

• Increase exercise frequency, intensity, and time very gradually.

• Don't hold your breath when exercising as this can cause a sudden, steep increase in blood pressure.

• Discuss the effects of your medication with your physician. If your physician has prescribed nitroglycerine, carry it with you during exercise.

Arthritis

• Begin an exercise program as early as possible in the course of the disease.

• Warm up thoroughly before each workout to loosen stiff muscles and lower the risk of injury.

• Avoid high-impact activities that may damage arthritic joints; consider swimming or water aerobics.

• In strength training, pay special attention to muscles that support and protect affected joints; add weight very gradually.

• Stretch regularly.

Osteoporosis

• If possible, choose low-impact, weight-bearing activities to help safely maintain bone density.

• To prevent fractures, avoid any activity or movement that stresses the back or carries a risk of falling.

• Weight train to improve strength and balance and reduce the risk of falls and fractures, but avoid lifting heavy weights.

---

blindness, and severe problems of the nervous and circulatory systems. Exercise prevents the development of type 2 diabetes, the most common form of the disease. Exercise burns excess sugar and makes cells more sensitive to insulin. Exercise also helps keep body fat at healthy levels. (Obesity is a key risk factor for type 2 diabetes.) For people who have diabetes, physical activity is an important part of treatment.

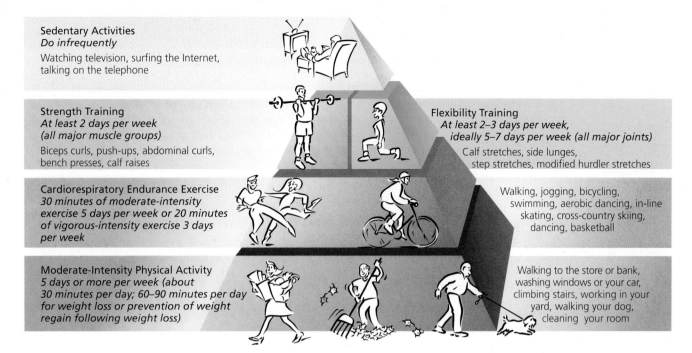

FIGURE 10.2 Physical activity pyramid.

Improved Psychological and Emotional Wellness

People who are physically active experience many social, psychological, and emotional benefits, including the following:

• *Reduced stress.* In response to stressors, physically fit people experience milder physical responses and less emotional distress than sedentary individuals. Regular exercise can also relieve sleeping problems.

• *Reduced anxiety and depression.* Sedentary adults are much more likely to feel fatigue and depression than those who are physically active.

• *Improved self-image.* Performing physical activities provides proof of skill and self-control, thus enhancing your self-concept.

• *Learning and memory.* Exercise enhances the formation and survival of new nerve cells and the connections between nerves, which in turn improve memory and learning.

• *Enjoyment.* Exercise is fun. It offers a way to interact with other people. Physically fit people can perform everyday tasks with ease. They have plenty of energy and can lead lives that are full and varied.

Improved Immune Function

Exercise can have either positive or negative effects on the immune system, the physiological processes that protect us from disease. Moderate endurance exercise boosts immune function, whereas excessive training depresses it. Physically fit people get fewer colds and upper respiratory tract infections than people who are not fit.

Prevention of Injuries and Low-Back Pain

Increased muscle strength provides protection against injury because it helps people maintain good posture and appropriate body mechanics when carrying out everyday activities such as walking, lifting, and carrying. Good muscle endurance in the abdomen, hips, lower back, and legs supports the back in proper alignment and helps prevent low-back pain.

Improved Wellness for Life

Although people differ in the maximum levels of fitness they can achieve through exercise, the wellness benefits of exercise are available to everyone (see the box "Exercise for People with Special Health Concerns"). Exercising regularly may be the single most important thing you can do now to improve the quality of your life in the future.

DESIGNING YOUR EXERCISE PROGRAM

The best exercise program has two primary characteristics: It promotes your health, and it's fun for you to do. Exercise does not have to be a chore. On the contrary, it can provide some of the most pleasurable moments of your day, once you make it a habit.

Figure 10.2 shows a physical activity pyramid to guide you in meeting goals for physical activity. If you are sedentary, start at the bottom of the pyramid and gradually

Exercise to Develop and Maintain Cardiorespiratory Endurance and Body Composition

Frequency of training	3–5 days per week.
Intensity of training	55/65–90% of maximum heart rate or 40/50–85% of heart rate reserve or maximum oxygen uptake reserve. The lower intensity values (55–64% of maximum heart rate and 40–49% of heart rate reserve) are most applicable to individuals who are quite unfit. For average individuals, intensities of 70–85% of maximum heart rate or 60–80% of heart rate reserve are appropriate; see page 396 for instructions for determining target heart rate.
Time (duration) of training	20–60 total minutes of continuous or intermittent (in sessions lasting 10 or more minutes) aerobic activity. Duration is dependent on the intensity of activity; thus, low-intensity activity should be conducted over a longer period of time (30 minutes or more). Low-to-moderate-intensity activity of longer duration is recommended for nonathletic adults.
Type (mode) of activity	Any activity that uses large-muscle groups, can be maintained continuously, and is rhythmic and aerobic in nature—for example, walking-hiking, running-jogging, cycling-bicycling, cross-country skiing, aerobic dance, stair climbing, swimming, and skating.

Exercise to Develop and Maintain Muscular Strength and Endurance, Flexibility, and Body Composition

Resistance training	One set of 8–10 exercises that condition the major muscle groups should be performed at least 2 days per week. Most people should complete 8–12 repetitions of each exercise to the point of fatigue; practicing other repetition ranges (for example, 3–5 or 12–15) also builds strength and endurance; for older and frailer people (approximately 50–60 and older), 10–15 repetitions with a lighter weight may be more appropriate. Multiple-set regimens will provide greater benefits if time allows. Any mode of exercise that is comfortable throughout the full range of motion is appropriate (for example, free weights, bands, or machines).
Flexibility training	Static stretches should be performed for the major muscle groups at least 2–3 days per week, ideally 5–7 days per week. Stretch to the point of tightness, holding each stretch for 15–30 seconds; perform 2–4 repetitions of each stretch.

SOURCE: Adapted from American College of Sports Medicine. 2006. *ACSM's Guidelines for Exercise Testing and Prescription,* 7th ed. Philadelphia: Lippincott Williams & Wilkins.

QUESTIONS FOR CRITICAL THINKING AND REFLECTION

Which benefits of exercise are most important to you, and why? For example, is there a history of heart disease or diabetes in your family? Have you thought about how regular exercise could reduce your risks for specific diseases?

increase the moderate-intensity physical activity in your daily life. You don't have to exercise vigorously, but you should experience a moderate increase in your heart and breathing rates. If weight management is a concern for you, begin by achieving the goal of 30 minutes per day and then gradually raise your activity level to 60 minutes per day or more.

For even greater benefits, move up to the next two levels of the pyramid, which illustrate parts of a formal exercise program. The American College of Sports Medicine has established guidelines for an exercise program that includes cardiorespiratory endurance (aerobic) exercise, strength training, and flex-

ibility training (Table 10.1). Such a program will develop all the health-related components of physical fitness. For a summary of the health and fitness benefits of different levels of physical activity, see Figure 10.3.

First Steps

Are you thinking about starting a formal exercise program? A little planning can help make it a success.

Medical Clearance Previously inactive men over 40 and women over 50 should get a medical examination before beginning an exercise program. Diabetes, asthma, heart disease, and extreme obesity are conditions that may call for a modified program. If you have an increased risk of heart disease because of smoking, high blood pressure, or obesity, get a physical checkup, including an **electrocardiogram (ECG or EKG)**, before beginning an exercise program.

Basic Principles of Physical Training To put together an effective exercise program, you should first understand the basic principles of physical training.

SPECIFICITY To develop a fitness component, you must perform exercises that are specifically designed for that component. Weight training, for example, develops muscular strength, but is less effective for developing flexibility. A well-rounded exercise program includes exercises

	Lifestyle physical activity 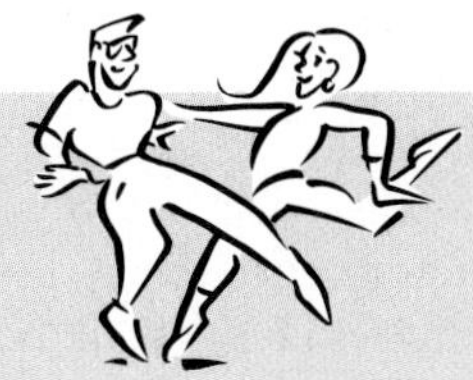	Moderate exercise program 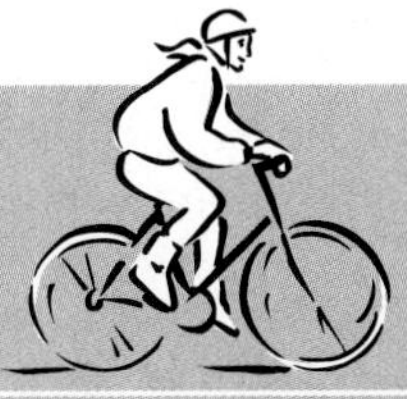	Vigorous exercise program 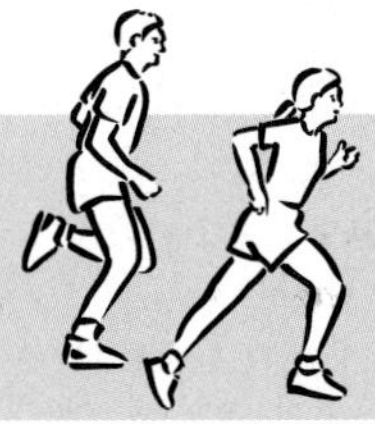
Description	Moderate physical activity—an amount of activity that uses about 150 calories per day	Cardiorespiratory endurance exercise (30 minutes, 5 days per week); strength training (at least 2 nonconsecutive days per week) and stretching exercises (2 or more days per week)	Cardiorespiratory endurance exercise (20 minutes, 3 days per week); interval training; strength training (3–4 days per week); and stretching exercises (5–7 days per week)
Sample activities or program	*One of the following:* • Walking to and from work, 15 minutes each way • Cycling to and from class, 15 minutes each way • Yard work for 30 minutes • Dancing (fast) for 30 minutes • Playing basketball for 20 minutes	• Walking for 30 minutes, 5 days per week • Weight training, 1 set of 8 exercises, 2 days per week • Stretching exercises, 3 days per week	• Jogging for 45 minutes, 3 days per week • Intervals: running 400 m at high effort, 4 sets, 2 days per week • Weight training, 3 sets of 10 exercises, 3 days per week • Stretching exercises, 6 days per week
Health and fitness benefits	Better blood cholesterol levels, reduced body fat, better control of blood pressure, improved metabolic health, and enhanced glucose metabolism; improved quality of life; reduced risk of some chronic diseases Greater amounts of activity can help prevent weight gain and promote weight loss	All the benefits of lifestyle physical activity, plus improved physical fitness (increased cardiorespiratory endurance, muscular strength and endurance, and flexibility) and even greater improvements in health and quality of life and reductions in chronic disease risk	All the benefits of lifestyle physical activity and a moderate exercise program, with greater increases in fitness and somewhat greater reductions in chronic disease risk Participating in a vigorous exercise program may increase risk of injury and overtraining

FIGURE 10.3 Health and fitness benefits of different amounts of physical activity and exercise.

geared to each component of fitness, to different parts of the body, and to specific activities or sports.

PROGRESSIVE OVERLOAD When the amount of exercise, also called **overload**, is progressively increased, fitness continues to improve. Too little exercise will have no effect on fitness; too much may cause injury. The amount of overload needed to maintain or improve a particular level of fitness is determined in four dimensions: Frequency, Intensity, Time, and Type. These dimensions of overload, represented by the acronym FITT, are described individually as they apply to the health-related components of fitness discussed in this chapter.

REVERSIBILITY The body adjusts to lower levels of physical activity in the same way it adjusts to higher levels—the principle of **reversibility**. Try to exercise consistently, and don't quit if you miss a few workouts.

INDIVIDUAL DIFFERENCES There are limits to the potential for improvement and large individual differences in our ability to improve fitness, achieve a desirable body composition, and perform and learn sports skills. But physical training improves fitness and wellness regardless of heredity.

Selecting Activities If you have been inactive, you should begin slowly by gradually increasing the amount of moderate physical activity in your life (the bottom of the activity pyramid). Once your body adjusts to your new level

TERMS

electrocardiogram (ECG or EKG) A recording of the changes in electrical activity of the heart.

overload The amount of stress placed on the body; a gradual increase in the amount of overload causes adaptations that improve fitness.

reversibility The training principle that fitness improvements are lost when demands on the body are lowered.

of activity, you can choose additional activities for your exercise program.

Be sure the activities you choose contribute to your overall wellness and make sense for you. Are you competitive? If so, try racquetball, basketball, or squash. Do you prefer to exercise alone? Then consider cross-country skiing or road running. Have you been sedentary? A walking program may be a good place to start. If you think you may have trouble sticking with an exercise program, find a structured activity that you can do with a buddy or a group. Be realistic about the constraints presented by some sports, such as accessibility, expense, and time.

Cardiorespiratory Endurance Exercises

Exercises that condition your heart and lungs should have a central role in your fitness program.

Frequency The optimal workout schedule for endurance training is 3–5 days per week. Beginners should start with 3 and work up to 5 days. Training more than 5 days a week often leads to injury for recreational athletes.

Intensity Intensity is the crucial factor in attaining a significant training effect—that is, in increasing the body's cardiorespiratory capacity. A primary purpose of endurance training is to increase **maximal oxygen consumption** ($\dot{V}O_{2max}$). $\dot{V}O_{2max}$ represents the maximum ability of the cells to use oxygen and is considered the best measure of cardiorespiratory capacity. Intensity of training is the crucial factor in improving $\dot{V}O_{2max}$.

One of the easiest ways to determine exactly how intensely you should work involves measuring your heart rate. It is not necessary or desirable to exercise at your maximum heart rate—the fastest heart rate possible before exhaustion sets in—in order to improve your cardiorespiratory capacity. Beneficial effects occur at lower heart rates with a much lower risk of injury. **Target heart rate range** is the range of rates within which you should exercise to obtain cardiorespiratory benefits. To determine the intensity at which you should exercise, refer to the box "Determining Your Target Heart Rate Range."

Time (Duration) A total time of 20–60 minutes is recommended; exercise can take place in a single session or several sessions lasting 10 or more minutes. The total duration of exercise depends on its intensity. To improve cardiorespiratory endurance during a low- to moderate-intensity activity such as walking or slow swimming, you should exercise for 45–60 minutes. For high-intensity exercise performed at the top of your target heart rate zone, a duration of 20 minutes is sufficient. Start with less vigorous activities and gradually increase intensity.

Type The best exercises for developing cardiorespiratory endurance stress a large portion of the body's muscle mass for a prolonged period of time. These include walking, jogging, running, swimming, bicycling, and aerobic dancing. Many popular sports and recreational activities, such as racquetball, tennis, basketball, and soccer, are also good if the skill level and intensity of the game are sufficient to provide a vigorous workout.

The Warm-Up and Cool-Down It is always important to warm up before you exercise and to cool down afterward. Warming up enhances your performance and decreases your chances of injury. A warm-up session should include low-intensity movements similar to those in the activity that will follow. For example, hit forehands and backhands before a tennis game or jog slowly for 400 meters before progressing to an 8-minute mile.

Experts recommend that you stretch *after* the active part of your warm-up, when your body temperature has been elevated. Studies have found that stretching prior to exercise can temporarily decrease muscle strength and power, so if a high-performance workout is your goal, it is best to stretch after a workout.

Cooling down after exercise is important to restore the body's circulation to its normal resting condition. When you are at rest, a relatively small percentage of your total blood volume is directed to muscles, but during exercise, as much as 90% of the heart's output is directed to them. During recovery from exercise, it is important to continue exercising at a low level to provide a smooth transition to the resting state.

> **5–10** minutes of warming up and cooling down is adequate for a 30-minute workout of brisk walking.
>
> —Mayo Clinic, 2007

Developing Muscular Strength and Endurance

Any program designed to promote health should include exercises that develop muscular strength and endurance (see the box "Gender Differences in Muscular Strength").

Determining Your Target Heart Rate Range

Your target heart rate is the range of rates at which you should exercise to experience cardiorespiratory benefits. Your target heart rate range is based on your maximum heart rate, which can be estimated from your age. (If you are a serious athlete or face possible cardiovascular risks from exercise, you may want to have your maximum heart rate determined more accurately through a treadmill test in a physician's office, hospital, or sports medicine laboratory.) Your target heart rate is a range: The lower value corresponds to moderate-intensity exercise, and the higher value is associated with high-intensity exercise. Target heart rate ranges are shown in the table.

You can monitor the intensity of your workouts by measuring your pulse either at your wrist or at one of your carotid arteries, located on either side of your Adam's apple. Your pulse rate drops rapidly after exercise, so begin counting immediately after you have finished exercising. You will obtain the most accurate results by counting beats for 10 seconds and then multiplying by 6 to get your heart rate in beats per minute (bpm). The 10-second counts corresponding to each target heart rate range are also shown in the table.

Age (years)	Target Heart Rate Range (bpm)*	10-Second Count (beats)*
20–24	127–180	21–30
25–29	124–176	20–29
30–34	121–171	20–28
35–39	118–167	19–27
40–44	114–162	19–27
45–49	111–158	18–26
50–54	108–153	18–25
55–59	105–149	17–24
60–64	101–144	16–24
65+	97–140	16–23

*Target heart rates lower than those shown here are appropriate for individuals with a very low initial level of fitness. Ranges are based on the following formula: Target heart rate = 0.65 to 0.90 of maximum heart rate, assuming maximum heart rate = 220 − age.

Types of Strength Training Exercises Muscular strength and endurance can be developed in many ways, from weight training to calisthenics. Common exercises such as curl-ups, push-ups, pull-ups, and wall-sitting (leaning against a wall in a seated position and supporting yourself with your leg muscles) maintain the muscular strength of most people if they practice them several times a week. To condition and tone your whole body, choose exercises that work the major muscles of the shoulders, chest, back, arms, abdomen, and legs.

To increase muscular strength and endurance, you must do **resistance exercise**—exercises in which your muscles must exert force against a significant amount of resistance. Resistance can be provided by weights, exercise machines, or your own body weight. **Isometric (static) exercises** involve applying force without movement, such as when you contract your abdominal muscles. This static type of exercise is valuable for toning and strengthening muscles. Isometrics can be practiced anywhere and do not require any equipment. For maximum strength gains, hold an isometric contraction maximally for 6 seconds; do five to ten repetitions. Don't hold your breath—that can restrict blood flow to your heart and brain. Within a few weeks, you will notice the effect of this exercise. Isometrics are particularly useful when recovering from an injury.

Isotonic (dynamic) exercises involve applying force with movement, as in weight training exercises such as the bench press. These are the most popular type of exercises for increasing muscle strength and seem to be most valuable for developing strength that can be transferred to other forms of physical activity.

Choosing Equipment Weight machines are preferred by many people because they are safe, convenient, and easy to use. You just set the resistance, sit down at the machine, and start working. Machines make it easy to isolate and work specific muscles. Free weights require more care, balance, and coordination to use, but they strengthen your body in ways that are more adaptable to real life. When using free weights, you need to use a spotter, someone who stands by to assist in case you lose control over a weight.

Choosing Exercises A complete weight training program works all the major muscle groups: neck, upper back, shoulders, arms, chest, abdomen, lower back, thighs, buttocks, and calves. Different exercises work different muscles, so it usually takes about eight to ten exercises to get a complete workout for general fitness—for example, bench presses to develop the chest, shoulders, and upper arms; pull-ups to work the biceps and upper back; squats to develop the legs and buttocks; toe raises to work the calves; and so on.

Frequency For general fitness, the American College of Sports Medicine recommends a frequency of at least 2 nonconsecutive days per week. This allows your muscles one or more days of rest between workouts to avoid soreness and injury. If you enjoy weight training and would like to train more often, try working different muscle groups on alternate days.

Intensity and Time The amount of weight (resistance) you lift in weight training exercises is equivalent to intensity

Men are generally stronger than women because they typically have larger bodies overall and a larger proportion of their total body mass is made up of muscle. But when strength is expressed per unit of muscle tissue, men are only 1–2% stronger than women in the upper body and about equal to women in the lower body. Individual muscle cells are larger in men, but the functioning of the cells is the same in both sexes.

Two factors that help explain these disparities are testosterone levels and the speed of nervous control of muscle. Testosterone promotes the growth of muscle tissue in both males and females, but testosterone levels are about 6–10 times higher in men than in women, so men develop larger muscles. Also, because the male nervous system can activate muscles faster, men tend to have more power.

Some women are concerned that they will develop large muscles from strength training. Because of hormonal differences, most women do not develop large muscles unless they train intensely over many years or take steroids. A study of average women who weight trained 2–3 days per week for 8 weeks found that the women gained about 1.75 pounds of muscle and lost about 3.5 pounds of fat. Another study followed women who trained with weights for 2 years. Not only did the women reduce their overall body fat levels but they ended up with less fat around their midsection.

Losing muscle over time is a much greater health concern for women than small gains in muscle weight in response to strength training, especially as any gains in muscle weight are typically more than balanced with loss of fat weight. Both men and women lose muscle mass and power as they age, but because men start out with more muscle when they are young and don't lose power as quickly as women, older women tend to have greater impairment of muscle function than older men. This may partially explain the higher incidence of life-threatening falls in older women.

Healthy People 2010 sets a national health objective of increasing to 30% the proportion of adults who perform strength training exercises on 2 or more days per week. In 2008, however, the CDC reported that only 22% of men and 17% of women met this goal, underscoring the need for additional programs and campaigns that promote this form of exercise.

SOURCES: Fahey, T. D. 2010. *Basic Weight Training for Men and Women*, 6th ed. New York: McGraw-Hill; Centers for Disease Control and Prevention. 2006. Trends in strength training—United States, 1998–2004. *Morbidity and Mortality Weekly Report* 55(28): 769–772.

---

in cardiorespiratory endurance training; the number of repetitions of each exercise is equivalent to time. In order to improve fitness, you must do enough repetitions of each exercise to temporarily fatigue your muscles. The number of repetitions needed to cause fatigue depends on the amount of resistance: the heavier the weight, the fewer repetitions to reach fatigue. In general, a heavy weight and a low number of repetitions (1–5) build strength, whereas a light weight and a high number of repetitions (20–25) build endurance. For a general fitness program to build both strength and endurance, try to do 8–12 repetitions of each exercise; a few exercises, such as abdominal crunches and calf raises, may require more.

To start, choose a weight that you can move easily through 8–12 repetitions. Add weight when you can do more than 12 repetitions of an exercise. If adding weight means you can do only 7 or 8 repetitions before your muscles fatigue, stay with that weight until you can again complete 12 repetitions. If you can do only 4–6 repetitions after adding weight, or if you can't maintain good form, you've added too much and should take some off.

For developing strength and endurance for general fitness, a single set (group) of each exercise is sufficient, provided you use enough resistance (weight) to fatigue your muscles. Doing more than one set of each exercise may increase strength development, and most serious weight trainers do at least three sets of each exercise. If you do more than one set of an exercise, rest long enough between sets to allow your muscles to recover. You should warm up before every weight training session and cool down afterward.

A Caution About Supplements No nutritional supplement or drug will change a weak person into a strong person. Those changes require regular training that stresses the body and causes physiological adaptations. Supplements or drugs that promise quick, large gains in strength usually don't work and are often either dangerous, expensive, or both (see the box "Drugs and Supplements for Improved Athletic Performance"). Over-the-counter supplements are not carefully regulated, and their long-term effects have not been systematically studied.

Flexibility Exercises

Flexibility, or stretching, exercises are important for maintaining the normal range of motion in the major joints of the body. Some exercises, such as running, can actually decrease flexibility because they require only a partial range of motion. Like a good weight training program, a good stretching program includes exercises for all the major muscle groups and joints of the body: neck, shoulders, back, hips, thighs, hamstrings, and calves.

QUICK STATS

15% of tested supplements contained substances that would cause an athlete to fail a drug test.

—International Olympic Committee, 2004

When Alex Rodriguez, third baseman for the New York Yankees, admitted taking a banned substance in a 2009 interview, he was only the latest in a long string of athletes who have succumbed to the lure of performance-enhancing drugs, includin cyclist Floyd Landis, sprinter Marion Jones, and former Giants hitter Barry Bonds.

Professional and Olympic athletes aren't the only ones using performance-enhancing drugs. About 2–6% of high school and college students report having used anabolic steroids, and over-the-counter dietary supplements are much more popular. Many such substances are ineffective and expensive, and many are also dangerous.

Anabolic Steroids These synthetic derivatives of testosterone are taken to increase strength, power, speed, endurance, muscle size, and aggressiveness. **Anabolic steroids** have dangerous side effects, including disruption of the body's hormone system, liver disease, acne, breast development and testicular shrinkage in males, masculinization in women and children, and increased risk of heart disease and cancer. Evidence links steroid use and risk of heart attack, stroke, and sudden death. Steroid users who inject the drugs face the same health risks as other injection drug users, including increased risk of HIV infection.

Adrenal Androgens This group of drugs, which includes dehydroepiandrosterone (DHEA) and androstenedione, are typically taken to stimulate muscle growth and aid in weight control. The few studies of these agents done on humans show that they are of very little value in improving athletic performance, and they have side effects similar to those of anabolic steroids, especially when taken in high doses.

Ephedra and Other Stimulants These drugs may be taken to increase training intensity, to suppress hunger, to reduce fatigue, and to promote weight loss. They raise heart rate and blood pressure and, at high doses, may increase the risk of heart attack, stroke, and heat-related illness. Several stimulants, including ephedra and phenylpropanolamine, have been banned by the FDA.

Erythropoietin (EPO) A naturally occurring hormone that boosts the concentration of red blood cells, EPO is used by athletes to improve performance. EPO can cause blood clots and death.

Creatine Monohydrate Creatine is thought to improve performance in short-term, high-intensity, repetitive exercise and decrease the risk of injury. People vary in their responses to creatine. The long-term effects of creatine use, especially among young people, are not well established.

Protein, Amino Acid, and Polypeptide Supplements Little research supports the use of such supplements, even in athletes on extremely heavy training regimens. The protein requirements of athletes are not much higher than those of sedentary individuals, and most people take in more than enough protein in their diets. By substituting supplements for food sources of protein, people may risk deficiencies in other key nutrients typically found in such foods, including iron and B vitamins.

Chromium Picolinate Sold over the counter, chromium picolinate is a more easily digested form of the trace mineral chromium. Although often marketed as a means to build muscle and reduce fat, most studies have found no positive effects. Long-term use of high dosages may have serious health consequences.

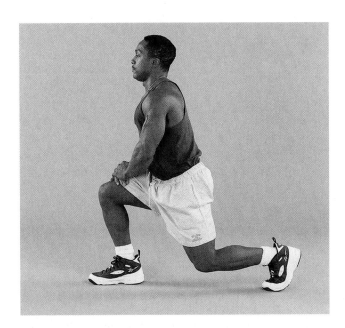

When performed regularly, stretching exercises help maintain or improve the range of motion in joints. For each exercise, stretch to the point of tightness in the muscle and hold the position for 15–30 seconds.

Proper Stretching Technique Stretching should be performed statically. Ballistic stretching ("bouncing") is dangerous and counterproductive. In active stretching, a muscle is stretched under a person's own power by contracting the opposing muscles. In passive stretching, an outside force or resistance provided by yourself, a partner, gravity, or a weight helps elongate the targeted muscle. You can achieve a greater range of motion and a more intense stretch using passive stretching, but there is a greater risk of injury. The safest and most convenient technique may be active static stretching with a passive assist. For example, you might do a seated stretch of your calf muscles both by contracting the muscles on the top of your shin and by grabbing your feet and pulling them toward you.

Frequency Do stretching exercises at least 2–3 days per week, ideally 5–7 days per week. If you stretch after

anabolic steroids Synthetic male hormones used to increase muscle size and strength.

TERMS

cardiorespiratory endurance exercise or strength training, during your cool-down, you may develop more flexibility, because your muscles are warmer then and can be stretched farther.

Intensity and Time   For each exercise, stretch to the point of tightness in the muscle, and hold the position for 15–30 seconds. Rest for 30–60 seconds, then repeat, trying to stretch a bit farther. Relax and breathe easily as you stretch. You should feel a pleasant, mild stretch as you let the muscles relax; stretching should not be painful. Do 2–4 repetitions of each exercise. A complete flexibility workout usually takes about 20–30 minutes.

Increase your intensity gradually over time. Improved flexibility takes many months to develop. There are large individual differences in joint flexibility. Don't feel you have to compete with others during stretching workouts.

Training in Specific Skills

The final component in your fitness program is learning the skills required for the sports or activities in which you choose to participate. The first step in learning a new skill is getting help. Sports like tennis, golf, sailing, and skiing require mastery of basic movements and techniques, so instruction from a qualified teacher can save you hours of frustration and increase your enjoyment of the sport. Skill is also important in conditioning activities such as jogging, swimming, and cycling. Even if you learned a sport as a child, additional instruction now can help you refine your technique.

Putting It All Together

Now that you know the basic components of a fitness program, you can put them all together in a program that works for you. Refer to Figure 10.4 for a summary of the FITT principle for the health-related fitness components.

GETTING STARTED AND STAYING ON TRACK

Once you have a program that fulfills your basic fitness needs and suits your personal tastes, adhering to a few basic principles will help you improve at the fastest rate, have more fun, and minimize the risk of injury.

Selecting Instructors, Equipment, and Facilities

One of the best places to get help is an exercise class, where an expert instructor can help you learn the basics of training and answer your questions. A qualified personal trainer can also get you started on an exercise program or a new form of training. Make sure that your instructor or trainer has proper qualifications, such as a college degree in exercise physiology or physical education and certification by the American College of Sports Medicine (ACSM), National Strength and Conditioning Association (NSCA), or another professional organization.

Many Web sites provide fitness programs, including ongoing support and feedback via e-mail. Many of these sites charge a fee, so it is important to review the sites, decide which ones seem most appropriate, and if possible go through a free trial period before subscribing. Also remember to consider the reliability of the information at fitness Web sites, especially those that also advertise or sell products.

If you plan to purchase equipment, try to buy the best you can afford. Good equipment will enhance your enjoyment and decrease your risk of injury. Appropriate safety equipment, such as pads and helmets for in-line skating, is particularly important. Before you invest in a new piece of equipment, try it out at a local gym to make sure that you'll use it regularly. Footwear is an important piece of equipment for almost any activity (see the box "Choosing Exercise Footwear").

	Cardiorespiratory endurance training	Strength training	Flexibility training
Frequency	3–5 days per week	At least 2 nonconsecutive days per week	2–3 days per week (minimum); 5–7 days per week (ideal)
Intensity	55/65–90% of maximum heart rate	Sufficient resistance to fatigue muscles	Stretch to the point of tension
Time	20–60 minutes in sessions lasting 10 minutes or more	8–12 repetitions of each exercise, 1 or more sets	2–4 repetitions of each exercise, held for 15–30 seconds
Type	Continuous rhythmic activities using large muscle groups	Resistance exercises for all major muscle groups	Stretching exercises for all major joints

FIGURE 10.4   A summary of the FITT principle for the health-related components of fitness.

Choosing Exercise Footwear

When choosing athletic shoes, first consider the activity you've chosen for your exercise program. Shoes appropriate for different activities have very different characteristics. For example, running shoes typically have highly cushioned midsoles, rubber outsoles with elevated heels, and a great deal of flexibility in the forefoot. The heels of walking shoes tend to be lower, less padded, and more beveled than those designed for running. For aerobic dance, shoes must be flexible in the forefoot and have straight, nonflared heels to allow for safe and easy lateral movements. Court shoes also provide substantial support for lateral movements; they typically have outsoles made from white rubber that will not damage court surfaces.

Also consider the location and intensity of your workouts. If you plan to walk or run on trails, choose shoes with water-resistant, highly durable uppers and more outsole traction. If you work out intensely or have a relatively high body weight, you'll need thick, firm midsoles to avoid bottoming-out the cushioning system of your shoes.

Foot type is another important consideration. If your feet tend to roll inward excessively, you may need shoes with additional stability features on their inner side to counteract this movement. If your feet tend to roll outward excessively, you may need highly flexible and cushioned shoes that promote foot motion. For aerobic dancers with feet that tend to roll inward or outward, mid-cut to high-cut shoes may be more appropriate than low-cut aerobic shoes or cross-trainers (shoes designed to be worn for several different activities). Compared with men, women have narrower feet overall and narrower heels relative to the forefoot. Most women will get a better fit if they choose shoes that are specifically designed for women's feet rather than those that are downsized versions of men's shoes.

For successful shoe shopping, keep the following strategies in mind:

- Shop at an athletic shoe or specialty store that has personnel trained to fit athletic shoes and a large selection of styles and sizes.

- Shop late in the day or following a workout. Your foot size increases over the course of the day and as a result of exercise.

- Wear socks like those you plan to wear during exercise. If you have an old pair of athletic shoes, bring them with you. The wear pattern on your old shoes can help you select a pair with extra support or cushioning where you need it.

- Ask for help. Trained salespeople know which shoes are designed for your foot type and your level of activity. They can also help fit your shoes properly.

- Don't insist on buying shoes in what you consider to be your typical shoe size. Sizes vary from shoe to shoe. In addition, foot sizes change over time, and many people have one foot that is larger or wider than the other.

- Try on both shoes, and wear them for 10 or more minutes. Try walking on a noncarpeted surface. Approximate the movements of your activity: walk, jog, run, jump, and so on.

- Check the fit and style carefully:

  Is the toe box roomy enough? Your toes will spread out when your foot hits the ground or you push off. There should be at least one thumb's width of space from the longest toe to the end of the toe box.

  Do the shoes have enough cushioning? Do your feet feel supported when you bounce up and down? Try bouncing on your toes and on your heels.

  Do your heels fit snugly into the shoe? Do they stay put when you walk, or do they rise up?

  Are the arches of your feet right on top of the shoes' arch supports?

  Do the shoes feel stable when you twist and turn on the balls of your feet? Try twisting from side to side while standing on one foot.

  Do you feel any pressure points?

- If the shoes are not comfortable in the store, don't buy them. Don't expect athletic shoes to stretch over time in order to fit your feet properly.

- If you exercise at dawn or dusk, choose shoes with reflective sections for added visibility and safety.

- Replace athletic shoes about every 3 months or 300–500 miles of jogging or walking.

If you are thinking of joining a health club or fitness center, be sure to choose one that has the right programs and equipment available at the times you will use them. Also make sure the facility is certified; look for the displayed names American College of Sports Medicine (ACSM); National Strength and Conditioning Association (NSCA); American Council on Exercise (ACE); Aerobics and Fitness Association of America (AFAA); or International Health, Racquet, and Sportsclub Association (IHRSA). These trade associations have established standards to help protect consumer health, safety, and rights. Ask for a free trial workout, a 1-day pass, or an inexpensive 1- to 2-week trial membership before committing to a long-term contract. Be wary of promotional gimmicks and high-pressure sales tactics.

Eating and Drinking for Exercise

Most people do not need to change their eating habits when they begin a fitness program. In almost every case, a well-balanced diet contains all the energy and nutrients needed to sustain an exercise program. A balanced diet is also the key to improving your body composition when you begin to exercise more. One of the promises of a fitness program is a decrease in body fat and an increase in muscular body mass. The best way to control body fat is to follow a diet containing adequate but not excessive calories and to be physically active.

One of the most important principles to follow when exercising is to drink enough water. Sweating during exercise depletes the body's water supply and can lead to dehydration if fluids are not replaced. Serious dehydration can cause reduced blood volume, accelerated heart rate, elevated body temperature, muscle cramps, heat stroke, and other serious problems.

During heavy or prolonged exercise or exercise in hot weather, thirst alone isn't a good indication of how much fluid you need to drink. As a rule of thumb, drink at least 2 cups (16 ounces) of fluid 2 hours before exercise and then drink enough during exercise to match fluid loss in sweat—at least 1 cup of fluid every 20–30 minutes of exercise, more in hot weather or if you sweat heavily. To determine if you're drinking the right amount of fluid, weigh yourself before and after an exercise session: Any weight loss is due to fluid loss that needs to be replaced. Any weight gain is due to over-consumption of fluid.

Bring a bottle of water when you exercise so you can replace your fluids when they're depleted. For exercise sessions lasting less than 60–90 minutes, cool water is an excellent fluid replacement. For longer workouts, a sports drink that contains water and small amounts of electrolytes (sodium, potassium, and magnesium) and simple carbohydrates (sugar, usually in the form of sucrose or glucose) is recommended.

Managing Your Fitness Program

How can you tell when you're in shape? When do you stop improving and start maintaining? How can you stay motivated? If your program is going to become an integral part of your life, and if the principles behind it are going to serve you well in the future, these are key questions.

Start Slowly, Get in Shape Gradually   An exercise program can be divided into three phases:

- *Beginning phase.* The body adjusts to the new type and level of activity.
- *Progress phase.* Fitness increases.
- *Maintenance phase.* The targeted level of fitness is sustained over the long term.

Start slowly to give your body time to adapt to the stress of exercise. Choose activities carefully; if you have been sedentary or are overweight, try an activity such as walking or swimming that won't jar the body or strain your joints.

Exercising Consistently   Steady fitness improvement comes when you overload your body consistently over a long period of time. The best way to ensure consistency is to keep a training journal in which you record the details of your workouts: how far you ran, how much weight you lifted, how many laps you swam, and so on. This record will help you evaluate your progress and plan your workout sessions intelligently. Don't increase your exercise volume by more than 5–10% per week.

Assessing Your Fitness   When are you in shape? It depends. One person may be out of shape running a mile in 5 minutes; another may be in shape running a mile in 12 minutes. Your ultimate level of fitness depends on your goals, your program, and your natural ability. The important thing is to set goals that make sense for you. If you are interested in finding out exactly how fit you are before you begin a program, the best approach is to get an assessment from a sports medicine laboratory.

Preventing and Managing Athletic Injuries   It is important to learn how to deal with injuries so they don't derail your fitness program (Table 10.2). Some injuries

THINKING ABOUT THE ENVIRONMENT

Wherever you see people exercising, you will see bottled water in abundance. For several years, however, a debate has been raging about the quality and safety of commercially bottled water. In recent months, new evidence has emerged showing that most bottled waters are no better for you than regular tap water, and some bottled waters may actually be bad for you.

In a 2008 analysis, the Environmental Working Group (EWG) found 38 different contaminants in ten popular brands of bottled water. Contaminants included heavy metals such as arsenic, pharmaceutical residues and other pollutants commonly found in urban wastewater, and a variety of industrial chemicals.

In recent years, government and private agencies have revealed that many commercially bottled water products are really just tap water drawn from municipal water systems. These products are priced many times higher than water from a residential tap. They also provide no benefit over standard tap water.

Further, plastic water bottles have become a huge solid waste problem, as millions of bottles end up in landfills each day. Once in a landfill, many kinds of plastic bottles will never decompose at all; at best, some types of plastic take years to biodegrade.

Experts say that when you're exercising, the cheapest and safest way to stay hydrated is to drink filtered tap water. If you need to carry water with you, buy a reusable container (preferably made of stainless steel) that can be cleaned and sterilized after each use. If you drink from plastic bottles, be sure they are recyclable and dispose of them by recycling.

Table 10.2 Care of Common Exercise Injuries and Discomforts

Injury	Symptoms	Treatment
Blister	Accumulation of fluid in one spot under the skin	Don't pop or drain it unless it interferes too much with your daily activities. If it does pop, clean the area with antiseptic and cover with a bandage. Do not remove the skin covering the blister.
Bruise (contusion)	Pain, swelling, and discoloration	R-I-C-E: rest, ice, compression, elevation.
Fracture and/or dislocation	Pain, swelling, tenderness, loss of function, and deformity	Seek medical attention, immobilize the affected area, and apply cold.
Joint sprain	Pain, tenderness, swelling, discoloration, and loss of function	R-I-C-E. Apply heat when swelling has disappeared. Stretch and strengthen affected area.
Muscle cramp	Painful, spasmodic muscle contractions	Gently stretch for 15–30 seconds at a time and/or massage the cramped area. Drink fluids and increase dietary salt intake if exercising in hot weather.
Muscle soreness or stiffness	Pain and tenderness in the affected muscle	Stretch the affected muscle gently; exercise at a low intensity; apply heat. Nonsteroidal anti-inflammatory drugs, such as ibuprofen, help some people.
Muscle strain	Pain, tenderness, swelling, and loss of strength in the affected muscle	R-I-C-E; apply heat when swelling has disappeared. Stretch and strengthen the affected area.
Plantar fasciitis	Pain and tenderness in the connective tissue on the bottom of your feet	Apply ice, take nonsteroidal anti-inflammatory drugs, and stretch. Wear night splints when sleeping.
Shin splint	Pain and tenderness on the front of the lower leg; sometimes also pain in the calf muscle	Rest; apply ice to the affected area several times a day and before exercise; wrap with tape for support. Stretch and strengthen muscles in the lower legs. Purchase good-quality footwear and run on soft surfaces.
Side stitch	Pain on the side of the abdomen	Stretch the arm on the affected side as high as possible; if that doesn't help, try bending forward while tightening the abdominal muscles.
Tendinitis	Pain, swelling, and tenderness of the affected area	R-I-C-E; apply heat when swelling has disappeared. Stretch and strengthen the affected area.

SOURCE: Fahey, T. D., P. M. Insel, and W. T. Roth. 2009. *Fit and Well: Core Concepts and Labs in Physical Fitness and Wellness,* 8th ed. New York: McGraw-Hill. Copyright © 2009 The McGraw-Hill Companies, Inc.

require medical attention. Consult a physician for head and eye injuries, possible ligament injuries, broken bones, and internal disorders such as chest pain, fainting, and intolerance to heat. Also seek medical attention for apparently minor injuries that do not get better within a reasonable amount of time.

For minor cuts and scrapes, stop the bleeding and clean the wound with soap and water. Treat soft tissue injuries (muscles and joints) with the R-I-C-E principle:

Rest: Stop using the injured area as soon as you experience pain, protect it from further injury, and avoid any activity that causes pain.

Ice: Apply ice to the injured area to reduce swelling and alleviate pain. Apply ice immediately for 10–20 minutes, and repeat every few hours until the swelling disappears. Let the injured part return to normal temperature between icings, and do not apply ice to one area for more than 20 minutes (10 minutes if you are using a cold gel pack).

Compression: Wrap the injured area with an elastic or compression bandage between icings. If the area starts throbbing or begins to change color, the bandage may be wrapped too tightly. Do not sleep with the bandage on.

Elevation: Raise the injured area above heart level to decrease the blood supply and reduce swelling.

After about 36–48 hours, apply heat, if the swelling has completely disappeared, to help relieve pain, relax muscles, and reduce stiffness. Immerse the affected area in warm water or apply warm compresses, a hot water bottle, or a heating pad.

To prevent injuries in the future, follow a few basic guidelines:

- Stay in condition; haphazard exercise programs invite injury.
- Warm up thoroughly before exercise.
- Use proper body mechanics when lifting objects or executing sports skills.
- Don't exercise when you're ill or overtrained (experiencing extreme fatigue due to overexercising).
- Use the proper equipment.
- Don't return to your normal exercise program until athletic injuries have healed.

Have you ever suffered an injury while exercising? If so, how did you treat the injury? Compare your treatment with the guidelines given in this chapter. Did you do the right things? What can you do to avoid such injuries in the future?

You can minimize the risk of injury by following safety guidelines, using proper technique and equipment, respecting signals from your body that something may be wrong, and treating any injuries that occur. Warm up, cool down, and drink plenty of fluids before, during, and after exercise. Use special caution in extreme heat or humidity (over 80°F and/or 60% humidity): Exercise slowly, rest frequently in the shade, wear clothing that "breathes," and drink plenty of fluids; slow down or stop if you begin to feel uncomfortable. During hot weather, it's best to exercise in the early morning or evening, when temperatures are lowest.

Staying with Your Program   Once you have attained your desired level of fitness, you can maintain it by exercising regularly at a consistent intensity, 3 to 5 days a week. In general, if you exercise at the same intensity over a long period, your fitness will level out and can be maintained easily.

Adapt your program to changes in environment or schedule. Don't use wet weather or a new job as an excuse to give up your fitness program. If you walk in the summer, dress appropriately and walk in the winter as well. If you can't go out because of darkness or an unsafe neighborhood, walk in a local shopping mall or on campus or join a gym and walk on a treadmill.

What if you run out of steam? Although good health is an important *reason* to exercise, it's a poor *motivator* for consistent adherence to an exercise program. It's a good idea to have a meaningful goal, anything from fitting into the same-size jeans you used to wear to successfully skiing down a new slope.

Varying your program is another key strategy. Some people alternate two or more activities—swimming and jogging, for example—to improve a particular component of fitness. The practice, called **cross-training**, can help prevent boredom and overuse injuries. Try new activities, especially ones that you will be able to do for the rest of your life.

TERMS

cross-training   Participating in two or more activities to develop a particular component of fitness.

TIPS FOR TODAY AND THE FUTURE
Physical activity and exercise offer benefits in nearly every area of wellness. Even a low-to-moderate level of activity provides valuable health benefits.

RIGHT NOW YOU CAN
- Go outside and take a brisk 15-minute walk.
- Look at your calendar for the rest of the week and write in some physical activity—such as walking, running, or playing Frisbee—on as many days as you can. Schedule the activity for a specific time and stick to it.
- Call a friend and invite him or her to start planning a regular exercise program with you.

IN THE FUTURE YOU CAN
- Schedule a session with a qualified personal trainer who can evaluate your current fitness level and help you set personalized fitness goals.
- Create seasonal workout programs for the summer, spring, fall, and winter. Develop programs that are varied but consistent with your overall fitness goals.

SUMMARY

• The five components of physical fitness most important to health are cardiorespiratory endurance, muscular strength, muscular endurance, flexibility, and body composition.

• Exercise improves the functioning of the heart and the ability of the cardiorespiratory system to carry oxygen to the body's tissues. It also increases the efficiency of the body's metabolism and improves body composition.

• Exercise lowers the risk of cardiovascular disease, cancer, osteoporosis, and diabetes. It improves immune function and psychological health and helps prevent injuries and low-back pain.

• Everyone should accumulate at least 30–60 minutes per day of moderate endurance-type physical activity. Additional health and fitness benefits can be achieved through longer or more vigorous activity.

• Cardiorespiratory endurance exercises stress a large portion of the body's muscle mass. Endurance exercise should be performed 3–5 days per week for a total of 20–60 minutes per day. Intensity can be evaluated by measuring the heart rate.

• Warming up before exercising and cooling down afterward improve your performance and decrease your chances of injury.

Planning a Personal Exercise Program

Although most people recognize the importance of incorporating exercise into their lives, many find it difficult to do. No single strategy will work for everyone, but the general steps outlined here should help you create an exercise program that fits your goals, preferences, and lifestyle. A carefully designed contract and program plan can help you convert your vague wishes into a detailed plan of action. And the strategies for program compliance outlined here and in Chapter 1 can help you enjoy and stick with your program for the rest of your life.

Step 1: Set Goals

Setting specific goals to accomplish by exercising is an important first step in a successful fitness program because it establishes the direction you want to take. Your goals might be specifically related to health, such as lowering your blood pressure and risk of heart disease, or they might relate to other aspects of your life, such as improving your tennis game or the fit of your clothes. If you can decide why you're starting to exercise, it can help you keep going.

Step 2: Select Activities

As discussed in the chapter, the success of your fitness program depends on the consistency of your involvement. Select activities that encourage your commitment: The right program will be its own incentive to continue; poor activity choices provide obstacles and can turn exercise into a chore.

When choosing activities for your fitness program, consider the following:

- Is this activity fun? Will it hold my interest over time?

- Will this activity help me reach the goals I have set?

- Will my current fitness and skill level enable me to participate fully in this activity?

- Can I easily fit this activity into my daily schedule? Are there any special requirements (facilities, partners, equipment, etc.) that I must plan for?

- Can I afford any special costs required for equipment or facilities?

- If you have special exercise needs due to a particular health problem: Does this activity conform to those exercise needs? Will it enhance my ability to cope with my specific health problem?

Using the guidelines listed above, select a number of sports and activities.

Step 3: Make a Commitment

To affirm your commitment, sign a contract like the one shown in Chapter 1 and have a friend sign it as a witness. By completing a written contract, you will make a firm commitment and will be more likely to follow through until you meet your goals.

Step 4: Begin and Maintain Your Program

Start out slowly to allow your body time to adjust. Be realistic and patient—meeting your goals will take time. The following guidelines may help you start and stick with your program:

- Set aside regular periods for exercise. Choose times that fit in best with your schedule, and stick to them. Allow an adequate amount of time for warm-up, cool-down, and a shower.

- Take advantage of any opportunity for exercise that presents itself (for example, walk to class, take the stairs instead of the elevator).

- Do what you can to avoid boredom. Do stretching exercises or jumping jacks to music, or watch the evening news while riding your stationary bicycle.

- Exercise with a group that shares your goals and general level of competence.

- Vary the program. Change your activities periodically. Alter your route or distance if biking or jogging. Change racquetball partners, or find a new volleyball court.

- Establish minigoals or a point system, and work rewards into your program. Until you reach your main goals, a series of small rewards will help you stick with your program. Rewards should be things you enjoy that are easily obtainable.

Step 5: Record and Assess Your Progress

Keeping a record that notes the daily results of your program will help remind you of your ongoing commitment to your program and give you a sense of accomplishment. Create daily and weekly program logs that you can use to track your progress. Record the activity frequency, intensity, time, and type. Keep your log handy, and fill it in immediately after each exercise session. Post it in a visible place to remind you of your activity schedule and to provide incentive for improvement.

SOURCE: Adapted from Kusinitz, I., and M. Fine. 1995. *Your Guide to Getting Fit*, 3rd ed. Mountain View, Calif.: Mayfield.

- Exercises that develop muscular strength and endurance involve exerting force against a significant resistance. A strength training program for general fitness typically involves one set of 8–12 repetitions of 8–10 exercises, at least 2 nonconsecutive days per week.

- A good stretching program includes exercises for all the major muscle groups and joints of the body. Do a series of active, static stretches 2–3 days per week, ideally 5–7 days per week. Hold each stretch for 15–30 seconds; do two to four repetitions. Stretch when muscles are warm.

- Instructors, equipment, and facilities should be chosen carefully to enhance enjoyment and prevent injuries.

- A well-balanced diet contains all the energy and nutrients needed to sustain a fitness program. When exercising, remember to drink enough fluids.

- Rest, ice, compression, and elevation (R-I-C-E) are treatments for muscle and joint injuries.

FOR MORE INFORMATION

BOOKS

Fahey, T. 2010. *Basic Weight Training for Men and Women*, 7th ed. New York: McGraw-Hill. *Weight training and plyometric exercises for fitness, weight control, and improved sports performance.*

Fahey, T., P. Insel, and W. Roth. 2009. *Fit and Well: Core Concepts and Labs in Physical Fitness and Wellness*, 8th ed. New York: McGraw-Hill. *A comprehensive guide to developing a complete fitness program.*

Fenton, M. 2008. *The Complete Guide to Walking, New and Revised: For Health, Weight Loss, and Fitness.* Guildford, Conn.: Lyons Press. *Discusses walking as a fitness method and a way to avoid diseases such as diabetes.*

Gotlin, R. 2007. *Sport Injuries Guidebook.* Champaign, Ill.: Human Kinetics. *Provides information and care instructions on many types of sports-related injuries.*

Nelson, A. G., et al. 2006. *Stretching Anatomy.* Champaign, Ill.: Human Kinetics. *A guide to stretching that features highly detailed illustrations of the muscles affected by each exercise.*

Nieman, D. C. 2007. *Exercise Testing and Prescription. A Health-Related Approach,* 6th ed. New York: McGraw-Hill. *A comprehensive discussion of the effects of exercise and exercise testing and prescription.*

ORGANIZATIONS, HOTLINES, AND WEB SITES

American Academy of Orthopaedic Surgeons. Provides fact sheets on many fitness and sports topics, including how to begin a program, how to choose equipment, and how to prevent and treat many types of injuries.

http://orthoinfo.aaos.org

American College of Sports Medicine. Provides brochures, publications, and audio- and videotapes on the positive effects of exercise.

http://www.acsm.org

American Heart Association: MyStart! Provides practical advice for people of all fitness levels plus an online fitness diary.

http://www.americanheart.org/presenter.jhtml?identifier=3040839

CDC Physical Activity Information. Provides information on the benefits of physical activity and suggestions for incorporating moderate physical activity into daily life.

http://www.cdc.gov/nccdphp/dnpa

Disabled Sports USA. Provides sport and recreation services to people with physical or mobility disorders.

http://www.dsusa.org

Federal Trade Commission: Consumer Protection—Diet, Health, and Fitness. Provides several brochures with consumer advice about purchasing exercise equipment.

http://www.ftc.gov/bcp/menus/consumer/health.shtm

MedlinePlus: Exercise and Physical Fitness. Provides links to news and reliable information about fitness and exercise from government agencies and professional associations.

http://www.nlm.nih.gov/medlineplus/
exerciseandphysicalfitness.html

National Institute on Drug Abuse: Anabolic Steroid Abuse. Provides information and links about the dangers of anabolic steroids.

http://www.steroidabuse.org

President's Council on Physical Fitness and Sports (PCPFS). Provides information on PCPFS programs and publications.

http://www.fitness.gov
http://www.presidentschallenge.org

SmallStep.gov. Provides resources for increasing activity and improving diet through small changes in daily habits.

http://www.smallstep.gov

World Health Organization (WHO): Move for Health. Provides information about the WHO initiative to promote increased physical activity.

http://www.who.int/moveforhealth/en/

SELECTED BIBLIOGRAPHY

American College of Sports Medicine. 2006. *ACSM's Guidelines for Exercise Testing and Prescription,* 7th ed. Philadelphia: Lippincott Williams & Wilkins.

American College of Sports Medicine. 2006. *ACSM's Resource Manual for Guidelines for Exercise Testing and Prescription,* 5th ed. Philadelphia: Lippincott Williams & Wilkins.

American Heart Association. 2008. *Heart Disease and Stroke Statistics—2008 Update.* Dallas: American Heart Association.

Armstrong, L. E., et al. 2007. American College of Sports Medicine position stand: Exertional heat illness during training and competition. *Medicine and Science in Sports and Exercise* 39(3): 556–572.

Brooks, G. A., et al. 2005. *Exercise Physiology: Human Bioenergetics and Its Applications,* 4th ed. New York: McGraw-Hill.

Brownson, R. C., T. K. Boehmer, and D. A. Luke. 2005. Declining rates of physical activity in the United States: What are the contributors? *Annual Review of Public Health* 26: 421–443.

Carnathon, M. R., M. Gulati, and P. Greenland. 2006. Prevalence and cardiovascular disease correlates of low cardiorespiratory fitness in adolescents and adults. *Journal of the American Medical Association* 294(23): 2981–2988.

Centers for Disease Control and Prevention. 2008. Prevalence of self-reported physically active adults—United States, 2007. *Morbidity and Mortality Weekly Report* 57(48): 1297–1300.

Dishman, R. K., et al. 2006. Neurobiology of exercise. *Obesity* (Silver Spring) 14(3): 345–356.

Dugan, S. 2005. Safe exercise for women. *ACSM Fit Society Page,* Winter.

Dunn, A. L., et al. 2005. Exercise treatment for depression: Efficacy and dose response. *American Journal of Preventive Medicine* 28(1): 1–8.

Fahey, T. D., P. M. Insel, and W. T. Roth. 2009. *Fit and Well: Core Concepts and Labs in Physical Fitness and Wellness,* 8th ed. New York: McGraw-Hill.

Fenicchia, L. M., et al. 2004. Influence of resistance exercise training on glucose control in women with type 2 diabetes. *Metabolism* 53(3): 284–289.

Franco, O. H., et al. 2005. Effects of physical activity on life expectancy with cardiovascular disease. *Archives of Internal Medicine* 165(20): 2355–2360.

Gunter, M. J., and M. F. Leitzmann. 2006. Obesity and colorectal cancer: Epidemiology, mechanisms and candidate genes. *Journal of Nutritional Biochemistry* 17(3): 145–156.

Hart, L. 2006. Exercise therapy for nonspecific low-back pain: A meta-analysis. *Clinical Journal of Sports Medicine* 16(2): 189–190.

Haskell, W. L., et al. 2007. Physical activity and public health: Updated recommendations for adults from the American College of Sports Medicine and the American Heart Association. *Circulation* 116(9): 1081–1093.

Larson, E. B., et al. 2006. Exercise is associated with reduced risk for incident dementia among persons 65 years of age and older. *Annals of Internal Medicine* 144(2): 73–81.

LaRoche, D. P., and D. A. Connolly. 2006. Effects of stretching on passive muscle tension and response to eccentric exercise. *American Journal of Sports Medicine* 34(6): 1000–1007.

Nattiv, A., et al. 2007. American College of Sports Medicine position stand: The female athlete triad. *Medicine and Science in Sports and Exercise* 39(10): 1867–1882.

Nelson, M. E., et al. 2007. Physical activity and public health in older adults: Recommendations from the American College of Sports Medicine and the American Heart Association. *Medicine and Science in Sports and Exercise* 39(8): 1435–1445.

Pescatello, L. S., et al. 2004. American College of Sports Medicine position stand: Exercise and hypertension. *Medicine and Science in Sports and Exercise* 36(3): 533–553.

Sawka, M. N., et al. 2007. American College of Sports Medicine position stand: Exercise and fluid replacement. *Medicine and Science in Sports and Exercise* 39(2): 377–390.

Shehab, R., et al. 2006. Pre-exercise stretching and sports-related injuries: Knowledge, attitudes and practices. *Clinical Journal of Sports Medicine* 16(3): 228–231.

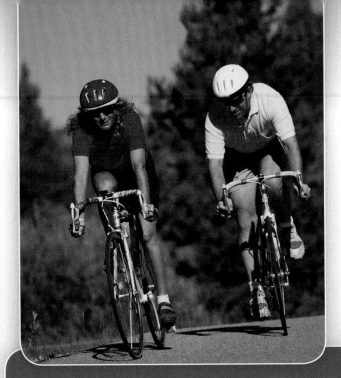

LOOKING AHEAD>>>>>

AFTER READING THIS CHAPTER, YOU SHOULD BE ABLE TO:

- Discuss different methods for assessing body weight and body composition
- Explain the health risks associated with overweight and obesity
- Explain factors that may contribute to a weight problem, including genetic, physiological, lifestyle, and psychosocial factors
- Describe lifestyle factors that contribute to weight gain and loss, including the roles of diet, exercise, and emotional factors
- Identify and describe the symptoms of eating disorders and the health risks associated with them
- Design a personal plan for successfully managing body weight

WEIGHT MANAGEMENT

11

Achieving and maintaining a healthy body weight is a serious public health challenge and a source of distress for many Americans. Under standards developed by the National Institutes of Health (NIH), about 66% of American adults are overweight, including more than 34% who are obese (Figure 11.1). In the United States, the number of obese adults doubled between 1980 and 2004, although obesity rates have begun leveling off since 2003. Even so, experts say that by 2015, 75% of adults will be overweight and 41% will be obese. By 2030, it is estimated that the entire American adult population will be overweight or obese. And while millions struggle to lose weight, others fall into dangerous eating patterns such as binge eating or self-starvation.

Although not completely understood, managing body weight is not a mysterious process. It's simply a matter of balancing calories consumed with calories expended in daily activities—in other words, eating a moderate diet and exercising regularly. Successful weight management requires the long-term coordination of many aspects of a wellness lifestyle, including proper nutrition, adequate physical activity, and stress management.

This chapter explores the factors that contribute to the development of overweight and to eating disorders. It also takes a closer look at weight management through lifestyle behaviors and suggests specific strategies for reaching and maintaining a healthy weight.

BASIC CONCEPTS OF WEIGHT MANAGEMENT

If you are like most people, you are concerned about your weight. But at what point does being overweight present a health risk? And how thin is too thin?

Body Composition

The human body can be divided into fat-free mass and body fat. Fat-free mass is composed of all the body's non-

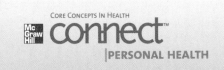

http://www.mcgrawhillconnect.com/personalhealth

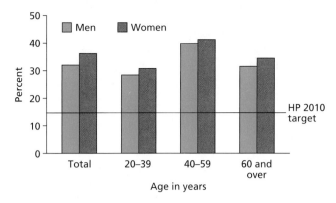

FIGURE 11.1 Obesity prevalence, by age and sex, of American adults, 2005–2006. *Healthy People 2010 sets a target obesity prevalence of not greater than 15% for all adults.*

SOURCE: Ogden, C. L., et al. 2007. Obesity among adults in the United States. No change since 2003–2004. *NCHS Data Brief No. 1.* Hyattsville, MD: National Center for Health Statistics.

fat tissues: bone, water, muscle, connective tissue, organ tissues, and teeth. There are two types of body fat:

• **Subcutaneous fat** includes *lipids,* or fats, incorporated in the nerves, brain, heart, lungs, liver, and mammary glands. These fat deposits, which are crucial for normal body functioning, make up approximately 3–5% of total body weight in men and 8–12% in women. The larger percentage in women is due to fat deposits in the breasts, uterus, and other sites specific to females.

• **Visceral fat** exists primarily within *adipose tissue,* or fat cells, often located just below the skin and around major organs. The amount of visceral fat varies from person to person based on many factors, including gender, age, heredity, metabolism, diet, and activity level. When we talk about wanting to lose weight, most of us are referring to visceral fat.

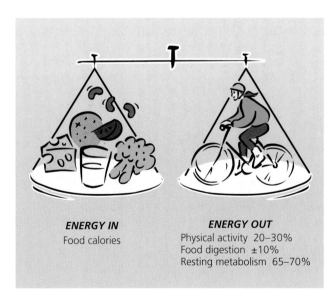

ENERGY IN
Food calories

ENERGY OUT
Physical activity 20–30%
Food digestion ±10%
Resting metabolism 65–70%

FIGURE 11.2 The energy balance equation.

A pound of body fat is equal to 3500 calories. This means that having only an extra 10 calories per day will equal a one-pound weight gain over the course of a year. In 10 years, this would amount to a 10-pound weight gain. What is most important for health is not total weight but rather the proportion of the body's total weight that is fat—the **percent body fat.**

For example, two women may both be 5 feet, 5 inches tall and weigh 130 pounds. But one woman, an endurance runner, may have only 15% of her body weight as fat, whereas the other woman, who is sedentary, may have 34% body fat. Although 130 pounds is not considered overweight for women of this height by most standards, the sedentary woman may be overfat. Because most people use the word "overweight" to describe the condition of having too much body fat, we use it in this chapter, although "overfat" is actually a more accurate term.

Energy Balance

The key to keeping a healthy ratio of fat to fat-free mass is maintaining an energy balance (Figure 11.2). You take in energy (calories) from the food you eat. Your body uses energy (calories) to maintain vital body functions (resting metabolism), to digest food, and to fuel physical activity. When energy in equals energy out, you maintain your current weight. To change your weight and body composition, you must tip the energy balance equation in a particular direction. If you take in more calories daily than your body burns, the excess calories will be stored as fat and you will gain weight over time. If you eat fewer calories than you burn each day, you will lose some of the stored fat and probably lose weight.

Our environment is rich in large portion sizes; high-fat, high-calorie foods; and palatable, easily available, and inexpensive foods. Unfortunately, we've decreased work-related physical activity, decreased activity associated with

subcutaneous fat   The fats incorporated in various tissues of the body; critical for normal body functioning.

visceral fat   The fat inside the abdominal wall in and around the internal organs. An excess leads to a greater risk of heart disease, insulin resistance, and metabolic syndrome.

percent body fat   The percentage of total body weight that is composed of fat.

TERMS

daily living, and increased time spent in sedentary pastimes like TV watching and computer use. The good news, however, is that you control both parts of the energy balance equation.

Evaluating Body Weight and Body Composition

Overweight is usually defined as total body weight above the recommended range for good health (as determined by large-scale population surveys). **Obesity** is defined as a more serious degree of overweight. Many methods are available for measuring and evaluating body weight and percent body fat.

Height-Weight Charts In the past, many people relied on height-weight charts to evaluate body weight. Based on insurance company statistics, these charts list a range of ideal or recommended body weights associated with the lowest mortality for people of a particular sex, age, and height. Although easy to use, height-weight charts can be highly inaccurate for some people, and they provide only an indirect measure of body fat.

Body Mass Index Body mass index (BMI) is a measure of body weight that is useful for classifying the health risks of body weight if you don't have access to more sophisticated methods. Though more accurate than height-weight tables, BMI is also based on the concept that weight should be proportional to height. Easy to calculate and rate, BMI is a fairly accurate measure of the health risks of body weight for average people. However, because BMI does not distinguish between fat weight and fat-free weight, it can be very inaccurate for some groups, including short people (under 5 feet tall), muscular athletes, and older adults with little muscle mass. If you are in one of these groups, use one of the methods described in the next section for estimating percent body fat to assess whether your current weight and body composition are healthy. BMI is also not particularly useful for tracking changes in body composition—gains in muscle mass and losses of fat. Women are likely to have more body fat for a given BMI than men.

You can look up your BMI by using the chart in Figure 11.3, or use the following formula to calculate it more precisely.

1. Divide your body weight in pounds by 2.2 to convert the amount to kilograms.
2. Multiply your height in inches by 0.0254 to convert the amount to meters.
3. Multiply the result of step 2 by itself to get the square of the height measurement.
4. Divide the result of step 1 by the result of step 3 to determine your BMI.

	<18.5 Underweight		18.5–24.9 Normal						25–29.9 Overweight					30–34.9 Obesity (Class I)					35–39.9 Obesity (Class II)					≥40 Extreme obesity
BMI	17	18	19	20	21	22	23	24	25	26	27	28	29	30	31	32	33	34	35	36	37	38	39	40
Height												Body Weight (pounds)												
4' 10"	81	86	91	96	101	105	110	115	120	124	129	134	139	144	148	153	158	163	168	172	177	182	187	192
4' 11"	84	89	94	99	104	109	114	119	124	129	134	139	144	149	154	159	163	168	173	178	183	188	193	198
5'	87	92	97	102	108	113	118	123	128	133	138	143	149	154	159	164	169	174	179	184	190	195	200	205
5' 1"	90	95	101	106	111	117	122	127	132	138	143	148	154	159	164	169	175	180	185	191	196	201	207	212
5' 2"	93	98	104	109	115	120	126	131	137	142	148	153	159	164	170	175	181	186	191	197	202	208	213	219
5' 3"	96	102	107	113	119	124	130	136	141	147	153	158	164	169	175	181	186	192	198	203	209	215	220	226
5' 4"	99	105	111	117	122	128	134	140	146	152	157	163	169	175	181	187	192	198	204	210	216	222	227	233
5' 5"	102	108	114	120	126	132	138	144	150	156	162	168	174	180	186	192	198	204	210	216	222	229	235	241
5' 6"	105	112	118	124	130	136	143	149	155	161	167	174	180	186	192	198	205	211	217	223	229	236	242	248
5' 7"	109	115	121	128	134	141	147	153	160	166	173	179	185	192	198	204	211	217	224	230	236	243	249	256
5' 8"	112	118	125	132	138	145	151	158	165	171	178	184	191	197	204	211	217	224	230	237	244	250	257	263
5' 9"	115	122	129	136	142	149	156	163	169	176	183	190	197	203	210	217	224	230	237	244	251	258	264	271
5' 10"	119	126	133	139	146	153	160	167	174	181	188	195	202	209	216	223	230	237	244	251	258	265	272	279
5' 11"	122	129	136	143	151	158	165	172	179	187	194	201	208	215	222	230	237	244	251	258	265	273	280	287
6'	125	133	140	148	155	162	170	177	184	192	199	207	214	221	229	236	243	251	258	266	273	280	288	295
6' 1"	129	137	144	152	159	167	174	182	190	197	205	212	220	228	235	243	250	258	265	273	281	288	296	303
6' 2"	132	140	148	156	164	171	179	187	195	203	210	218	226	234	242	249	257	265	273	281	288	296	304	312
6' 3"	136	144	152	160	168	176	184	192	200	208	216	224	232	240	248	256	264	272	280	288	296	304	312	320
6' 4"	140	148	156	164	173	181	189	197	206	214	222	230	238	247	255	263	271	280	288	296	304	312	321	329

FIGURE 11.3 Body mass index (BMI). To determine your BMI, find your height in the left column. Move across the appropriate row until you find the weight closest to your own. The number at the top of the column is the BMI at that height and weight.

SOURCE: Ratings from National Heart, Lung, and Blood Institute. 1998. *Clinical Guidelines on the Identification, Evaluation, and Treatment of Overweight and Obesity in Adults: The Evidence Report.* Bethesda, Md.: National Institutes of Health.

Table 11.1	Percentage of Body Fat as the Criterion for Obesity

Category	Percent Body Fat	
	Males	Females
Normal	12–20%	20–30%
Borderline	21–25%	31–33%
Obese	>25%	>33%

SOURCE: Bray, G. A. 2003. *Contemporary Diagnosis and Management of Obesity and the Metabolic Syndrome*, 3rd ed. Newton, Pa.: Handbooks in Health Care.

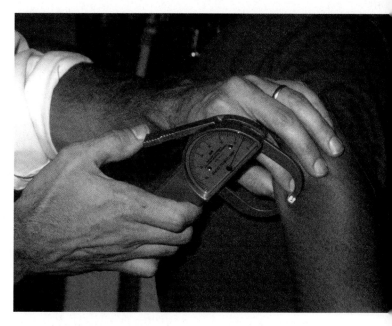

Calipers are used to perform skinfold measurements, which is a simple and inexpensive way to determine body fat levels. To assure accuracy, skinfold measurements must be done by someone with appropriate training.

Under standards issued by the National Institutes of Health, a BMI between 18.5 and 24.9 is considered healthy; a person with a BMI of 25 or above is classified as overweight, and a person with a BMI of 30 or above is classified as obese. A person with a BMI below 18.5 is classified as underweight, although low BMI values may be healthy in some cases if they are not the result of smoking, an eating disorder, or an underlying disease; a BMI of 17.5 or less is sometimes used as a diagnostic criterion for the eating disorder anorexia nervosa.

Body Composition Analysis   The most accurate and direct way to evaluate body composition is to determine percent body fat. See Table 11.1 for body composition ratings based on percent body fat.

HYDROSTATIC (UNDERWATER) WEIGHING AND BOD POD   In hydrostatic weighing, a person is submerged and weighed under water. Percent body fat can be calculated from body density. Muscle has a higher density and fat a lower density than water, so people with more fat tend to float and weigh less under water, while lean people tend to sink and weigh more under water. A specialized body composition analysis device called the Bod Pod uses air instead of water. A person sits in a chamber, and computerized pressure sensors determine the amount of air displaced by the person's body.

SKINFOLD MEASUREMENTS   The skinfold thickness technique measures the thickness of fat under the skin. Measurements are taken at several sites and plugged into formulas that calculate body fat percentages.

ELECTRICAL IMPEDANCE ANALYSIS   In this method, electrodes are attached to the body and a harmless electrical current is transmitted from electrode to electrode. The electrical conduction through the body favors the path of the fat-free tissues over the fat tissues. A computer can calculate fat percentages from measurements of current.

Excess Body Fat and Wellness

The amount of fat in the body—and its location—can have profound effects on health.

The Health Risks of Excess Body Fat   Obesity doubles mortality rates and can reduce life expectancy by 10–20 years. If the current trends continue, scientists believe that the average American's life expectancy will soon decline by 5 years. Obesity is associated with unhealthy cholesterol and triglyceride levels, impaired heart function, and death from cardiovascular disease. Other health risks include hypertension, many kinds of cancer, impaired immune function, gallbladder and kidney diseases, skin problems, impotence, sleep and breathing disorders, back pain, arthritis, and other bone and joint disorders. Obesity is also associated with complications of pregnancy, menstrual irregularities, urine leakage (stress incontinence), and increased surgical risk.

There is a strong association between excess body fat and diabetes mellitus, a disease that causes a disruption of normal metabolism. The pancreas normally secretes the hormone insulin, which stimulates cells to take up blood

overweight   Body weight that falls above the recommended range for good health.

obesity   The condition of having an excess of nonessential body fat; having a body mass index of 30 or greater or having a percent body fat greater than about 25% for men and 33% for women.

body mass index (BMI)   A measure of relative body weight that takes height into account and is highly correlated with more direct measures of body fat; calculated by dividing total body weight (in kilograms) by the square of height (in meters).

TERMS

Symptoms of diabetes

- Frequent urination
- Extreme thirst and hunger
- Unexplained weight loss
- Extreme fatigue
- Blurred vision
- Frequent infections
- Slow wound healing
- Tingling or numbness in hands and feet
- Dry, itchy skin

Note: In the early stages, diabetes often has no symptoms.

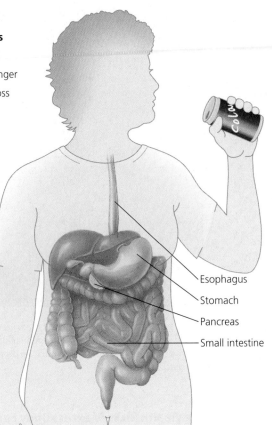

Esophagus
Stomach
Pancreas
Small intestine

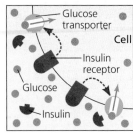

Normal
Insulin binds to receptors on the surface of a cell and signals special transporters in the cell to transport glucose inside.

Glucose transporter
Cell
Insulin receptor
Glucose
Insulin

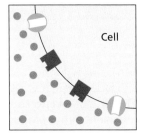

Type 1 diabetes
The pancreas produces little or no insulin. Thus, no signal is sent instructing the cell to transport glucose, and glucose builds up in the bloodstream.

Cell

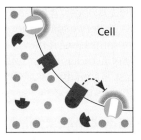

Type 2 diabetes
The pancreas produces too little insulin and/or the body's cells are resistant to it. Some insulin binds to receptors on the cell's surface, but the signal to transport glucose is blocked. Glucose builds up in the bloodstream.

Cell

FIGURE 11.4 Diabetes mellitus. During digestion, carbohydrates are broken down in the small intestine into glucose, a simple sugar that enters the bloodstream. The presence of glucose signals the pancreas to release insulin, a hormone that helps cells take up glucose; once inside a cell, glucose can be converted to energy. In diabetes, this process is disrupted, resulting in a buildup of glucose in the bloodstream.

sugar (glucose) to produce energy (Figure 11.4). In diabetes, this process is disrupted, causing a buildup of glucose in the bloodstream. Diabetes is associated with kidney failure; nerve damage; circulation problems and amputations; retinal damage and blindness; and increased rates of heart attack, stroke, and hypertension (see the box "Diabetes").

The risks from obesity increase with its severity, and they are much more likely to occur in people who are more than twice their desirable body weight. The NIH recommends weight loss for people whose BMI places them in the obese category and for those who are overweight *and* have two or more major risk factors for disease. If your BMI is 25 or above, consult a physician for help in determining a healthy BMI for you.

The Nurses' Health Study, in which Harvard researchers have followed more than 120,000 women since 1976, has found that even mildly to moderately overweight women have an 80% increased risk of developing CHD compared to leaner women. This study also confirmed that to reduce the risk of dying prematurely of any cause, maintaining a desirable body weight is important. But it is also important to realize that small weight losses—5% to 10% of total body weight—can lead to significant health improvements.

Body Fat Distribution and Health The distribution of body fat is also an important indicator of health. Men and postmenopausal women tend to store fat in the upper regions of their bodies, particularly in the abdominal area (the apple shape). Premenopausal women usually store fat in hips, buttocks, and thighs (the pear shape). Excess fat in the abdominal area increases risk of high blood pressure, diabetes, early-onset heart disease, stroke, certain types of cancer, and mortality. It appears that abdominal fat is more easily mobilized and sent into the bloodstream, increasing disease-related blood fat levels.

The risks from body fat distribution are usually assessed by measuring waist circumference (the distance around the abdomen at the level of the hip bone, known as the iliac crest). A total waist measurement of more than

QUICK STATS

Using standard height-weight ratios, a person who is 5'9" tall and weighs 203 pounds is obese.

—NCHS, 2007

Types of Diabetes

About 24 million Americans (or 8% of the population) have one of two major forms of diabetes. About 5–10% of people with diabetes have the more serious form, known as *type 1 diabetes*. In this type of diabetes, the pancreas produces little or no insulin, so daily doses of insulin are required. Type 1 diabetes occurs when the body's immune system, triggered by a viral infection or some other environmental factor, mistakenly destroys the insulin-producing cells in the pancreas. It usually strikes before age 30.

The remaining 90–95% of Americans with diabetes have *type 2 diabetes*, and the prevalence is rising dramatically. This condition can develop slowly, and about 25% of affected individuals are unaware of their condition. In type 2 diabetes, the pancreas doesn't produce enough insulin, cells are resistant to insulin, or both. This condition is usually diagnosed in people over age 40, although there has been a tenfold increase in type 2 diabetes in children in the past two decades. About one-third of people with type 2 diabetes must take insulin; others may take medications that increase insulin production or stimulate cells to take up glucose.

A third type of diabetes occurs in about 7% of women during pregnancy. *Gestational diabetes* usually disappears after pregnancy, but more than half of women who experience it eventually develop type 2 diabetes.

The term *pre-diabetes* describes blood glucose levels that are higher than normal but not high enough for a diagnosis of full-blown diabetes. About 57 million Americans have pre-diabetes, and most people with the condition will develop type 2 diabetes unless they adopt preventive lifestyle measures. Pre-diabetes poses a risk to health beyond just the development of diabetes: Blood glucose levels in the pre-diabetes range increase the risk of heart attack or stroke by 50%. The insulin resistance and elevated glucose levels associated with pre-diabetes (and diabetes) are among the defining risk factors of metabolic syndrome.

The major factors involved in the development of diabetes are age, obesity, physical inactivity, a family history of diabetes, and lifestyle. Excess body fat reduces cell sensitivity to insulin, and insulin resistance is almost always a precursor of type 2 diabetes.

Ethnic background also plays a role. According to statistics released by the CDC in 2008, the rate of diagnosed diabetes cases is highest among Native Americans and Alaska Natives (16.5%), followed by blacks (11.8%), Hispanics (10.4%), Asian Americans (7.5%), and white Americans (6.6%). Across all races, about 25% of Americans age 60 and older have diabetes.

Prevention

It is estimated that 90% of cases of type 2 diabetes could be prevented if people adopted healthy lifestyle behaviors, including regular physical activity, a moderate diet, and modest weight loss. For people with pre-diabetes, lifestyle measures are more effective than medication for delaying or preventing the development of diabetes. Studies of people with pre-diabetes show that just a 5–7% weight loss can lower diabetes onset by nearly 60%. Exercise (endurance and/or strength training) makes cells more sensitive to insulin and helps stabilize blood glucose levels; it also helps keep body fat at healthy levels.

A moderate diet to control body fat is perhaps the most important dietary recommendation for the prevention of diabetes. However, the composition of the diet may also be important. Studies have linked diets low in fiber and high in sugar, refined carbohydrates, saturated fat, red meat, and high-fat dairy products to increased risk of diabetes; diets rich in whole grains, fruits, vegetables, legumes, fish, and poultry may be protective. Specific foods linked to higher risk of diabetes include soft drinks, white bread, white rice, french fries, processed meats, and sugary desserts.

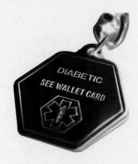

Treatment

There is no cure for diabetes, but it can be successfully managed by keeping blood sugar levels within safe limits through diet, exercise, and, if necessary, medication. Blood sugar levels can be monitored using a home test; close monitoring and control of glucose levels can significantly reduce the rate of serious complications. New drug therapies include inhibitors known as DDP-4, which lower blood sugar without causing weight gain.

Nearly 90% of people with type 2 diabetes are overweight when diagnosed, including 55% who are obese. An important step in treatment is to lose weight; even a small amount of weight loss can be beneficial. People with diabetes should get their carbohydrate from whole grains, fruits, vegetables, and low-fat dairy products; carbohydrate and mono-unsaturated fat together should provide 60–70% of total daily calories. Regular exercise and a healthy diet are often sufficient to control type 2 diabetes.

Warning Signs and Testing

Be alert for the warning signs of diabetes:

- Frequent urination
- Extreme hunger or thirst
- Unexplained weight loss
- Extreme fatigue
- Blurred vision
- Frequent infections
- Cuts and bruises that are slow to heal
- Tingling or numbness in hands or feet
- Generalized itching with no rash

The best way to avoid complications is to recognize these symptoms and get early diagnosis and treatment. Type 2 diabetes is often asymptomatic in the early stages, however, so routine screening is recommended for people over age 45 and anyone younger who is at high risk. Screening involves a blood test to check glucose levels after either a period of fasting or the administration of a set dose of glucose. A fasting glucose level of 126 mg/dl or higher indicates diabetes; a level of 100–125 mg/dl indicates pre-diabetes.

40 inches for men and 35 inches for women is associated with a significantly increased risk of disease. Large waist circumference can be a marker for increased risk of diabetes, high blood pressure, and CVD even in people with a BMI in the normal range.

Body Image The collective picture of the body as seen through the mind's eye, **body image** consists of perceptions, images, thoughts, attitudes, and emotions. A negative body image is characterized by dissatisfaction with the body in general or some part of the body in particular. Recent surveys indicate that the majority of Americans, many of whom are not actually overweight, are unhappy with their body weight or with some aspect of their appearance.

Losing weight or getting cosmetic surgery does not necessarily improve body image. However, improvements in body image may occur in the absence of changes in weight or appearance. Many experts now believe that body image issues must be dealt with as part of treating obesity and eating disorders.

Problems Associated with Very Low Levels of Body Fat

Health experts have generally viewed very low levels of body fat—less than 8–12% for women and 3–5% for men—as a threat to wellness. Extreme leanness has been linked with reproductive, circulatory, and immune system disorders. Extremely lean people may experience muscle wasting and fatigue; they are also more likely to suffer from dangerous eating disorders.

In physically active women and girls, particularly those involved in sports where weight and appearance are important (ballet, gymnastics, skating, and distance running, for example), a condition called the **female athlete triad** may develop. The triad consists of three interrelated disorders: abnormal eating patterns (and excessive exercising), followed by **amenorrhea** (absence of menstruation), followed by decreased bone density (premature osteoporosis). Prolonged amenorrhea can cause bone density to erode to a point that a woman in her twenties will have the bone density of a woman in her sixties. Left untreated, the triad can lead to decreased physical performance, increased incidence of bone fractures, disturbances of heart rhythm and metabolism, and even death.

What Is the Right Weight for You?

BMI, percent body fat, and waist circumference measurement can best serve as general guides or estimates for body weight. To answer the question of what you should weigh, let your lifestyle be your guide. Don't focus on a particular weight as your goal. Instead, focus on living a lifestyle that includes eating moderate amounts of healthful foods, getting plenty of exercise, thinking positively, and learning to cope with stress. Then let the pounds fall where they may. For most people, the result will be close to the recommended weight ranges discussed earlier. For some, their weight will be somewhat higher than societal standards—but right for them. By letting a healthy lifestyle determine your weight, you can avoid developing unhealthy patterns of eating and a negative body image.

FACTORS CONTRIBUTING TO EXCESS BODY FAT

Body weight and body composition may be determined by multiple factors that may vary with each individual.

Genetic Factors

Estimates of the genetic contribution to obesity vary widely, from about 25% to 40% of an individual's body fat. Genes influence body size and shape, body fat distribution, and metabolic rate. Genetic factors also affect the ease with which weight is gained as a result of overeating and where on the body extra weight is added. If both parents are obese, their children have an 80% risk of being obese; children with only one obese parent face a 40% risk of becoming obese. In studies that compared adoptees and their biological parents, the weights of the adoptees were found to be more like those of the biological parents than the adoptive parents, again indicating a strong genetic link.

Hereditary influences, however, must be balanced against the contribution of environmental factors. Not all children of obese parents become obese, and normal-weight parents may have overweight children. The *tendency* to develop obesity may be inherited, but the expression of this tendency is affected by environmental influences.

QUESTIONS FOR CRITICAL THINKING AND REFLECTION

Calculate your BMI using the formula given in this chapter, then compare it with the BMIs of some classmates. Do the results surprise you? How well do you think BMI reflects body composition? Why do you think it is such a commonly used measure?

Environmental factors can make weight management even more difficult for many people. In this case, it is the man-made environment, not the natural one, that creates obstacles to a healthy lifestyle:

- A noisy environment can make it difficult to sleep, and poor sleep quality has been associated with weight gain, difficulty in losing weight, and other conditions such as depression and high blood pressure.

- In some urban and high-poverty areas, it is not always easy to make ideal food choices because fresh, healthy foods may be more expensive or harder to obtain than cheaper, less healthy fast food or junk food.

- People who live in unsafe environments, such as some inner-city areas, may not get as much physical activity as they need, simply because there are not enough safe places to walk or exercise.

As you create your own weight-management program, remember to account for environmental factors that may interfere with your efforts. Creative solutions may be needed to keep your program on track.

The message you should take from this research is that genes are not destiny. It is true that some people have a harder time losing weight and maintaining weight loss than others. However, with increased exercise and attention to diet, even those with a genetic tendency toward obesity can maintain a healthy body weight.

Physiological Factors

Metabolism is the sum of all the vital processes by which food energy and nutrients are made available to and used by the body. The largest component of metabolism, **resting metabolic rate (RMR)**, is the energy required to maintain vital body functions, including respiration, heart rate, body temperature, and blood pressure, while the body is at rest. As shown in Figure 11.2, RMR accounts for about 65–70% of daily energy expenditure. The energy required to digest food accounts for an additional ±10% of daily energy expenditure. The remaining 20–30% is expended during physical activity.

Both heredity and behavior affect metabolic rate. Men, who have a higher proportion of muscle mass than women, have a higher RMR because muscle tissue is more metabolically active than fat. Also, some individuals inherit a higher or lower RMR than others. A higher RMR means that a person burns more calories while at rest and can therefore take in more calories without gaining weight.

Weight loss or gain also affects metabolic rate. When a person loses weight, both RMR and the energy required to perform physical tasks decrease. The reverse occurs when weight is gained. Exercise has a positive effect on metabolism. When people exercise, they slightly increase their RMR—the number of calories their bodies burn at rest. They also increase their muscle mass, which is associated with a higher metabolic rate. The exercise itself also burns calories, raising total energy expenditure. The higher the energy expenditure, the more the person can eat without gaining weight.

Lifestyle Factors

Although genetic and physiological factors may increase risk for excess body fat, they are not sufficient to explain the increasingly high rate of obesity seen in the United States. The gene pool has not changed in the past 40 years, but the rate of obesity among Americans has more than doubled. Clearly, other factors are at work—particularly lifestyle factors such as increased eating and decreased physical activity.

Eating   Americans have access to plenty of calorie-dense foods, and many have eating habits that contribute to weight gain. (See the box "Are Diet Sodas Bad for You?"). Most overweight adults admit to eating more than they should of high-fat, high-sugar, high-calorie foods. Americans eat out more frequently now than in the past, and we rely more heavily on fast food and packaged convenience foods. Restaurant and convenience food portion sizes tend to be large, and the foods themselves are likely to be high in fat, sugar, and calories and low in nutrients. Studies have consistently found that people underestimate portion sizes by as much as 25%.

Physical Activity   Activity levels among Americans are declining, beginning in childhood and continuing throughout life. Many schools have cut back on physical education classes and recess. Most adults drive to work, sit all day, and then relax in front of the TV at night. Modern conveniences such as remote controls, elevators, and power mowers have also reduced daily physical activity.

body image   The mental representation a person holds about his or her body at any given moment in time, consisting of perceptions, images, thoughts, attitudes, and emotions about the body.

female athlete triad   A condition consisting of three interrelated disorders: abnormal eating patterns (and excessive exercising) followed by lack of menstrual periods (amenorrhea) and decreased bone density (premature osteoporosis).

amenorrhea   The absence of menstruation.

resting metabolic rate (RMR)   The energy required to maintain vital body functions, including respiration, heart rate, body temperature, and blood pressure, while the body is at rest.

A can of regular soda contains about 150 calories. High consumption of sugary soda has previously been linked with obesity and diabetes in children and adolescents and with high blood pressure in adults. Further, some studies have shown that the added sweeteners in soft drinks are linked to increased triglycerides in the blood, leading to a greater risk of heart disease.

Why does drinking more soda lead to obesity and insulin resistance? Researchers have attributed this effect to the following factors:

• Consuming more calories in general

• The high fructose corn syrup content in sodas

• Lower feelings of satiety (satisfaction)

• The general effect of eating a diet that is high in refined carbohydrates, including sugar

Many weight-conscious people have changed to diet soda in the hope that this is a healthier, calorie-free alternative to regular soda. Recent research indicates that drinking more than one soft drink a day, even if it is diet soda, may be associated with an increased incidence of metabolic syndrome, which is a cluster of risk factors linked to the development of diabetes, heart disease, and stroke. The syndrome includes high blood pressure, elevated triglyceride levels, low levels of HDL ("good" cholesterol), high fasting blood sugar levels, and excessive waist circumference.

The link between diet soft drink consumption and metabolic syndrome was clear even when researchers accounted for other factors, such as saturated fat and fiber in the diet, total calories, physical activity, and smoking.

Compared to people who did not drink soda, researchers found that people who consumed more than one soft drink per day—regular or diet—were associated with the following:

• 44% more likely to develop metabolic syndrome

• 31% more likely to be obese

• 25% more likely to have higher-than-average blood pressure

• 18% more likely to have high blood pressure

Some research has suggested that the artificial sweeteners in diet drinks make a person more prone to eat sweet, higher-calorie foods. Another theory is that the caramel content in both regular and diet sodas may play a role in insulin resistance.

On the other hand, some contradictory studies show the benefit of diet soda consumption in overweight individuals and suggest that other factors could explain the development of risk factors for heart disease. Regardless, everyone agrees that more research should be done before a final verdict on diet soda consumption is reached.

Meanwhile, nutritionists say that this is a wake-up call for diet soda drinkers, suggesting that a zero-calorie beverage cannot undo the damage of an unhealthy diet.

Psychosocial Factors

Many people have learned to use food as a means of coping with stress and negative emotions. Eating can provide a powerful distraction from difficult feelings—loneliness, anger, boredom, anxiety, shame, sadness, inadequacy. It can be used to combat low moods, low energy levels, and low self-esteem. When food and eating become the primary means of regulating emotions, binge eating or other disturbed eating patterns can develop.

Obesity is strongly associated with socioeconomic status. The prevalence of obesity goes down as income level goes up. More women than men are obese at lower income levels, but men are somewhat more obese at higher levels. These differences may reflect the greater sensitivity and concern for a slim physical appearance among upper-income women, as well as greater access to information about nutrition, to low-fat and low-calorie foods, and to opportunities for physical activity. It may also reflect the greater acceptance of obesity among certain ethnic groups, as well as different cultural values related to food choices.

In some families and cultures, food is used as a symbol of love and caring. It is an integral part of social gatherings and celebrations. In such cases, it may be difficult to change established eating patterns because they are linked to cultural and family values.

ADOPTING A HEALTHY LIFESTYLE FOR SUCCESSFUL WEIGHT MANAGEMENT

Permanent weight loss is not something you start and stop. You need to adopt healthy behaviors that you can maintain throughout your life.

Diet and Eating Habits

In contrast to dieting, which involves some form of food restriction, the term *diet* refers to your daily food choices. Everyone has a diet, but not everyone is dieting. You need to develop a diet that you enjoy and that enables you to maintain a healthy body composition. Use MyPyramid as the basis for a healthy diet (see Chapter 9). For weight management, pay special attention to total calories, portion sizes, energy density, fat and carbohydrate intake, and eating habits.

Total Calories MyPyramid suggests approximate daily energy intakes based on gender, age, and activity level. However, energy balance may be a more important consideration for weight management than total calories consumed (refer back to Figure 11.2). To maintain your

QUESTIONS FOR CRITICAL THINKING AND REFLECTION
How do you view your own body composition? Where do you think you've gotten your ideas about how your body should look and perform? In light of what you've read in this chapter, do the ideals and images promoted in our culture seem reasonable? Do they seem healthy?

current weight, the total number of calories you eat must equal the number you burn. To lose weight, you must decrease your calorie intake and/or increase the number of calories you burn; to gain weight, the reverse is true. (One pound of body fat represents 3500 calories.)

The best approach for weight loss is combining an increase in physical activity with moderate calorie restriction. Don't go on a crash diet. To maintain weight loss, you will probably have to maintain some degree of the calorie restriction you used to lose the weight. Therefore, you need to adopt a level of food intake that provides all the essential nutrients that you can live with over the long term. For most people, maintaining weight loss is more difficult than losing the weight in the first place.

Portion Sizes Overconsumption of total calories is closely tied to portion sizes. Many Americans are unaware that the portions of packaged foods and of foods served at restaurants have increased in size, and most of us significantly underestimate the amount of food we eat. Limiting portion sizes is critical for maintaining good health. To counteract portion distortion, weigh and measure your food at home for a few days. In addition, check the serving sizes listed on packaged foods. When eating out, try to order the smallest-sized items on the menu. Don't supersize your meals and snacks; although huge servings may seem like the best deal, it is more important to order just what you need.

Energy (Calorie) Density To cut back on calories and still feel full, you should favor foods that are low in energy density, foods that have more volume and bulk—that is, they are relatively heavy but have few calories. For example, for the same 100 calories, you could eat 21 baby carrots or 4 pretzel twists; you are more likely to feel full after eating the serving of carrots because it weighs 10 times as much as the serving of pretzels (10 ounces versus 1 ounce).

Fresh fruits and vegetables, with their high water and fiber content, are low in energy density, as are whole-grain foods. Fresh fruits contain less calories and more fiber than fruit juices or drinks. Meat, ice cream, potato chips, croissants, crackers, and cakes and cookies are examples of foods high in energy density. Strategies for lowering the energy density of your diet include the following:

- Eat fruit with breakfast and for dessert.

- Add extra vegetables to sandwiches, casseroles, stir-fry dishes, pizza, pasta dishes, and fajitas.
- Start meals with a bowl of broth-based soup; include a green salad or fruit salad.
- Snack on fresh fruits and vegetables rather than crackers, chips, or other energy-dense snack foods.

Limit serving sizes of energy-dense foods such as butter, mayonnaise, cheese, chocolate, fatty meats, croissants, and snack foods that are fried, high in added sugars (including reduced-fat products), or contain trans fats.

It is also important to watch out for processed foods, which can be high in fat and sodium. Even processed foods labeled "fat-free" or "reduced fat" may be high in calories; such products may contain sugar and fat substitutes.

Eating Habits Equally important to weight management is the habit of eating small, frequent meals—four to five meals per day, including breakfast and snacks—on a regular schedule. Skipping meals leads to excessive hunger, feelings of deprivation, and increased vulnerability to binge eating or snacking. In addition to establishing a regular pattern of eating, set some rules to govern your food choices. Rules for breakfast might be these, for example: Choose a sugar-free, high-fiber cereal with fat-free milk on most days; have a hard-boiled egg (no more than 3 per week); save pancakes and waffles for special occasions, unless they are whole-grain. The ultimate goal is to eat in moderation; no foods need to be entirely off-limits, though some should be eaten judiciously.

Physical Activity and Exercise

Physical activity and exercise burn calories and keep the metabolism geared to using food for energy instead of storing it as fat. Making significant cuts in food intake in order to lose weight is a difficult strategy to maintain; increasing your physical activity is a much better approach. Regular physical activity protects against weight gain, is essential for maintaining weight loss, and improves quality of life. The sooner you establish good habits, the better. The key to success is making exercise an integral part of the lifestyle you can enjoy now and in the future.

> **Americans get about 17%** of their total daily calories at breakfast, but experts say 25% would be better.
>
> **—USDA, 2006**
>
> QUICK STATS

Thinking and Emotions

The way you think about yourself and your world influences, and is influenced by, how you feel and how you act. Often, people with low self-esteem mentally compare the actual self to an internally held picture of an "ideal

Exercise, Body Image, and Self-Esteem

If you gaze into the mirror and wish you could change the way your body looks, consider getting some exercise—not to reshape your contours but to firm up your body image and enhance your self-esteem. In a recent study, 82 adults completed a 12-week aerobic exercise program and had 12 months of follow-up. Compared with the control group, these participants improved their fitness and also benefited psychologically in tests of mood, anxiety, and self-concept. These same physical and psychological benefits were still significant at the 1-year follow-up.

One reason for the findings may be that people who exercise regularly often gain a sense of mastery and competence that enhances their self-esteem and body image. In addition, exercise contributes to a more toned look, which many adults prefer. Research suggests that physically active people are more comfortable with their body and their image than sedentary people are. In one workplace study, 60 employees were asked to complete a 36-session stretching program whose main purpose was to prevent muscle strains at work. At the end of the program, besides the signifi-

cant increase by all participants in measurements of flexibility, their perceptions of their bodies improved and so did their overall sense of self-worth.

Similar results were obtained in a Norwegian study, in which 219 middle-aged people at risk for heart disease were randomly assigned to one of four groups: diet, diet plus exercise, exercise, and no intervention. The greater the participation of individuals in the exercise component of the program, the higher were their scores in perceived competence/self-esteem and coping.

---

self," an image based on perfectionistic goals and beliefs about how they and others should be. The more these two pictures differ, the larger the impact on self-esteem and the more likely the presence of negative emotions.

Besides the internal picture we carry of ourselves, all of us carry on an internal dialogue about events happening to us and around us. This *self-talk* can be either self-deprecating or positively motivating, depending on our beliefs and attitudes. Having realistic beliefs and goals, and practicing positive self-talk and problem solving support a healthy lifestyle.

Coping Strategies

Appropriate coping strategies help you deal with the stresses of life; they are also an important lifestyle factor in weight management. Those who overeat might use food to alleviate loneliness or to serve as a pickup for fatigue, as an antidote to boredom, or as a distraction from problems. Some people even overeat to punish themselves for real or imagined transgressions. Those who recognize that they are misusing food can consciously attempt to find new coping strategies and begin to use food appropriately—to fuel life's activities, to foster growth, and to bring pleasure, but *not* as a way to manage stress.

APPROACHES TO OVERCOMING A WEIGHT PROBLEM

What should you do if you are overweight? You have several options.

Doing It Yourself

If you need to lose weight, focus on adopting the healthy lifestyle described throughout this book. The right weight for you will naturally evolve. Combine modest cuts in energy

QUESTIONS FOR CRITICAL THINKING AND REFLECTION

Have you ever used food as an escape when you were stressed out or distraught? Were you aware of what you were doing at the time? How can you avoid using food as a coping mechanism in the future?

intake with exercise, and avoid very-low-calorie diets. (In general, a low-calorie diet should have 1200–1500 calories per day.) By producing a negative energy balance of 250–1000 calories per day, you will produce the recommended weight loss of 0.5–2.0 pounds per week. Realize that most low-calorie diets cause a rapid loss of body water at first. When this phase passes, weight loss declines, and dieters are often misled into believing that their efforts are not working. They then give up, not realizing that smaller, mostly fat, losses later in the diet are actually better than the initial larger, mostly fluid losses. Reasonable weight loss is 8–10% of body weight over 6 months. A registered dietitian or nutritionist can recommend an appropriate plan for you when you want to lose weight on your own.

Americans spend **$40 billion** annually on weight-loss products and programs.

—*Business Week*, 2008

STATS

Dietary Supplements and Diet Aids

Dietary supplements marketed for weight loss are subject to fewer regulations than OTC medications. The Federal

Lifestyle Strategies for Successful Weight Management

Food Choices

• Follow the recommendations in MyPyramid for eating a moderate, varied diet.

• Favor foods with a *low energy density* and a *high nutrient density.*

• Check food labels for serving sizes, calories, and nutrient levels.

• Watch for hidden calories. Reduced-fat foods often have as many calories as their full-fat versions. Fat-based condiments like butter, margarine, mayonnaise, and salad dressings provide about 100 calories per tablespoon; added sugars such as jams, jellies, and syrup are also packed with calories.

• Drink fewer calories in the form of soda, fruit drinks, sports drinks, alcohol, and specialty coffees and teas.

• For problem foods, try eating small amounts under controlled conditions. Go out for a scoop of ice cream, for example, rather than buying half a gallon for your freezer.

Planning and Serving

• Keep a log of what you eat. Before you begin your program, your log will provide a realistic picture of your current diet and what changes you can make. Once you start your program, a log will keep you focused on your food choices and portion sizes.

• Eat 4–5 meals/snacks daily, *including breakfast,* to distribute calories throughout your day. Fix more meals yourself and eat out less often. Keep low-calorie snacks on hand to combat the "munchies": baby carrots, popcorn, and fresh fruits and vegetables are good choices.

• When shopping, make a list and stick to it. Don't shop when you're hungry. Avoid aisles that contain problem foods.

• Consume the majority of your daily calories during the day, not in the evening.

• Serve meals on small plates and in small bowls to help you eat smaller portions without feeling deprived.

• Eat only in specifically designated spots.

• When you eat, just eat—don't do anything else, such as reading or watching TV.

• Avoid late-night eating, a behavior specifically associated with weight gain among college students.

• Eat slowly. Take small bites and chew food thoroughly. Pay attention to every bite, and enjoy your food.

• When you're done eating, remove your plate. Cue yourself that the meal is over; drink a glass of water, suck on a mint, chew gum, or brush your teeth.

Special Occasions

• When you eat out, choose a restaurant where you can make healthy food choices. Ask the server not to put bread and butter on the table before the meal, and request that sauces and salad dressings be served on the side. If portion sizes are large, take half your food home for a meal later in the week.

• If you cook a large meal for friends, send leftovers home with your guests.

• If you're eating at a friend's, eat a little and leave the rest. Don't eat to be polite.

• Take care during the winter holidays. Research indicates that people gain less than they think during the winter holidays (about a pound) but that the weight isn't lost during the rest of the year, leading to slow, steady weight gain.

Physical Activity and Stress Management

• Increase your level of daily physical activity. If you have been sedentary for a long time or are seriously overweight, increase your level of activity slowly.

• Begin a formal exercise program that includes cardiorespiratory endurance exercise, strength training, and stretching.

• Develop techniques for handling stress. Try walking, or use a relaxation technique. Practice positive self-talk. Get adequate sleep.

• Develop strategies for coping with nonhunger cues to eat, such as boredom, sleepiness, or anxiety. Try calling a friend, taking a shower, or reading a magazine.

• Tell family members and friends that you're changing your eating and exercise habits. Ask them to be supportive.

Visit the Small Steps site for more tips (www.smallstep.gov).

Trade Commission reports that more than half of advertisements for weight-loss products made representations that are likely to be false.

Formula Drinks and Food Bars Canned diet drinks, powders used to make shakes, and diet food bars and snacks are designed to achieve weight loss by substituting for some or all of a person's daily food intake. However, most people find it difficult to use these products for long periods, and muscle loss and other serious health problems may result if they are used as the sole source of nutrition for an extended period. Use of such products sometimes results in rapid short-term weight loss, but the

weight is typically regained because users don't learn to change their eating and lifestyle behaviors.

Herbal Supplements Herbs are marketed as dietary supplements, so there is little information about effectiveness, proper dosage, drug interactions, and side effects. The FDA has banned the sale of ephedra (*ma huang*), stating that it presented a significant and unreasonable risk to human health. Ephedrine, the active ingredient in ephedra, is structurally similar to amphetamine and was widely used in weight-loss supplements. It may suppress appetite, but adverse effects have included elevated blood pressure, panic attacks, seizures, insomnia, and increased

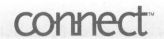

Is Any Diet Best for Weight Loss?

Many popular weight-loss plans promote specific food choices and macronutrient (protein, fat, carbohydrate) combinations as best for weight loss. Research findings have been mixed, but two points are clear. Total calorie intake matters, and the best diet is probably the one you can stick with.

Low-Carbohydrate Diets

Some low-carb diets advocate fewer than 10% of total calories from carbohydrates, compared to the 45–65% recommended by the Food and Nutrition Board. Some suggest daily carbohydrate intake below the 130 grams needed to provide essential carbohydrates in the diet. Small studies have found that low-carbohydrate diets can help with short-term weight loss and be safe for relatively short periods of time—although unpleasant effects such as bad breath, constipation, and headache are fairly common.

Some low-carb diets tend to be very high in protein and saturated fat and low in fiber, whole grains, vegetables, and fruits (and thus lack some essential nutrients). Such diets have been linked to an increased risk of heart disease, high blood pressure, and cancer. Other low-carb diets, though still emphasizing protein, limit saturated fats, allow most vegetables after an initial period, and advocate switching to "healthy carbs." These diets are healthier than the more extreme versions.

Low-Fat Diets

Many experts advocate diets that are relatively low in fat, high in carbohydrates, and moderate in protein. Critics of these diets blame them for rising rates of obesity. However, low-fat diets combined with physical activity can be safe and effective for many people.

The debate has highlighted the importance of total calorie intake and the quality of carbohydrate choices. A low-fat diet is not a license to consume excess calories, even in low-fat foods.

How Do Popular Diets Measure Up?

A 2005 study followed participants in four popular diets that emphasize different strategies—Weight Watchers (restricted portion sizes and calories), Atkins (low-carbohydrate, high-fat), Zone (relatively high protein, moderate fat and carbohydrate), and Ornish (very low fat). Each of these diets modestly reduced body weight and heart disease risk factors. There was no significant difference in weight loss at 1 year among the diets, and the more closely people adhered to each diet, the more weight they lost. Dropout rates were high—about 50% for Atkins and Ornish and 35% for Weight Watchers and Zone.

Energy Balance Counts: The National Weight Control Registry

Important lessons about energy balance can be drawn from the National Weight Control Registry, an ongoing study of people who have lost significant amounts of weight and kept it off. The average participant in the registry has lost 71 pounds and kept the weight off for more than 5 years. Nearly all participants use a combination of diet and exercise to manage their weight. Most consume diets moderate in calories and relatively low in fat and fried foods; they monitor their body weight and their food intake frequently. Participants engage in an average of 60 minutes of moderate physical activity daily. The National Weight Control Registry study illustrates that to lose weight and keep it off, you must decrease daily calorie intake and/or increase daily physical activity—and continue to do so over your lifetime.

SOURCES: Battle of the diet books II. 2006. *Nutrition Action Healthletter*, July/August; Dansinger, M. L., et al. 2005. Comparison of the Atkins, Ornish, Weight Watchers, and Zone diets for weight loss and heart disease risk reduction. *Journal of the American Medical Association* 293(1): 43–53; Hays, N. P., et al. 2004. Effects of an ad libitum low-fat, high-carbohydrate diet on body weight, body composition, and fat distribution in older men and women. *Archives of Internal Medicine* 164(2): 210–217. Hill, J., and R. Wing. 2003. The National Weight Control Registry. *Permanente Journal* 7(3): 34–37. Bravata, D. M., et al. 2003. Efficacy and safety of low-carbohydrate diets. *Journal of the American Medical Association* 289: 1837–1850; Foster, G. D., et al. 2003. A randomized trial of low-carbohydrate diet for obesity. *New England Journal of Medicine* 348: 2082–2090.

---

risk of heart attack or stroke, particularly when combined with another stimulant, such as caffeine. The FDA banned the synthetic stimulant phenylpropanolamine for similar reasons.

Other Supplements Fiber is another common ingredient in OTC diet aids, promoted for appetite control. However, dietary fiber acts as a bulking agent in the large intestine, not the stomach, so it doesn't have a pronounced effect on appetite. Other popular dietary supplements include conjugated linoleic acid, carnitine, chromium, pyruvate, calcium, B vitamins, chitosan, and a number of products labeled "fat absorbers," "fat blockers," and "starch blockers." Research has not found these products to be effective, and many have potentially adverse side effects.

Weight-Loss Programs

Weight-loss programs come in a variety of types, including noncommercial support organizations, commercial programs, Web sites, and clinical programs.

Noncommercial Weight-Loss Programs Noncommercial programs such as TOPS (Take Off Pounds Sensibly) and Overeaters Anonymous (OA) mainly provide group support. They do not advocate any particular diet but do recommend seeking professional advice for creating an individualized plan. These types of programs are generally free. Your physician or a registered dietitian can also provide information and support for weight loss.

Commercial Weight-Loss Programs Commercial weight-loss programs typically provide group support, nutrition education, physical activity recommendations, and behavior modification advice. Some also make available packaged foods to assist in following dietary advice.

A 2005 study evaluated major commercial weight-loss programs, including Weight Watchers, NutriSystem, Jenny Craig, and L A Weight Loss for 12 weeks or more with a 1-year follow-up assessment. Results showed Weight Watchers to be the only moderately priced commercial program with a mean loss of 5% of initial weight. A responsible and safe weight-loss program should have the following features:

- The recommended diet should be safe and balanced, include all the food groups, and meet the DRIs for all nutrients. Physical activity and exercise should be strongly encouraged.

- The program should promote slow, steady weight loss averaging 0.5–2.0 pounds per week.)

- If a participant plans to lose more than 20 pounds, has any health problems, or is taking medication on a regular basis, physician evaluation and monitoring should be recommended. The staff of the program should include qualified counselors and health professionals.

- The program should include plans for weight maintenance after the weight-loss phase is over.

- The program should provide information on all fees and costs, including those of supplements and prepackaged foods, as well as data on risks and expected outcomes of participating in the program.

A strong commitment and a plan for maintenance are especially important because only about 10–15% of program participants maintain their weight loss—the rest gain back all or more than they had lost. One study of participants found that regular exercise was the best predictor of maintaining weight loss, whereas frequent television viewing was the best predictor of weight gain.

Clinical Weight-Loss Programs   Medically supervised clinical programs are usually located in a hospital or other medical setting. Designed to help those who are severely obese, these programs typically involve a closely monitored very-low-calorie diet. The cost of a clinical program is usually high, but insurance will often cover part of the fee.

Prescription Drugs

The medications most often prescribed for weight loss are appetite suppressants that reduce feelings of hunger or increase feelings of fullness. Appetite suppressants usually work by increasing levels of catecholamine or serotonin, two brain chemicals that affect mood and appetite and may cause sleeplessness, nervousness, and euphoria. Sibutramine (Meridia) acts on both the serotonin and catecholamine systems; it may trigger increases in blood

pressure and heart rate. Headaches, constipation or diarrhea, dry mouth, and insomnia are other side effects.

A new drug, rimonabant (Acomplia) has been used successfully in Europe and is now awaiting FDA approval for use in the United States. It suppresses appetite by acting on certain brain receptors. Studies show that rimonabant may lead to greater weight loss than other drugs and may help users keep weight off for a longer time. Side effects include mild diarrhea, dizziness, and nausea, although studies show that some users also suffer psychological side effects such as depression and suicidal thoughts.

Studies have generally found that appetite suppressants produce modest weight loss—about 5–22 pounds above the loss expected with nondrug obesity treatments. Individuals respond very differently, however, and some experience more weight loss than others. Unfortunately, weight loss tends to level off or reverse after 4–6 months on a medication, and many people regain the weight they've lost when they stop taking the drug.

Prescription drugs are recommended only for people who have been unable to lose weight with nondrug options and who have a BMI over 30 (or over 27 if two or more additional risk factors such as diabetes and high blood pressure are present).

Surgery

It is estimated that 23 million Americans have a BMI greater than 35 (obese) and 8 million have a BMI greater than 40 (severely obese). Severe obesity is a serious medical condition that is often complicated by other health problems such as diabetes, sleep disorders, heart disease, and arthritis. Surgical intervention may be necessary as a treatment of last resort. According to the NIH, gastric bypass surgery is recommended for patients with a BMI greater than 40, or greater than 35 with obesity-related illnesses.

Gastric bypass surgery modifies the gastrointestinal tract by changing either the size of the stomach or how the intestine drains, thereby reducing food intake. However, surgery is not without risks. A 2006 study found that patients with poor cardiorespiratory fitness prior to surgery experienced more postoperative complications, including stroke, kidney failure, and even death, than patients with higher fitness levels.

BODY IMAGE

Developing a positive body image is an important aspect of psychological wellness and an important component of successful weight management.

Severe Body Image Problems

A person can become preoccupied with a perceived defect in appearance, thereby damaging self-esteem and interfering with relationships. Adolescents and adults who have a negative body image are more likely to diet restrictively, eat compulsively, or develop some other form of disordered eating.

When dissatisfaction becomes extreme, the condition is called *body dysmorphic disorder (BDD)*. BDD affects about 2% of Americans, males and females in equal numbers; BDD usually begins before age 18 but can begin in adulthood. Sufferers are overly concerned with physical appearance, often focusing on slight flaws that are not obvious to others. Low self-esteem is common. Individuals with BDD may spend hours every day thinking about their flaws and looking at themselves in mirrors; they may desire and seek repeated cosmetic surgeries. BDD is related to obsessive-compulsive disorder and can lead to depression, social phobia, and suicide if left untreated. An individual with BDD needs to get professional evaluation and treatment; medication and therapy can help people with BDD.

In some cases, body image may bear little resemblance to fact. A person suffering from the eating disorder anorexia nervosa typically has a severely distorted body image—she believes herself to be fat even when she has become emaciated. Distorted body image is also a hallmark of *muscle dysmorphia,* a disorder experienced by some bodybuilders and other active people in which they see themselves as small and out of shape despite being very muscular. Those who suffer from muscle dysmor-

phia may let obsessive bodybuilding interfere with their work and relationships. They may also use steroids and other potentially dangerous muscle-building drugs.

Acceptance and Change

There are limits to the changes that can be made to body weight and body shape, both of which are influenced by heredity. The changes that can and should be made are lifestyle changes.

Knowing when the limits to healthy change have been reached—and learning to accept those limits—is crucial for overall wellness. Obesity is a serious health risk, but weight management needs to take place in a positive and realistic atmosphere. For an obese person, losing as few as 10 pounds can reduce blood pressure and improve mood. The hazards of excessive dieting and overconcern about body weight need to be countered by a change in attitude. A reasonable weight must take into account a person's weight history, social circumstances, metabolic profile, and psychological well-being.

EATING DISORDERS

Problems with body weight and weight control are not limited to excessive body fat. A growing number of people, especially adolescent girls and young women, experience **eating disorders**, characterized by severe disturbances in body image, eating patterns, and eating-related behaviors. The major eating disorders are anorexia nervosa, bulimia nervosa, and binge-eating disorder. Disordered eating affects an estimated 10 million American females and 1 million males. About 90% of eating disorders begin during adolescence. In recent years, however, cases of eating disorders have increased among children as young as 8.

Anorexia Nervosa

A person with **anorexia nervosa** does not eat enough food to maintain a reasonable body weight. Anorexia affects about 3 million people, 95% of them female. Although it can occur later, anorexia typically develops between the ages of 12 and 18.

Characteristics of Anorexia Nervosa People with anorexia have an intense fear of gaining weight or becoming fat. Their body image is so distorted that even when

?

QUESTIONS FOR CRITICAL THINKING AND REFLECTION

Describe your own body image, in the fewest words possible. What satisfies you most and least about your body? Do you think your self-image is in line with the way others see you?

Gender, Ethnicity, and Body Image

Body Image and Gender

Women are much more likely than men to be dissatisfied with their bodies, often wanting to be thinner than they are. In one study, only 30% of eighth-grade girls reported being content with their bodies, while 70% of their male classmates expressed satisfaction with their looks.

One reason that girls and women are dissatisfied with their bodies is that they are influenced by the media—particularly advertisements and women's fashion magazines. Most teen girls report that the media influence their idea of the perfect body and their decision to diet. Some 75% of normal-weight women think they are overweight, and 90% overestimate their body size.

The image of the ideal woman presented in the media is often unrealistic and even unhealthy. In a review of BMI data for Miss America pageant winners since 1922, researchers noted a significant decline in BMI over time, with an increasing number of recent winners having BMIs in the "underweight" category. The average fashion model is 4–7 inches taller and almost 50 pounds lighter than the average American woman.

Our culture may be promoting an unattainable masculine ideal as well. Researchers studying male action figures such as GI Joe from the past 40 years noted that they have become increasingly muscular. A recent Batman action figure, if projected onto a man of average height, would result in someone with a 30-inch waist, 57-inch chest, and 27-inch biceps.

Body Image and Ethnicity

Although some groups espouse thinness as an ideal body type, others do not. In many traditional African societies, for example, full-figured women's bodies are seen as symbols of health, prosperity, and fertility. African American teenage girls have a much more positive body image than do white girls; in one survey, two-thirds of them defined beauty as "the right attitude," whereas white girls were more preoccupied with weight and body shape.

Nevertheless, recent evidence indicates that African American women are as likely to engage in disordered eating behavior, especially binge eating and vomiting, as their Latina, American Indian, and white counterparts.

Avoiding Body Image Problems

To minimize your risk of developing a body image problem, keep the following strategies in mind:

- Focus on healthy habits and good physical health.

- Focus on good psychological health and put concerns about physical appearance in perspective.

- Practice body acceptance. You can influence your body size and type to some degree through lifestyle, but the basic fact is that some people are genetically designed to be bigger or heavier than others.

- Find things to appreciate in yourself besides an idealized body image. What you can do is more important than how you look.

- See the beauty and fitness industries for what they are. Realize that one of their goals is to prompt dissatisfaction with yourself so that you will buy their products.

---

emaciated they think they are fat. People with anorexia may engage in compulsive behaviors or rituals that help keep them from eating, though some may also binge and **purge.** They often use vigorous and prolonged exercise to reduce body weight as well. Although they may express a great interest in food, even taking over the cooking responsibilities for the rest of the family, their own diet becomes more and more extreme. People with anorexia often hide or hoard food without eating it.

Anorexic people are typically introverted, emotionally reserved, and socially insecure. They are often model children who rarely complain and are anxious to please others and win their approval. Although school performance is typically above average, they are often critical of themselves and not satisfied with their accomplishments. For people with anorexia nervosa, their entire sense of self-esteem may be tied up in their evaluation of their body shape and weight.

Health Risks of Anorexia Nervosa Because of extreme weight loss, females with anorexia often stop menstruating, become intolerant of cold, and develop low blood pressure and heart rate. They develop dry skin that is often covered by fine body hair like that of an infant. Their hands and feet may swell and take on a blue tinge.

Anorexia nervosa has been linked to a variety of medical complications, including disorders of the cardiovascular, gastrointestinal, endocrine, and skeletal systems. When body fat is virtually gone and muscles are severely wasted, the body turns to its own organs in a desperate search for protein. Death can occur from heart failure caused by electrolyte imbalances. About one in ten women with anorexia dies of starvation, cardiac arrest, or other medical complications—the highest death rate for any psychiatric disorder. Depression is also a serious risk, and about half the fatalities related to anorexia are suicides.

eating disorder A serious disturbance in eating patterns or eating-related behavior, characterized by a negative body image and concerns about body weight or body fat.

anorexia nervosa An eating disorder characterized by a refusal to maintain body weight at a minimally healthy level and an intense fear of gaining weight or becoming fat; self-starvation.

purging The use of vomiting, laxatives, excessive exercise, restrictive dieting, enemas, diuretics, or diet pills to compensate for food that has been eaten and that the person fears will produce weight gain.

TERMS

Bulimia Nervosa

A person suffering from **bulimia nervosa** engages in recurrent episodes of binge eating followed by purging. Bulimia is often difficult to recognize because sufferers conceal their eating habits and usually maintain a normal weight, although they may experience weight fluctuations of 10–15 pounds. Although bulimia usually begins in adolescence or young adulthood, it has begun to emerge at increasingly younger (11–12 years) and older (40–60 years) ages.

Characteristics of Bulimia Nervosa   During a binge, a bulimic person may rapidly consume thousands of calories. This is followed by an attempt to get rid of the food by purging, usually by vomiting or using laxatives or diuretics. During a binge, bulimics feel as though they have lost control and cannot stop or limit how much they eat. Some binge and purge only occasionally; others do so many times every day.

People with bulimia may appear to eat normally, but they are rarely comfortable around food. Binges usually occur in secret and can become nightmarish—raiding the kitchen for food, going from one grocery store to another to buy food, or even stealing food. During the binge, food acts as an anesthetic, and all feelings are blocked out. Afterward, bulimics feel physically drained and emotionally spent. They usually feel deeply ashamed and disgusted with both themselves and their behavior and terrified that they will gain weight from the binge.

Major life changes such as leaving for college, getting married, having a baby, or losing a job can trigger a binge-purge cycle. At such times, stress is high and the person may have no good outlet for emotional conflict or tension. As with anorexia, bulimia sufferers are often insecure and depend on others for approval and self-esteem. They may hide difficult emotions such as anger and disappointment from themselves and others. Binge eating and purging become a way of dealing with feelings.

Health Risks of Bulimia Nervosa   The binge-purge cycle of bulimia places a tremendous strain on the body. Contact with vomited stomach acids erodes tooth enamel. Repeated vomiting or the use of laxatives, in combination with deficient calorie intake, can damage the liver and kidneys and cause cardiac arrhythmia. Chronic hoarseness and esophageal tearing with bleeding may also result

from vomiting. More rarely, binge eating can lead to rupture of the stomach. Although less often associated with suicide or premature death than anorexia, bulimia is associated with increased depression, excessive preoccupation with food and body image, and sometimes disturbances in cognitive functioning.

Binge-Eating Disorder

Binge-eating disorder affects about 2% of American adults. It is characterized by uncontrollable eating, usually followed by feelings of guilt and shame with weight gain. Common eating patterns are eating more rapidly than normal, eating until uncomfortably full, eating when not hungry, and preferring to eat alone. Binge eaters may eat large amounts of food throughout the day, with no planned mealtimes. Many people with binge-eating disorder mistakenly see rigid dieting as the only solution to their problem. However, rigid dieting usually causes feelings of deprivation and a return to overeating.

Compulsive overeaters rarely eat because of hunger. Instead, food is used as a means of coping with stress, conflict, and other difficult emotions or to provide solace and entertainment. People who do not have the resources to deal effectively with stress may be more vulnerable to binge-eating disorder. Inappropriate overeating often begins during childhood. In some families, eating may be used as an activity to fill otherwise empty time. Parents may reward children with food for good behavior or withhold food as a means of punishment, thereby creating distorted feelings about the use of food.

Binge eaters are almost always obese, so they face all the health risks associated with obesity. In addition, binge eaters may have higher rates of depression and anxiety.

Borderline Disordered Eating

Eating habits and body image run a continuum from healthy to seriously disordered. Where each of us falls along that continuum can change depending on life stresses, illnesses, and many other factors. People with borderline disordered eating have some symptoms of eating disorders but do not meet the full diagnostic criteria for anorexia, bulimia, or binge-eating disorder. Behaviors such as excessive dieting, occasional bingeing or purging, or the inability to control eating turn food into the enemy and create havoc in the lives of millions of Americans.

How do you know if you have disordered eating habits? When thoughts about food and weight dominate your life, you have a problem. If you're convinced that your worth as a person hinges on how you look and how much you weigh, it's time to get help. Other danger signs include frequent feelings of guilt after a meal or snack, any use of vomiting or laxatives after meals, or overexercising or severely restricting your food intake to compensate for what you've already eaten.

TERMS

bulimia nervosa   An eating disorder characterized by recurrent episodes of binge eating and purging—overeating and then using compensatory behaviors such as vomiting, laxatives, and excessive exercise to prevent weight gain.

binge-eating disorder   An eating disorder characterized by binge eating and a lack of control over eating behavior in general.

If you suspect you have an eating problem, don't go it alone or delay getting help, as disordered eating habits can develop into a full-blown eating disorder. Check with your student health or counseling center—nearly all colleges have counselors and medical personnel who can help you or refer you to a specialist if needed.

Treating Eating Disorders

The treatment of eating disorders must address both problematic eating behaviors and the misuse of food to manage stress and emotions. Anorexia nervosa treatment first involves averting a medical crisis by restoring adequate body weight; then the psychological aspects of the disorder can be addressed. The treatment of bulimia nervosa or binge-eating disorder involves first stabilizing the eating patterns, then identifying and changing the patterns of thinking that led to disordered eating, and then improving coping skills. Concurrent problems, such as depression or anxiety, must also be addressed.

In 2006, a study published in the *Journal of the American Medical Association* showed that the antidepressant Prozac, which is widely used to treat anorexia, worked no better than a placebo in preventing recurrence in women recovering from the disorder. However, the anti-seizure drug topiramate has shown promise in the treatment of bulimia by reducing the urges to binge and purge.

Treatment of eating disorders usually involves a combination of psychotherapy and medical management. The therapy may be carried out individually or in a group; sessions involving the entire family may be recommended. A support or self-help group can be a useful adjunct to such treatment.

QUESTIONS FOR CRITICAL THINKING AND REFLECTION

Do you know someone you suspect may suffer from an eating disorder? Does the advice in this chapter seem helpful to you? Do you think you could follow it? Why or why not? Have you ever experienced disordered eating patterns yourself? If so, can you identify the reasons for it?

TIPS FOR TODAY AND THE FUTURE

Many approaches work, but the simplest formula for weight management is moderate food intake coupled with regular exercise.

RIGHT NOW YOU CAN
- Assess your weight-management needs. Do you need to gain weight, lose weight, or stay at your current weight?
- List five things you can do to add more physical activity (not exercise) to your daily routine.
- Identify the foods you regularly eat that may be sabotaging your ability to manage your weight.

IN THE FUTURE YOU CAN
- Make an honest assessment of your current body image. Is it accurate and fair, or is it unduly negative and unhealthy? If your body image presents a problem, consider getting professional advice on how to view yourself realistically.
- Keep track of your energy needs to determine whether your energy balance equation is correct. Use this information as part of your long-term weight-management efforts.

SUMMARY

- Body composition is the relative amounts of fat-free mass and fat in the body. *Overweight* and *obesity* refer to body weight or the percentage of body fat that exceeds what is associated with good health.

- The key to weight management is maintaining a balance of calories in (food) and calories out (resting metabolism, food digestion, and physical activity).

- Standards for assessing body weight and body composition include body mass index (BMI) and percent body fat.

- Too much or too little body fat is linked to health problems; the distribution of body fat can also be a significant risk factor.

- An inaccurate or negative body image is common and can lead to psychological distress.

- Factors involved in the regulation of body weight and body fat include heredity and metabolic rate.

- Nutritional guidelines for weight management include consuming a moderate number of calories; limiting portion sizes, energy density, and the intake of fat, simple sugars, refined carbohydrates, and protein to recommended levels; and developing an eating schedule and rules for food choices.

A Weight-Management Program

The behavior management plan described in Chapter 1 provides an excellent framework for a weight-management program. Following are some suggestions about specific ways you can adapt that general plan to controlling your weight.

Motivation and Commitment

Make sure you are motivated and committed before you begin. Failure at weight loss is a frustrating experience that can make it more difficult to lose weight in the future. Think about why you want to lose weight. Self-focused reasons, such as to feel good about yourself or to have a greater sense of well-being, are often associated with success. Trying to lose weight for others or out of concern for how others view you is a poor foundation for a weight-loss program. Make a list of your reasons for wanting to lose weight, and post it in a prominent place.

Setting Goals

Choose a reasonable weight you think you would like to reach over the long term, and be willing to renegotiate it as you get further along. Break down your long-term weight and behavioral goals into a series of short-term goals. Develop a new way of behaving by designing small, manageable steps that will get you to where you want to go.

Creating a Negative Energy Balance

When your weight is constant, you are burning approximately the same number of calories as you are taking in. To tip the energy balance toward weight loss, you must either consume fewer calories, or burn more calories through physical activity, or both. One pound of body fat represents 3500 calories. To lose weight at the recommended rate of 0.5–2.0 pounds per week, you must create a negative energy balance of 1750–7000 calories per week or 250–1000 calories per day. To generate a negative energy balance, it's usually best to begin by increasing activity level rather than decreasing your calorie consumption.

Physical Activity

Consider how you can increase your energy output simply by increasing routine physical activity, such as walking or taking the stairs. (Chapter 10 lists activities that use about 150 calories.) If you are not already involved in a regular exercise routine aimed at increasing endurance and building or maintaining muscle mass, seek help from someone who is competent to help you plan and start an appropriate exercise routine. If you are already doing regular physical exercise, evaluate your program according to the guidelines in Chapter 10.

Don't try to use exercise to spot reduce. Leg lifts, for example, contribute to fat loss only to the extent that they burn calories; they don't burn fat just from your legs. You can make parts of your body appear more fit by exercising them, but the only way you can reduce fat in any specific part of your body is to create an overall negative energy balance.

Diet and Eating Habits

If you can't generate a large enough negative energy balance solely by increasing physical activity, you may want to supplement exercise with modest cuts in your calorie intake. Don't think of this as going on a diet; your goal is to make small changes in your diet that you can maintain for a lifetime. Focus on cutting your intake of saturated and trans fats and added sugars and on eating a variety of nutritious foods in moderation. Don't skip meals, fast, or go on a very-low-calorie diet or a diet that is unbalanced.

Making changes in eating habits is another important strategy for weight management. If your program centers on a conscious restriction of certain food items, you're likely to spend all your time thinking about the forbidden foods. Focus on *how* to eat rather than *what* to eat. Refer to the box "Lifestyle Strategies for Successful Weight Management" for suggestions.

Self-Monitoring

Keep a record of your weight and behavior change progress. Try keeping a record of everything you eat. Write down what you plan to eat, in what quantity, *before* you eat. You'll find that just having to record something that is not OK to eat is likely to stop you from eating it. If you also note what seems to be triggering your urges to eat (for example, you feel bored, or someone offered you something), you'll become more aware of your weak spots and be better able to take corrective action. Also, keep track of your daily activities and your formal exercise program so you can monitor increases in physical activity.

Putting Your Plan into Action

- Examine the environmental cues that trigger poor eating and exercise habits, and devise strategies for dealing with them. For example, you may need to remove problem foods from your house temporarily or put a sign on the refrigerator reminding you to go for a walk instead of having a snack. Anticipate problem situations, and plan ways to handle them more effectively.

- Create new environmental cues that will support your new healthy behaviors. Put your walking shoes by the front door. Move fruits and vegetables to the front of the refrigerator.

- Get others to help. Talk to friends and family members about what they can do to support your efforts. Find a buddy to join you in your exercise program.

- Give yourself lots of praise and rewards. Think about your accomplishments and achievements and congratulate yourself. Plan special nonfood treats for yourself, such as a walk or a movie. Reward yourself often and for anything that counts toward success.

- If you slip, tell yourself to get back on track immediately, and don't waste time on self-criticism. Think positively instead of getting into a cycle of guilt and self-blame. Don't demand too much of yourself.

- Don't get discouraged. Be aware that although weight loss is bound to slow down after the first loss of body fluid, the weight loss at this slower rate is more permanent than earlier, more dramatic, losses.

- Remember that weight management is a lifelong project. You need to adopt reasonable goals and strategies that you can maintain over the long term.

- Activity guidelines for weight management emphasize daily physical activity and regular sessions of cardiorespiratory endurance exercise and strength training.

- Weight management requires developing positive, realistic self-talk and self-esteem and a repertoire of appropriate techniques for handling stress and other emotional and physical challenges.

- People can be successful at long-term weight loss on their own, by combining diet and exercise.

- OTC diet aids and supplements and formal weight-loss programs should be assessed for safety and efficacy.

- Professional help is needed in cases of severe obesity; medical treatments include prescription drugs, surgery, and psychological therapy.

- Dissatisfaction with weight and shape are common to all eating disorders. Anorexia nervosa is characterized by self-starvation, distorted body image, and an intense fear of gaining weight. Bulimia nervosa is characterized by recurrent episodes of uncontrolled binge eating and frequent purging. Binge-eating disorder involves binge eating without regular use of compensatory purging.

FOR MORE INFORMATION

BOOKS

Dillon, E. 2006. *Issues That Concern You: Obesity.* New York: Greenhaven Press. *A collection of perspectives on the causes of obesity, its management, and its impact on individuals and society.*

Gaesser, G. A., and K. Kratina. 2006. *It's the Calories, Not the Carbs.* Victoria, B.C.: Trafford. *Provides a detailed look at the facts behind successful weight loss by shunning fad diets and practicing sound energy balance.*

Hensrud, D. D. 2005. *Mayo Clinic Healthy Weight for Everyone.* Rochester, Minn.: Mayo Clinic. *Provides guidelines for successful weight management.*

Milchovich, S. K., and B. Dunn-Long. 2007. *Diabetes Mellitus: A Practical Handbook,* 9th. ed. Boulder, Colo.: Bull. *A user-friendly guide to diabetes.*

ORGANIZATIONS, HOTLINES, AND WEB SITES

American Diabetes Association. Provides information, a free newsletter, and referrals to local support groups; the Web site includes an online diabetes risk assessment.

http://www.diabetes.org

FDA Center for Food Safety and Applied Nutrition: Dietary Supplements. Provides background facts and information on the current regulatory status of dietary supplements, including compounds marketed for weight loss.

http://www.cfsan.fda.gov/~dms/supplmnt.html

Federal Trade Commission (FTC): Project Waistline. Provides advice for evaluating advertising about weight-loss products.

http://www.ftc.gov/bcp/conline/edcams/waistline/index.html

National Heart, Lung, and Blood Institute (NHLBI): Aim for a Healthy Weight. Provides information and tips on diet and physical activity, as well as a BMI calculator.

http://www.nhlbi.nih.gov/health/public/heart/obesity/lose_wt

National Institute of Diabetes and Digestive and Kidney Diseases (NIDDK). Provides information and referrals for problems related to obesity, weight control, and nutritional disorders.

http://win.niddk.nih.gov/

SmallStep.gov. Provides resources for increasing activity and improving diet through small changes in daily habits.

http://www.smallstep.gov

U.S. Consumer Gateway: Health—Dieting and Weight Control. Provides links to government sites with advice on evaluating claims about weight-loss products and programs.

http://www.consumer.gov/health.htm

USDA Food and Nutrition Information Center: Weight and Obesity. Provides links to recent reports and studies on the issue of obesity among Americans.

http://www.nal.usda.gov/fnic/reports/obesity.html

Resources for people concerned about eating disorders:

Eating Disorder Referral and Information Center
http://www.edreferral.com

MedlinePlus: Eating Disorders
http://www.nlm.nih.gov/medlineplus/eatingdisorders.html

National Association of Anorexia Nervosa and Associated Disorders
847-831-3438 (referral line)
http://www.anad.org

National Eating Disorders Association
800-931-2237
http://www.nationaleatingdisorders.org

SELECTED BIBLIOGRAPHY

Adams, K. F., et al. 2006. Overweight, obesity, and mortality in a large prospective cohort of persons 50 to 71 years old. *New England Journal of Medicine* 355(8): 763–778.

Baker, B. 2006. Weight loss and diet plans. *American Journal of Nursing* 106(6): 52–59.

Behn, A., and E. Ur. 2006. The obesity epidemic and its cardiovascular consequences. *Current Opinions in Cardiology* 21(4): 353–360.

Centers for Disease Control and Prevention. 2006. *Diabetes Care.* Atlanta, Ga.: U.S. Department of Health and Human Services, Centers for Disease Control and Prevention.

Centers for Disease Control and Prevention. 2008. *National Diabetes Fact Sheet: General Information and National Estimates on Diabetes in the United States, 2007.* Atlanta, Ga: U.S. Department of Health and Human Services, Centers for Disease Control and Prevention.

Chandon, P., and B. Wansink. 2007. The biasing health halos of fast-food restaurant health claims: Lower calorie estimates and higher side-dish consumption intentions. *Journal of Consumer Research* 34(3): 301–314.

Dhingra, R., et al. 2007. Soft drink consumption and risk of developing cardiometabolic risk factors and the metabolic syndrome in middle-aged adults in the community. *Circulation* 116(5): 480–488.

Drewnowski, A., and F. Bellisle. 2007. Liquid calories, sugar and body weight. *American Journal of Clinical Nutrition* 85(3): 651–661.

Flegal, K. M., et al. 2005. Excess deaths associated with underweight, overweight, and obesity. *Journal of the American Medical Association* 293(15): 1861–1867.

Hamilton, M., et al. 2007. Role of low energy expenditure and sitting in obesity, metabolic syndrome, type 2 diabetes, and cardiovascular disease. *Diabetes* 56(11): 2655–2667.

Kumanyika, S. K, et al. 2008. Population-based prevention of obesity: The need for comprehensive promotion of healthful eating, physical activity, and energy balance: A scientific statement from American Heart Association Council on Epidemiology and Prevention, Interdisciplinary Committee for Prevention (formerly the Expert Panel on Population and Prevention Science). *Circulation* 118(4): 428–464.

McCullough, P. A., et al. 2006. Cardiorespiratory fitness and short-term complications after bariatric surgery. *CHEST* 130: 517–525.

Muenning, P., et al. 2006. Gender and the burden of disease attributable to obesity. *American Journal of Public Health* 96(9): 1662–1668.

O'Brien, P., et al. 2006. Treatment of mild to moderate obesity with laparoscopic adjustable gastric banding or an intensive medical program. *Annals of Internal Medicine* 144(9): 625–633.

Ogden, C. L., et al. 2007. Obesity among adults in the United States: No change since 2003–2004. *National Center for Health Statistics Data Brief* 1: 1–8.

Olshansky, S. J., et al. 2005. A potential decline in life expectancy in the United States in the 21st century. *New England Journal of Medicine* 352(11): 1138–1145.

Tsai, A. G., and T. A. Wadden. 2005. Systematic review: An evaluation of major commercial weight loss programs in the United States. *Annals of Internal Medicine* 142(1): 56–66.

van Dam, R. M., et al. 2006. The relationship between overweight in adolescence and premature death in women. *Annals of Internal Medicine* 145(2): 91–97.

Vorona, R. D., et al. 2005. Overweight and obese patients in a primary care population report less sleep than patients with a normal body mass index. *Archives of Internal Medicine* 165: 25–30.

Wang, Y., and M. A. Beydoun. 2007. The obesity epidemic in the United States—gender, age, socioeconomic, racial/ethnic and geographical characteristics: A systematic review and meta-regression analysis. *Epidemiologic Reviews* 29: 6–28.

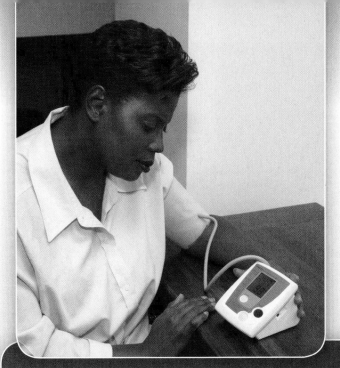

LOOKING AHEAD>>>>>

AFTER READING THIS CHAPTER, YOU SHOULD BE ABLE TO:

- List the major components of the cardiovascular system and describe how blood is pumped and circulated throughout the body

- Describe the controllable and uncontrollable risk factors associated with cardiovascular disease

- Discuss the major forms of cardiovascular disease and how they develop

- Explain what cancer is and how it spreads

- List and describe common cancers—their risk factors, signs and symptoms, treatments, and approaches to prevention

- List the steps you can take to lower your personal risk of cardiovascular disease and cancer

CARDIOVASCULAR DISEASE AND CANCER

12

Cardiovascular disease (CVD) affects about 80 million Americans and is the leading cause of death in the United States, claiming one life every 37 seconds—about 2400 Americans every day. Heart attacks and strokes are the number-one and number-three causes of death, respectively, making them the most common life-threatening manifestations of CVD. Cancer is the second leading cause of death in the United States, claiming about 565,000 lives annually—about 1500 each day. Although age, genetics, and the environment play roles in the development of CVD and cancers, these diseases are primarily lifestyle diseases, linked to many controllable lifestyle factors. This chapter describes the forms and causes of these two diseases and provides information about how you can reduce your risk of developing and dying from CVD or cancer.

THE CARDIOVASCULAR SYSTEM

The **cardiovascular system** consists of the heart and blood vessels (Figure 12.1); together, they move blood throughout the body.

The heart is a four-chambered, fist-sized muscle located just beneath the sternum (breastbone). It pumps deoxygenated (oxygen-poor) blood to the lungs and delivers oxygenated (oxygen-rich) blood to the rest of the body. Blood actually travels through two separate circulatory systems (Figure 12.2): The right side of the heart pumps blood to the lungs in what is called **pulmonary circulation,** and the left side pumps blood through the rest of the body in **systemic circulation.**

Waste-laden, oxygen-poor blood travels the **venae cavae,** into the heart's right upper chamber, or **atrium.** After the right atrium fills, it contracts and pumps blood into

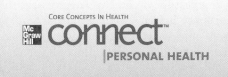

http://www.mcgrawhillconnect.com/personalhealth

the heart's right lower chamber, or **ventricle.** When the right ventricle is full, it contracts and pumps blood through the pulmonary artery into the lungs. There, blood picks up oxygen and discards carbon dioxide. Cleaned, oxygenated blood then flows from the lungs through the pulmonary veins into the left atrium. After this chamber fills, it contracts and pumps blood into the left ventricle, which then pumps blood through the **aorta**—the body's largest artery—for distribution to the rest of the body's blood vessels. The period of the heart's contraction is called **systole;** the period of relaxation is called **diastole.**

Blood vessels are classified by size and function. **Veins** carry blood to the heart. **Arteries** carry blood away from the heart. Veins have thin walls, but arteries have thick elastic walls that enable them to

TERMS

cardiovascular disease (CVD) The collective term for various diseases of the heart and blood vessels.

cardiovascular system The system that circulates blood through the body; consists of the heart and blood vessels.

pulmonary circulation The part of the circulatory system governed by the right side of the heart; the circulation of blood between the heart and the lungs.

systemic circulation The part of the circulatory system governed by the left side of the heart; the circulation of blood between the heart and the rest of the body.

vena cava Either of two large veins through which blood is returned to the right atrium of the heart.

atria The two upper chambers of the heart in which blood collects before passing to the ventricles.

ventricles The two lower chambers of the heart that pump blood through arteries to the lungs and other parts of the body.

aorta The large artery that receives blood from the left ventricle and distributes it to the body.

systole Contraction phase of the heart.

diastole Relaxation phase of the heart.

veins Vessels that carry blood to the heart.

arteries Vessels that carry blood away from the heart.

capillaries Very small blood vessels that serve to exchange oxygen and nutrients between the blood and the tissues.

coronary arteries A system of arteries branching from the aorta that provides blood to the heart muscle.

platelets Cell fragments in the blood that are necessary for the formation of blood clots.

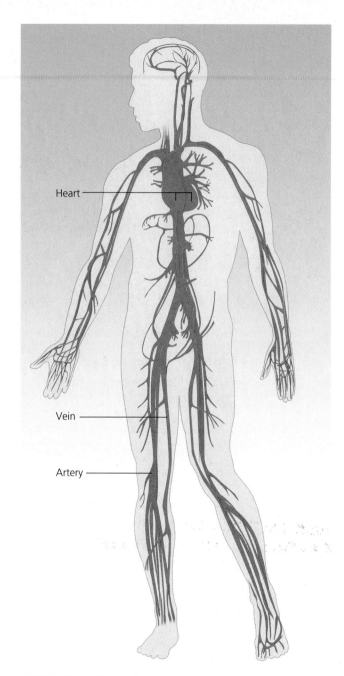

FIGURE 12.1 The cardiovascular system.

expand and relax with the volume of blood being pumped through them. After leaving the heart, the aorta branches into smaller and smaller vessels. The smallest arteries branch still further into **capillaries,** tiny vessels only one cell thick. The capillaries deliver oxygen and nutrient-rich blood to the tissues and pick up oxygen-poor, waste-laden blood. From the capillaries, this blood empties into small veins and then into larger veins that return it to the heart to repeat the cycle. Two large vessels, the right and left **coronary arteries,** branch off the aorta and supply the heart muscle with oxygenated blood. Blockage of a coronary artery is a leading cause of heart attacks.

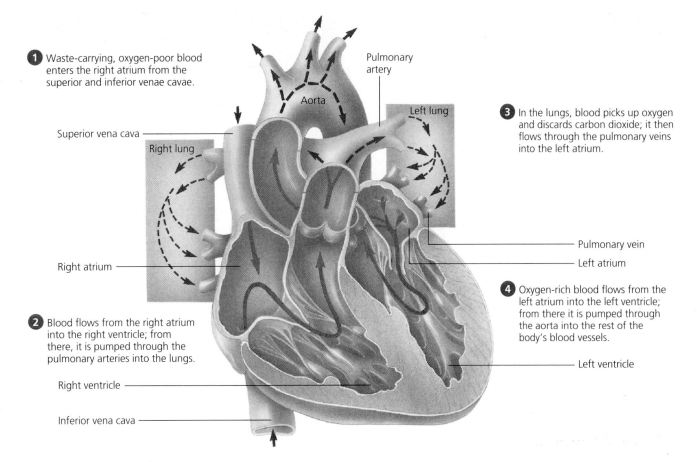

**① **Waste-carrying, oxygen-poor blood enters the right atrium from the superior and inferior venae cavae.

Pulmonary artery

Aorta

Left lung

**③ **In the lungs, blood picks up oxygen and discards carbon dioxide; it then flows through the pulmonary veins into the left atrium.

Superior vena cava

Right lung

Pulmonary vein

Left atrium

Right atrium

**④ **Oxygen-rich blood flows from the left atrium into the left ventricle; from there it is pumped through the aorta into the rest of the body's blood vessels.

**② **Blood flows from the right atrium into the right ventricle; from there, it is pumped through the pulmonary arteries into the lungs.

Right ventricle

Left ventricle

Inferior vena cava

FIGURE 12.2   Circulation in the heart.

RISK FACTORS FOR CARDIOVASCULAR DISEASE

Researchers have identified a variety of factors associated with an increased risk of developing CVD. They are grouped into two categories: major risk factors and contributing risk factors. Some risk factors are linked to controllable aspects of lifestyle and can therefore be changed. Others are beyond your control.

Major Risk Factors That Can Be Changed

The American Heart Association (AHA) has identified six major risk factors for CVD that can be changed: tobacco use,

high blood pressure, unhealthy blood cholesterol levels, physical inactivity, overweight and obesity, and diabetes.

Tobacco Use   About one in five deaths from CVD is attributable to smoking. People who smoke a pack of cigarettes a day have twice the risk of heart attack as nonsmokers; smoking two or more packs a day triples the risk. When smokers have heart attacks, they are two to three times more likely than nonsmokers to die from them. Cigarette smoking also doubles the risk of stroke.

Smoking harms the cardiovascular system in several ways. It damages the lining of arteries. It reduces the level of high-density lipoproteins (HDL), or "good" cholesterol and raises the levels of triglycerides and low-density lipoproteins (LDL), or "bad" cholesterol. Nicotine increases blood pressure and heart rate. The carbon monoxide in cigarette smoke displaces oxygen in the blood, reducing the oxygen available to the body. Smoking causes **platelets** to stick together in the blood stream, leading to clotting, and it also speeds the development of fatty deposits in the arteries.

You don't have to smoke to be affected. The risk of death from coronary heart disease increases up to 30% among those exposed to environmental tobacco smoke (ETS) at home or at work. Researchers estimate that about 35,000 nonsmokers die from heart disease each year as a result of exposure to ETS.

QUESTIONS FOR CRITICAL THINKING AND REFLECTION

How often do you give thought to the health of your heart? Are there certain situations, for example, that make you aware of your heart rate, or make you wonder how strong your heart is?

High Blood Pressure High blood pressure, or **hypertension,** is a risk factor for many forms of cardiovascular disease, including heart attacks and strokes, and is itself considered a form of CVD.

Blood pressure, the force exerted by the blood on the vessel walls, is created by the pumping action of the heart. High blood pressure occurs when too much force is exerted against the walls of the arteries. Many factors affect blood pressure, such as exercise or excitement. Short periods of high blood pressure are normal, but chronic high blood pressure is a health risk.

Blood pressure is measured with a stethoscope and an instrument called a *sphygmomanometer.* It is expressed as two numbers—for example, 120 over 80—and measured in millimeters of mercury. The first number is the systolic blood pressure; the second is the diastolic blood pressure. A normal blood pressure reading for a healthy adult is below 120 systolic and below 80 diastolic; CVD risk increases when blood pressure rises above 120 over 80. High blood pressure in adults is defined as equal to or greater than 140 over 90 (Table 12.1).

High blood pressure results from an increased output of blood by the heart or from increased resistance to blood flow in the arteries. The latter condition can be caused by constriction of smooth muscle surrounding the arteries or by **atherosclerosis,** a disease process that causes arteries to become clogged and narrowed. High blood pressure also scars and hardens arteries, making them less elastic and further increasing blood pressure. When a person has high blood pressure, the heart must work harder than normal to force blood through the narrowed and stiffened arteries, straining both the heart and arteries. High blood pressure is often called a silent killer, because it usually has no symptoms. A person may have high blood pressure for years without realizing it. But during that time, it damages vital organs and increases the risk of heart attack, congestive heart failure, stroke, kidney failure, and blindness.

PREVALENCE Hypertension is common, and its incidence increases with age. The rate of hypertension is highest in

| Table 12.1 | Blood Pressure Classification for Healthy Adults |

Category[a]	Systolic (mm Hg)		Diastolic (mm Hg)
Normal[b]	below 120	and	below 80
Prehypertension	120–139	or	80–89
Hypertension[c]			
Stage 1	140–159	or	90–99
Stage 2	160 and above	or	100 and above

[a]When systolic and diastolic pressure fall into different categories, the higher category should be used to classify blood pressure status.

[b]The risk of death from heart attack and stroke begins to rise when blood pressure is above 115/75.

[c]Based on the average of two or more readings taken at different physician visits. In persons over 50, systolic blood pressure greater than 140 is a much more significant CVD risk factor than diastolic blood pressure.

SOURCE: *The Seventh Report of the Joint National Committee on Prevention, Detection, Evaluation, and Treatment of High Blood Pressure.* 2003. Bethesda, Md.: National Heart, Lung, and Blood Institute. National Institutes of Health (NIH Publication No. 03-5233).

African Americans (41%), in whom, compared with other groups, the disorder is often more severe, more resistant to treatment, and more likely to be fatal at an early age.

Primary hypertension cannot be cured, but it can be controlled. Because hypertension has no early warning signs, it's crucial to have your blood pressure tested at least once every 2 years (more often if you have other CVD risk factors). Lifestyle changes are recommended for everyone with prehypertension and hypertension. These changes include weight reduction, regular exercise, a healthy diet, and moderation of alcohol use. The DASH diet is recommended; it emphasizes eating more fruits, vegetables, and whole grains and increasing potassium and fiber intake. Even small increases in fruit and vegetable intake can create measurable drops in blood pressure. Sodium restriction is also helpful for most people with hypertension. The 2005 Dietary Guidelines for Americans recommend restricting sodium consumption to less than 2300 mg (about 1 teaspoon of salt) per day. People with hypertension, African Americans, and middle-aged and older adults should aim to consume no more than 1500 mg of sodium per day. For people whose blood pressure isn't adequately controlled with lifestyle changes, medication is prescribed.

Recent research has shed new light on the importance of lowering blood pressure to improve cardiovascular

About 32% of Americans with high blood pressure aren't aware of their condition.

—American Heart Association, 2009

QUICK STATS

TERMS

hypertension Sustained abnormally high blood pressure.

atherosclerosis A form of CVD in which the inner layers of artery walls are made thick and irregular by plaque deposits; arteries become narrow, and blood supply is reduced.

lipoproteins Protein-and-lipid substances in the blood that carry fats and cholesterol; classified according to size, density, and chemical composition.

low-density lipoprotein (LDL) A lipoprotein containing a moderate amount of protein and a large amount of cholesterol, "bad" cholesterol.

high-density lipoprotein (HDL) A lipoprotein containing relatively little cholesterol that helps transport cholesterol out of the arteries and thus protects against heart diseases; "good" cholesterol.

health. Death rates from CVD begin to rise when blood pressure is above 115 over 75, well below the traditional 140 over 90 cutoff for hypertension. People with blood pressure in the prehypertension range are at increased risk of heart attack and stroke as well as at significant risk of developing full-blown hypertension.

High Cholesterol   Cholesterol is a fatty, waxlike substance that circulates through the bloodstream and is an important component of cell membranes, sex hormones, vitamin D, the fluid that coats the lungs, and the protective sheaths around nerves. Adequate cholesterol is essential for the proper functioning of the body. Excess cholesterol, however, can clog arteries and increase the risk of CVD. Your liver manufactures cholesterol; you also get cholesterol from the foods you eat.

GOOD VERSUS BAD CHOLESTEROL   Cholesterol is carried in the blood in protein-lipid packages called **lipoproteins. Low-density lipoproteins (LDLs)** shuttle cholesterol from the liver to the organs and tissues that require it. LDL is known as "bad" cholesterol because if there is more than the body can use, the excess is deposited in the blood vessels. If coronary arteries are blocked, the result may be a heart attack; if an artery carrying blood to the brain is blocked, a stroke may occur. **High-density lipoproteins (HDLs)**, or "good" cholesterol, shuttle unused cholesterol back to the liver for recycling. By removing cholesterol from blood vessels, HDL helps protect against atherosclerosis.

RECOMMENDED BLOOD CHOLESTEROL LEVELS   The risk for cardiovascular disease increases with higher blood cholesterol levels, especially LDL. The National Cholesterol Education Program (NCEP) recommends lipoprotein testing at least once every 5 years for all adults, beginning at age 20. The recommended test measures total cholesterol, LDL cholesterol, HDL cholesterol, and triglycerides (another blood fat). In general, high LDL, total cholesterol, and triglyceride levels combined with low HDL levels, are associated with a higher risk for CVD. You can reduce this risk by lowering LDL, total cholesterol, and triglycerides. Raising HDL is important because a high HDL level seems to offer protection from CVD even in cases where total cholesterol is high. This seems to be especially true for women.

As shown in Table 12.2, LDL levels below 100 mg/dl (milligrams per deciliter) and total cholesterol levels below 200 mg/dl are desirable. An estimated 99 million American adults have total cholesterol levels of 200 mg/dl or higher. The CVD risk associated with elevated cholesterol levels also depends on other factors. For example, an above-optimal level of LDL would be of more concern for an individual who also smokes and has high blood pressure than for someone without these additional CVD risk factors, and it is especially a concern for diabetics.

BENEFITS OF CONTROLLING CHOLESTEROL   Important dietary changes for reducing LDL levels include increasing fiber

Table 12.2	Cholesterol Guidelines
Total cholesterol (mg/dl)	
Less than 200	Desirable
200–239	Borderline high
240 or more	High
LDL cholesterol (mg/dl)	
Less than 100	Optimal
100–129	Near optimal/above optimal
130–159	Borderline high
160–189	High
190 or more	Very high
HDL cholesterol (mg/dl)	
Less than 40	Low (undesirable)
60 or more	High (desirable)
Triglycerides (mg/dl)	
Less than 150	Normal
150–199	Borderline high
200–499	High
500 or more	Very high

SOURCE: Expert Panel on Detection, Evaluation, and Treatment of High Blood Cholesterol in Adults. 2001. Executive Summary of the Third Report of the National Cholesterol Education Program (NCEP) Expert Panel on Detection, Evaluation, and Treatment of High Blood Cholesterol in Adults (Adult Treatment Panel III). *Journal of the American Medical Association* 285(19).

intake and substituting unsaturated for saturated and trans fats. Decreasing saturated and trans fats is particularly important because they promote the production of cholesterol by the liver. Exercising regularly and eating more fruits, vegetables, fish, and whole grains also help. You can raise your HDL levels by exercising regularly, losing weight if you are overweight, quitting smoking, and altering the amount and type of fat you consume.

> A **10%** decrease in total cholesterol levels could reduce the prevalence of coronary heart disease by 30%.
> —**American Heart Association, 2009**
>
> QUICK STATS

Physical Inactivity   An estimated 40–60 million Americans are so sedentary that they are at high risk for developing CVD. Exercise is thought to be the closest thing we have to a magic bullet against heart disease. It lowers CVD risk by helping to decrease blood pressure and resting heart rate, increase HDL levels, maintain desirable weight, improve the condition of blood vessels, and prevent or control diabetes. One study found that women who accumulated at least 3 hours of brisk walking each week cut their risk of heart attack and stroke by more than 50%.

Obesity   The risk of death from CVD is two to three times more likely in obese people (BMI ≥ 30) than it is in

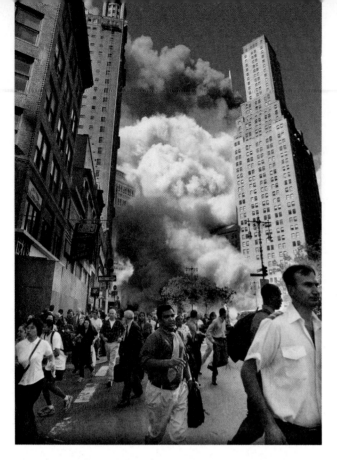

Acute stress is associated with heart rhythm problems and deaths. The rate of arrhythmias in patients with underlying heart disease doubled in the month after the September 11, 2001, terrorist attacks.

Diabetes Diabetes is a disorder characterized by elevated blood glucose levels due to an insufficient supply or inadequate action of insulin. Diabetes doubles the risk of CVD for men and triples the risk for women. Diabetics tend to have higher rates of other CVD risk factors, including hypertension, obesity, and unhealthy blood lipid levels (typically, high triglyceride levels and low HDL levels). The elevated blood glucose and insulin levels that occur in diabetes can damage the endothelial cells that line the arteries, making them more vulnerable to atherosclerosis; diabetics also often have platelet and blood coagulation abnormalities that increase the risk of heart attacks and strokes. People with pre-diabetes also face a significantly increased risk of CVD.

65% of people with diabetes die from some form of CVD.

—**American Heart Association, 2009**

QUICK STATS

In people with pre-diabetes, a healthy diet and exercise are more effective than medication at preventing diabetes. For people with diabetes, a healthy diet, exercise, and careful control of glucose levels are recommended to decrease chances of developing complications. Even people whose diabetes is under control face a high risk of CVD, so control of other risk factors is critical.

Contributing Risk Factors That Can Be Changed

Other factors that can be changed have been identified as contributing to CVD risk, including triglyceride levels and psychological and social factors.

High Triglyceride Levels Like cholesterol, **triglycerides** are blood fats that are obtained from food and manufactured by the body. High triglyceride levels are a reliable predictor of heart disease, especially if associated with other risk factors. Factors contributing to elevated triglyceride levels include excess body fat, physical inactivity, cigarette smoking, type 2 diabetes, excess alcohol intake, very high carbohydrate diets, and certain diseases and medications.

A full lipid profile should include testing and evaluation of triglyceride levels (see Table 12.2). For people with borderline high triglyceride levels, increased physical activity, reduced intake of added sugars, and weight reduction can help bring levels down into the healthy range; for people with high triglyceride levels, drug therapy may be recommended. Being moderate in the use of alcohol and quitting smoking are also important.

Psychological and Social Factors Many of the psychological and social factors that influence other areas of wellness are also important risk factors for CVD.

lean people (BMI 18.5–24.9), and for every 5-unit increment of BMI, a person's risk of death from coronary heart disease increases by 30%. Excess body fat is strongly associated with hypertension, high cholesterol levels, insulin resistance, diabetes, physical inactivity, and increasing age. With excess weight, there is also more blood to pump and the heart has to work harder. This causes chronically elevated pressures within the heart chambers that can lead to ventricular **hypertrophy** (enlargement), and eventually the heart muscle can start to fail.

Physical activity and physical fitness have a strong positive influence on cardiovascular health in those who are overweight and obese. People who are obese but have at least moderate cardiorespiratory fitness may have lower rates of cardiovascular disease than their normal-weight but unfit peers. For someone who is overweight, even modest weight reduction—5–10% of body weight—can reduce CVD risk.

TERMS

hypertrophy Abnormal enlargement of an organ secondary to an increase in cell size.

triglyceride A type of blood fat that can be a predictor of heart disease.

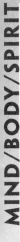

Anger, Hostility, and Heart Disease

People with a quick temper, a persistently hostile outlook, and a cynical, mistrusting attitude toward life are more likely to develop heart disease than those with a calmer, more trusting attitude. People who are angry frequently, intensely, and for long periods experience the stress response much more often than more relaxed individuals. Over the long term, the effects of stress may damage arteries and promote CVD.

Are You Too Hostile?

To help answer that question, Duke University researcher Redford Williams, M.D., has devised a short self-test. It's not a scientific evaluation, but it does offer a rough measure of hostility. Are the following statements true or false for you?

1. I often get annoyed at checkout cashiers or the people in front of me when I'm waiting in line.
2. I usually keep an eye on the people I work or live with to make sure they do what they should.
3. I often wonder how homeless people can have so little respect for themselves.

4. I believe that most people will take advantage of you if you let them.
5. The habits of friends or family members often annoy me.
6. When I'm stuck in traffic, I often start breathing faster and my heart pounds.
7. When I'm annoyed with people, I really want to let them know it.
8. If someone does me wrong, I want to get even.
9. I'd like to have the last word in any argument.
10. At least once a week, I have the urge to yell at or even hit someone.

According to Williams, five or more "true" statements suggest that you're excessively hostile and should consider taking steps to mellow out.

Managing Your Anger

Begin by monitoring your angry responses and looking for triggers—people or situations that typically make you angry. Familiarize yourself with the patterns of thinking that lead to angry or hostile feelings, and then try to head

them off before they develop into full-blown anger. If you feel your anger starting to build, try reasoning with yourself by asking the following questions:

1. *Is this really important enough to get angry about?*
2. *Am I really justified in getting angry?*
3. *Is getting angry going to make a real and positive difference in this situation?*

If you answer yes to all three questions, then calm but assertive communication may be an appropriate response. If your anger isn't reasonable, try distracting yourself or removing yourself from the situation. Exercise, humor, social support, and other stress-management techniques can also help (see Chapter 3 for additional anger-management tips). Your heart—and the people around you—will benefit from your calmer, more positive outlook.

SOURCES: Virginia Williams and Redford Williams, 1999, *Lifeskills: Lifeskills: 8 Simple Ways to Build Stronger Relationships, Communicate More Clearly, and Improve Your Health,* New York: Times Books. Reprinted by permission.

STRESS Excessive stress can strain the heart and blood vessels over time and contribute to CVD. When you experience stress, stress hormones activate the sympathetic nervous system, which causes the fight-or-flight response and increases heart rate and blood pressure in anticipation of physical activity. If you are healthy, you can tolerate the cardiovascular responses that take place during stress, but if you already have CVD, stress can lead to abnormal heart rhythms (arrhythmias), heart attacks, and sudden cardiac death.

CHRONIC HOSTILITY AND ANGER Certain traits in the hard-driving Type A personality—hostility, cynicism, and anger—are associated with increased risk of heart disease. Men prone to anger have two to three times the heart attack risk of calmer men and are much more likely to develop CVD at young ages.

SUPPRESSING PSYCHOLOGICAL DISTRESS Suppressing anger and other negative emotions may also be hazardous to a healthy heart. People who hide psychological distress appear to have higher rates of heart disease than people who experience similar distress but share it with others. People with such "Type D" personalities tend to be pessimistic, negative, and unhappy and to suppress these feelings.

DEPRESSION Depression appears to increase the risk of CVD in healthy people and the risk of adverse cardiac events in those who already have heart disease. Depression also causes physiological changes; for example, it elevates basal levels of stress hormones, which induce a variety of stress-related responses.

ANXIETY Chronic anxiety and anxiety disorders (such as phobias and panic disorder) are associated with up to a threefold increased risk of coronary heart disease, heart attack, and sudden cardiac death. People with anxiety are more likely to have a subsequent adverse cardiac event after having a heart attack.

SOCIAL ISOLATION Social isolation and low social support (living alone, or having few friends or family members) are associated with an increased incidence of coronary heart disease (CHD) and poorer outcomes after the first diagnosis of CHD. A strong social support network is a major antidote to stress. Friends and family members can also promote and support a healthy lifestyle.

LOW SOCIOECONOMIC STATUS Low socioeconomic status and low educational attainment also increase risk for CVD. These associations are probably due to a variety of factors, including lifestyle and access to health care.

Women and CVD

On average, women live 10–15 more years free of coronary heart disease than men do. But heart disease is the leading cause of death among women, and it has killed more women than men every year since 1984.

Polls indicate that women vastly underestimate their risk of dying of a heart attack and, in turn, overestimate their risk of dying of breast cancer. In reality, nearly 1 in 3 women dies of CVD, whereas 1 in 30 dies of breast cancer. Minority women face the highest risk of developing CVD, but their awareness of heart disease as a killer of women is lower than that of white women. To help raise awareness of CVD in women, the American Heart Association launched the "Go Red for Women" campaign; visit their Web site for more information (http://www.goredforwomen.org/).

Risk factors for CVD are similar for men and women and include age, family history, smoking, hypertension, high cholesterol, and diabetes. There are some gender differences, however. HDL appears to be an even more powerful predictor of CAD risk in women than it is in men. Also, women with diabetes have a greater risk of having CVD events like heart attack and stroke than men with diabetes.

Estrogen: A Heart Protector?

The hormone estrogen, produced naturally by a woman's ovaries until menopause, improves blood lipid concentrations and other CVD risk factors. For the past several decades, many U.S. physicians encouraged menopausal women to take hormone replacement therapy (HT) to relieve menopause symptoms and presumably reduce the risk of CVD. However, studies found that HT may actually *increase* a woman's risk for heart disease and certain other health problems, including breast cancer. Some newer studies have found a reduced risk of CVD in women who start HT in the early stages of menopause (usually the mid-40s), suggesting that outcomes may depend on several factors, including the timing of hormone use. The U.S. Preventive Services Task Force and the American Heart Association currently recommend that HT not be used to protect against CVD.

For younger women, the most common form of hormonal medication is oral contraceptives (OCs). Typical OCs contain estrogen and progestin in relatively low doses and are generally considered safe for most nonsmoking women. But women who smoke and use OCs are up to 32 times more likely to have a heart attack than nonsmoking OC users.

Postmenopausal Women: At Risk

When women have heart attacks, they are more likely than men to die within a year. One reason is that because women develop heart disease at older ages, they are more likely to have other health problems that complicate treatment. Women have smaller hearts and arteries than men, possibly making diagnosis and treatment more difficult. There may also be unknown biological or psychosocial risk factors contributing to women's mortality.

Also, medical personnel appear to evaluate and treat women less aggressively than men. Women with positive stress tests and those whose evaluation raises concern about a heart attack are less likely to be referred to further testing than are men. In addition, studies of heart attack patients have found that women usually have to wait longer than men to receive clot-dissolving drugs in an emergency room.

Women presenting with CHD are just as likely as men to report chest pain, but are also likely to report non-chest-pain symptoms, which may obscure their diagnosis. These additional symptoms include fatigue, weakness, shortness of breath, nausea, vomiting, and pain in the abdomen, neck, jaw, and back. Women are also more likely to have pain at rest, during sleep, or with mental stress.

Careful diagnosis of cardiac symptoms is also key in cases of stress-induced cardiomyopathy ("broken heart syndrome"), which occurs much more commonly in women. In this condition, a severe stress response stuns the heart, producing heart-attack-like symptoms and decreased pumping function of the heart, but no damage to the heart muscle. Typically, the condition reverses quickly, and correct diagnosis is important to avoid unnecessary invasive procedures.

Alcohol and Drugs   Although moderate drinking may have health benefits for some people, drinking too much alcohol raises blood pressure and can increase the risk of stroke and heart failure. Stimulant drugs, particularly cocaine, can also cause serious cardiac problems, including heart attack, stroke, and sudden cardiac death. Injection drug use can cause infection of the heart and stroke.

Major Risk Factors That Can't Be Changed

A number of major risk factors for CVD cannot be changed. They include heredity, aging, being male, and ethnicity.

Heredity   Multiple genes contribute to the development of CVD and its associated risk factors, such as high cholesterol, hypertension, diabetes, and obesity. Having a favorable set of genes decreases your risk of developing CVD; having an unfavorable set of genes increases your risk. Risk, however, is modifiable by lifestyle factors.

Aging   About 70% of all heart attack victims are age 65 or older, and about 75% who suffer fatal heart attacks are over 65. For people over 55, the incidence of stroke more than doubles in each successive decade. However, even people in their thirties and forties, especially men, can have heart attacks.

Being Male   Although CVD is the leading killer of both men and women in the United States, men face a greater risk of heart attack than women, especially earlier in life. Until age 55, men also have a greater risk of hypertension. By age 75, the gender gap nearly disappears (see the box "Women and CVD").

DIMENSIONS OF DIVERSITY

African Americans are at substantially higher risk for death from CVD than other groups. The rate of hypertension among African Americans is among the highest of any group in the world. Blacks tend to develop hypertension at an earlier age than whites, and their average blood pressures are much higher. African Americans have a higher risk of stroke, have strokes at younger ages, and, if they survive, have more significant stroke-related disabilities. Some experts recommend that blacks be treated with antihypertensive drugs at an earlier stage—when blood pressure reaches 130/80 rather than the typical 140/90 cutoff for hypertension.

A number of genetic and biological factors may contribute to CVD in African Americans. They may be more sensitive to dietary sodium, leading to greater blood pressure elevation in response to a given amount of sodium. African Americans may also experience less dilation of blood vessels in response to stress, an attribute that also raises blood pressure.

Heredity also plays a large role in the tendency to develop diabetes, another important CVD risk factor that is more common in blacks than whites. However, Latinos are even more likely to develop diabetes and insulin resistance, and at a younger age, than African Americans. There is variation within the Latino population, however, with a higher prevalence of diabetes occurring among Mexican Americans and Puerto Ricans and a relatively lower prevalence among Cuban Americans.

Another factor that likely contributes to the high incidence of CVD among ethnic minority groups is low income. Economic deprivation usually means reduced access to adequate health care and health insurance. Also associated with low income is low educational attainment, which often means less information about preventive health measures, such as diet and stress management. And people with low incomes tend to smoke more, use more salt, and exercise less than those with higher incomes.

Discrimination may also play a role in CVD. Physicians and hospitals may treat the medical problems of ethnic minorities differently than those of whites. Discrimination, along with low income and other forms of deprivation, may also increase stress, which is linked with hypertension and CVD. In terms of access to care, factors such as insurance coverage and availability of high-tech cardiac equipment in hospitals used most often by minorities may also play a role.

CVD risk in ethnic groups is further affected by immigration and one's place of birth. Upon immigration to the United States, an Asian's risk for CVD tends to increase and reflect that of a typical American more than a typical Asian, perhaps in part because Asian immigrants often abandon their traditional (and healthier) diets.

However, birthplace (and its associated lifestyle factors) also seems to be a strong determinant of risk. One study found that among New Yorkers born in the Northeast, blacks and whites have nearly identical risk of CVD. But black New Yorkers who were born in the South have a sharply higher risk, and black New Yorkers born in the Caribbean have a significantly lower risk. Researchers speculate that instead of abandoning their traditional diets and lifestyles, blacks from the South instead bring these traditions with them. Some risk factors for CVD, including smoking and a high-fat diet, are more common in the South. When combined with urban stress, these factors create a lifestyle that is far from heart-healthy.

All Americans are advised to have their blood pressure checked regularly, exercise, eat a healthy diet, manage stress, and avoid smoking. These general preventive strategies may be particularly helpful for ethnic minorities. Tailoring your lifestyle to your particular ethnic risk may also be helpful in some cases. Discuss your particular risk profile with your physician to help identify lifestyle changes most appropriate for you.

Ethnicity　Rates of heart disease vary among ethnic groups in the United States, with African Americans having much higher rates of hypertension, heart disease, and stroke than other groups. Puerto Rican Americans, Cuban Americans, and Mexican Americans are also more likely to suffer from high blood pressure and angina (a warning sign of heart disease) than non-Hispanic white Americans. Asian Americans historically have had far lower rates of CVD than white Americans.

Inflammation and C-Reactive Protein　Inflammation plays a key role in the development of CVD. When an artery is injured by smoking, cholesterol, hypertension, or other factors, the body's response is to produce inflammation. A substance called *C-reactive protein (CRP)* is released into the bloodstream during the inflammatory response, and high levels of CRP indicate a substantially elevated risk of heart attack and stroke. CRP may also be harmful to the coronary arteries themselves.

Lifestyle changes and certain drugs can reduce CRP levels. Statin drugs, widely prescribed to lower cholesterol, also decrease inflammation and reduce CRP levels; this may be one reason that statin drugs seem to lower CVD risk even in people with normal blood lipid levels.

Possible Risk Factors Currently Being Studied

In recent years, a number of other possible risk factors for cardiovascular disease have been identified.

Insulin Resistance and Metabolic Syndrome　As people gain weight and engage in less physical activity, their muscles, fat, and liver become less sensitive to the effect of insulin—a condition known as insulin resistance

QUICK STATS

Nearly 48% of
Americans with CVD are 60 years old or older.

—American Heart Association, 2009

Table 12.3	Defining Characteristics of Metabolic Syndrome*	
Abdominal obesity (waist circumference)		
Men		>40 in (>102 cm)
Women		>35 in (>88 cm)
Triglycerides		≥150 mg/dl
HDL cholesterol		
Men		<40 mg/dl
Women		<50 mg/dl
Blood pressure		≥130/≥85 mm Hg
Fasting glucose		≥110 mg/dl

*A person is diagnosed with metabolic syndrome if she or he has three or more of the risk factors listed here.

SOURCE: National Cholesterol Education Program. 2001. *ATP III Guidelines At-A-Glance Quick Desk Reference.* Bethesda, Md.: National Heart, Lung, and Blood Institute. NIH Publication No. 01-3305.

(or pre-diabetes). As the body becomes increasingly insulin resistant, the pancreas must secrete more and more insulin to keep glucose levels within a normal range. Eventually, however, even high levels of insulin may become insufficient, and blood glucose levels will also start to rise (hyperglycemia), resulting in type 2 diabetes.

Those who have insulin resistance tend to have several other related risk factors; as a group, this cluster of abnormalities is called metabolic syndrome or insulin resistance syndrome (Table 12.3). Metabolic syndrome significantly increases the risk of CVD—more so in women than in men. It is estimated that nearly 35% of the adult U.S. population has metabolic syndrome.

To reduce your risk for metabolic syndrome, choose a healthy diet and get plenty of exercise. The amount and type of carbohydrate intake is also important: Diets high in carbohydrates, especially high-glycemic-index foods, can raise levels of glucose and triglycerides and lower HDL, thus contributing to the development or worsening of metabolic syndrome and CVD, particularly in people who are already sedentary and overweight. For people prone to insulin resistance, eating more unsaturated fats, protein, vegetables, and fiber while limiting added sugars and starches may be beneficial.

Homocysteine Elevated levels of homocysteine, an amino acid circulating in the blood, are associated with an increased risk of CVD. Homocysteine appears to damage the lining of blood vessels, resulting in inflammation and the development of fatty deposits in artery walls. These changes can lead to the formation of clots and blockages in arteries, which in turn can cause heart attacks and strokes. High homocysteine levels are also associated with cognitive impairment, such as memory loss. Men generally have higher homocysteine levels than women, as do individuals with diets low in folic acid, vitamin B-12, and vitamin B-6. If your homocysteine level is high, it may be helpful to follow a diet rich in fruits, vegetables, and whole grains.

MAJOR FORMS OF CARDIOVASCULAR DISEASE

According to the CDC, heart diseases killed more than 650,000 Americans in 2005. Figure 12.3 shows the death rates among various ethnic groups due to heart disease in 2005, the most recent year for which data is available. The main forms of CVD are atherosclerosis, heart disease and heart attack, stroke, peripheral arterial disease (PAD), congestive heart failure, congenital heart disease, rheumatic heart disease, and heart valve problems. Many forms are interrelated and have elements in common; we treat them separately here for the sake of clarity. Hypertension, which is both a major risk factor and a form of CVD, was described earlier in the chapter.

> The estimated annual financial burden of CVD is **$475.3 billion.**
>
> —American Heart Association, 2009

FIGURE 12.3 Heart disease death rates of Americans, 2005. Deaths due to various forms of heart disease per 100,000 people.

SOURCE: National Center for Health Statistics. 2008. Update. *Health, United States, 2007.* Hyattsville, Md.: National Center for Health Statistics.

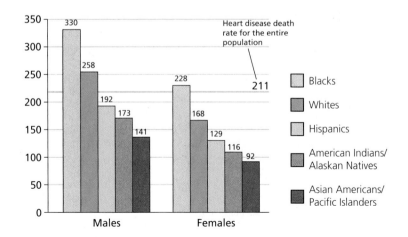

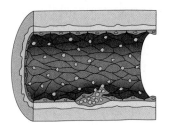 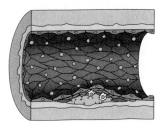 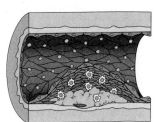 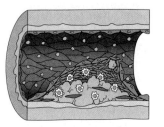

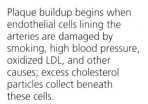

Plaque buildup begins when endothelial cells lining the arteries are damaged by smoking, high blood pressure, oxidized LDL, and other causes; excess cholesterol particles collect beneath these cells.

In response to the damage, platelets and other types of cells collect at the site; a fibrous cap forms, isolating the plaque within the artery wall. An early-stage plaque is called a fatty streak.

Chemicals released by cells in and around the plaque cause further inflammation and buildup; an advanced plaque contains LDL, white blood cells, connective tissue, smooth muscle cells, platelets, and other compounds.

The narrowed artery is vulnerable to blockage by clots. The risk of blockage and heart attack rises if the fibrous cap cracks (probably due to destructive enzymes released by white blood cells within the plaque).

FIGURE 12.4 Stages of plaque development.

QUESTIONS FOR CRITICAL THINKING AND REFLECTION

What risk factors do you have for cardiovascular disease? Which ones are factors you have control over, and which are factors you can't change? If you have risk factors you cannot change (such as a family history of CVD), were you aware that you can make lifestyle adjustments to reduce your risk? Do you think you will make them?

Atherosclerosis

Atherosclerosis is a form of arteriosclerosis, or thickening and hardening of the arteries. In atherosclerosis, arteries become narrowed by deposits of fat, cholesterol, and other substances. The process begins when the endothelial cells (cells that line the arteries) become damaged, most likely through a combination of factors such as smoking, high blood pressure, high insulin or glucose levels, and deposits of oxidized LDL particles. The body's response to this damage results in inflammation and changes in the artery lining that create a sort of magnet for LDL, platelets, and other cells; these cells build up and cause a bulge in the wall of the artery. As these deposits, called **plaques**, accumulate on artery walls, the arteries lose their elasticity and their ability to expand and contract, restricting blood flow. Once narrowed by a plaque, an artery is vulnerable to blockage by blood clots (Figure 12.4).

If the heart, brain, and/or other organs are deprived of blood and the oxygen it carries, the effects of atherosclerosis can be deadly. Coronary arteries, which supply the heart with blood, are particularly susceptible to plaque buildup, a condition called **coronary heart disease (CHD)**, or *coronary artery disease (CAD)*. The blockage of a coronary artery causes a heart attack. If a cerebral artery (leading to the brain) is blocked, the result is a stroke. If an artery in a limb becomes narrowed or blocked, it causes *peripheral arterial disease*, a condition that causes pain and sometimes loss of the affected limb.

The main risk factors for atherosclerosis are cigarette smoking, physical inactivity, high levels of blood cholesterol, high blood pressure, and diabetes. Atherosclerosis often begins in childhood.

Heart Disease and Heart Attack

When one of the coronary arteries becomes blocked, a **heart attack,** or *myocardial infarction (MI)*, results. Although a heart attack may come without warning, it is usually the end result of a long-term disease process. Heart attack symptoms may include chest pain or pressure, arm, neck, or jaw pain, difficulty breathing, excessive sweating, nausea and vomiting, and loss of consciousness. Most people having a heart attack suffer chest pain, but about one-third of heart attack victims do not. Women, ethnic minorities, older adults, and people with diabetes are the most likely groups to experience heart attack without chest pain.

Angina Arteries narrowed by disease may still be open enough to deliver blood to the heart. At times, however—during stress or exertion, for example—the heart needs more oxygen than can flow through narrowed arteries. When the need for oxygen exceeds the supply, chest pain,

plaque A deposit of fatty (and other) substances on the inner wall of the arteries.

coronary heart disease (CHD) Heart disease caused by atherosclerosis in the arteries that supply blood to the heart muscle; also called *coronary artery disease*.

heart attack Damage to, or death of, heart muscle, resulting from a failure of the coronary arteries to deliver enough blood to the heart; also known as *myocardial infarction (MI)*.

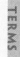

TERMS

called **angina pectoris,** may occur. Angina pain is usually felt as an extreme tightness in the chest and heavy pressure behind the breastbone or in the shoulder, neck, arm, hand, or back. Angina may be controlled in a number of ways (with drugs and surgical or nonsurgical procedures), but its course is unpredictable. Over a period ranging from hours to years, the narrowing may go on to full blockage and a heart attack.

Arrhythmias and Sudden Cardiac Death   The pumping of the heart is controlled by electrical impulses from the sinus node, located in the right atrium, that maintain a regular heartbeat of 60–100 beats per minute. If this electrical conduction system is disrupted, the heart may beat too quickly, too slowly, or in an irregular fashion, a condition known as **arrhythmia.** Arrhythmia can cause symptoms ranging from imperceptible to severe and even fatal.

   Sudden cardiac death, also called *cardiac arrest,* is most often caused by an arrhythmia called *ventricular fibrillation,* a kind of quivering of the ventricle that makes it ineffective in pumping blood. If ventricular fibrillation continues for more than a few minutes, it is generally fatal. Cardiac defibrillation, in which an electrical shock is delivered to the heart, can be effective in jolting the heart into a more efficient rhythm. Automated external defibrillators (AEDs) are

becoming increasingly available in public places for use by the general public. (Training in the use of AEDs is available from organizations such as the American Red Cross and the American Heart Association.) Some arrhythmias cause no problems and resolve without treatment; more serious arrhythmias are usually treated with medication or a surgically implanted pacemaker or defibrillator that delivers electrical stimulation to the heart to create a more normal rhythm.

Helping a Heart Attack Victim   Most people who die from a heart attack do so within 2 hours from the time they experience the first symptoms. If you or someone you are with has any of the warning signs of heart attack listed in the box "What to Do in Case of a Heart Attack, Stroke, or Cardiac Arrest," take immediate action. Many experts also suggest that the heart attack victim chew and swallow one adult aspirin tablet (325 mg) as soon as possible after symptoms begin; aspirin has an immediate anticlotting effect.

   If the victim loses consciousness, a qualified person should immediately start administering emergency **cardiopulmonary resuscitation (CPR).** Damage to the heart muscle increases with time. If the person receives emergency care quickly enough, a clot-dissolving agent can be injected to break up a clot in the coronary artery.

Detecting and Treating Heart Disease   Currently, the most common initial screening tool for CAD is the stress, or exercise, test, in which a patient runs or walks on a treadmill or pedals a stationary cycle while being monitored for abnormalities with an **electrocardiogram (ECG or EKG).** Certain characteristic changes in the heart's electrical activity while under stress can reveal particular heart problems, such as restricted blood flow. Exercise testing can also be performed in conjunction with imaging techniques such as nuclear medicine or echocardiography that provide pictures of the heart, which can help pinpoint problems.

   If symptoms or noninvasive tests such as **magnetic resonance imaging (MRI)** or positron emission tomography (PET) suggest coronary artery disease, the next step is usually a coronary **angiogram,** performed in a cardiac catheterization lab. In this test, a catheter (a small plastic tube) is threaded into an artery, usually in the groin, and

TERMS

angina pectoris   Pain in the chest, and often in the left arm and shoulder, caused by the heart muscle not receiving enough blood.

arrhythmia   A change in the normal pattern of the heartbeat.

sudden cardiac death   A nontraumatic, unexpected death from sudden cardiac arrest, most often due to arrhythmia; in most instances, victims have underlying heart disease.

cardiopulmonary resuscitation (CPR)   A technique involving mouth-to-mouth breathing and/or chest compression to keep oxygen flowing to the brain.

electrocardiogram (ECG or EKG)   A test to detect abnormalities by evaluating the electrical activity in the heart.

magnetic resonance imaging (MRI)   A computerized imaging technique that uses a strong magnetic field and radio frequency signals to examine a thin cross section of the body.

angiogram   A picture of the arterial system taken after injecting a dye that is opaque to X rays; also called *arteriogram.*

balloon angioplasty   A technique in which a catheter with a deflated balloon on the tip is inserted into an artery; the balloon is then inflated at the point of obstruction in the artery, pressing the plaque against the artery wall to improve blood supply; also known as *percutaneous coronary intervention (PCI).*

coronary bypass surgery   Surgery in which a vein is grafted from a point above to a point below an obstruction in a coronary artery, improving the blood supply to the heart.

stroke   An impeded blood supply to some part of the brain resulting in the destruction of brain cells; also called *cerebrovascular accident.*

QUESTIONS FOR CRITICAL THINKING AND REFLECTION

Has anyone you know ever had a heart attack? If so, was the onset gradual or sudden? Were appropriate steps taken to help the person (for example, did anyone call 911, give CPR, or use an AED)? Do you feel comfortable dealing with a cardiac emergency? If not, what can you do to improve your readiness?

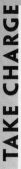

What to Do in Case of a Heart Attack, Stroke, or Cardiac Arrest

TAKE CHARGE

Heart Attack Warning Signs

Some heart attacks are sudden and intense—the "movie heart attack," where no one doubts what's happening. But most heart attacks start slowly, with mild pain or discomfort. Often people affected aren't sure what's wrong and wait too long before getting help. Here are signs that can mean a heart attack is happening:

• **Chest discomfort.** Heart attacks often involve discomfort in the chest that lasts more than a few minutes, or that goes away and comes back. It can feel like uncomfortable pressure, squeezing, fullness, or pain.

• **Discomfort in other areas of the upper body.** Symptoms can include pain or discomfort in one or both arms, the back, neck, jaw, or stomach.

• **Shortness of breath.** May occur with or without chest discomfort.

• **Other signs:** These may include breaking out in a cold sweat, nausea, vomiting, or lightheadedness.

If you or someone you're with has chest discomfort, especially with one or more of the other signs, don't wait longer than a few minutes (no more than 5) before calling for help.

Calling 9-1-1 is almost always the fastest way to get lifesaving treatment. Emergency medical services staff can begin treatment when they arrive—up to an hour sooner than if someone gets to the hospital by car. Patients with chest pain who arrive by ambulance usually receive faster treatment at the hospital, too.

If you can't access the emergency medical services (EMS), have someone drive you to the hospital right away. If you're the one having symptoms, don't drive yourself, unless you have absolutely no other option.

Stroke Warning Signs

The American Stroke Association says these are the warning signs of stroke:

• Sudden numbness or weakness of the face, arm, or leg, especially on one side of the body

• Sudden confusion, trouble speaking or understanding

• Sudden trouble seeing in one or both eyes

• Sudden trouble walking, dizziness, or loss of balance or coordination

• Sudden, severe headache with no known cause

If you or someone with you has one or more of these signs, call 9-1-1 immediately. If given within 3 hours of the start of symptoms, a clot-busting drug can reduce long-term disability for the most common type of stroke.

Signs of Cardiac Arrest

Cardiac arrest strikes immediately and without warning. Here are the signs:

• Sudden loss of responsiveness. No response to gentle shaking. No movement or coughing.

• No normal breathing. The victim does not take a normal breath for several seconds.

• No signs of circulation. No pulse or blood pressure.

If cardiac arrest occurs, call 9-1-1 and begin CPR immediately. If an automated external defibrillator (AED) is available and someone trained to use it is nearby, involve her or him.

For more on emergency care for cardiac arrest, see the inside back cover.

SOURCE: American Heart Association. 2005. *Heart Attack, Stroke, and Cardiac Arrest Warning Signs.* Reprinted with permission. www .americanheart.org. Copyright © 2007 American Heart Association.

---

advanced through the aorta to the coronary arteries. The catheter is then placed into the opening of the coronary artery and a special dye is injected. The dye can be seen moving through the arteries under moving X ray, and any narrowings or blockages can be identified. If a problem is found, it is commonly treated with **balloon angioplasty,** which involves placing a small wire in the artery and feeding a deflated balloon over it. The balloon is advanced to the site of the narrowing and then inflated, flattening the fatty plaque and widening the arterial opening. This is generally followed by placement of a stent, a small metal tube that helps keep the artery open.

Other treatments, ranging from medication to major surgery, are also available. Along with a low-fat diet, regular exercise, and smoking cessation, one frequent recommendation for people at high risk for CVD is to take a low-dose aspirin tablet every day. Aspirin has an anticlotting effect,

discouraging platelets in the blood from sticking to arterial plaques and forming clots; it also reduces inflammation.

In cases of a more severe blockage, **coronary bypass surgery** may be performed. Cardiothoracic surgeons remove a healthy blood vessel, usually a vein from one of the patient's legs, and graft it from the aorta to one or more coronary arteries to bypass a blockage.

Stroke

A **stroke,** also called a *cerebrovascular accident (CVA),* occurs when the blood supply to the brain is cut off.

795,000 Americans suffer strokes each year.

—**American Heart Association, 2009**

QUICK STATS

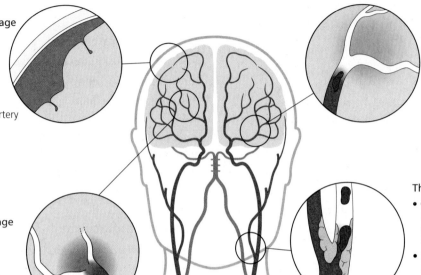

HEMORRHAGIC STROKE
- 13% of strokes
- Caused by ruptured blood vessels followed by blood leaking into tissue
- Usually more serious than ischemic stroke

ISCHEMIC STROKE
- 87% of strokes
- Caused by blockages in brain blood vessels; potentially treatable with clot-busting drugs
- Brain tissue dies when blood flow is blocked

Subarachnoid hemorrhage
- A bleed into the space between the brain and the skull
- Develops most often from an *aneurysm*, a weakened, ballooned area in the wall of an artery

Embolic stroke
- Caused by *emboli*, blood clots that travel from elsewhere in the body to the brain blood vessels
- 25% of embolic strokes are related to atrial fibrillation

Intracerebral hemorrhage
- A bleed from a blood vessel inside the brain
- Often caused by high blood pressure and the damage it does to arteries

Thrombotic stroke
- Caused by *thrombi*, blood clots that form where an artery has been narrowed by atherosclerosis
- Most often develops when part of a thrombus breaks away and causes a blockage in a downstream artery

FIGURE 12.5   Types of stroke.

SOURCE: Excerpted from *Harvard Health Letter*, April 2000. Reprinted with permission obtained via The Copyright Clearance Center.

Types of Strokes   There are two major types of strokes (Figure 12.5).

ISCHEMIC STROKE   An **ischemic stroke** is caused by a blockage in a blood vessel. There are two types of ischemic strokes: A *thrombotic stroke* is caused by a **thrombus,** a blood clot that forms in a cerebral artery that has been narrowed or damaged by atherosclerosis; an *embolic stroke* is caused by an **embolus,** a wandering blood clot that is carried in the bloodstream and may become wedged in a cerebral artery. Many embolic strokes are linked to a type of abnormal heart rhythm called *atrial fibrillation.* Ischemic strokes account for 87% of all strokes.

HEMORRHAGIC STROKE   A **hemorrhagic stroke** occurs when a blood vessel in the brain bursts, spilling blood into the surrounding tissue. Cells normally nourished by the artery are deprived of blood and cannot function. In addition, accumulated blood from the burst vessel may put pressure on surrounding brain tissue, causing damage and even death. There are two types of hemorrhagic strokes: An *intracerebral hemorrhage* occurs when a blood vessel ruptures within the brain; a *subarachnoid hemorrhage* occurs when a blood vessel on the brain's surface ruptures and bleeds into the space between the brain and the skull. Hemorrhages can be caused by head injuries or the bursting of a malformed blood vessel or an **aneurysm,** a blood-filled pocket that bulges out from a weak spot in an artery

wall. Aneurysms in the brain may remain stable and never break. But when they do, the result is a stroke. Aneurysms may be caused or worsened by hypertension.

The Effects of a Stroke   The interruption of the blood supply to any area of the brain prevents the nerve cells there from functioning—in some cases causing death. Stroke survivors usually have some lasting disability. A stroke may cause paralysis, walking disability, speech impairment, memory loss, and changes in behavior. The severity of the stroke and its long-term effects depend on which brain cells have been injured, how widespread the damage is, how effectively the body can restore the blood supply, and how rapidly other areas of the brain can take over.

Detecting and Treating Stroke   Effective treatment requires the prompt recognition of symptoms and correct diagnosis of the type of stroke. Many people have strokes, however, without knowing it. These "silent strokes" do not cause any noticeable symptoms while they are occurring. Although they may be mild, silent

Only **16%** of Americans know all five warning signs of a stroke.

—CDC, 2008

STATS

strokes leave their victims at a higher risk for subsequent and more serious strokes later in life. They also contribute to loss of mental and cognitive skills.

Some stroke victims have a **transient ischemic attack (TIA),** or ministroke, days, weeks, or months before they have a full-blown stroke. A TIA produces temporary stroke-like symptoms, such as weakness or numbness in an arm or a leg, speech difficulty, or dizziness. These symptoms are brief, often lasting just a few minutes, and do not cause permanent damage. TIAs should be taken as warning signs of a stroke, however, and anyone with a suspected TIA should get immediate medical help.

A person with stroke symptoms should be rushed to the hospital. A **computed tomography (CT)** scan, which uses a computer to construct an image of the brain from X rays, can assess brain damage and determine the type of stroke. Newer techniques using MRI and ultrasound are becoming increasingly available and should improve the speed and accuracy of stroke diagnosis.

If tests reveal that a stroke is caused by a blood clot—and if help is sought within a few hours of the onset of symptoms—the person can be treated with the same kind of clot-dissolving drugs that are used to treat coronary artery blockages. If the clot is dissolved quickly enough, brain damage is minimized and symptoms may disappear.

If tests reveal that a stroke was caused by a cerebral hemorrhage, drugs may be prescribed to lower the blood pressure, which will usually be high. Careful diagnosis is crucial, because administering clot-dissolving drugs to a person suffering a hemorrhagic stroke would cause more bleeding and potentially more brain damage.

If detection and treatment of stroke come too late, rehabilitation is the only treatment. Although damaged or destroyed brain tissue does not normally regenerate, nerve cells in the brain can make new pathways, and some functions can be taken over by other parts of the brain. Some people recover completely in a matter of days or weeks, but most stroke victims who survive must adapt to some disability.

Congestive Heart Failure

When the heart has been damaged by high blood pressure or other disease conditions and cannot maintain its regular pumping rate and force, fluids begin to back up into body tissue. When extra fluid seeps through capillary walls, edema (swelling) results, usually in the legs and ankles, but sometimes in other parts of the body as well. Fluid can collect in the lungs and interfere with breathing, particularly when a person is lying down. This condition is called **pul-**

monary edema, and the entire process is known as **congestive heart failure.** Treatment includes reducing the workload on the heart, modifying salt intake, and using drugs that help the body eliminate excess fluid. When medical therapy is ineffective, heart transplant is a solution for some patients with severe heart failure, but the need greatly exceeds the number of hearts available.

Other Forms of Heart Disease

Other, less common, disorders and diseases also affect the heart.

Congenital Heart Defects About 36,000 children born each year in the United States have a malformation of the heart or major blood vessels. These conditions are collectively referred to as **congenital heart defects,** and they cause about 3600 deaths a year. The most common congenital defects are holes in the wall that divides the chambers of the heart and *coarctation of the aorta,* a narrowing, or constriction, of the aorta. Most of the common congenital defects can now be accurately diagnosed and treated with medication or surgery.

Hypertrophic cardiomyopathy (HCM) occurs in 1 out of every 500 people and is the most common cause of sudden death among athletes younger than age 35. The disease

TERMS

ischemic stroke Impeded blood supply to the brain caused by the obstruction of a blood vessel by a clot.

thrombus A blood clot in a blood vessel that usually remains at the point of its formation.

embolus A blood clot that breaks off from its place of origin in a blood vessel and travels through the bloodstream.

hemorrhagic stroke Impeded blood supply to the brain caused by the rupture of a blood vessel.

aneurysm A sac formed by a distention or dilation of the artery wall.

transient ischemic attack (TIA) A small stroke; usually a temporary interruption of blood supply to the brain, causing numbness or difficulty with speech.

computed tomography (CT) The use of computerized X ray images to create a cross-sectional depiction (scan) of tissue density.

pulmonary edema The accumulation of fluid in the lungs.

congestive heart failure A condition resulting from the heart's inability to pump out all the blood that returns to it; blood backs up in the veins leading to the heart, causing an accumulation of fluid in various parts of the body.

congenital heart defect A defect or malformation of the heart or its major blood vessels, present at birth.

hypertrophic cardiomyopathy (HCM) An inherited condition in which there is an enlargement of the heart muscle, especially between the two ventricles.

causes the heart muscle to become hypertrophic (enlarged). People with hypertrophic cardiomyopathy are at high risk for sudden death, mainly due to serious arrhythmias. Hypertrophic cardiomyopathy may be identified by a **murmur,** then diagnosed using echocardiography. Possible treatments include medication and a pacemaker or internal defibrillator.

Rheumatic Heart Disease   **Rheumatic fever,** a consequence of certain types of untreated streptococcal throat infections, is a leading cause of heart disease worldwide. Rheumatic fever can permanently damage the heart muscle and heart valves, a condition called *rheumatic heart disease (RHD)*. Symptoms of strep throat include the sudden onset of a sore throat, painful swallowing, fever, swollen glands, headache, nausea, and vomiting. If left untreated, up to 3% of strep infections progress into rheumatic fever.

Heart Valve Disorders   Congenital defects and certain types of infections can cause abnormalities in the valves between the chambers of the heart. The most common heart valve disorder is **mitral valve prolapse (MVP),** which occurs in about 3% of the population. Most people with MVP have no symptoms; they have the same ability to exercise and live as long as people without MVP. Treatment for MVP is usually unnecessary, although surgery may be needed in the rare cases where leakage through the faulty valve is severe.

PROTECTING YOURSELF AGAINST CARDIOVASCULAR DISEASE

CVD can begin very early in life. For example, fatty streaks (very early atherosclerosis) can be seen on the aorta in children younger than age 10. Reducing CVD risk factors when you are young can pay off with many extra years of life and health.

Eat Heart-Healthy

For most Americans, eating a heart-healthy diet involves cutting total fat intake, substituting unsaturated fats for saturated and trans fats, and increasing intake of whole grains and fiber.

Decreased Fat and Cholesterol Intake   The National Cholesterol Education Program (NCEP) recommends that all Americans over age 2 adopt a diet in which total fat consumption is no more than 30% of total daily calories, with no more than one-third of total fat calories (10% of total daily calories) coming from saturated fat. For people with heart disease or high LDL levels, the NCEP recommends a total fat intake of 25–35% of total daily calories and a saturated fat intake of less than 7% of total calories. The NCEP recommends that most Americans limit dietary cholesterol intake to no more than 300 mg per day; for people with heart disease or high LDL levels, the suggested daily limit is 200 mg. Animal products contain cholesterol as well as saturated fat; vegetable products do not contain cholesterol.

Increased Fiber Intake   Fiber traps the bile acids the liver needs to manufacture cholesterol and carries them to the large intestine, where they are excreted. It slows the production of proteins that promote blood clotting. Fiber may also interfere with the absorption of dietary fat and may help you cut total food intake because foods rich in fiber tend to be filling.

To get the recommended 25–38 grams of dietary fiber per day, eat whole grains, fruits, and vegetables. Good sources of fiber include oatmeal, some breakfast cereals, barley, legumes, and most fruits and vegetables.

Decreased Sodium Intake and Increased Potassium Intake   The recommended limit for sodium intake is 2300 mg per day; for population groups at special risk, including those with hypertension, middle-aged and older adults, and African Americans, the recommended limit is 1500 mg per day. Potassium is also important in controlling blood pressure. Good food sources include leafy green vegetables like spinach and beet greens, root vegetables like white and sweet potatoes, vine fruits like cantaloupe and honeydew melon, winter squash, bananas, many dried fruits, and tomato sauce.

Moderate Alcohol Consumption (For Some)   The Dietary Guidelines for Americans state that moderate alcohol consumption may lower the risk of CHD among middle-aged and older adults. For most people under age 45, however, the risks of alcohol use probably outweigh any health benefit.

Other Dietary Factors   Researchers have identified other dietary factors that may affect CVD risk:

- *Omega-3 fatty acids.* Found in fish, shellfish, and some plant foods (nuts and canola, soybean, and flaxseed oils), omega-3 fatty acids may reduce clotting, abnormal heart rhythms, and inflammation and have other heart-healthy effects, such as lowering triglycerides. The American Heart Association recommends eating fish two or more times a week.
- *Plant stanols and sterols.* Plant stanols and sterols, found in some types of trans fat–free margarines and other products, reduce the absorption of cholesterol in the body and help lower LDL levels.
- *Folic acid, vitamin B-6, and vitamin B-12.* These vitamins lower homocysteine levels, and folic acid has also been found to reduce the risk of hypertension.
- *Calcium.* Diets rich in calcium may help prevent hypertension and possibly stroke by reducing insulin resistance and platelet aggregation.

- *Soy protein.* Replacing some animal proteins with soy protein may help lower LDL cholesterol.
- *Healthy carbohydrates.* Healthier carbohydrate choices, including whole grains, fruits, and nonstarchy vegetables, typically provide more nutrients and have a lower glycemic index than refined grains and starchy foods. Choosing healthy carbohydrates is important for people with insulin resistance, pre-diabetes, or diabetes.
- *Total calories.* Reducing energy intake can improve cholesterol and triglyceride levels as much as reducing fat intake does. Reduced calorie intake also helps control body weight.

DASH A diet plan that reflects many of the recommendations described above was released as part of a study called Dietary Approaches to Stop Hypertension, or DASH. The DASH study found that a diet low in fat and high in fruits, vegetables, and low-fat dairy products reduces blood pressure. It also follows the recommendations for lowering the risk of heart disease, cancer, and osteoporosis.

Exercise Regularly

You can significantly reduce your risk of CVD with a moderate amount of physical activity. The American Heart Association recommends strength training in addition to aerobic exercise for building and maintaining cardiovascular health. Strength training helps lower blood pressure, reduce body fat, and improve lipid levels and glucose metabolism.

Avoid Tobacco

The number-one risk factor for CVD that you can control is smoking. If you smoke, quit. If you don't, don't start. If you find yourself breathing in ETS, take steps to prevent or stop the exposure.

Know and Manage Your Blood Pressure

If you have no CVD risk factors, have your blood pressure measured by a trained professional at least once every 2 years; yearly tests are recommended if you have other risk factors. If your blood pressure is high, follow your physician's advice on how to lower it.

Know and Manage Your Cholesterol Levels

All people age 20 and over should have their cholesterol checked at least once every 5 years. The NCEP recommends a fasting lipoprotein profile that measures total cholesterol, HDL, LDL, and triglyceride levels. Once you know your baseline numbers, you and your physician can develop an LDL goal and lifestyle plan.

Develop Effective Ways to Handle Stress and Anger

To reduce the psychological and social risk factors for CVD, develop effective strategies for handling the stress in your life. Shore up your social support network, and try some of the techniques described in Chapter 2 for managing stress.

WHAT IS CANCER?

Cancer is the abnormal, uncontrolled multiplication of cells, which, if left untreated, can ultimately cause death.

Tumors

Most cancers take the form of tumors, although not all tumors are cancerous. A **tumor** (or *neoplasm*) is simply a mass of tissue that serves no physiological purpose. **Benign** (noncancerous) **tumors** are made up of cells similar to the surrounding normal cells and are enclosed in a membrane

TERMS

murmur An abnormal heart sound indicating turbulent blood flow through a valve or hole in the heart.

rheumatic fever A disease, mainly of children, characterized by fever, inflammation, and pain in the joints; often damages the heart valves and muscle, a condition called *rheumatic heart disease.*

mitral valve prolapse (MVP) A condition in which the mitral valve billows out during ventricular contraction, possibly allowing leakage of blood from the left ventricle into the left atrium.

cancer Abnormal, uncontrolled cellular multiplication.

tumor A mass of tissue that serves no physiological purpose; also called a *neoplasm.*

benign tumor A tumor that is not cancerous.

that prevents them from penetrating neighboring tissues. They are dangerous only if their physical presence interferes with body functions. A benign brain tumor, for example, can cause death if it blocks the blood supply to the brain.

The term **malignant tumor** is synonymous with cancer. A malignant tumor can invade surrounding structures, including blood vessels, the **lymphatic system,** and nerves. It can also spread to distant sites via the blood and lymphatic circulation, producing invasive tumors in almost any part of the body. A few cancers, like leukemia (cancer of the blood), do not produce a mass but still have the fundamental property of rapid, uncontrolled cell multiplication; for this reason, such diseases are considered to be a form of cancer.

Every case of cancer begins as a change in a cell that allows it to grow and divide when it should not. Normally (in adults), cells divide and grow at a rate just sufficient to replace dying cells. In contrast, a malignant cell divides without regard for normal control mechanisms and gradually produces a mass of abnormal cells, or a tumor. It takes about a billion cells to make a mass the size of a pea, so a single tumor cell must go through many divisions, often taking years, before the tumor grows to a noticeable size.

Eventually a tumor produces a sign or symptom. In the breast, for example, a tumor may be felt as a lump and diagnosed as cancer by an X ray or **biopsy.** In less accessible locations, like the lung, ovary, or intestine, a tumor may be noticed only after considerable growth has taken place and may then be detected only by an indirect symptom—for instance, a persistent cough or unexplained bleeding or pain. In the case of leukemia, there is no lump, but the changes in the blood will eventually be noticed as increasing fatigue, infection, or abnormal bleeding.

Metastasis

Metastasis, the spreading of cancer cells, occurs because cancer cells do not stick to each other as strongly as normal cells do and therefore may not remain at the site of the *primary tumor* (the original location). They break away and can pass through the lining of lymph or blood vessels to invade nearby tissue. They can also travel to different parts of the body where they establish new cancer cells. This traveling and seeding process is called *metastasizing,* and the new tumors are called *secondary tumors,* or *metastases.* The ability of cancer cells to metastasize makes early cancer detection critical. To control the cancer, every cancerous cell must be removed. Once cancer cells enter either the lymphatic system or the bloodstream, it is extremely difficult to stop their spread to other organs of the body.

Types of Cancer

The behavior of tumors arising in different body organs is characteristic of the tissue of origin. (Figure 12.6 shows the major cancer sites and the incidence of each type.) Malignant tumors are classified according to the types of cells that give rise to them:

- **Carcinomas** arise from **epithelia,** tissues that cover external body surfaces, line internal tubes and cavities, and form the secreting portion of glands. They are the most common type of cancers; major sites include the skin, breast, uterus, prostate, lungs, and gastrointestinal tract.

- **Sarcomas** arise from connective and fibrous tissues such as muscle, bone, cartilage, and the membranes covering muscles and fat.

- **Lymphomas** are cancers of the lymph nodes, part of the body's infection-fighting system.

- **Leukemias** are cancers of the blood-forming cells, which reside chiefly in the **bone marrow.**

Cancers vary greatly in how easily they can be detected and how well they respond to treatment. For example, certain types of skin cancer are easily detected, grow slowly, and are very easy to remove; virtually all of these cancers are cured. Cancer of the pancreas, on the other hand, is very difficult to detect or treat, and very few patients survive the disease.

TERMS

malignant tumor A tumor that is cancerous and capable of spreading.

lymphatic system A system of vessels that returns proteins, lipids, and other substances from fluid in the tissues to the circulatory system.

biopsy The removal and examination of a small piece of body tissue; a needle biopsy uses a needle to remove a small sample, but some biopsies require surgery.

metastasis The spread of cancer cells from one part of the body to another.

carcinoma Cancer that originates in epithelial tissue (skin, glands, and lining of internal organs).

epithelia Tissue that covers a surface or lines a tube or cavity of the body, enclosing and protecting other parts of the body.

sarcoma Cancer arising from bone, cartilage, or striated muscle.

lymphoma A tumor originating from lymphatic tissue.

leukemia Cancer of the blood or the blood-forming cells.

bone marrow Soft vascular tissue in the interior cavities of bones that produces blood cells.

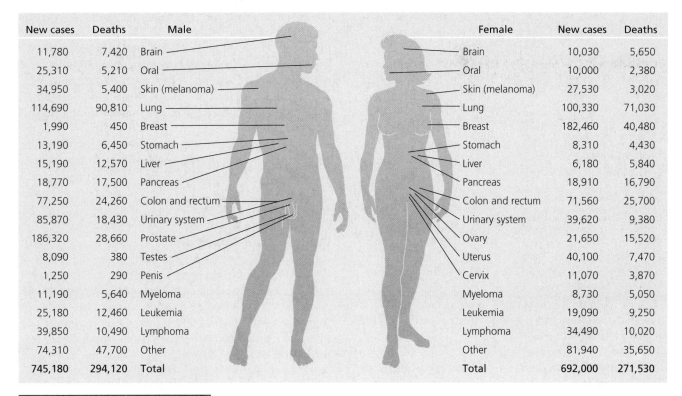

New cases	Deaths	Male	Female	New cases	Deaths
11,780	7,420	Brain	Brain	10,030	5,650
25,310	5,210	Oral	Oral	10,000	2,380
34,950	5,400	Skin (melanoma)	Skin (melanoma)	27,530	3,020
114,690	90,810	Lung	Lung	100,330	71,030
1,990	450	Breast	Breast	182,460	40,480
13,190	6,450	Stomach	Stomach	8,310	4,430
15,190	12,570	Liver	Liver	6,180	5,840
18,770	17,500	Pancreas	Pancreas	18,910	16,790
77,250	24,260	Colon and rectum	Colon and rectum	71,560	25,700
85,870	18,430	Urinary system	Urinary system	39,620	9,380
186,320	28,660	Prostate	Ovary	21,650	15,520
8,090	380	Testes	Uterus	40,100	7,470
1,250	290	Penis	Cervix	11,070	3,870
11,190	5,640	Myeloma	Myeloma	8,730	5,050
25,180	12,460	Leukemia	Leukemia	19,090	9,250
39,850	10,490	Lymphoma	Lymphoma	34,490	10,020
74,310	47,700	Other	Other	81,940	35,650
745,180	294,120	Total	Total	692,000	271,530

VITAL STATISTICS

FIGURE 12.6 Cancer cases and deaths by site and sex. The *New Cases* column indicates the number of cancers that occur annually in each site; the *Deaths* column indicates the number of cancer deaths that are annually attributed to each type.

SOURCE: American Cancer Society. 2008. *Cancer Facts and Figures, 2008.* Atlanta: American Cancer Society.

The Incidence of Cancer

Each year, more than 1.4 million people in the United States are diagnosed with cancer. Most will be cured, or be able to live years longer. In fact, the American Cancer Society (ACS) estimates that the 5-year survival rate for all cancers diagnosed between 1996 and 2003 is 66%. These statistics exclude more than 1 million cases of the curable types of skin cancer. At current U.S. rates, however, nearly 1 in 2 men and more than 1 in 3 women will develop cancer at some point in their lives.

Death rates from cancer are not declining as fast as those from heart disease, in large part because of the differing effects that quitting smoking has on disease risk. Heart-related damage of smoking reverses more quickly and more significantly than the cancer-related damage from smoking. Smoking-related gene mutations cannot be reversed, although other mechanisms can sometimes control cellular changes. If heart disease death rates continue to decline faster than cancer death rates, cancer may overtake heart disease as the leading cause of death among Americans of all ages.

The American Cancer Society estimates that 90% of skin cancer could be prevented by protecting the skin from the rays of the sun and 87% of lung cancer could be prevented by avoiding exposure to tobacco smoke. Thou-sands of cases of colon, breast, and uterine cancer could be prevented by improving the diet and controlling body weight. Regular screenings and self-examinations have the potential to save an additional 100,000 lives per year.

COMMON CANCERS

In this section we look at some of the most common cancers and their causes, prevention, and treatment.

Lung Cancer

Lung cancer is the most common cause of cancer death in the United States, responsible for about 162,000 deaths

QUESTIONS FOR CRITICAL THINKING AND REFLECTION
Most people think of cancer as a death sentence, but is that necessarily true? Have you or anyone you know had an experience with cancer? If so, what was the outcome? Have you ever considered whether you might be at risk for some type of cancer? Have you taken any steps to reduce your risk?

each year. Since 1987 lung cancer has surpassed breast cancer as the leading cause of cancer death in women.

Risk Factors The chief risk factor for lung cancer is tobacco smoke, which currently accounts for 30% of all cancer deaths and 87% of lung cancer deaths. When smoking is combined with exposure to other carcinogens, such as asbestos particles or certain pollutants, the risk of cancer can be multiplied by a factor of 10 or more. Environmental tobacco smoke (ETS) is a human carcinogen; even brief exposure can cause serious harm. It is estimated that ETS causes about 3000 lung cancer deaths each year in nonsmokers.

Detection and Treatment Lung cancer is difficult to detect at an early stage and hard to cure even when detected early. Symptoms of lung cancer do not usually appear until the disease has advanced to the invasive stage. Signals such as a persistent cough, chest pain, or recurring bronchitis may be the first indication of a tumor's presence. A diagnosis can usually be made by CT scanning, chest X rays, or analysis of the cells in sputum. If caught early, localized cancers can be treated with surgery. But because only about 16% of lung cancers are detected before they spread, radiation and **chemotherapy** are often used in addition to surgery. For cases detected early, 49% of patients are alive 5 years after diagnosis; but overall, the 5-year survival rate is only 15%. One form of lung cancer, known as small-cell lung cancer and accounting for about 13% of cases, can be treated fairly successfully with chemotherapy—alone or in combination with radiation. A large percentage of cases go into **remission,** which in some cases lasts for years.

Colon and Rectal Cancer

Although there are effective screening methods for colorectal cancer, it is the third most common type of cancer.

Risk Factors Age is a key risk factor for colon and rectal cancer, with more than 90% of cases diagnosed in people age 50 and older. Heredity also plays a role. Many cancers arise from preexisting **polyps,** small growths on the wall of the colon that may gradually develop into malignancies. The tendency to form colon polyps appears to be determined by specific genes, so many colon cancers may be due to inherited gene mutations.

Excessive alcohol use and smoking may increase the risk of colorectal cancer. Regular physical activity appears to reduce a person's risk, whereas obesity increases risk. A diet rich in red and processed meats increases risk, whereas eating fruits, vegetables, and whole grains is associated with lower risk. However, research findings on whether dietary fiber prevents colon cancer have been mixed. Studies have suggested a protective role for folic acid, magnesium, vitamin D, and calcium; in contrast, high intake of refined carbohydrates, simple sugars, and smoked meats and fish may increase risk.

Use of oral contraceptives or hormone replacement therapy may reduce risk in women. Regular use of nonsteroidal anti-inflammatory drugs such as aspirin and ibuprofen may decrease the risk of colon cancer and other cancers of the digestive tract.

Detection and Treatment If identified early, precancerous polyps and early-stage cancers can be removed before they become malignant or spread. Because polyps may bleed as they progress, the standard warning signs of colon cancer are bleeding from the rectum and a change in bowel habits. Regular screening tests are recommended beginning at age 50 (earlier for people with a family history of the disease). A yearly stool blood test can detect small amounts of blood in the stool long before obvious bleeding would be noticed. More involved screening tests are recommended at 5- or 10-year intervals.

Surgery is the primary treatment for colon and rectal cancer. Radiation and chemotherapy may be used before surgery to shrink a tumor or after surgery to destroy any remaining cancerous cells. The survival rate is 90% for colon and rectal cancers detected early and 64% overall.

Breast Cancer

Breast cancer is the most common cancer in women and causes almost as many deaths in women as lung cancer. In the United States, about 1 woman in 7 will develop breast cancer during her lifetime, and 1 woman in 30 will die from the disease. About 182,000 American women are diagnosed with breast cancer each year and about 41,000 women die from it each year. Less than 1% of breast cancer cases occur in women under age 30, but a woman's risk doubles every 5 years between ages 30 and 45 and then increases more slowly, by 10–15% every 5 years after age 45. More than 75% of breast cancers are diagnosed in women over 50.

Risk Factors There is a strong genetic factor in breast cancer. A woman who has two close relatives with breast cancer is four to six times more likely to develop the disease than a woman who has no close relatives with it. However, even though genetic factors are important, only about 15% of cancers occur in women with a family history of breast cancer.

Other risk factors include early onset of menstruation, late onset of menopause, having no children or having a first child after age 30, current use of hormone replacement therapy (HT), obesity, and alcohol use. Estrogen may be a unifying element for many of these risk factors. Estrogen circulates in a woman's body in high concentrations between puberty and menopause. Fat cells also produce estrogen, and estrogen levels are higher in obese women. Alcohol can interfere with estrogen metabolism in the liver and increase estrogen levels in the blood. Estrogen promotes the growth of cells in responsive sites, including the breast and the uterus, so any factor that increases estrogen exposure may raise breast cancer risk. A dramatic drop in rates of breast cancer from 2001 to 2004 was attributed in part to reduced use of HT by women over 50 beginning in July 2002. Millions of women stopped taking the hormones after research linked HT with an increased risk of breast cancer and heart disease.

Eating a low-fat, vegetable-rich diet, exercising regularly, limiting alcohol intake, and maintaining a healthy body weight can minimize the chance of developing breast cancer. Long-term use of aspirin and other non-steroidal anti-inflammatory drugs reduces risk, possibly by affecting estrogen synthesis.

Early Detection   A cure is most likely if breast cancer is detected early, so regular screening is a good investment, even for younger women. The ACS advises a three-part personal program for the early detection of breast cancer:

- The ACS recommends a **mammogram** (low-dose breast X ray) every year for women over 40. Studies show that magnetic resonance imaging (MRI) may be better than mammography at detecting breast abnormalities in some women.

- Women between ages 20 and 39 should have a clinical breast exam every 3 years, and women age 40 and older should have one every year before their scheduled mammogram.

- Breast self-exam (BSE) allows a woman to become familiar with her breasts, so she can alert her health care provider to any changes. Women who choose to do breast self-exams should begin at age 20 (see the box "How to Perform a Breast Self-Exam").

Breast pain or tenderness is usually associated with benign conditions such as menstruation rather than breast cancer. The first physical signs of breast cancer are more likely to be a lump, swelling, or thickening; skin irritation or dimpling; or nipple pain, scaliness, or retraction. Although most breast lumps are benign, any breast lump should be brought to the attention of a health care provider.

Treatment   If a lump is detected, it may be scanned by **ultrasonography** and biopsied to see if it is cancerous. In 90% of cases, the lump is found to be a cyst or other harmless growth, and no further treatment is needed. If the lump contains cancer cells, a variety of surgeries may be called for, ranging from a lumpectomy (removal of the lump and surrounding tissue) to a mastectomy (removal of the breast).

If the tumor is discovered before it has spread to the adjacent lymph nodes, the patient has about a 98% chance of surviving more than 5 years. The survival rate for all stages is 89% at 5 years and 80% at 10 years.

New Strategies for Treatment and Prevention   A number of new drugs have been developed for the treatment or prevention of breast cancer. A family of drugs called selective estrogen-receptor modulators, or SERMs, act like estrogen in some tissues of the body but block estrogen's effects in others. One SERM, tamoxifen, has long been used in breast cancer treatment because it blocks the action of estrogen in breast tissue. In 1998, the FDA approved the use of tamoxifen to reduce the risk of breast cancer in healthy women who are at high risk for the disease. Another SERM currently being tested as a potential preventive agent is raloxifene, an osteoporosis drug that has fewer side effects than tamoxifen.

For advanced cancer, treatment with trastuzumab, a monoclonal antibody, is an option for some women. Monoclonal antibodies are a special type of antibody that is produced in the laboratory and designed to bind to a specific cancer-related target.

Prostate Cancer

The prostate gland is situated at the base of the bladder in men, and completely surrounds the male's urethra. It produces seminal fluid; if enlarged, it can block the flow of urine. Prostate cancer is the most common cancer in men and the second leading cause of cancer death in men. More than 186,000 new cases are diagnosed each year, and more than 28,000 American men die from the disease each year.

TERMS

chemotherapy   The treatment of cancer with chemicals that selectively destroy cancerous cells.

remission   A period during the course of cancer in which there are no symptoms or other evidence of disease.

polyp   A small, usually harmless, mass of tissue that projects from the inner surface of the colon or rectum.

mammogram   Low-dose X ray of the breasts used to check for early signs of breast cancer.

ultrasonography   An imaging method in which sound waves are bounced off body structures to create an image on a TV monitor; also called *ultrasound*.

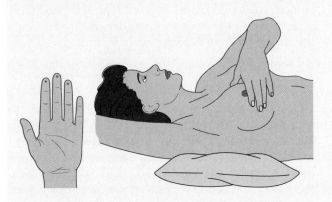

How to Perform a Breast Self-Exam

The best time for a woman to examine her breasts is when the breasts are not tender or swollen. Women who examine their breasts should have their technique reviewed during their periodic health exams by their health care professional.

Women with breast implants can do BSE. It may be helpful to have the surgeon help identify the edges of the implant so that you know what you are feeling. There is some thought that the implants push out the breast tissue and may actually make it easier to examine. Women who are pregnant or breast-feeding can also choose to examine their breasts regularly.

It is acceptable for women to choose not to do BSE or to do BSE once in a while. Women who choose not to do BSE should still be aware of the normal look and feel of their breasts and report any changes to their doctor right away.

How to Examine Your Breasts

• Lie down and place your right arm behind your head. The exam is done while lying down, not standing up. This is because when lying down the breast tissue spreads evenly over the chest wall and is as thin as possible, making it much easier to feel all the breast tissue.

• Use the finger pads of the three middle fingers on your left hand to feel for lumps in the right breast. Use overlapping dime-sized circular motions of the finger pads to feel the breast tissue.

• Use three different levels of pressure to feel all the breast tissue. Light pressure is needed to feel the tissue closest to the skin; medium pressure to feel a little deeper; and firm pressure to feel the tissue closest to the chest and ribs. A firm ridge in the lower curve of each breast is normal. If you're not sure how hard to press, talk with your doctor or nurse. Use each pressure level to feel the breast tissue before moving on to the next spot.

• Move around the breast in an up-and-down pattern starting at an imaginary line drawn straight down your side from the underarm and moving across the breast to the middle of the chest bone (sternum or breastbone). Be sure to check the entire breast area going down until you feel only ribs and up to the neck or collar bone (clavicle).

• There is some evidence to suggest that the up-and-down pattern (sometimes called the vertical pattern) is the most effective pattern for covering the entire breast, without missing any breast tissue.

• Repeat the exam on your left breast, using the finger pads of the right hand.

• While standing in front of a mirror with your hands pressing firmly down on your hips, look at your breasts for any changes of size, shape, contour, or dimpling, or redness or scaliness of the nipple or breast skin. (The pressing down on the hips position contracts the chest wall muscles and enhances any breast changes.)

• Examine each underarm while sitting up or standing and with your arm only slightly raised so you can easily feel in this area. Raising your arm straight up tightens the tissue in this area and makes it harder to examine.

This procedure for doing breast self-exam is different than in previous recommendations. These changes represent an extensive review of the medical literature and input from an expert advisory group. These is evidence that this position (lying down), area felt, pattern of coverage of the breast, and use of different amounts of pressure increase a woman's ability to find abnormal areas.

SOURCE: American Cancer Society's Web site www.cancer.org, 2008. Copyright © 2008 American Cancer Society, Inc. Reprinted with permission.

Risk Factors   Age is the strongest predictor of the risk, with about 64% of cases of prostate cancer diagnosed in men over age 65. Inherited genetic predisposition may be responsible for 5–10% of cases, and men with a family history of the disease should be particularly vigilant about screening. African American men have the highest rate of prostate cancer of any group in the world; both genetic and lifestyle factors may be involved. Diets high in calories, dairy products, and animal fats and low in plant foods have also been implicated as possible culprits, as have obesity, inactivity, and a history of sexually transmitted diseases. Type 2 diabetes and insulin resistance are also associated with pros-

tate cancer. Soy foods, tomatoes, and cruciferous vegetables are being investigated for their possible protective effects.

Detection   Warning signs of prostate cancer can include changes in urinary frequency, weak or interrupted urine flow, painful urination, and blood in the urine. Techniques for early detection include a digital rectal examination and the **prostate-specific antigen (PSA) blood test.** Annual screening tests for early detection are recommended, beginning at age 50 for men at average risk and age 45 for men at high risk, including African Americans and those with a family history of the disease.

PSA testing has been a subject of controversy among experts for several years because of its tendency to yield misleading results, leading to further testing that can lead to harm. This is especially a concern for older men (over 75), who are more likely to die of other causes even if they have slow-growing prostate cancer. The American Cancer Society recommends that physicians discuss PSA and other prostate-cancer tests with their male patients and offer the tests to any man over age 50 (or younger if the patient is at high risk for the disease).

Ultrasound is used increasingly as a follow-up, to detect lumps too small to be felt and to determine their size, shape, and properties. A needle biopsy of suspicious lumps can be performed to determine if the biopsied cells are malignant.

Treatment   Treatments vary based on the stage of the cancer and the age of the patient. A small, slow-growing tumor in an older man may be treated with watchful waiting, because he is more likely to die from another cause before his cancer becomes life threatening; however, a recent study shows that older men who undergo treatment live longer than those who don't. More aggressive treatment would be indicated for younger men or those with more advanced cancers. Treatment usually involves radical prostatectomy, in which the prostate is removed surgically. Although radical surgery has an excellent cure rate, it is major surgery and often results in **incontinence** and/or erectile dysfunction. A less invasive alternative involves surgical implantation of radioactive seeds that destroy the tumor and much of the normal prostate tissue but leave surrounding tissue relatively untouched. Survival rates for all stages of this cancer have improved steadily since 1940; the 5-year survival rate is now nearly 100%.

Cancers of the Female Reproductive Tract

Because the uterus, cervix, and ovaries are subject to similar hormonal influences, the cancers of these organs can be discussed as a group.

Cervical Cancer   Cancer of the cervix occurs frequently in women in their thirties or even twenties. Most cases of cervical cancer stem from infection by the human papillomavirus (HPV), a group of about 100 related viruses that cause both common warts and genital warts. When certain types of HPV are introduced into the cervix, usually by an infected sex partner, the virus infects cervical cells, causing the cells to divide and grow. If unchecked, this growth can develop into cervical cancer.

Cervical cancer is associated with multiple sex partners. The regular use of condoms can reduce the risk of transmitting HPV. Studies also suggest that women whose sexual partners are circumcised may be at reduced risk because circumcised men are less likely to be infected with HPV and to pass it to their partners.

Because only a very small percentage of HPV-infected women ever get cervical cancer, other factors must be involved. Two of the most important seem to be smoking and infection with genital herpes. Some studies show that past exposure to the bacterium that causes the STD chlamydia may be a risk factor for cervical cancer that operates independently of HPV.

Screening for the changes in cervical cells that precede cancer is done chiefly by means of the **Pap test.** During a pelvic exam, loose cells are scraped from the cervix and examined under a microscope to see whether they are normal. If cells are abnormal but not yet cancerous, a condition commonly referred to as *cervical dysplasia*, the Pap test is repeated at intervals. Sometimes cervical cells spontaneously return to normal, but in about one-third of cases, the cellular changes progress toward malignancy. If this happens, the abnormal cells must be removed, either surgically or by destroying them with a cryoscopic (ultracold) probe or localized laser treatment. Without timely surgery, the malignant patch of cells goes on to invade the wall of the cervix and spreads to adjacent lymph nodes and to the uterus. At this stage, chemotherapy may be used with radiation to kill the fast-growing cancer cells, but chances for a complete cure are lower.

Because the Pap test is highly effective, all sexually active women and women between ages 18 and 65 should be tested. The recommended schedule for testing depends on risk factors, the type of Pap test performed, and whether the Pap test is combined with HPV testing.

In 2006, the federal government approved a vaccine, called Gardasil, that protects against four types of HPV viruses, including two that cause about 70% of cervical cancer cases. Studies show the vaccine also protects against cancers of the vagina and vulva. The vaccine is recommended for all girls age 11–12; the recommendation also allows for vaccination of girls as young as 9 and women

prostate-specific antigen (PSA) blood test   A diagnostic test for prostate cancer that measures blood levels of prostate-specific antigen (PSA).

incontinence   The inability to control the flow of urine.

Pap test   A scraping of cells from the cervix for examination under a microscope to detect cancer.

through age 26. The drug is not yet known to be effective for boys or men, but it may be recommended when more information becomes available.

Uterine, or Endometrial, Cancer   Cancer of the lining of the uterus, or endometrium, most often occurs after the age of 55. The risk factors are similar to those for breast cancer, including prolonged exposure to estrogen, early onset of menstruation, late menopause, never having been pregnant, and obesity. Type 2 diabetes is also associated with increased risk. The use of oral contraceptives, which combine estrogen and progestin, appears to provide protection.

Endometrial cancer is usually detectable by pelvic examination. It is treated surgically, commonly by hysterectomy, or removal of the uterus. Radiation treatment, hormones, and chemotherapy may be used in addition to surgery. When the tumor is detected at an early stage, about 95% of patients are alive and disease-free 5 years later. When the disease has spread beyond the uterus, the 5-year survival rate is less than 67%.

Ovarian Cancer   Although ovarian cancer is rare compared with cervical or uterine cancer, it causes more deaths than the other two combined. There are often no warning signs of developing ovarian cancer. Early clues may include increased abdominal size and bloating, urinary urgency, and pelvic pain. It cannot be detected by Pap tests or any other simple screening method and is often diagnosed only late in its development, when surgery and other therapies are unlikely to be successful.

The risk factors are similar to those for breast and endometrial cancer: increasing age (most ovarian cancer occurs after age 60), never having been pregnant, a family history of breast or ovarian cancer, obesity, and specific genetic mutations. A high number of ovulations appears to increase the chance that a cancer-causing genetic mutation will occur, so anything that lowers the number of lifetime ovulation cycles—pregnancy, breastfeeding, or use of oral contraceptives—reduces a woman's risk of ovarian cancer. A diet rich in fruits and vegetables may be associated with reduced risk.

Women with symptoms or who are at high risk because of family history or because they harbor a mutant gene should have thorough pelvic exams at regular intervals. Ovarian cancer is treated by surgical removal of both ovaries, the fallopian tubes, and the uterus. Radiation and chemotherapy are sometimes used in addition to surgery.

Skin Cancer

Skin cancer is the most common cancer of all when cases of the highly curable forms are included in the count. (Usually these forms are not included, precisely because they are easily treated.) Of the more than 1 million cases of skin cancer diagnosed each year, 62,500 are of the most

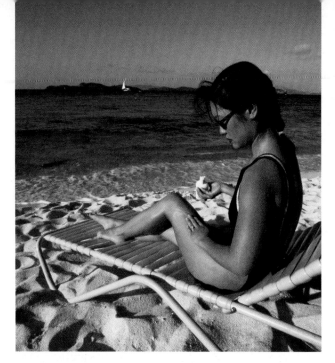

Tanning, either under direct sunlight or in a tanning bed, is a known cause of skin cancer.

serious type, **melanoma.** Treatments are usually simple and successful when the cancers are caught early.

Risk Factors   Almost all cases of skin cancer can be traced to excessive exposure to **ultraviolet (UV) radiation** from the sun, including longer-wavelength ultraviolet A (UVA) and shorter-wavelength ultraviolet B (UVB) radiation. UVB radiation causes sunburns and can damage the eyes and the immune system. UVA is less likely to cause an immediate sunburn, but by damaging connective tissue it leads to premature aging of the skin. (Tanning lamps and tanning-salon beds emit mostly UVA radiation.) Both UVA and UVB radiation have been linked to the development of skin cancer, and the National Toxicology Program has declared both solar and artificial sources of UV radiation, including sunlamps and tanning beds, to be known human carcinogens.

Both severe, acute sun reactions (sunburns) and chronic low-level sun reactions (suntans) can lead to skin cancer. People with fair skin have less natural protection against skin damage from the sun and a higher risk of developing skin cancer; people with naturally dark skin have a considerable degree of protection. Caucasians are about 10 times more likely than African Americans to develop melanoma, but African Americans and Latinos are still at risk.

Severe sunburns in childhood have been linked to a greatly increased risk of skin cancer in later life, so children in particular should be protected. According to the American Academy of Dermatology, the risk of skin cancer doubles in people who have had five or more sunburns in their lifetime. Because of damage to the ozone layer of the atmosphere, there is a chance that we may all be exposed to increasing amounts of UV radiation in the future.

Other risk factors for skin cancer include having many moles, particularly large ones; spending time at high altitudes; and a family history of the disease.

Types of Skin Cancer There are three main types of skin cancer, named for the types of skin cells from which they develop. **Basal cell** and **squamous cell carcinomas** together account for about 95% of the skin cancers diagnosed each year. They are usually found in chronically sun-exposed areas, such as the face, neck, hands, and arms. They usually appear as pale, waxlike, pearly nodules or red, scaly, sharply outlined patches. These cancers are often painless, although they may bleed, crust, and form an open sore on the skin.

Melanoma is by far the most dangerous skin cancer because it spreads so rapidly. It can occur anywhere on the body, but the most common sites are the back, chest, abdomen, and lower legs. A melanoma usually appears at the site of a preexisting mole. The mole may begin to enlarge, become mottled or varied in color (colors can include blue, pink, and white), or develop an irregular surface or irregular borders. Tissue invaded by melanoma may also itch, burn, or bleed easily.

Prevention One of the major steps you can take to protect yourself against all forms of skin cancer is to avoid lifelong overexposure to sunlight. Blistering, peeling sunburns from unprotected sun exposure are particularly dangerous, but suntans—whether from sunlight or tanning lamps—also increase your risk of developing skin cancer later in life. People of every age, especially babies and children, need to be protected from the sun with sunscreens and protective clothing (see the box "Choosing and Using Sunscreens and Sun-Protective Clothing").

Detection and Treatment Make it a habit to examine your skin regularly. Most of the spots, freckles, moles, and blemishes on your body are normal; you were born with some of them, and others appear and disappear throughout your life. But if you notice an unusual growth, discoloration, sore that does not heal,

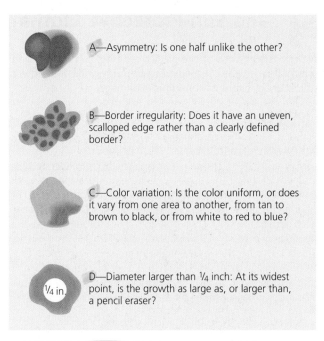

A—Asymmetry: Is one half unlike the other?

B—Border irregularity: Does it have an uneven, scalloped edge rather than a clearly defined border?

C—Color variation: Is the color uniform, or does it vary from one area to another, from tan to brown to black, or from white to red to blue?

D—Diameter larger than ¼ inch: At its widest point, is the growth as large as, or larger than, a pencil eraser?

FIGURE 12.7 The ABCD test for melanoma. To see a variety of photos of melanoma and benign moles, visit the National Cancer Institute's Visuals Online site (http://visualsonline.cancer.gov).

or mole that undergoes a sudden or progressive change, see your physician or a dermatologist immediately.

The characteristics that may signal that a skin lesion is a melanoma—asymmetry, border irregularity, color change, and a diameter greater than ¼ inch—are illustrated in Figure 12.7. If you have an unusual skin lesion, your physician will examine it and possibly perform a biopsy. If the lesion is cancerous, it is usually removed surgically, a procedure that can almost always be performed in the physician's office using a local anesthetic.

Oral Cancer

Oral cancer—cancers of the lip, tongue, mouth, and throat—can be traced principally to cigarette, cigar, or pipe smoking, the use of spit tobacco, and the excessive consumption of alcohol. The incidence of oral cancer is twice as great in men as in women and most frequent in men over 40. Oral cancers have the virtue of being fairly

TERMS

melanoma A malignant tumor of the skin that arises from pigmented cells, usually a mole.

ultraviolet (UV) radiation Light rays of a specific wavelength emitted by the sun; most UV rays are blocked by the ozone layer in the upper atmosphere.

basal cell carcinoma Cancer of the deepest layers of the skin.

squamous cell carcinoma Cancer of the surface layers of the skin.

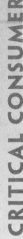

CRITICAL CONSUMER

Choosing and Using Sunscreens and Sun-Protective Clothing

With consistent use of the proper clothing, sunscreens, and common sense, you can lead an active outdoor life *and* protect your skin against most sun-induced damage.

Clothing

• Wear long-sleeved shirts and long pants. Dark-colored, tightly woven fabrics provide reasonable protection from the sun. Another good choice is clothing made from special sun-protective fabrics; these garments have an ultraviolet protection factor (UPF) rating, similar to the SPF for sunscreens. For example, a fabric with a UPF rating of 20 allows only one-twentieth of the sun's UV radiation to pass through. There are three categories of UPF protection: A UPF of 15–24 provides "good" UV protection; a UPF of 25–39 provides "very good" protection; and a UPF of 40–50 provides "excellent" protection. By comparison, typical shirts provide a UPF of only 5–9, a value that drops when clothing is wet.

• Consider washing some extra sun protection into your clothes. A new laundry additive adds UV protection to ordinary fabrics; it is recommended by the Skin Cancer Foundation.

• Wear a hat. Your face, ears, neck, and scalp are especially vulnerable to the sun's harmful effects, making hats an essential weapon in the battle against sun damage. A good choice is a broad-brimmed hat or a legionnaire-style cap that covers the ears and neck. Wear sunscreen on your face even if you are wearing a hat.

• Wear sunglasses. Exposure to UV rays can damage the eyes and cause cataracts.

Sunscreen

• Use a sunscreen and lip balm with a sun protection factor (SPF) of 15 or higher. (An SPF rating refers to the amount of time you can stay out in the sun before you burn, compared with not using sunscreen. For example, a product with an SPF of 15 would allow you to remain in the sun without burning 15 times longer, on average, than if you didn't apply sunscreen.) If you're fair-skinned, have a family history of skin cancer, are at high altitude, or will be outdoors for many hours, use a sunscreen with a high SPF (301).

• Choose a broad-spectrum sunscreen that protects against both UVA and UVB radiation. The SPF rating of a sunscreen currently applies only to UVB, but a number of ingredients, especially titanium dioxide and zinc oxide, are effective at blocking most UVA radiation. In 2006, the FDA approved a product called Anthelios SX that protects against both UVA and UVB radiation. Use a water-resistant sunscreen if you swim or sweat a great deal. If you have acne, look for a sunscreen that is labeled "non-comedogenic," which means that it will not cause pimples.

• In late 2007, the FDA proposed new regulations that would require more stringent testing and labeling of commercial sunscreen products. The new system would require products to be tested for UVA protection and would implement a 4-star rating system based on those tests. The higher a product's rating in stars, the more protection it would provide against UVA radiation. The FDA also proposed placing caps on SPF ratings (which indicate how well a product protects against UVB radi-

ation), to make those ratings more consistent and meaningful to consumers.

• Shake sunscreen before applying. Apply it 30 minutes before exposure to allow it time to bond to the skin. Reapply sunscreen frequently and generously to all sun-exposed areas (many people overlook their temples, ears, and sides and backs of their necks). Most people use less than half as much as they need to attain the full SPF rating. One ounce of sunscreen is enough to cover an average-size adult in a swimsuit. Reapply sunscreen 15–30 minutes after sun exposure begins and then every 2 hours after that and/or following activities, such as swimming, that could remove sunscreen.

• If you're taking medications, ask your physician or pharmacist about possible reactions to sunlight or interactions with sunscreens. Medications for acne, allergies, and diabetes are just a few of the products that can trigger reactions. If you're using sunscreen and an insect repellent containing DEET, use extra sunscreen (DEET may decrease sunscreen effectiveness).

• Don't let sunscreens give you a false sense of security. Most of the sunscreens currently on the market allow considerable UVA radiation to penetrate the skin, with the potential for causing skin cancers (especially melanoma), as well as wrinkles and other forms of skin damage.

Time of Day and Location

• Avoid sun exposure between 10 A.M. and 4 P.M., when the sun's rays are most intense. Clouds allow as much as 80% of UV rays to reach your skin. Stay in the shade when you can.

• Consult the day's UV Index, which predicts UV levels on a 0–10+ scale, to get a sense of the amount of sun protection you'll need; take special care on days with a rating of 5 or above. UV Index ratings are available in local newspapers, from the weather bureau, or from certain Web sites.

• Be aware that UV rays can penetrate at least 3 feet in water. Thus swimmers should wear water-resistant sunscreens. Snow, sand, water, concrete, and white-painted surfaces are also highly reflective.

Tanning Salons and Sunless Tanning Products

• Stay away from tanning salons! Despite advertising claims to the contrary, the lights used in tanning parlors are damaging to your skin. Tanning beds and lamps emit mostly UVA radiation, increasing your risk of premature skin aging (such as wrinkles) and skin cancer.

• If you really want a tan, consider using a sunless tanning product. Lotions, creams, and sprays containing the color additive dihydroxyacetone (DHA) are approved by the FDA for tanning. (The FDA has not approved so-called tanning accelerators and tanning pills because these products have not been proven to be safe or effective.) DHA is for external use only and should not be inhaled, swallowed, or used around the eyes. Tanning salons that offer spraying or misting with DHA need to ensure that customers are protected from exposure to the eyes, lips, and mucous membranes as well as internal exposure. Most sunless tanning products do not contain sunscreen, so if you use them in the sun, be sure to wear sunscreen.

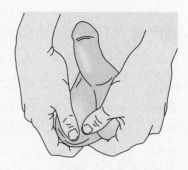
easy to detect, but they are often hard to cure. Furthermore, among those who survive, a significant number will develop another primary cancer of the head and neck. The primary methods of treatment are surgery and radiation.

Testicular Cancer

Testicular cancer is relatively rare, accounting for only 1% of cancer in men (about 8100 cases per year), but it is the most common cancer in men age 20–35. It is much more common among white Americans than Latinos, Asian Americans, or African Americans and among men whose fathers had testicular cancer. Men with undescended testicles are at increased risk for testicular cancer, and for this reason the condition should be corrected in early childhood. Men whose mothers took DES during pregnancy have an increased risk of undescended testicles and other genital anomalies. Thus, they may have a higher risk of testicular cancer. Self-examination may help in the early detection of testicular cancer (see the box "Testicle Self-Examination"). Tumors are treated by surgical removal of the testicle and, if the tumor has spread, by chemotherapy.

QUESTIONS FOR CRITICAL THINKING AND REFLECTION

Has anyone you know had cancer? If so, what type of cancer was it? What were its symptoms? Based on the information presented so far in this chapter, did the person have any of the known risk factors for the disease?

THE CAUSES OF CANCER

Although scientists do not know everything about what causes cancer, they have identified genetic, environmental, and lifestyle factors.

The Role of DNA

Heredity and genetics are important factors in a person's risk of cancer. Certain genes may predispose some people to cancer, and specific genetic mutations—changes in the normal makeup of a gene—have been associated with cancer.

QUICK STATS

5% of all cancers have a strong hereditary component.

—American Cancer Society, 2008

Some mutations are inherited, and others are caused by environmental agents, including radiation, certain viruses, and chemical substances in the air we breathe. An example of an inherited mutation is *BRCA1* (breast cancer gene 1): Women who inherit a damaged copy of this gene face a significantly increased risk of breast and ovarian cancer. Testing and identification of hereditary cancer risks can be helpful for some people, especially if it leads to increased attention to controllable risk factors and better medical screening.

Tobacco Use

Smoking is responsible for 80–90% of lung cancers and for about 30% of all cancer deaths. The U.S. Surgeon General has reported that tobacco use is a direct cause of several types of cancer besides lung and bronchial cancer, including cancer of the larynx, mouth, pharynx, esophagus, stomach, pancreas, kidneys, bladder, and cervix.

In a report released in 2008, the CDC stated that 2.4 million cases of tobacco-related cancer were diagnosed in the United States from 1999 to 2004. The report estimated that tobacco causes nearly 444,000 premature deaths annually in the United States—nearly one of every five deaths each year. The CDC estimates the economic burden of tobacco use at $193 billion annually, including the costs of health care and loss of productivity.

Dietary Factors

The foods you eat contain many biologically active compounds, and your food choices affect your cancer risk by both exposing you to potentially dangerous compounds and depriving you of potentially protective ones.

Dietary Fat and Meat   Diets high in fat and meat appear to contribute to certain cancers, including colon, stomach, and prostate. As is true with heart disease, certain types of fats may be riskier than others. Diets favoring omega-6 polyunsaturated fats are associated with a higher risk of certain cancers than are diets favoring the omega-3 forms of fat commonly found in fish and canola oil.

Alcohol   Alcohol is associated with an increased incidence of several cancers. An average alcohol intake of three drinks per day is associated with a doubling in the risk of breast cancer. Alcohol and tobacco interact as risk factors for oral cancer. Alcohol also increases the risk of colon cancer.

Fried Foods   Scientists have found high levels of the chemical acrylamide (a probable human carcinogen) in starch-based foods that had been fried or baked at high temperatures, especially french fries and certain types of snack chips and crackers.

Studies are ongoing, but the World Health Organization (WHO) has urged food companies to lower the acrylamide content of foods to reduce any risk to public health. The wisest course may be to eat a variety of foods and avoid overindulging in any single class of foods, particularly foods like french fries and potato chips, which may contain other unhealthy substances such as saturated and trans fats.

Fruits and Vegetables   Some essential nutrients act as **anticarcinogens.** For example, vitamin C, vitamin E, selenium, and the carotenoids (vitamin A precursors) may help block cancer by acting as antioxidants. Vitamin C may also block the conversion of nitrites (food preservatives) into cancer-causing agents. Many other anti-cancer agents in the diet fall under the broader heading of phytochemicals, substances in plants that help protect against chronic diseases. One of the first to be identified was sulforaphane, a potent anticarcinogen found in broccoli. Most fruits and vegetables contain beneficial phytochemicals. To increase your intake of these potential cancer fighters, eat a wide variety of fruits, vegetables, legumes, and grains.

Inactivity and Obesity

The American Cancer Society recommends maintaining a healthy weight throughout life by balancing caloric intake with physical activity, and by achieving and maintaining a healthy weight if you are currently overweight or obese. Being overweight or obese is linked with increased risk of several kinds of cancer, including breast and colon cancer.

Carcinogens in the Environment

Some carcinogens occur naturally in the environment, like viruses and the sun's UV rays. Others are manufactured or synthetic substances that show up occasionally in the general environment but more often in the work environments of specific industries.

Ingested Chemicals   The food industry uses preservatives and other additives to prevent food from becoming

THINKING ABOUT THE ENVIRONMENT
The American Cancer Society estimates that about 7% of cancer deaths stem from exposure to carcinogens in the environment. According to this estimate, about 5% of deaths result from occupational exposure to carcinogens; the remaining 2% result from man-made or naturally occurring pollutants in the larger environment.

These cancer-inducing or cancer-promoting agents come from a wide variety of sources. Radon, for example, is an invisible radioactive element that rises into the atmosphere from the ground in some areas. Exposure to radon is known to cause lung cancer, and radon is present in many buildings and homes. Asbestos, which is tightly controlled but still present in many older buildings, is another known carcinogen that affects people who are regularly exposed to it.

Other environmental carcinogens include some agricultural chemicals, industrial pollutants, and waste products that are not properly disposed of (such as certain materials used in electronic devices). While it isn't possible to avoid all these things completely, it is a good idea to be aware of them and minimize contact as much as possible.

anticarcinogen   An agent that destroys or otherwise blocks the action of carcinogens.

TERMS

Cancer Myths and Misperceptions

Almost daily, cancer receives wide-ranging media coverage as it affects the lives of its victims and as breakthroughs create new hope for a cure. During regular checkups, doctors and dentists routinely look for signs of cancer and are quick to discuss the risks of being stricken by cancer.

Remarkably, even as we are being inundated with information about cancer, studies show that most Americans do not understand basic facts about the disease. Indeed, many still believe myths about cancer that were disproved long ago. Such misperceptions are leading Americans to ignore good advice on cancer prevention and to continue lifestyle habits that increase the risk of cancer.

Healthier Cigarettes?

Scientists have concluded that "low-tar," "low-nicotine," and "light" cigarettes are no safer than regular cigarettes. In fact, some brands of light cigarettes contain just as much nicotine and additives as regular cigarettes. Further, users of light cigarettes tend to smoke more frequently and inhale more deeply than smokers of regular cigarettes—often in the misguided belief that their chosen brand won't hurt them. In a 2006 survey, 72% of women and 63% of men said they believed light cigarettes were not as harmful as regular cigarettes.

Similarly, many smokers have switched to smokeless tobacco products (such as chewing tobacco), thinking they pose no health risks. Smokeless tobacco products contribute to head, throat, and oral cancers.

Obesity and Cancer

A 2006 survey conducted for the American Cancer Society showed that only 8% of Americans are aware of the link between obesity and cancer. (Only about 15% of respondents knew their own BMI; most overweight and obese people surveyed did not view themselves as being too heavy.)

Although scientists aren't sure how body fat works to increase cancer risk, there is bountiful evidence that overweight and obese people are in greater danger of breast, prostate, colorectal, and other cancers.

Prevailing Myths

Many Americans accept some myths about cancer, such as the following:

• *Supplements prevent cancer.* Scientists say there is no evidence that any single vitamin, mineral, or herb can boost the immune system enough to ward off cancer.

• *Surgery causes cancer to spread.* For generations, physicians did not have the means to detect cancer until it was advanced. As a result, doctors often performed surgery to remove a tumor from one part of the body without realizing that the cancer had already metastasized. When cancer was found again in another part of the body, many patients assumed that their surgery had "disturbed" the cancer and caused it to spread. This myth prevails even today, although it was disproved long ago.

• *Stress causes cancer.* Stress has been linked to a variety of illnesses, but there is no evidence that it causes cancer.

• *Cancer cannot be prevented.* You can do a lot to prevent cancer, such as eating a healthy diet, exercising, controlling weight, and not smoking.

• *Cancer cannot be cured.* There are nearly 11 million cancer survivors in the United States. Treatments are more powerful than ever, and although some types of cancer are more lethal than others, there is hope for anyone whose cancer is detected early and who takes steps to get rid of it.

---

spoiled or stale. Some of these compounds are antioxidants and may actually decrease any cancer-causing properties the food might have. Other compounds, like the nitrates and nitrites found in processed meat, are potentially more dangerous. While nitrates and nitrites are not themselves carcinogenic, they can combine with dietary substances in the stomach and be converted to nitrosamines, which are highly potent carcinogens. Foods cured with nitrites, as well as those cured by salt or smoke, have been linked to esophageal and stomach cancer, and they should be eaten only in modest amounts.

Environmental and Industrial Pollution Pollutants in urban air have long been suspected of contributing to the incidence of lung cancer. The best available data indicate that less than 2% of cancer deaths are caused by general environmental pollution, such as substances in our air and water but exposure to carcinogenic materials in the workplace is a more serious problem. Occupational exposure to specific carcinogens may account for up to 5% of cancer deaths. With increasing industry and government regulation, we can anticipate that the industrial sources of cancer risk will continue to diminish, at least in the United States.

> Worldwide, **7.6 million** people died of cancer in 2007.
>
> —American Cancer Society, 2008

QUICK STATS

Radiation All sources of radiation are potentially carcinogenic, including medical X rays, radioactive substances

QUESTIONS FOR CRITICAL THINKING AND REFLECTION

What do you think your risks for cancer are? Do you have a family history of cancer, or have you been exposed to carcinogens? How about your diet and exercise habits? What can you do to reduce your risks?

Table 12.4	Screen Guidelines for the Early Detection of Cancer in Asymptomatic People

Site	Recommendation
Breast	• Yearly mammograms are recommended starting at age 40. The age at which screening should be stopped should be individualized by considering the potential risks and benefits of screening in the context of overall health status and longevity. • Clinical breast exam should be part of a periodic health exam about every 3 years for women in their twenties and thirties and every year for women 40 and older. • Women should know how their breasts normally feel and report any breast change promptly to their health care providers. Breast self-exam is an option for women starting in their twenties. • Screening MRI is recommended for women with an approximately 20–25% or greater lifetime risk of breast cancer, including women with a strong family history of breast or ovarian cancer and women who were treated for Hodgkin's disease.
Colon and rectum	Beginning at age 50, men and women should begin screening with one of the examination schedules below: • A fecal occult blood test (FOBT) or fecal immunochemical test (FIT) every year • A flexible sigmoidoscopy (FSIG) every 5 years • Annual FOBT or FIT and flexible sigmoidoscopy every 5 years* • A double-contrast barium enema every 5 years • A colonoscopy every 10 years *Combined testing is preferred over either annual FOBT or FIT, or FSIG every 5 years, alone. People who are at moderate or high risk for colorectal cancer should talk with a doctor about a different testing schedule.
Prostate	The PSA test and the digital rectal examination should be offered annually, beginning at age 50, to men who have a life expectancy of at least 10 years. Men at high risk (African American men and men with a strong family history of one or more first-degree relatives diagnosed with prostate cancer at an early age) should begin testing at age 45. For men at both average risk and high risk, information should be provided about what is known and what is uncertain about the benefits and limitations of early detection and treatment of prostate cancer so that they can make an informed decision about testing.
Uterus	Cervix: Screening should begin approximately 3 years after a woman begins having vaginal intercourse, but no later than 21 years of age. Screening should be done every year with regular Pap tests or every 2 years using liquid-based tests. At or after age 30, women who have had three normal test results in a row may get screened every 2 to 3 years. Alternatively, cervical cancer screening with HPV DNA testing and conventional or liquid-based cytology could be performed every 3 years. However, doctors may suggest a woman get screened more often if she has certain risk factors, such as HIV infection or a weak immune system. Women age 70 and older who have had three or more consecutive normal Pap tests in the past 10 years may choose to stop cervical cancer screening. Screening after total hysterectomy (with removal of the cervix) is not necessary unless the surgery was done as a treatment for cervical cancer. Endometrium: The American Cancer Society recommends that at the time of menopause all women should be informed about the risks and symptoms of endometrial cancer and strongly encouraged to report any unexpected bleeding or spotting to their physicians. Annual screening for endometrial cancer with endometrial biopsy beginning at age 35 should be offered to women with or at risk for hereditary nonpolyposis colon cancer (HNPCC).
Cancer-related checkup	For individuals undergoing periodic health examinations, a cancer-related checkup should include health counseling and, depending on a person's age and gender, might include examinations for cancers of the thyroid, oral cavity, skin, lymph nodes, testes, and ovaries, as well as for some nonmalignant diseases.

SOURCE: American Cancer Society's *Cancer Facts and Figures 2008*. Copyright © 2008 American Cancer Society, Inc. www.cancer.org. Reprinted with permission.

(radioisotopes), and UV rays from the sun. Successful efforts have been made to reduce the amount of radiation needed for mammograms, dental X rays, and other necessary medical X rays. UV radiation from the sun is also a potential carcinogen, and care should be taken to avoid excessive exposure.

DETECTING, DIAGNOSING, AND TREATING CANCER

Early cancer detection often depends on our willingness to be aware of changes in our own body and to make sure we keep up with recommended diagnostic tests.

Detecting Cancer

By being aware of the risk factors in your own life, your immediate family's cancer history, and your own history, you may bring a problem to the attention of a physician long before it would have been detected at a routine physical. In addition to self-monitoring, the ACS recommends routine cancer checkups, as well as specific screening tests for certain cancers (Table 12.4).

Diagnosing and Treating Cancer

Methods for determining the exact location, type, and degree of malignancy of a cancer continue to improve. A

Avoiding Cancer Quackery

As many as 80% of cancer patients report combining conventional treatments with some type of mind-body technique. A much smaller number of patients look for alternatives to the more conventional therapies. These may be therapies within the bounds of legitimate medical practice that have not yet proven themselves in clinical trials. Or, at the extreme, alternative therapies may be scientifically unsound and dangerous, as well as expensive.

Complementary therapies such as yoga, massage, meditation, music therapy, t'ai chi, and prayer can have positive physical and psychological benefits for patients and help them improve their quality of life as they deal with illness and the often difficult treatments for cancer. Mind-body practices can reduce pain and anxiety, improve sleep, and give people a sense of control and participation in their treatment; such practices may also enhance the immune system. Mind-body practices typically can be used in combination with conventional cancer therapies.

For other types of therapies, the National Cancer Institute suggests that patients and their families consider the following questions when making decisions about cancer treatment:

• *Has the treatment been evaluated in clinical trials?* Advances in cancer treatment are made through carefully monitored clinical trials. If a patient wants to try a new therapy, participation in a clinical trial may be a treatment option.

• *Do the practitioners of an approach claim that the medical community is trying to keep their cure from the public?* No one genuinely committed to finding better ways to treat a disease would knowingly keep an effective treatment secret or try to suppress such a treatment.

• *Does the treatment rely on nutritional or diet therapy as its main focus?* Although diet can be a key risk factor in the development of cancer, there is no evidence that diet alone can get rid of cancerous cells in the body.

• *Do those who endorse the treatment claim that it is harmless and painless and that it produces no unpleasant side effects?* Reputable researchers are working to develop less toxic cancer therapies, but because effective treatments for cancer must be powerful, they frequently have unpleasant side effects.

• *Does the treatment have a secret formula that only a small group of practitioners can use?* Scientists who believe they have developed an effective treatment routinely publish their results in reputable journals so they can be evaluated by other researchers.

Use special caution when evaluating cancer remedies promoted online; one recent study found that as many as one-third of cancer-related alternative medicine sites offered advice that was harmful or potentially dangerous.

One danger of alternative medicine is the very real possibility that proven therapies will be neglected while unproven, faddish alternative approaches are pursued; if alternate therapies delay proven therapies, lives may be lost. Another danger is that complementary therapies may counteract or affect conventional therapies; for example, some herbal supplements have been found to affect how cancer drugs are absorbed and used by the body. A recent study revealed that 70% of patients using complementary therapies do not inform their physicians. However, it is essential for physicians to have this information so any side effects or harmful interactions can be prevented.

SOURCES: American Cancer Society. 2006. *Complementary and Alternative Therapies* (http://www.cancer.org/docroot/ETO/ETO_5.asp; retrieved February 15, 2009); National Cancer Institute. 2006. *Complementary and Alternative Medicine in Cancer Treatment: Questions and Answers* (http://www.cancer.gov/cancertopics/factsheet/therapy/CAM; retrieved February 15, 2009).

biopsy may be performed to confirm the type of tumor. Several diagnostic imaging techniques have replaced exploratory surgery for some patients. They include MRIs, CT scanning, and ultrasonography.

For most cancers, surgery is the most useful treatment. Chemotherapy, or the use of cell-killing drugs to destroy rapidly growing cancer cells, work by interfering with DNA synthesis and replication in rapidly dividing cells. Chemotherapy drugs are often used in combinations or with surgery. In cancer radiation therapy, a beam of X rays or gamma rays is directed at the tu-

mor, and the tumor cells are killed. Occasionally, when an organ is small enough, radioactive seeds are surgically placed inside the cancerous organ to destroy the tumor and then removed later if necessary. Radiation destroys both normal and cancerous cells, but because it can be precisely directed at the tumor it is usually less toxic for the patient than either surgery or chemotherapy.

New and Experimental Techniques Many new and exciting possibilities for cancer therapy promise alternatives to the options of surgery, radiation, and chemotherapy. Although it is impossible to predict which of these new approaches will be most successful, researchers hope that cancer therapy overall will become increasingly safer and more effective. When existing treatments are not successful at curbing cancer, patients often turn to complementary and alternative medicine, and experts caution them to be wary of fraudulent approaches (see the box "Avoiding Cancer Quackery").

PREVENTING CANCER

As mentioned throughout this chapter, your lifestyle choices can radically lower your cancer risks.

- *Avoid tobacco.* The bloodstream carries carcinogens from tobacco smoke throughout the body, making smoking a risk for many forms of cancer other than lung cancer. The use of spit tobacco increases the risk of cancers of the mouth, larynx, throat, and esophagus. Exposure to ETS should also be avoided.

- *Control diet and weight.* Choose a low-fat, plant-based diet containing a wide variety of fruits, vegetables, and whole grains rich in phytochemicals. Drink alcohol only in moderation, if at all. Maintain a healthy weight.

- *Exercise.* Regular exercise is linked to lower rates of some cancers. It also helps control weight and reduce risk factors for other diseases.

- *Protect your skin.* Almost all cases of skin cancer are sun-related. Wear protective clothing when you're out in the sun, and use a sunscreen with an SPF rating of 15 or higher. Don't go to tanning salons.

- *Avoid environmental and occupational carcinogens.* Try to avoid exposure to cancer-causing agents in the environment, especially in the workplace.

- *Follow the American Cancer Society's recommendations for cancer screenings.*

TIPS FOR TODAY AND THE FUTURE
A growing body of research suggests that we can take an active role in preventing CVD and many cancers by adopting a wellness lifestyle.

RIGHT NOW YOU CAN
- Plan to replace one high-fat item in your diet with one that is high in fiber. For example, replace a doughnut with a bowl of whole-grain cereal.
- Check the cancer screening guidelines in this chapter and make sure you are up-to-date on your screenings.

IN THE FUTURE YOU CAN
- Take a class in cardiopulmonary resuscitation (CPR). A CPR certification equips you to help someone who is having a heart attack or experiencing cardiac arrest.
- Learn where to find information about daily UV radiation levels in your area, and learn how to interpret the information. Many local newspapers and television stations (and their Web sites) report current UV levels every day.
- Gradually add foods with abundant phytochemicals to your diet.

SUMMARY

- The cardiovascular system pumps and circulates blood throughout the body. The heart pumps blood to the lungs via the pulmonary artery and to the body via the aorta.

- The six major risk factors for CVD that can be changed are smoking, high blood pressure, unhealthy cholesterol levels, inactivity, overweight and obesity, and diabetes.

- Hypertension occurs when blood pressure exceeds normal limits most of the time. It weakens the heart, scars and hardens arteries, and can damage the eyes and kidneys.

- Physical inactivity, obesity, and diabetes are interrelated and are associated with high blood pressure and unhealthy cholesterol levels.

- Contributing risk factors that can be changed include high triglyceride levels and psychological and social factors.

- Risk factors for CVD that can't be changed include being over 65, being male, being African American, and having a family history of CVD.

- Atherosclerosis is a progressive hardening and narrowing of arteries that can lead to restricted blood flow and even complete blockage.

- Heart attacks are usually the result of a long-term disease process.

- A stroke occurs when the blood supply to the brain is cut off by a blood clot or hemorrhage.

- Congestive heart failure occurs when the heart's pumping action becomes less efficient and fluid collects in the lungs or in other parts of the body.

- CVD risk can be reduced by engaging in regular exercise, avoiding tobacco and environmental tobacco smoke, knowing and managing your blood pressure and cholesterol levels, and developing effective ways of handling stress and anger.

- A malignant tumor can invade surrounding structures and spread to distant sites via the blood and lymphatic system, producing additional tumors.

Modifying Your Diet for Heart Health and Cancer Prevention

Gradually modifying your diet to include less saturated and trans fat and more fruits and vegetables can help you avoid both CVD and cancer in the future. Begin by assessing your current diet: Keep a record in your health journal of everything you eat for a week. At the end of the week, you can evaluate your diet and start taking steps to modify it.

Reducing Saturated and Trans Fat in Your Diet

The American Heart Association recommends that no more than 10% of the calories in your diet come from saturated and trans fat. Foods high in these fats include meat, poultry skin, full-fat dairy products, coconut and palm oils, and products made with hydrogenated vegetable oils, such as deep-fried fast food and packaged baked goods. To find out if your diet is within the 10% recommendation, at the end of the week, record the grams of saturated and trans fat next to the foods you've listed in your health journal. This information is available on many food labels, in books, and on the Internet. For fast foods, use the appendix. Trans fat content can be more difficult to determine. Here are the average values per serving for a few trans fat–rich foods: french fries (large), 5 g; pound cake, 5 g; doughnut, 4 g; fried breaded chicken, 3 g; Danish pastry, 3 g; vegetable shortening, 3 g; sandwich cookies, 2 g; crackers, 2 g; margarine (stick), 2 g; margarine (tub), 1 g.

Once you have the grams of fat listed, add up what you consumed each day. For a 2000-calorie diet, the 10% limit corresponds to about 22 grams of saturated and trans fat (2000 × 10% = 200 calories; 200 divided by 9 calories per gram of fat = 22 grams.) If you're not able to get all the data you need, estimate by looking at the number of servings of food high in saturated or trans fat you consume in a day.

If your diet is higher in these fats than it should be, look at your food record to see if you are choosing high-fat foods more often than you should. To reduce your intake of saturated and trans fats, try making healthy substitutions:

- Vegetable oils or trans fat–free tub margarine rather than butter, stick margarine, or vegetable shortening

- Fruits, vegetables, rice cakes, unbuttered popcorn, or pretzels instead of chips, crackers, or cheese puffs

- Low-fat or fat-free milk, cheese, yogurt, or mayonnaise instead of the full-fat versions

- Fruit or a low-fat sweet (angel food cake, frozen yogurt, sorbet) instead of cakes, cookies, pastries, or regular ice cream

- Whole-grain breads and rolls, English muffins, or bagels instead of croissants, muffins, or coffee cake

- Lean meat, skinless poultry, or a veggie burger instead of ground beef, fried chicken, or lunch meats

- Baked potato or rice instead of french fries or onion rings

- Vegetarian chili or pasta with vegetables instead of pizza or macaroni and cheese

When you do eat high-fat foods, eat smaller portions, and balance your higher-fat choices with low-fat choices over the course of the day.

Increasing Fruits and Vegetables in Your Diet

Many fruits and vegetables contain phytochemicals, compounds that help slow, stop, or even reverse the process of cancer. For this reason, the National Cancer Institute (NCI) has developed the "Fruits and Veggies Matter" program to help Americans increase their consumption of fruits and vegetables to health-promoting levels. Take a look at the foods you've listed in your health journal for a week. Have you included five or more fruits and vegetables each day? If not, here are some tips from the NCI:

- Drink 100% juice every morning.

- Add raisins, berries, or sliced fruit to cereal; top bagels with tomato slices.

- Make a fruit smoothie from fresh or frozen fruit and orange juice or low-fat yogurt.

- Have vegetable soup or a salad with your lunch.

- Replace french fries or potato chips with cut-up vegetables.

- Try adding vegetables such as roasted peppers, cucumber slices, shredded carrots, avocado, or salsa to sandwiches.

- Drink tomato or vegetable juice instead of soda (monitor the sodium content of vegetable juices).

- At the salad bar, pile your plate with healthy fruits and vegetables and use low-fat or fat-free dressing.

- At dinner, choose a vegetarian main dish, such as stir-fry, or include two servings of vegetables.

- Substitute vegetables for meat in pasta, chili, and casseroles.

- Keep raw fruits and vegetables (apples, plums, carrots) on hand for snacks.

Some fruits and vegetables are particularly rich in phytochemicals; choose them as often as you can. They include cruciferous vegetables (e.g., broccoli, cauliflower, cabbage, bok choy, brussels sprouts); citrus fruits (e.g., oranges, lemons, grapefruit); berries (e.g., strawberries, raspberries); dark-green leafy vegetables (e.g., spinach, chard, romaine lettuce); and deep-yellow, orange, and red fruits and vegetables (e.g., carrots, red and yellow bell peppers, winter squash, cantaloupe, apricots).

SOURCES: American Heart Association, 2008. *Following a Healthy Eating Plan* (http://www.americanheart.org; retrieved February 24, 2009); National Cancer Institute. 2008. *Fruits and Veggies Matter* (http://www.fruitsandveggiesmatter.gov; retrieved February 24, 2009).

- Lung cancer kills more people than any other type of cancer. Tobacco smoke is the primary cause.

- Colon and rectal cancer is linked to age, heredity, obesity, and a diet rich in red meat and low in fruits and vegetables. Most colon cancers arise from preexisting polyps.

- Breast cancer affects about one in seven women in the United States. Although there is a genetic component to breast cancer, diet and hormones are also risk factors.

- Prostate cancer is chiefly a disease of aging; diet and lifestyle probably are factors in its occurrence.

- Cancers of the female reproductive tract include cervical, uterine, and ovarian cancer. The Pap test is an effective screening test for cervical cancer.

- Skin cancers occur as basal cell carcinoma, squamous cell carcinoma, and melanoma.

- Oral cancer is caused primarily by smoking, excess alcohol consumption, and use of spit tobacco.

- Testicular cancer can be detected early through self-examination.

- Some cancers are caused by inherited genetic mutations, but most mutations are the result of environmental and lifestyle factors, such as radiation, a poor diet, or smoking.

- Self-monitoring and regular screening tests are essential to early cancer detection.

- Methods of cancer diagnosis include magnetic resonance imaging, computed tomography, and ultrasound. Treatment methods usually consist of some combination of surgery, chemotherapy, and radiation.

FOR MORE INFORMATION

BOOKS

American Cancer Society. 2003. *Cancer: What Causes It. What Doesn't.* Atlanta: American Cancer Society. *Provides basic background information about cancer and its causes.*

Heller, M. 2005. *The DASH Diet Action Plan, Based on the National Institutes of Health Research: Dietary Approaches to Stop Hypertension.* Northbrook, Ill.: Amidon Press. *Provides background information and guidelines for adopting the DASH diet; also includes meal plans to suit differing caloric needs and recipes.*

McKinnell, R. G., et al. 2006. *The Biological Basis of Cancer,* 2nd ed. Boston: Cambridge University Press. *Examines the underlying causes of cancer and discusses actual cases of the disease and its impact on patients and families.*

Lipsky, M. S., et al. 2008. *American Medical Association Guide to Preventing and Treating Heart Disease.* New York: Wiley. *A team of doctors provides advice for heart health to consumers.*

Phibbs, B. 2007. *The Human Heart: A Basic Guide to Heart Disease.* Philadelphia: Lippincott Williams & Wilkins. *Provides information*

about heart disease, treatments, and recovery for patients and their families.

Rosenbaum, E., et al. 2008. *Everyone's Guide to Cancer Therapy,* rev. 5th ed. Riverside, N.J.: Andrews McMeel. *Reviewed by a panel of more than 100 oncologists; provides articles on the known causes, diagnoses, and treatments for many types of cancer.*

ORGANIZATIONS, HOTLINES, AND WEB SITES

American Academy of Dermatology. Provides information on skin cancer prevention.

http://www.aad.org

American Cancer Society. Provides a wide range of free materials on the prevention and treatment of cancer.

http://www.cancer.org

American Heart Association. Provides information on hundreds of topics relating to the prevention and control of cardiovascular disease; sponsors a general Web site as well as several sites focusing on specific topics.

http://www.americanheart.org (general information)
http://www.deliciousdecisions.org (dietary advice)
http://www.goredforwomen.org (information just for women)

Centers for Disease Control and Prevention: DES Update. Provides information about drugs containing DES and advice for exposed women and DES daughters and sons.

http://www.cdc.gov/DES

Clinical Trials. Information about clinical trials for new cancer treatments can be accessed at the following sites:

http://www.cancer.gov/clinicaltrials
http://www.centerwatch.com

Dietary Approaches to Stop Hypertension (DASH). Provides information about the design, diets, and results of the DASH study, including tips on how to follow the DASH diet at home.

http://www.nhlbi.nih.gov/health/public/heart/hbp/dash

EPA/Sunwise. Information about the UV Index and the effects of sun exposure, with links to sites with daily UV Index ratings for cities in the United States and other countries.

http://www.epa.gov/sunwise/uvindex.html

Food and Drug Administration, Center for Drug Evaluation and Research: Oncology Tools. Provides information about types of cancer, treatments, and clinical trials.

http://www.fda.gov/cder/cancer

Harvard School of Public Health: Disease Risk Index. Includes interactive risk assessments as well as tips for preventing common cancers.

http://www.diseaseriskindex.harvard.edu/update

The Human Heart: An On-Line Exploration. An online museum exhibit containing information on the structure and function of the heart, how to monitor your heart's health, and how to maintain a healthy heart.

http://www.fi.edu/learn/heart/index.html

National Cancer Institute. Provides information on treatment options, screening, and clinical trials.

http://www.cancer.gov

National Heart, Lung, and Blood Institute. Provides information on and interactive applications for a variety of topics relating to cardiovascular health and disease, including cholesterol, smoking, obesity, hypertension, and the DASH diet.

http://www.nhlbi.nih.gov
http://rover.nhlbi.nih.gov/chd

National Stroke Association. Provides information and referrals for stroke victims and their families; the Web site has a stroke risk assessment.

http://www.stroke.org

SELECTED BIBLIOGRAPHY

American Cancer Society. 2008. *Cancer Facts and Figures 2008.* Atlanta: American Cancer Society.

American Cancer Society. 2008. *Cancer Prevention and Early Detection Facts and Figures 2008.* Atlanta: American Cancer Society.

American Cancer Society. 2006. *Few Americans Know Connection Between Excess Weight and Cancer Risk, Survey Finds* (http://www.cancer.org/docroot/MED/content/MED_2_1x_Few_Americans_Know_Connection_Between_Excess_Weight_and_Cancer_Risk_Survey_Finds.asp; retrieved February 15, 2009).

American Heart Association. 2009. *Heart Disease and Stroke Statistics—2009 Update.* Dallas: American Heart Association.

Baker, S., and J. Kaprio. 2006. Common susceptibility genes for cancer: Search for the end of the rainbow. *British Medical Journal* 332(7550): 1150–1152.

Berger, J. S., et al. 2006. Aspirin for the primary prevention of cardiovascular events in women and men: A sex-specific meta-analysis of randomized controlled trials. *Journal of the American Medical Association* 295(3): 306–313.

Centers for Disease Control and Prevention. 2005. Health disparities experienced by black or African Americans—United States. *Morbidity and Mortality Weekly Report* 54(1): 1–3.

Centers for Disease Control and Prevention. 2008. Awareness of stroke warning symptoms—13 states and the District of Columbia, 2005. *Morbidity and Mortality Weekly Report* 57(18): 481–485.

Centers for Disease Control and Prevention. 2008. Surveillance for cancers associated with tobacco use—United States, 1999–2004. *Morbidity and Mortality Weekly Report Surveillance Summaries* 57(SS-08): 1–33.

Chao, A., et al. 2005. Meat consumption and risk of colorectal cancer. *Journal of the American Medical Association* 293(2): 172–182.

Colihan, D. 2008. *Silent Strokes Take a Toll.* (http://www.webmd.com/stroke/news/20080626/silent-strokes-take-a-toll; retrieved November 10, 2008).

de Torbal, A., et al. 2006. Incidence of recognized and unrecognized myocardial infarction in men and women aged 55 and older: The Rotterdam Study. *European Heart Journal* 27(6): 729–736.

Garland, S. 2006. Efficacy of a quadrivalent HPV (types 6, 11, 16, 18) L1 VLP vaccine against external genital disease: Future 1 analysis. *European Journal of Obstetrics, Gynecology, and Reproductive Biology,* August 16.

Genetics and breast cancer. 2004. *Journal of the American Medical Association* 292(4): 522.

Giovannucci, E., et al. 2008. 25-hydroxyvitamin D and risk of myocardial infarction in men; a prospective study. *Archives of Internal Medicine* 168(11): 1174–1180.

Harvard Medical School. 2008. The status of statins. *Harvard Women's Health Watch* 15(6): 1–3.

Jenkins, D. J., et al. 2006. Assessment of the longer-term effects of a dietary portfolio of cholesterol-lowering foods in hypercholesterolemia. *American Journal of Clinical Nutrition* 83(3): 582–591.

Kauff, N. D., et al. 2008. Risk-reducing salpingo-oophorectomy for the prevention of BRCA1- and BRCA2-associated breast and gynecologic cancer: A multicenter, prospective study. *Journal of Clinical Oncology* 26(8): 1331–1337.

Kroenke, C. H., et al. 2005. Weight, weight gain, and survival after breast cancer diagnosis. *Journal of Clinical Oncology* 23(7): 1370–1378.

Martinez, M. E. 2005. Primary prevention of colorectal cancer: Lifestyle, nutrition, exercise. *Recent Results in Cancer Research* 166: 177–211.

Mayo Clinic. 2006. Skin cancer epidemic. Take steps to avoid sun damage. *Mayo Clinic Health Letter* 24(4): 1–3.

Mayo Clinic. 2008. Breast imaging: Advances in earlier cancer detection. *Mayo Clinic Health Letter* 26(2): 1–3.

Meadows, M. 2005. Brain attack: A look at stroke prevention and treatment. *FDA Consumer,* March/April.

Mukamal, K. J., et al. 2005. Alcohol and risk of ischemic stroke in men: The role of drinking patterns and usual beverage. *Annals of Internal Medicine* 142(1): 11–19.

National Toxicology Program. 2005. *Report on Carcinogens,* Eleventh Edition. Research Triangle Park, N.C.: National Toxicology Program.

Osborn, N. K., and D. A. Ahlquist. 2005. Stool screening for colorectal cancer: Molecular approaches. *Gastroenterology* 128(1): 192–206.

Ostrom, M. P., et al. 2008. Mortality incidence and the severity of coronary atherosclerosis assessed by computed tomography angiography. *Journal of the American College of Cardiology* 52(16): 1335–1343.

Pickering, T. G., et al. 2008. Call to action on use and reimbursement for home blood pressure monitoring: A joint scientific statement from the American Heart Association, American Society of Hypertension, and Preventive Cardiovascular Nurses Association. *Hypertension* 52(1): 10–29.

Prostate cancer: Should you still have a PSA test? 2005. *University of California, Berkeley Wellness Letter,* January.

Putt, K. S., et al. 2006. Small-molecule activation of procaspase-3 to caspase-3 as a personalized anticancer strategy. *Nature Chemical Biology,* August.

Raggi, P., et al. 2008. Coronary artery calcium to predict all-cause mortality in elderly men and women. *Journal of the American College of Cardiology* 52(1): 17–23.

Ridker, P. M., et al. 2005. A randomized trial of low-dose aspirin in the primary prevention of cardiovascular disease in women. *New England Journal of Medicine,* 7 March [epub].

Ridker, P. M., et al. 2008. Rosuvastatin to prevent vascular events in men and women with elevated C-reactive protein. *New England Journal of Medicine* 359(21): 2195–2207.

Sesso, H. D., et al. 2008. Vitamins E and C in the prevention of cardiovascular disease in men: Physician's Health Study II randomized controlled trial. *Journal of the American Medical Association* 300(18): 2123–2133.

Terry, M. B., et al. 2004. Association of frequency and duration of aspirin use and hormone receptor status with breast cancer risk. *Journal of the American Medical Association* 291(20): 2433–2440.

Trimble, C. L., et al. 2005. Active and passive cigarette smoking and the risk of cervical neoplasia. *Obstetrics and Gynecology* 105(1): 174–181.

Turhan, H., et al. 2005. High prevalence of metabolic syndrome among young women with premature coronary artery disease. *Coronary Artery Disease* 16(1): 37–40.

University of California, Berkeley. 2008. Heart tests: low- to high-tech. University of California, Berkeley, Wellness Letter, August, 5.

U.S. Food and Drug Administration. 2008. *Controlling Cholesterol with Statins.* (http://www.dfa.gov/consumer/updates/statins051608.html; retrieved November 10, 2008).

U.S. Preventive Services Task Force. 2008. Screening for prostate cancer: U.S. Preventive Services Task Force recommendation statement. *Annals of Internal Medicine* 149(3): 185–191.

Van Gils, C. H., et al. 2005. Consumption of vegetables and fruits and risk of breast cancer. *Journal of the American Medical Association* 293(3): 183–193.

World Health Organization. 2005. *Cancer: Diet and Physical Activity's Impact* (http://www.who.int/dietphysicalactivity/publications/facts/cancer/en/; retrieved Feburary 15, 2009).

Yusuf, S., et al. 2005. Obesity and the risk of myocardial infarction in 27,000 participants from 52 countries: A case-control study. *Lancet* 366(9497): 1640–1649.

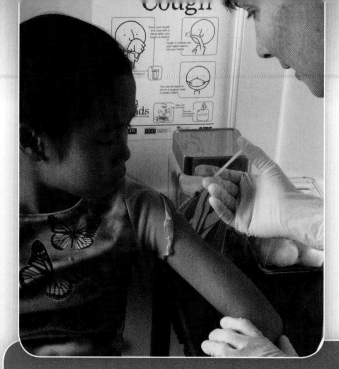

LOOKING AHEAD>>>>>

AFTER READING THIS CHAPTER, YOU SHOULD BE ABLE TO:

- Describe the step-by-step process by which infectious diseases are transmitted

- Explain how the immune system responds to an invading microorganism

- Identify the major types of pathogens and describe the common diseases they cause

- Explain how HIV infection affects the body and how it is transmitted, diagnosed, and treated

- Discuss the symptoms, risks, and treatments for the other major STDs

- Discuss steps you can take to prevent infections, including STDs, and strengthen your immune system

IMMUNITY AND INFECTION 13

The immune system works to keep the body from being overwhelmed, not just by external invaders that cause **infections,** but also by internal changes such as cancer. Most people don't notice these internal skirmishes unless they become sick. But people today are more knowledgeable about the complexities of immunity because they have heard about or had experience with HIV infection, which directly attacks the immune system. This chapter introduces you to the mechanisms of immunity and infection, and shows how to keep yourself well in a world of disease-causing microorganisms.

THE CHAIN OF INFECTION

Infectious diseases are transmitted from one person to another through a series of steps—a chain of infection. The infectious disease cycle begins with a **pathogen,** a microorganism that causes disease. HIV (the virus that causes AIDS) and the tuberculosis bacterium are examples of pathogens. The pathogen has a natural environment—called a **reservoir**—in which it typically lives. This reservoir can be a person, an animal, or an environmental component like soil or water. To transmit infection, the pathogen must leave the reservoir through some portal of exit. In the case of a human reservoir, portals of exit include saliva (for mumps, for example), the mucous membranes (for many sexually transmitted diseases), blood (for HIV and hepatitis), feces (for intestinal infections), and nose and throat discharges (for colds and influenza).

Transmission can occur directly or indirectly. In direct transmission, the pathogen is passed from one person to another without an intermediary; this usually requires fairly close association with an infected host, but not necessarily physical contact. For example, sneezing and coughing can discharge infectious particles into the air, where they can be inhaled by someone nearby. Most common respiratory infections and many intestinal infections are passed directly. Other means of direct transmission include sexual contact and contact with blood.

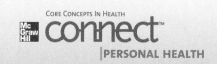

http://www.mcgrawhillconnect.com/personalhealth

In indirect transmission, animals or insects such as rats, ticks, and mosquitoes can serve as *vectors*, carrying the pathogen from one host to another. Pathogens can also be transmitted via contaminated soil, food, or water or from inanimate objects, such as eating utensils.

To infect a new host, a pathogen must have a portal of entry into the body. Pathogens can enter in one of three general ways: direct contact with or penetration of the skin, inhalation through the mouth or nose, or ingestion of contaminated food or water. Pathogens that enter the skin or mucous membranes can cause a local infection of the tissue, or they may penetrate into the bloodstream or lymphatic system, thereby causing a more extensive **systemic infection.** Agents that cause sexually transmitted diseases (STDs) usually enter the body through the mucous membranes lining the urethra (in males) or the cervix (in females). Organisms that are transmitted via respiratory secretions may cause upper respiratory infections or pneumonia, or they may enter the bloodstream and cause systemic infection. Foodborne and waterborne organisms enter the mouth and may attack the cells of the small intestine or the colon, causing diarrhea, or they may enter the bloodstream via the digestive system and travel to other parts of the body.

Once in the new host, a variety of factors determine whether the pathogen will be able to establish itself and cause infection. People with a strong immune system or resistance to a particular pathogen are less likely to become ill than people with poor immunity. If conditions are right, the pathogen will multiply and produce disease in the new host. In such a case, the new host may become a reservoir from which a new chain of infection can be started.

Interrupting the chain of infection at any point can prevent disease. Strategies for breaking the chain include a mix of public health measures and individual action.

For example, a pathogen's reservoir can be isolated or destroyed, as when a sick individual is placed under quarantine or when insects or animals carrying pathogens are killed. Public sanitation practices, such as sewage treatment and the chlorination of drinking water, can also kill pathogens. Transmission can be disrupted through strategies like hand washing and the use of face masks. Immunization and the treatment of infected hosts can stop the pathogen from multiplying, producing a serious disease, and being passed on to a new host.

THE BODY'S DEFENSE SYSTEM

Our bodies have very effective ways of protecting themselves against invasion by pathogens. The body's first line of defense is a formidable array of physical and chemical barriers. When these barriers are breached, the body's **immune system** comes into play.

Physical and Chemical Barriers

The skin, the body's largest organ, prevents many microorganisms from entering the body. Although many bacterial and fungal organisms live on the surface of the skin, very few can penetrate it except through a cut or break.

Wherever there is an opening in the body, or an area without skin, other barriers exist. The mouth is lined with mucous membranes, which contain cells designed to prevent the passage of unwanted organisms and particles. Body openings and the fluids that cover them (for example, tears, saliva, and vaginal secretions) are rich in antibodies and in enzymes that break down and destroy many microorganisms.

The respiratory tract is lined not only with mucous membranes but also with cells having hairlike protrusions called *cilia*. The cilia sweep foreign matter up and out of the respiratory tract. Particles that are not caught by this mechanism may be expelled from the system by a cough. If the ciliated cells are damaged or destroyed, a cough is the body's only way of ridding the airways of foreign particles.

? **QUESTIONS FOR CRITICAL THINKING AND REFLECTION**
Think about the last time you were sick with a cold, the flu, or an intestinal infection. Can you identify the reservoir from which the infection came? What vector, if any, transmitted the illness to you? Did you pass the infection to anyone else? If so, how?

TERMS

infection Invasion of the body by a microorganism.

pathogen A microorganism that causes disease.

reservoir A natural environment in which a pathogen typically lives.

systemic infection An infection spread by the blood or lymphatic system to large portions of the body.

immune system The body's collective physical and chemical defenses against foreign organisms and pathogens.

The Immune System

Once the body has been invaded by a foreign organism, an elaborate system of responses is activated. Two of these responses are the inflammatory response and the immune response.

Immunological Defenders   The immune response is carried out by different types of white blood cells, which are continuously being produced in the bone marrow. *Neutrophils,* one type of white blood cell, travel in the bloodstream to areas of invasion, attacking and ingesting pathogens. *Macrophages,* or "big eaters," take up stations in tissues and act as scavengers, devouring pathogens and worn-out cells. *Natural killer cells* directly destroy virus-infected cells and cells that have turned cancerous. *Dendritic cells,* which reside in tissues, eat pathogens and activate lymphocytes. *Lymphocytes,* of which there are several types, are white blood cells that travel in both the bloodstream and the lymphatic system. At various places in the lymphatic system there are lymph nodes (or glands), where macrophages and dendritic cells congregate and filter bacteria and other substances from the lymph. When these nodes are actively involved in fighting an invasion of microorganisms, they fill with cells; physicians use the location of swollen lymph nodes as a clue to the location and cause of an infection.

The two main types of lymphocytes are *T cells* and *B cells.* T cells are further differentiated into *helper T cells, killer T cells,* and *suppressor T cells.* B cells are lymphocytes that produce **antibodies.** The first time T cells and B cells encounter a specific invader, some of them are reserved as *memory T and B cells,* enabling the body to mount a rapid response should the same invader appear again in the future.

The immune system is built on a remarkable feature of these defenders: the ability to distinguish foreign cells from the body's own cells. Because lymphocytes are capable of great destruction, it is essential that they not attack the body itself. When they do, they cause **auto-immune diseases,** such as lupus and rheumatoid arthritis.

All the cells in your body display markers on their surfaces—tiny molecular shapes—that identify them as "self" to lymphocytes that encounter them. Invading microorganisms also display markers on their surface; lymphocytes identify these as foreign, or "nonself." Nonself markers that trigger the immune response are known as **antigens.** Antibodies have complementary surface markers that work with antigens like a lock and key. When an antigen appears in the body, it eventually encounters an antibody with a complementary pattern. The antibody locks onto the antigen, triggering a series of events designed to destroy the invading pathogen.

The Inflammatory Response   When the body has been injured or infected, one of the body's responses is the inflammatory response. Special cells in the area of invasion or injury release **histamine** and other substances that cause blood vessels to dilate and fluid to flow out of capillaries into the injured tissue. This produces increased heat, swelling, and redness in the affected area. White blood cells are drawn to the area and attack the invaders—in many cases, destroying them.

The Immune Response   The immune system has two types of responses to invading pathogens: natural (innate) and acquired (adaptive). In the natural immune response, immune system cells recognize pathogens as "foreign" and respond the same way no matter how many times a pathogen invades, essentially eating the invaders. In the acquired immune response, immune system cells develop a memory for the antigen. If the body is invaded again, they recognize the pathogen and mount a much more potent response. The immune response can be thought of as having four phases as depicted in Figure 13.1.

Immunity   After an infection, survival often confers **immunity;** that is, an infected person will never get the same illness again because some of the lymphocytes created

---

TERMS

antibody   A specialized protein, produced by white blood cells, that can recognize and neutralize specific microbes.

autoimmune disease   A disease in which the immune system attacks the person's own body.

antigen   A marker on the surface of a foreign substance that immune system cells recognize as nonself and that triggers the immune response.

histamine   A chemical responsible for the dilation and increased permeability of blood vessels in allergic reactions.

immunity   Mechanisms that defend the body against infection; specific defenses against specific pathogens.

acquired immunity   The body's ability to mobilize the cellular memory of an attack by a pathogen to throw off subsequent attacks; acquired through vaccination as well as the normal immune response.

incubation   The period when bacteria or viruses are actively multiplying inside the body's cells; usually a period without symptoms of illness.

cytokine   A chemical messenger produced by a variety of cell types that helps regulate many cell functions; immune system cells release cytokines that help amplify and coordinate the immune response.

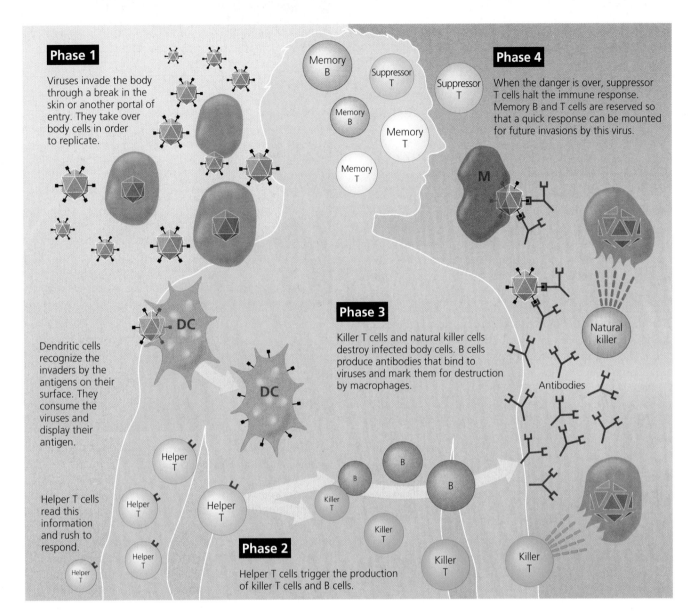

Phase 1

Viruses invade the body through a break in the skin or another portal of entry. They take over body cells in order to replicate.

Dendritic cells recognize the invaders by the antigens on their surface. They consume the viruses and display their antigen.

Helper T cells read this information and rush to respond.

Phase 2

Helper T cells trigger the production of killer T cells and B cells.

Phase 3

Killer T cells and natural killer cells destroy infected body cells. B cells produce antibodies that bind to viruses and mark them for destruction by macrophages.

Phase 4

When the danger is over, suppressor T cells halt the immune response. Memory B and T cells are reserved so that a quick response can be mounted for future invasions by this virus.

FIGURE 13.1 **The immune response.** Once invaded by a pathogen, the body mounts a complex series of reactions to eliminate the invader. Pictured here are the principal elements of the immune response to a virus.

during the second phase of the immune response are reserved as memory T and B cells. If the same antigen enters the body again, the memory T and B cells recognize and destroy it before it can cause illness. The ability of memory lymphocytes to remember previous infections is known as **acquired immunity.**

Symptoms and Contagion The immune system is operating at the cellular level at all times, maintaining its vigilance when you're well and fighting invaders when you're sick. During **incubation,** when viruses are multiplying in the body or when bacteria are actively multiplying before the immune system has gathered momentum, you may not have any symptoms of the illness, but you may be contagious. During the second and third phases

of the immune response, you may still be unaware of the infection, or you may "feel a cold coming on." Symptoms first appear during the *prodromal period,* which follows incubation. If the infected host has acquired immunity, the infection may be eradicated during the *incubation period* or the prodromal period. In this case, although you may have felt you were coming down with a cold, for example, it does not develop into a full-blown illness.

Many symptoms of an illness are actually due to the immune response of the body rather than to the actions or products of the invading organism. For example, fever is caused by the release and activation of certain **cytokines** in macrophages and other cells during the immune response. These cytokines travel in the bloodstream to the brain and cause the body's thermostat to be reset to a higher level.

27 common diseases can be prevented by vaccines.

—CDC, 2007

The resulting elevated temperature helps the body in its fight against pathogens by enhancing immune responses.

Immunization

The ability of the immune system to remember previously encountered organisms and retain its strength against them is the basis for **immunization.** When a person is immunized, the immune system is primed with an antigen similar to the pathogenic organism but not as dangerous. The body responds by producing antibodies, which prevent serious infection when and if the person is exposed to the disease organism itself. The preparations used to manipulate the immune system are known as **vaccines.** Most vaccines are made from microbes that have been weakened or killed in the laboratory but still retain their ability to stimulate the production of antibodies.

Vaccines confer what is known as *active immunity*—that is, the vaccinated person produces his or her own antibodies to the microorganism. Another type of injection confers *passive immunity.* In this case, a person exposed to a disease is injected with the antibodies themselves, produced by other human beings or animals who have recovered from the disease. Injections of *gamma globulin*—a product made from the blood plasma of many individuals containing all the antibodies they have ever made—are sometimes given to people to create a rapid but temporary immunity to a particular disease.

Worldwide, 2.1 million people (mostly young children) die annually of vaccine-preventable diseases.

—WHO, 2005

Allergy: The Body's Defense System Gone Haywire

Allergies result from a hypersensitive and overactive immune system. In someone with an allergy, the immune system mounts a response to a harmless substance such as pollen or animal dander. Allergy symptoms—stuffy nose, sneezing, wheezing, skin rashes, and so on—result primarily from the immune response rather than from **allergens,** the substances that provoke the response.

The Allergic Response   Most allergic reactions are due to the production of a special type of antibody known as

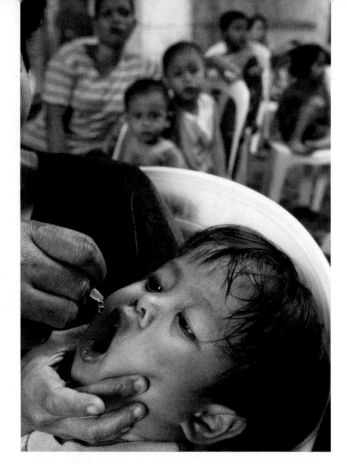

Oral vaccines have made it easier to immunize children in remote and impoverished areas of the world.

immunoglobulin E (IgE). Initial exposure to a particular allergen may cause little response, but it sensitizes the immune system. When the body is subsequently exposed to the allergen, the allergen binds to IgE, causing *mast cells* (another type of immune cell) to release large amounts of histamine and other compounds into surrounding tissues. Histamine has many effects, including increasing the inflammatory response and stimulating mucus production. In the nose, histamine may cause congestion and sneezing; in the eyes, itchiness and tearing; in the skin, redness, swelling, and itching; in the intestines, bloating and cramping; and in the lungs, coughing, wheezing, and shortness of breath. In some people, an allergen can trigger an asthma attack.

The most serious, but rare, kind of allergic reaction is **anaphylaxis,** which results from a release of histamine throughout the body. Anaphylactic reactions can be life-threatening because symptoms may include swelling of the throat, extremely low blood pressure, fainting, heart arrhythmia, and seizures. Anaphylaxis is a medical emergency, and treatment requires immediate injection of epinephrine.

Dealing with Allergies   If you suspect you might have an allergy, visit your physician or an allergy specialist. You may be able to avoid or minimize exposure to allergens by making changes in your environment or behavior. For example, removing carpets from the bedroom and using special bedding can reduce dust mite contact. There are also medications available for allergy sufferers. Many over-the-counter antihistamines are effective at controlling symptoms, and prescription corticosteroids delivered by aerosol markedly reduce allergy symptoms. A third approach is immunotherapy, in which a person is desensitized to a particular allergen through the administration of gradually increasing doses of the allergen over a period of months or years.

PATHOGENS AND DISEASE

When pathogens enter body tissue, they can cause illness and sometimes death to the host. Pathogens include bacteria, viruses, fungi, protozoa, parasitic worms, and prions (Figure 13.2 on page 324).

Bacteria

The most abundant living things on earth are **bacteria,** single-celled organisms that usually reproduce by splitting in two to create a pair of identical cells. We harbor both helpful and harmful bacteria on our skin and in our gastrointestinal and reproductive tracts. The human colon contains helpful bacteria that produce certain vitamins and help digest nutrients. Friendly bacteria also keep harmful bacteria in check by competing for food and resources and secreting substances toxic to pathogenic bacteria. Not all bacteria found in the body are beneficial, however.

Pneumonia Inflammation of the lungs, called *pneumonia,* may be caused by infection with bacteria, viruses, or fungi or by contact with chemical toxins or irritants. Pneumonia often follows another illness, such as a cold or the flu, but the symptoms are typically more severe—fever, chills, shortness of breath, increased mucus production, and cough. Pneumonia is the leading infectious cause of death worldwide and the eighth leading causes of death for Americans.

Pneumococcus bacteria are the most common cause of bacterial pneumonia; a vaccine is available and recommended for all adults age 65 and older and others at risk. Other bacteria that may cause pneumonia include *Streptococcus pneumoniae, Chlamydia pneumoniae,* and *mycoplasmas.* Outbreaks of infection with mycoplasmas are relatively common among young adults, especially in crowded settings such as dormitories.

Meningitis Infection of the *meninges,* the membranes covering the brain and spinal cord, is called *meningitis.*

Viral meningitis is usually mild and goes away on its own; bacterial meningitis, however, can be life-threatening and requires immediate treatment with antibiotics. Symptoms of meningitis include fever, a severe headache, stiff neck, sensitivity to light, and confusion. The disease is fatal in 10% of cases, and about 10–20% of people who recover have permanent hearing loss or other serious effects. A vaccine is available, but it is not effective against all strains of meningitis-causing bacteria. The CDC recommends routine vaccination of children 11–18 years old, previously unvaccinated adolescents at high school entry, and first-year college students who live in dormitories.

Strep Throat and Other Streptococcal Infections
The **streptococcus** bacterium can cause streptococcal pharyngitis, or strep throat, characterized by a red, sore throat with white patches on the tonsils, swollen lymph nodes, fever, and headache. It is typically spread through close contact with an infected person via sneezing or coughing. If left untreated, strep throat can develop into the more serious rheumatic fever. A particularly virulent type of streptococcus can invade the bloodstream, spread to other parts of the body, and produce dangerous systemic illness. It can also cause a serious but rare infection of the deeper layers of the skin, a condition called necrotizing fasciitis, or "flesh-eating strep."

Toxic Shock Syndrome and Other Staphylococcal Infections The spherical-shaped **staphylococcus** bacterium can cause infections ranging from minor skin

---

TERMS

immunization The process of conferring immunity to a pathogen by administering a vaccine.

vaccine A preparation of killed or weakened microorganisms, inactivated toxins, or components of microorganisms that is administered to stimulate an immune response; a vaccine protects against future infection by the pathogen.

allergy A disorder caused by the body's exaggerated response to foreign chemicals and proteins; also called *hypersensitivity.*

allergen A substance that triggers an allergic reaction.

anaphylaxis A severe systemic hypersensitive reaction to an allergen characterized by difficulty breathing, low blood pressure, heart arrhythmia, seizure, and sometimes death.

bacterium (plural, bacteria) A microscopic single-celled organism; about 100 bacterial species can cause disease in humans.

streptococcus Any of a genus (*Streptococcus*) of spherical bacteria; streptococcal species can cause skin infections, strep throat, rheumatic fever, pneumonia, scarlet fever, and other diseases.

staphylococcus Any of a genus (*Staphylococcus*) of spherical, clustered bacteria commonly found on the skin or in the nasal passages; staphylococcal species may enter the body and cause conditions such as boils, pneumonia, and toxic shock syndrome.

Type of Organism	Selected Pathogens	Associated Diseases
Bacteria Microscopic single-celled organisms 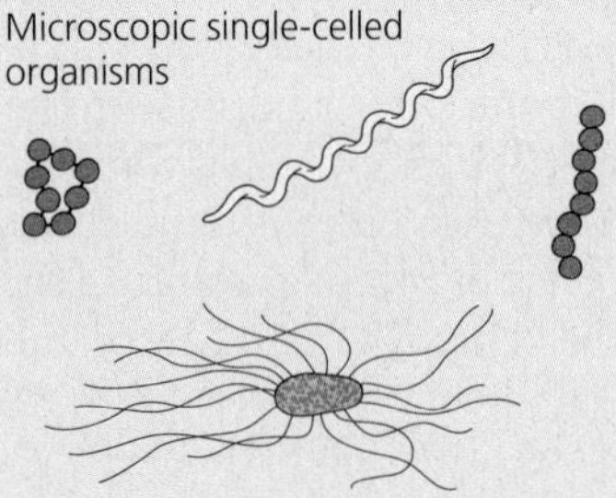	*Bordetella pertussis* *Borrelia burgdorferi* *Chlamydia* *Clostridium tetani* *Helicobacter pylori* *Legionella pneumophila* *Mycobacterium tuberculosis* Mycoplasma *Neisseria* Rickettsia Staphylococcus Streptococcus	Pertussis (whooping cough) Lyme disease Pneumonia (*C. pneumoniae*), chlamydia (*C. trachomatis*) Tetanus Peptic ulcers Legionnaire's disease Tuberculosis Pneumonia, ear infections, sore throat, urethritis Gonorrhea (*N. gonorroeae*), meningitis (*N. meningitidis*) Rocky Mountain spotted fever, typhus Boils and other skin infections, toxic shock syndrome Strep throat, skin infections, pneumonia, rheumatic fever and rheumatic heart disease, necrotizing fascitis
Viruses Infectious agents consisting of a protein shell enclosing DNA or RNA 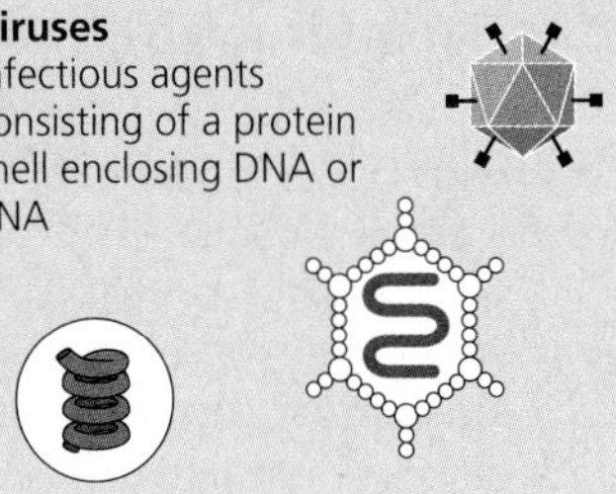	Coronavirus, rhinovirus Epstein-Barr virus Hepatitis viruses Herpes simplex 1 and 2 Human immunodeficiency virus Human papillomaviruses Influenza viruses A and B Paramyxovirus Rhabdovirus Togavirus Varicella-zoster	Severe acute respiratory syndrome (SARS), common cold Infectious mononucleosis Hepatitis (inflammation of the liver) Cold sores, genital herpes HIV/AIDS Warts, cervical cancer Flu Measles, mumps Rabies Rubella Chicken pox, shingles
Fungi Single- or multicelled organisms (e.g., yeasts, molds) 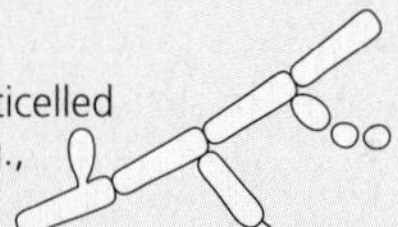	*Candida albicans* *Cryptococcus neoformans* Dermatophyte fungi *Histoplasma capsulatum* *Coccidioides immitis*	Yeast infections, thrush Pneumonia, meningitis Athlete's foot, jock itch, ringworm, nail infections Histoplasmosis Coccidioidomycosis
Protozoa Single-celled organisms 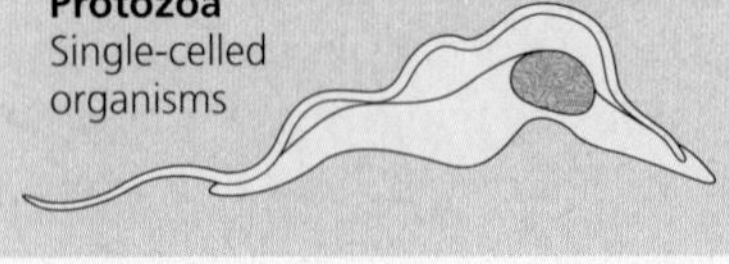	*Entamoeba histolytica* *Giardia lamblia* *Plasmodia* *Trichomonas vaginalis* *Trypanosoma brucei*	Amoebic dysentery Giardiasis Malaria Trichomoniasis African sleeping sickness
Parasitic worms Worms that feed and live on or in a host 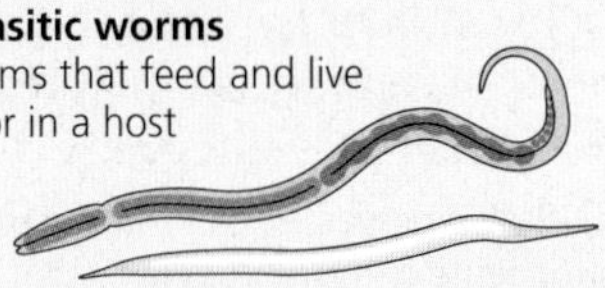	*Ancylostoma duodenale* *Ascaris lumbricoides* Beef, pork, or fish tapeworms *Enterobius vermicularis* *Necator americanus* Schistosoma	Ancylostomiasis (hookworm infection) Ascariasis (roundworm infection) Tapeworm infection Pinworm infection Hookworm infection Cercarial dermatitis (swimmer's itch), schistosomiasis
Prions Proteinaceous infectious particles	PrP^{Sc}	Creutzfeldt-Jakob disease (CJD)

FIGURE 13.2   Pathogens and associated infectious diseases.

infections to very serious conditions such as blood infections and pneumonia. The strain known as methicillin-resistant *Staphylococcus aureus* (MRSA) has become the most common cause of skin infections treated in emergency rooms (see the box "MRSA: The Superbug?" *Staphylococcus aureus* is also responsible for many cases of toxic shock syndrome (TSS). The bacteria produce a deadly toxin that causes shock (potentially life-threatening low blood pressure), high fever, a peeling skin rash, and inflammation of several organ systems.

Tuberculosis   Caused by the bacterium *Mycobacterium tuberculosis*, **tuberculosis (TB)** is a chronic bacterial infection that usually affects the lungs. TB is spread via the respiratory route. Symptoms include coughing, fatigue, night sweats, weight loss, and fever. Ten to 15 million Americans have been infected with, and therefore con-

TERMS

tuberculosis (TB)   A chronic bacterial infection that usually affects the lungs.

antibiotics   Synthetic or naturally occurring substances used as drugs to kill bacteria.

In recent years, an antibiotic-resistant strain of staph—called methicillin-resistant *Staphylococcus aureus* (MRSA)—has changed the public's perception of staph as a relatively harmless germ. Medical experts have dubbed MRSA a "superbug" because it is highly resistant to several first-line medicines normally used to treat staph infections. These drugs include methicillin, penicillin, oxacillin, and amoxicillin, among others.

MRSA is not only virulent, it can be deadly. The CDC estimates that more Americans died from MRSA infections (18,650) than from AIDS (16,000) in 2005. That year, the CDC says that more than 94,000 Americans suffered from severe, invasive MRSA infections. Other estimates, however, are higher.

About 85% of MRSA infections affect patients in health care facilities or who have recently left a health care setting. Health care–associated MRSA victims typically have undergone an invasive surgical procedure or have an immune system weakened by illness or treatment for another disease. Experts say

invasive MRSA is now the leading cause of surgical site infections, bloodstream infections, and pneumonia in hospitals and nursing homes.

Although less common, MRSA also affects people who have not been exposed to a health care facility; such infections are called *community-associated MRSA (CA-MRSA)* infections. CA-MRSA usually is not invasive, and instead, take the form of surface abscesses and pus-filled lesions. Even though their numbers are low, community-based infections are a growing concern because they may indicate that MRSA is gaining strength.

In the age of antibiotics, it's hard to imagine being infected by a germ that can't be killed. But epidemiologists say the overuse of antibiotics is one of the main reasons that bugs such as MRSA have become so strong. When people take antibiotics inappropriately or incorrectly, bacteria have an opportunity to adapt and can become resistant to antibiotics.

Doctors also say that MRSA is a powerful reminder that frequent hand

washing may be the most effective way to avoid infections—not just from MRSA, but from a host of other germs. Other simple but important methods for preventing infections also apply to MRSA: When washing your hands, use lots of soap and scrub briskly for at least 15 seconds. If soap and water aren't available, carry an alcohol-based hand sanitizer with you and use it often. Keep your hands away from your face. If you have an open wound, keep it clean, dry, and covered with a bandage. Don't share items such as towels, razors, and tweezers; they can harbor germs and spread infection. If you have a skin lesion that resembles a spider bite, have it checked by a physician right away.

SOURCES: Centers for Disease Control and Prevention. 2007. Invasive MRSA (http://www.cdc.gov/ncidod/dhqp/ar_mrsa_Invasive_FS.html; retrieved February 16, 2009); Klevens, R. M., et al. 2007. Invasive methicillin-resistant *Staphylococcus aureus* infections in the United States. *Journal of the American Medical Association* 298(15): 1763–1771.

tinue to carry, *M. tuberculosis.* Only about 10% of people with latent TB infections actually develop an active case of the disease. In the United States, active TB is most common among people infected with HIV, recent immigrants from countries where TB is endemic, and those who live in the inner cities. Many strains of tuberculosis respond to antibiotics, but only over a course of treatment lasting 6–12 months. Failure to complete treatment can lead to relapse and the development of strains of antibiotic-resistant bacteria. From 2000 to 2004, 20% of TB bacteria isolated in labs were multidrug resistant (MDR) and 2% were extensively drug resistant (XDR). XDR TB is geographically widespread, occurring even in the United States, and is a serious threat to public health.

Tickborne Infections Lyme disease is spread by the bite of a tick of the genus *Ixodes* that is infected with the spiral-shaped bacterium *Borrelia burgdorferi.* Symptoms of Lyme disease vary but typically occur in three stages. In the first stage, about 80% of victims develop a bull's-eye-shaped red rash expanding from the area of the bite, usually about 2 weeks after the bite occurs. The second stage occurs weeks to months later in 10–20% of untreated patients; symptoms may involve the nervous and cardiovascular systems and can include impaired coordination, partial facial paralysis, and heart rhythm abnormalities. Months or years after the tick bite some untreated people

may develop chronic or recurring arthritis. Lyme disease is preventable by avoiding contact with ticks or by removing a tick before it has had the chance to transmit the infection. Rocky Mountain spotted fever is also transmitted via tick bites and is characterized by sudden onset of fever, headache, and muscle pain, followed by development of a spotted rash.

Ulcers About 25 million Americans suffer from ulcers, sores in the lining of the stomach or the first part of the small intestine (duodenum). Up to 90% of ulcers are caused by infection with the bacterium *Helicobacter pylori.* Ulcer symptoms include gnawing or burning pain in the abdomen, nausea, and loss of appetite. If tests show the presence of *H. pylori,* antibiotics often cure the infection and the ulcers.

Antibiotic Treatments **Antibiotics** are both naturally occurring and synthetic substances that can kill bacteria. Most antibiotics work in a similar fashion: They interrupt the production of new bacteria by damaging some part of their reproductive cycle or by causing faulty parts of new bacteria to be made. Antibiotics are among the most widely prescribed and effective drugs.

When antibiotics are misused or overused, the pathogens they are designed to treat can become resistant to their effects. When exposed to antibiotics, resistant bacteria can grow and flourish, while the antibiotic-sensitive bacteria die off. Antibiotic-resistant strains of many common bacteria have developed, including strains of gonorrhea (an STD) and salmonellosis (a foodborne illness). One strain of tuberculosis is resistant to seven different antibiotics. Antibiotic resistance is a major factor contributing to the recent rise in problematic infectious diseases.

Resistance is promoted when people fail to take the full course of an antibiotic or when they inappropriately take antibiotics for viral infections. Another source of resistance is the use of antibiotics in agriculture, which is estimated to account for 50–80% of the 25,000 tons of antibiotics used annually in the United States.

You can help prevent the development of antibiotic-resistant strains of bacteria by using antibiotics properly:

- Don't take an antibiotic every time you get sick. They are mainly helpful for bacterial infections; they are ineffective against viruses.

- Use antibiotics as directed, and finish the full course of medication even if you begin to feel better. This helps ensure that all targeted bacteria are killed off.

- Never take an antibiotic without a prescription.

Viruses

Viruses lack all the enzymes essential to energy production and protein synthesis in normal animal cells, and they cannot grow or reproduce by themselves; they are parasites, taking what they need for growth and reproduction from the cells they invade. Once a virus is inside the host cell, it sheds its protein covering, and its genetic material takes control of the cell and manufactures more viruses like itself. Illnesses caused by viruses are the most common forms of contagious disease.

The Common Cold   Although generally brief, lasting only 1–2 weeks, colds are nonetheless irritating and often interfere with one's normal activities. A cold may be caused by any of more than 200 different viruses that attack the lining of the nasal passages. Cold viruses are almost always transmitted by hand-to-hand contact. To lessen your risk of contracting a cold, wash your hands frequently; if you touch someone else, avoid touching your face until after you've washed your hands. If you catch a cold, over-the-counter cold remedies may help treat your symptoms but do not directly attack the viral cause. Avoid multisymptom cold remedies. Because these products include drugs to treat

symptoms you may not even have, you risk suffering from side effects from medications you don't need. It's better to treat each symptom separately:

Antibiotics will not help a cold unless a bacterial infection such as strep throat is also present, and overuse of antibiotics leads to the development of drug resistance. The jury is still out on whether other remedies, including zinc gluconate lozenges, echinacea, and vitamin C, will relieve symptoms or shorten the duration of a cold.

Influenza   Commonly called the flu, **influenza** is an infection of the respiratory tract caused by the influenza virus. Compared to the common cold, influenza is a more serious illness, usually including a fever and extreme fatigue. Most people who get the flu recover within 1–2 weeks, but some develop potentially life-threatening complications, such as pneumonia. The highest rates of infection occur in children. Influenza is highly contagious and is spread via respiratory droplets.

Vaccination can be appropriate for anyone age 6 months or older who wants to reduce his or her risk of the flu. A number of medications are used to treat influenza and to reduce the risk of illness from influenza.

Chicken Pox, Cold Sores, and Other Herpesvirus Infections   The **herpesviruses** are a large group of viruses. Once infected, the host is never free of the virus. The virus lies latent within certain cells and becomes active periodically, producing symptoms. The family of herpesviruses includes varicella-zoster virus, which causes chicken pox and shingles; herpes simplex virus (HSV) types 1 and 2, which cause cold sores and the STD herpes; and Epstein-Barr virus (EBV), which causes infectious mononucleosis. Two herpesviruses that can cause severe infections in people with a suppressed immune system are cytomegalovirus (CMV), which infects the lungs, brain, colon, and eyes, and human herpesvirus 8 (HHV-8), which has been linked to Kaposi's sarcoma.

Viral Hepatitis   Viral **hepatitis** is a term used to describe several different infections that cause inflammation of the liver. Hepatitis is usually caused by one of the three most common hepatitis viruses. Hepatitis A virus (HAV) causes the mildest form of the disease and is usually transmitted by food or water contaminated by sewage or an infected person. Hepatitis B virus (HBV) is usually transmitted sexually. Hepatitis C virus (HCV) can also be transmitted sexually, but it is much more commonly passed through direct contact with infected blood via injection drug use or, prior to the development of screening tests,

The Next Influenza Pandemic— When, Not If?

IN FOCUS

There are three main types of influenza viruses, designated A, B, and C. Influenza C usually causes only mild illness and has not been associated with widespread outbreaks. Types A and B, however, are responsible for **epidemics** of respiratory illness that occur almost every winter.

Through replication errors and gene sharing, influenza viruses undergo constant change, enabling them to evade the immune system and thereby make people susceptible to influenza throughout life. A person infected with influenza does develop antibodies, but as the antigens change, the antibodies no longer recognize the virus, and reinfection can occur. Small changes in antigens are why the flu vaccine is reformulated each year. Fortunately, if the changes are small, the immune system may at least partially recognize the virus, giving many people some immune protection against the new strain.

Occasionally, an influenza A virus undergoes a sudden, dramatic change. If the new virus spreads easily from person to person, a worldwide epidemic, called a **pandemic,** can occur because few people have any antibody protection against the virus. During the twentieth century, three major influenza pandemics occurred in humans:

- 1918–1919 ("Spanish flu"): About 20–40% of the world's population became ill, and as many as 40 million people died, including more than 500,000 Americans.

- 1957–1958 ("Asian flu")

- 1968–1969 ("Hong Kong flu")

Many experts believe that an influenza pandemic is overdue, inevitable, and possibly imminent. Conditions that allow the mingling of flu viruses— including wild and domestic birds, humans, and other flu carriers living in crowded conditions and close proximity—exist in many parts of the world.

Scientists have been monitoring the progress of a strain of avian influenza A(H5N1). The H5N1 strain doesn't pass easily to or between humans. However, when it infects humans, it is deadly. Through mid-2006, outbreaks of H5N1 avian influenza were reported among migratory birds and poultry flocks in several countries in Asia, Africa, the Middle East, and Europe, with 63% of cases occurring in Indonesia and Vietnam. Where those outbreaks occurred, people who came into close contact with infected birds became ill or died. As of February 11, 2009, 407 people worldwide had been diagnosed with H5N1 infection and 254 of those victims died.

Scientists are studying the virus to determine how many mutations it would take to allow H5N1 to pass easily between humans. The avian flu virus is resistant to at least two antiviral medications commonly used to treat influenza, and scientists are trying to confirm whether the virus resists other currently available antiviral drugs, as well. In 2007, the Food and Drug Administration approved the first avian flu vaccine for use in humans; others are in development.

---

blood transfusions. HBV and, to a lesser extent, HCV can also be passed from a pregnant woman to her child. There are effective vaccines for hepatitis A and B.

Symptoms of acute hepatitis infection can include fatigue, **jaundice,** abdominal pain, loss of appetite, nausea, and diarrhea. Most people recover from hepatitis A within a month or so. However, 5–10% of people infected with HBV and 85–90% of people infected with HCV become chronic carriers of the virus, capable of infecting others for the rest of their lives. Some chronic carriers remain asymptomatic, while others slowly develop chronic liver disease, cirrhosis, or liver cancer. An estimated 4 million Americans and 500 million people worldwide may be chronic carriers of hepatitis.

The extent of HCV infection has only recently been recognized, and most infected people are unaware of their condition. To ensure proper treatment and prevention, testing for HCV may be recommended for people at risk, including people who have ever injected drugs (even once), who received a blood transfusion or a donated organ prior to July 1992, who have engaged in high-risk sexual behavior, or who have had body piercing, tattoos, or acupuncture involving unsterile equipment. If you are considering getting a tattoo or body piercing, choose the artist carefully and follow aftercare directions.

Human Papillomavirus (HPV) The more than 100 different types of HPV cause a variety of warts, including common warts on the hands, plantar warts on the soles of the feet, and genital warts. Depending on their location, warts may be removed using over-the-counter preparations or professional methods such as laser surgery or

TERMS

virus A very small infectious agent composed of nucleic acid (DNA or RNA) surrounded by a protein coat; lacks an independent metabolism and reproduces only within a host cell.

influenza Infection of the respiratory tract by the influenza virus, which is highly infectious and adaptable; the form changes so easily that every year new strains arise, making treatment difficult; commonly known as the flu.

herpesvirus A family of viruses responsible for cold sores, mononucleosis, chicken pox, and the STD known as herpes; frequently causes latent infections.

epidemic The occurrence in a particular community or region of more than the expected number of cases of a particular disease.

pandemic A disease epidemic that is unusually severe or widespread; often used to refer to worldwide epidemics affecting a large proportion of the population.

hepatitis Inflammation of the liver, which can be caused by infection, drugs, or toxins.

jaundice Increased bile pigment levels in the blood, characterized by yellowing of the skin and the whites of the eyes.

PATHOGENS AND DISEASE **327**

cryosurgery. Because HPV infection is chronic, warts can reappear despite treatment. HPV causes the majority of cases of cervical cancer; a vaccine is available and recommended for girls and women age 9–26.

Treating Viral Illnesses Antiviral drugs typically work by interfering with some part of the viral life cycle; for example, they may prevent a virus from entering body cells or from successfully reproducing within cells. Antivirals are currently available to fight infections caused by HIV, influenza, herpes simplex, varicella-zoster, HBV, and HVC. Most other viral diseases must simply run their course.

Fungi

A **fungus** is an organism that absorbs food from organic matter. Only about 50 fungi out of many thousands of species cause disease in humans, and these diseases are usually restricted to the skin, mucous membranes, and lungs.

Candida albicans is a common fungus found naturally in the vagina of most women. When excessive growth occurs, the result is itching and discomfort, commonly known as a yeast infection. Other common fungal conditions, including athlete's foot, jock itch, and ringworm, affect the skin. Fungi can also cause systemic diseases that are severe, life-threatening, and extremely difficult to treat. Fungal infections can be especially deadly in people with an impaired immune system.

Protozoa

Another group of pathogens is single-celled organisms known as **protozoa**. Millions of people in developing countries suffer from protozoal infections.

Malaria, caused by a protozoan of the genus *Plasmodium,* is a major killer worldwide; each year, there are 350–500 million new cases of malaria and more than 1 million deaths, mostly among infants and children, and drug-resistant strains of malaria have emerged, requiring new medicines.

Other protozoal diseases include **giardiasis**, a single-celled parasite that lives in the intestines of humans and animals and is characterized by nausea, diarrhea, bloating, and abdominal cramps; *trichomoniasis,* a common, treatable, vaginal infection; *trypanosomiasis,* known as African sleeping sickness; and *amoebic dysentery.*

Parasitic Worms

The **parasitic worms** are the largest organisms that can enter the body to cause infection. The tapeworm, for example, can grow to a length of many feet. Worms cause a variety of relatively mild infections. Pinworm, the most common worm infection in the United States, primarily affects young children. Worm infections generally originate from contaminated food or drink and can be controlled by careful attention to hygiene.

Prions

In recent years, several fatal degenerative disorders of the central nervous system have been linked to **prions,** or *proteinaceous infectious particles.* Unlike all other infectious agents, prions appear to lack DNA or RNA and to consist only of protein; their presence in the body does not trigger an immune response. Prions have an abnormal shape and form deposits in the brain. Prions are associated with a class of diseases known as *transmissible spongiform encephalopathies (TSEs),* which are characterized by sponge-like holes in the brain; symptoms of TSEs include loss of coordination, weakness, dementia, and death. Known prion diseases include Creutzfeldt-Jakob disease (CJD) in humans; bovine spongiform encephalopathy (BSE), or mad cow disease, in cattle; and scrapie in sheep. Some prion diseases are inherited or the result of spontaneous genetic mutations, whereas others are the result of eating infected tissue or being exposed to prions during medical procedures such as organ transplants.

Emerging Infectious Diseases

Emerging infectious diseases are those infections whose incidence in humans has increased or threatens to increase in the near future. They include both known diseases that have experienced a resurgence, such as tuberculosis and cholera, and diseases that were previously unknown or confined to specific areas, such as the Ebola and West Nile viruses.

Selected Infections of Concern

Although the chances of the average American contracting an exotic infection are very low, emerging infections represent a challenge to all nations in the future.

WEST NILE VIRUS A mini-outbreak of encephalitis in New York in 1999 led to identification of this virus, which had previously been restricted to Africa, the Middle East, and parts of Europe. Between 1999 and 2007, the virus spread across the United States and caused more than 27,605 illnesses and 1086 deaths. West Nile virus is carried by birds and then passed to humans when mosquitoes bite first an infected bird and then a person. Most people who are bitten have few or no symptoms, but the virus can cause permanent brain damage or death in some.

SEVERE ACUTE RESPIRATORY SYNDROME (SARS) In February 2003, SARS appeared in southern China and quickly spread to more than 15 countries; it is a form of pneumonia that is fatal in about 5–15% of cases. SARS is caused by a new type of coronavirus found in wildlife that may have crossed the species barrier. It has reemerged several times since 2003, and by 2004 had been responsible for more than 8000 illnesses and 800 deaths.

ROTAVIRUS The leading viral cause of gastroenteritis, an intestinal inflammation that results in vomiting and diarrhea, rotavirus infects almost every child at one time or another and kills about 600,000 children each year, mostly in developing countries. Left untreated, rotavirus-induced diarrhea can become severe and lead to dehydration, which can be fatal. Rotavirus spreads through poor hygiene and sanitation practices.

ESCHERICHIA COLI O157:H7 This potentially deadly strain of *E. coli,* transmitted in contaminated food, can cause bloody diarrhea and kidney damage. Outbreaks have been linked to contaminated spinach, lettuce, alfalfa sprouts, unpasteurized juice, petting zoos, and public swimming pools. An estimated 70,000 cases and 61 deaths occur in the United States each year.

HANTAVIRUS Since first being recognized in 1993, over 300 cases of hantavirus pulmonary syndrome (HPS) have been reported in the United States. HPS is caused by the rodentborne Sin Nombre virus (SNV) and is spread primarily through airborne viral particles from rodent urine, droppings, or saliva. It is characterized by a dangerous fluid buildup in the lungs and is fatal in about 45% of cases.

EBOLA Human outbreaks of the often fatal Ebola hemorrhagic fever (EHF) have occurred only in Africa. The Ebola virus is transmitted by contact with infected blood or other body secretions. Because symptoms appear quickly and 70% of victims die, usually within a few days, the virus tends not to spread widely.

Factors Contributing to Emerging Infections

What's behind this rising tide of infectious diseases? One factor is drug resistance. New or increasing drug resistance has been found in organisms that cause malaria, tuberculosis, gonorrhea, influenza, AIDS, and pneumococcal and staphylococcal infections. Some bacterial strains now appear to be resistant to all available antibiotics.

Another factor is poverty. More than 1 billion people live in extreme poverty, and half the world's population have no regular access to essential drugs. Population growth, urbanization, overcrowding, and migration (including the movement of refugees) also spread infectious diseases.

A poor public health infrastructure is often associated with poverty and social upheaval, but problems such as contaminated water supplies can occur even in industrial countries. Natural disasters such as hurricanes also disrupt the public health infrastructure, leaving survivors with contaminated water and food supplies and no shelter from disease-carrying insects.

Travel, commerce, and food production and distribution practices also contribute, as do human behaviors. More than 500 million travelers cross national borders each year, and international tourism and trade open the world to infectious agents. SARS was quickly spread throughout the world by infected air travelers. Food now

---

THINKING ABOUT THE ENVIRONMENT

Many environmental factors contribute to the spread of infectious diseases. Here are a few examples:

- In poverty-stricken regions, many people become ill as a result of unsanitary conditions and a lack of clean drinking water.

- Unsustainable development practices, such as clearing forests and draining wetlands, disturb the ecosystem and force many disease-carrying vectors (such as vermin and insects) out of their natural habitats and into contact with people.

- A shift in rainfall patterns (perhaps caused by global warming) may allow mosquito-borne diseases such as malaria to spread from the tropics into the temperate zones. Since many species of mosquito in North America can carry malaria, such changes could make malaria a health threat to the United States.

travels long distances to our table, and microbes are transmitted along with it. Mass production of food increases the likelihood that a chance contamination can lead to mass illness. The widespread use of injectable drugs rapidly transmits HIV infection and hepatitis. Changes in sexual behavior over the past 30 years have led to a proliferation of old and new STDs. The use of day-care facilities for children has led to increases in the incidence of several infections that cause diarrhea.

Finally, the deliberate release of deadly infectious agents is an ongoing concern. In 2001, infectious anthrax spores sent through the mail sickened 11 and killed 5 people in the United States. Potential bioterrorism agents that the CDC categorizes as a highest concern are those that can be easily disseminated or transmitted from person to person and that have a high mortality rate and the potential for a major public health impact; these include anthrax, smallpox, plague, botulism, and viral hemorrhagic fevers such as Ebola.

Other Immune Disorders: Cancer and Autoimmune Diseases

Sometimes, as in the case of cancer, the body comes under attack by its own cells. The immune system can often detect cells that have recently become cancerous and then destroy them just as it would a foreign microorganism. But if the immune system breaks down, the cancer cells may multiply out of control before the immune system recognizes the danger.

Another immune disorder occurs when the body confuses its own cells with foreign organisms. This is what happens in autoimmune diseases such as rheumatoid arthritis and systemic lupus erythematosus. In this type of malady, the immune system seems to be too sensitive and begins to misapprehend itself as nonself. For reasons not well understood, these conditions are much more common in women than in men.

SUPPORTING YOUR IMMUNE SYSTEM

Pathogens threaten everyone's wellness, but you can take steps to prevent them from compromising your health. Here are some general guidelines for keeping pathogens at bay:

- Eat a balanced diet and maintain a healthy weight.
- Get enough sleep. Most people need 6–8 hours every night.
- Exercise, but not when you're sick.
- Don't smoke.
- If you drink alcohol, do so only in moderation.
- Wash your hands frequently. Use hand sanitizer when soap and water aren't available.
- Avoid contact with people who are contagious with an infectious disease.

QUESTIONS FOR CRITICAL THINKING AND REFLECTION
Have you ever had any of the illnesses described in the preceding section? How were you exposed to the disease? Could you have taken any precautions to avoid it?

- Practice safer sex and don't inject drugs.
- Make sure you have received all your recommended vaccinations.

THE MAJOR STDS

Sexually transmitted diseases (STDs) are infectious diseases that are spread from person to person mainly through sexual activity. STDs are a particularly insidious group of illnesses because a person can be infected and able to transmit the disease, yet not look or feel sick; this is why the term *sexually transmitted infection (STI)* is often used synonymously with STD. The following seven STDs pose a major health threat:

- HIV/AIDS
- Hepatitis
- Syphilis
- Chlamydia
- Gonorrhea
- Herpes
- Human papillomavirus (HPV)

These diseases are considered major threats because they are serious in themselves, cause serious complications if left untreated, and pose risks to a fetus or newborn. STDs often result in long-term consequences, including chronic pain, infertility, stillbirths, genital cancers, and death.

The United States has the highest rate of STDs of any developed nation; at current rates, half of all young people will acquire an STD by age 25. A 2007 report from the Centers for Disease Control and Prevention (CDC) showed that many of the most common STDs are on the rise in the United States. In 2008, the CDC estimated that 65 million Americans were infected with an STD, and about 19 million Americans become newly infected with an STD each year.

HIV Infection and AIDS

The **human immunodeficiency virus (HIV)** causes **acquired immunodeficiency syndrome (AIDS)**, a disease that ultimately kills most of its victims, especially in parts of the world where adequate treatment is not available. An estimated total of 65 million people have been infected since the epidemic began—nearly 1% of the world's population—and tens of millions of those people have died (see the box "HIV/AIDS Around the World" on p. 332). Currently, about 33 million people are infected with HIV/

AIDS worldwide, and most of these people will die within the next 10 years.

Many experts believe that the global HIV epidemic peaked in the late 1990s, at about 3 million new infections per year, compared with an estimated 2.7 new infections in 2007. Despite a slowing of the epidemic, however, AIDS remains the primary cause of death in Africa and continues to be a major cause of mortality around the world. In the United States, about 1.1 million people have been infected with HIV and about 56,000 new HIV infections were reported in 2006. Nearly 550,000 Americans have died from AIDS since the start of the epidemic in 1981. Today, about 25% of HIV-infected Americans are unaware of their condition.

What Is HIV Infection? **HIV infection** is a chronic disease that progressively damages the body's immune system, making an otherwise healthy person less able to resist a variety of infections and disorders. Normally, when a virus or other pathogen enters the body, it is targeted and destroyed by the immune system. But HIV attacks the immune system itself, invading and taking over **CD4 T cells** and other essential elements of the immune system. HIV enters a human cell and converts its own genetic material, RNA, into DNA. It then inserts this DNA into the chromosomes of the host cell. The viral DNA takes over the CD4 cell, causing it to produce new copies of HIV; it also makes the CD4 cell incapable of performing its immune functions.

Immediately following infection with HIV, billions of infectious particles are produced every day. For a time, the immune system keeps pace, also producing billions of new cells. Unlike the virus, however, the immune system cannot make new cells indefinitely; as long as the virus keeps replicating, it wins in the end. The destruction of the immune system is signaled by the loss of CD4 T cells. As CD4 cells decline, an infected person may begin to experience mild to moderately severe symptoms. A person is diagnosed with full-blown AIDS when he or she develops one of the conditions defined as a marker for AIDS or when the number of CD4 cells in the blood drops below a certain level (200/μl). People with AIDS are vulnerable to a number of serious **opportunistic (secondary) infections.**

The first weeks after being infected with HIV are called the *primary infection* phase. People have large amounts of HIV in the bloodstream, making them much more infectious than they will be several months later when they enter the chronic infection stage.

The next phase of HIV infection is the chronic **asymptomatic** (symptom-free) stage. This period can last from 2 to 20 years, with an average of 11 years in untreated adults.

During this time the virus progressively infects and destroys the cells of the immune system. People infected with HIV can transmit the disease to others, even if they are symptom-free.

Transmitting the Virus HIV lives only within cells and body fluids, not outside the body. It is transmitted by blood and blood products, semen, vaginal and cervical secretions, and breast milk. It cannot live in air, in water, or on objects or surfaces such as toilet seats, eating utensils, or telephones. The three main routes of HIV transmission are (1) from specific kinds of sexual contact, (2) from direct exposure to infected blood, and (3) from an HIV-infected woman to her fetus during pregnancy or childbirth or to her infant during breastfeeding.

HIV is more likely to be transmitted by unprotected anal or vaginal intercourse than by other sexual activities. During vaginal intercourse, male-to-female transmission is more likely to occur than female-to-male transmission. HIV has been found in preejaculatory fluid, so transmission can occur before ejaculation. Being the receptive partner during unprotected anal intercourse is the riskiest of all sexual activities. Oral-genital contact carries some risk of transmission, although less than anal or vaginal intercourse.

The presence of lesions, blisters, or inflammation from other STDs in the genital, anal, or oral areas makes it two to nine times easier for the virus to be passed. Spermicides may also cause irritation and increase the risk of HIV transmission. Recent studies of the widely used spermicide nonoxynol-9 (N-9) found that frequent use may cause vaginal and rectal irritation, increasing the risk of transmission of HIV and other STDs. The risk of HIV transmission during oral sex increases if a person has poor oral hygiene, has oral sores, or has brushed or flossed just before or after oral sex. Studies have found that circumcised males have a lower risk of HIV infection than uncircumcised males.

TERMS

sexually transmitted disease (STD) A disease that can be transmitted by sexual contact; some can also be transmitted by other means.

human immunodeficiency virus (HIV) The virus that causes HIV infection and AIDS.

acquired immunodeficiency syndrome (AIDS) A generally fatal, incurable, sexually transmitted viral disease.

HIV infection A chronic, progressive viral infection that damages the immune system.

CD4 T cell A type of white blood cell that helps coordinate the activity of the immune system; the primary target for HIV infection.

opportunistic (secondary) infection An infection caused when organisms take the opportunity presented by a primary (initial) infection to multiply and cause a new, different infection.

asymptomatic Showing no signs or symptoms of a disease.

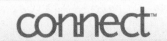

HIV/AIDS Around the World

In 2006, the world marked the twenty-fifth year since AIDS, a previously unknown disease, was diagnosed in 5 young gay men in Los Angeles. We now know that HIV originated in Africa about five decades earlier. HIV is now a worldwide scourge, with 65 million people infected and 25 million deaths since the epidemic began. Although some developments in efforts to address the epidemic have been promising, the number of people living with AIDS increased in every region of the world between 2004 and 2006.

The vast majority of cases—95%—have occurred in developing countries, where heterosexual contact is the primary means of transmission, responsible for 85% of all adult infections. In the developed world, HIV is increasingly becoming a disease that disproportionately affects the poor and ethnic minorities. Worldwide, women are the fastest-growing group of newly infected people; half of adults living with HIV in 2007 were women. In addition, an estimated 2 million children are living with HIV infection and about 12 million children are AIDS orphans.

Sub-Saharan Africa remains the hardest hit of all areas of the world. Two-thirds of all adults and children with HIV live in this region, and three-quarters of all deaths due to AIDS in 2007 occurred here. However, because the epidemic started about 10 years later in Asia than in Africa, experts expect an explosion of new cases in Asia. And because Asia accounts for more than 50% of the world's population, the pool of people at risk is much larger than in Africa. India has overtaken South Africa as the country with the largest number of people living with HIV infection. HIV is also spreading rapidly in Eastern Europe, and former Soviet countries have seen a fiftyfold increase in HIV infection in the last decade.

Efforts to combat AIDS are complicated by political, economic, and cultural barriers. Education and prevention programs are often hampered by resistance from social and religious institutions and by the taboo on openly discussing sexual issues. Condoms are not commonly used in many countries, and women in many societies do not have sufficient control over their lives to demand that men use condoms during sex. Prevention approaches that have had success include STD treatment and education, public education campaigns about safer sex, and syringe exchange programs for injection drug users.

In countries where there is a substantial imbalance in the social power of men and women, empowering women is a crucial priority in reducing the spread of HIV. In particular, reducing sexual violence against women, allowing women property and inheritance rights, and increasing women's access to education and employment are essential.

International efforts are under way to make condoms more available by lowering their price and to develop effective antiviral creams that women can use without the knowledge of their partners. Other potential strategies for fighting the spread of HIV include the widespread use of drugs to suppress genital herpes simplex, an extremely common STD that can dramatically increase transmission of HIV. Also, the practice of male circumcision might be useful in reducing the spread of HIV (and chlamydia, discussed later in this chapter). Recent research has shown a 60% reduction in HIV transmission among circumcised men compared with uncircumcised men, even when controlling for other factors.

In developed nations such as the United States, new drugs are easing AIDS symptoms and lowering viral levels dramatically for some patients. In the past few years, a small but growing number of people in poor countries have gained access to antiviral drugs because of the introduction of inexpensive generic drugs and increasing international funding for HIV treatment. Still, the vast majority of people with HIV remain untreated.

Direct contact with the blood of an infected person is another major route of HIV transmission. Needles used to inject drugs (including heroin, cocaine, and anabolic steroids) are routinely contaminated by the blood of the user. Nearly 20% of all new U.S. cases of HIV are caused, directly or indirectly, by sharing drug injection equipment contaminated with HIV. HIV has also been transmitted in blood and blood products used in the medical treatment of injuries and illnesses, resulting in about 14,000 cases of AIDS in the United States. Nearly all of these cases occurred in the early days of the AIDS epidemic, before effective screening tests were available. All blood in licensed U.S. blood banks and plasma centers is now thoroughly screened for HIV.

The final major route of HIV transmission is mother-to-child, also called *vertical*, or *perinatal, transmission*, which can occur during pregnancy, childbirth, or breastfeeding. About 25–30% of infants born to untreated HIV-infected mothers are also infected with the virus; testing and treatment can dramatically lower this infection rate.

Populations of Special Concern for HIV Infection

Among Americans with AIDS, the most common means of HIV exposure is sexual activity between men; heterosexual contact and injection drug use (IDU) are the next most common (Figure 13.3). Although HIV transmission occurs through specific individual behaviors, disproportionately high rates of infection in certain groups are tied to social, cultural, and economic factors. In 2008, the CDC estimated that 75% of HIV-positive Americans were men; the remaining 25% were women. HIV in the United States is increasingly becoming a disease that affects ethnic minorities, women, and the poor. Women, especially African American women and Latinas, make up an increasingly large proportion of all U.S. AIDS cases. Overall, African American men and women are vastly overrepresented among people newly diagnosed with AIDS.

Another group of people at increased risk for HIV infection are young men who have sex with men. There are probably several factors underlying this trend. Young gay men are less likely than older men to have experienced

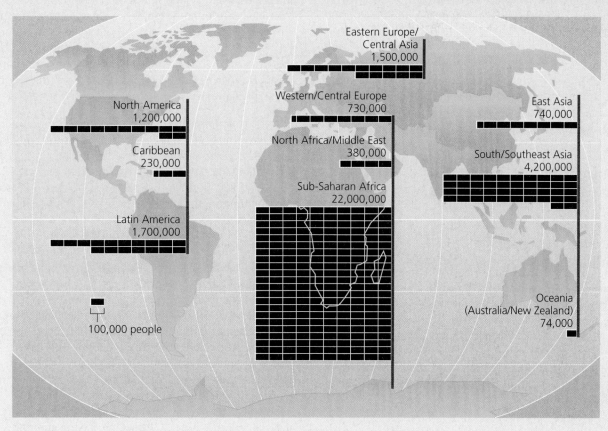

Approximate number of people living with HIV/AIDS in 2007.

SOURCE: Joint United Nations Programme on HIV/AIDS (UNAIDS). 2008. *2008 Report on the Global AIDS Epidemic*. Geneva: UNAIDS.

Estimated HIV Prevalence by Transmission Category, 2006

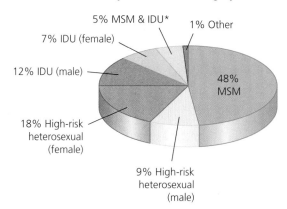

* MSM = Men who have sex with men
  IDU = Injection drug users

FIGURE 13.3   Routes of HIV transmission among Americans

SOURCE: Centers for Disease Control and Prevention. 2008. *New Estimates of U.S. HIV Prevalence, 2006.* (http://www.cdc.gov/hiv/topics/surveillance/resources/factsheets/pdf/prevalence.pdf; retrieved February 17, 2009).

watching friends die from AIDS and thus are more removed from the reality of the disease. They may be less afraid of acquiring HIV because of advances in treatment and a false belief that a cure is just around the corner.

96% of new HIV infections occur in low- and middle-income countries.

—UNAIDS, 2007

Another population of concern is men who have sex with men but still identify themselves as heterosexual. They are just as likely to be infected with HIV as are openly gay and bisexual men, but they are much less likely to know their HIV status and so may be more likely to transmit HIV to a male or female partner.

Symptoms of HIV Infection   Within a few days or weeks of infection with HIV, some people will develop the flulike symptoms of primary HIV infection. People who have engaged in behavior that places them at risk for HIV infection and who then experience such symptoms should immediately inform their physician of their risk status. Standard tests for HIV will usually be negative in the very early stages of infection, so specialized tests such as the **HIV RNA assay**, which directly measures the amount of virus in the body, must be used. Immediate treatment is sometimes given to help preserve immune function, slow the progress of the disease, and reduce transmission of HIV to others.

Other than the initial flulike symptoms, most people in the first months or years of HIV infection have few if any symptoms. As the immune system weakens, however, a variety of symptoms can develop—persistent swollen lymph nodes; lumps, rashes, sores, or other growths on or under the skin or on the mucous membranes of the eyes, mouth, anus, or nasal passages; persistent yeast infections; unexplained weight loss; fever and drenching night sweats; dry cough and shortness of breath; persistent diarrhea; easy bruising and unexplained bleeding; profound fatigue; memory loss; difficulty with balance; tremors or seizures; changes in vision, hearing, taste, or smell; difficulty in swallowing; changes in mood and other psychological symptoms; and persistent or recurrent pain. Obviously, many of these symptoms can also occur with a variety of other illnesses.

HIV RNA assay A test used to determine the viral load (the amount of HIV in the blood).

***Pneumocystis* pneumonia** A fungal infection common in people infected with HIV.

Kaposi's sarcoma A form of cancer characterized by purple or brownish lesions that are generally painless and occur anywhere on the skin; usually appears in men infected with HIV.

HIV antibody test A blood test to determine whether a person has been infected by HIV; becomes positive within weeks or months of exposure.

ELISA (enzyme-linked immunosorbent assay) A blood test that detects the presence of antibodies to HIV.

Western blot A blood test that detects the presence of HIV antibodies; a more accurate and more expensive test used to confirm positive results from an ELISA test.

HIV-positive A diagnosis resulting from the presence of HIV in the bloodstream; also referred to as *seropositive*.

reverse transcriptase inhibitor An antiviral drug used to treat HIV infection that works by inhibiting reverse transcriptase, the enzyme that converts viral RNA to DNA.

protease inhibitor A drug that inhibits the action of any of the protein-splitting enzymes known as proteases. Protease inhibitors have been developed to block the action of HIV protease and thus prevent the replication of HIV.

entry inhibitor An antiviral drug that blocks the entry of HIV into cells by inhibiting the fusion of viral and cell membranes.

People with HIV infection are highly susceptible to infections. The most common one in the United States is ***Pneumocystis* pneumonia**, a fungal infection. **Kaposi's sarcoma**, a previously rare form of cancer, is common in HIV-infected men. Women with HIV infection often have frequent and difficult-to-treat vaginal yeast infections. Cases of tuberculosis (TB) are increasingly being reported in people with HIV.

Diagnosing HIV Infection The most common HIV tests check for antibodies to the virus. **HIV antibody tests** are used because they are accurate and relatively inexpensive. Standard testing involves an initial test called an **ELISA**; if it is positive, a second test—either a **Western blot** or immunoflourescence assay—is done to confirm the results.

Babies born to HIV-infected mothers may carry HIV antibodies, passed from their mother, without being infected with HIV. Antibodies can pass through the placenta to a fetus, but in the majority of cases, even without treatment, an infant does not acquire HIV. Thus, an infant may test positive on an HIV antibody test but actually be uninfected. Further tests such as the HIV RNA assay must be done to determine if an infant is actually infected.

If a person is diagnosed as **HIV-positive**, the next step is to determine the disease's severity to plan appropriate treatment. The immune system's status can be gauged by measuring CD4 T-cells every few months. The infection itself can be monitored by tracking the the amount of virus in the body through HIV RNA assay. A new diagnostic test that may help guide treatment decisions is called HIV Replication Capacity. This test shows how fast HIV from a patient's blood sample can reproduce itself.

The CDC currently recommends universal HIV testing at least once as part of routine medical care for everyone age 13–64. People at greater risk should be tested periodically (see the box "Getting an HIV Test").

A diagnosis of AIDS is made if a person is HIV-positive and either has developed an infection defined as an AIDS indicator or has a severely damaged immune system (as measured by CD4 T-cell counts).

Treatment Although there is no known cure for HIV infection, medications can significantly alter the course of the disease and extend life. The drop in the number of U.S. AIDS deaths that has occurred since 1996 is in large part due to the increasing use of combinations of new drugs.

ANTIVIRAL DRUGS Antiviral drugs in current use to combat HIV fall into several categories based on how they block HIV replication. **Reverse transcriptase inhibitors,** including the widely used drug zidovudine (AZT), work by inhibiting the enzyme reverse transcriptase, which HIV uses to integrate its genetic material into human cells. **Protease inhibitors** target the enzyme HIV protease, which the virus uses to create a protein coat for each new copy of itself. **Entry inhibitors** block HIV from entering and infecting cells.

Getting an HIV Test

You should strongly consider being tested if any of the following apply to you or any past or current sexual partners: You have had unprotected sex (vaginal, anal, or oral) with more than one partner or with a partner who was not in a mutually monogamous relationship with you; you have used or shared needles, syringes, or other paraphernalia for injecting drugs (including steroids); you received a transfusion of blood or blood products between 1978 and 1985; or you have ever been diagnosed with an STD.

You can either visit a physician or health clinic or take a home test. If the test is performed by a physician or clinician, you will get one-on-one counseling about the test and your results. The home test is a good alternative for people at low risk who just want to be sure.

Physician or Clinic Testing

Your physician, student health clinic, Planned Parenthood, public health department, or local AIDS association can arrange your HIV test. It usually costs $50–$100, but public clinics often charge little or nothing. The standard test involves drawing a sample of blood that is sent to a laboratory for analysis for the presence of antibodies; if the first stage of testing is positive, a confirmatory test is done. This standard test takes 1–2 weeks, and you'll be asked to phone or come in personally to obtain your results, which should also include appropriate counseling.

Alternative tests are available at some clinics. The Orasure test uses oral fluid, collected by placing a treated cotton pad in the mouth; urine tests are also available. New rapid tests are also available at some locations. These tests use blood or oral fluid and can provide results in as little as 20 minutes. If a rapid test is positive for HIV infection, a confirmatory test will be performed.

Before you get an HIV test, be sure you understand what will be done with the results. Results from confidential tests may still become part of your medical record and/or be reported to state and federal public health agencies. If you decide you want to be tested anonymously, check with your physician or counselor about how to obtain an anonymous test or use a home test.

Home Testing

Home test kits for HIV are available; they cost about $40–70. (Avoid testing kits that are not FDA-approved; unapproved kits are sold over the Internet. As of this printing, the only FDA-approved home test kit for HIV was manufactured by Home Access.) To use a home test, you prick a finger with a supplied lancet, blot a few drops of blood onto blotting paper, and mail it to the company's laboratory. Anyone testing positive is routed to a trained counselor, who can provide emotional and medical support. The results of home test kits are anonymous.

Understanding the Results

A negative test result means that no antibodies were found in your sample. However, it usually takes at least a month after exposure to HIV (and possibly as long as 6 months in some people) for antibodies to appear. Therefore, an infected person may get a false-negative result. If you test negative but your risk of infection is high, ask about obtaining an HIV RNA assay, which allows very early diagnosis, and about the appropriateness of retesting in a few months.

A positive result means that you are infected. It is important to seek medical care and counseling immediately. You need to know more about your medical options; the possible psychological, social, and financial repercussions; and how to avoid spreading the disease. Rapid progress is being made in treating HIV, and treatments are potentially much more successful when begun early.

For more information about HIV testing and a national directory of testing sites, visit the CDC National HIV Testing Resources site (www.hivtest.org). You can also find a test center near you by using your mobile phone. Text-message your ZIP code to 566948. The CDC will automatically respond with a text message listing HIV test centers in your area.

Treatment with combinations of drugs, referred to as *highly active antiretroviral therapy,* or *HAART,* can reduce HIV in the blood to undetectable levels in many people. However, latent virus is still present in the body and HIV-infected people on HAART carry potentially transmissible HIV in their body fluids.

Antiviral medications are sometimes used to prevent infection in people who have been exposed to HIV, a practice called Postexposure Prophylaxis (PEP). PEP is recommended for health care workers with exposure to blood, victims of sexual assault, and for people who are at risk from recent unprotected sex or contact with a contaminated needle.

TREATMENTS FOR OPPORTUNISTIC INFECTIONS In addition to antiviral drugs, most patients with low CD4 T-cell counts also take a variety of antibiotics to help prevent opportunistic infections such as pneumonia and tuberculosis. A person with advanced HIV infection may need to take 20 or more pills every day.

HIV AND PREGNANCY Early-stage HIV infection does not appear to significantly affect a woman's chance of becoming pregnant. Without treatment, 25–30% of infants born to HIV-infected women are themselves infected with the virus. The risk of an infected mother transmitting HIV to her baby can be reduced to less than 2% by treating the mother during her pregnancy and labor, giving the baby antiretroviral drugs during the first weeks of life, avoiding breastfeeding, and delivering the baby by cesarean section if necessary.

TREATMENT CHALLENGES The average cost of treatment for an HIV-infected person in the United States is $2100–4000 per month. These costs are tremendous even for relatively wealthy countries, but 95% of people with HIV infection

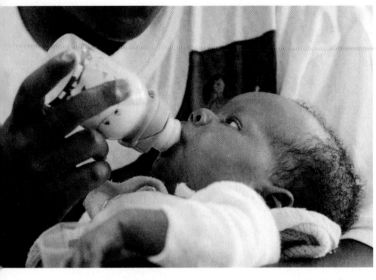

Currently available treatments can significantly increase the chance that this baby, born to an HIV-infected mother, will be free of the virus.

High Risk

Unprotected anal sex is the riskiest sexual behavior, especially for the receptive partner.

Unprotected vaginal intercourse is the next riskiest, especially for women, who are much more likely to be infected by an infected male partner than vice versa.

Oral sex is probably considerably less risky than anal and vaginal intercourse but can still result in HIV transmission.

Sharing of sex toys can be risky because they can carry blood, semen, or vaginal fluid.

Use of a condom reduces risk considerably but not completely for any type of intercourse. Anal sex with a condom is riskier than vaginal sex with a condom; oral sex with a condom is less risky, especially if the man does not ejaculate.

Hand-genital contact and deep kissing are less risky but could still theoretically transmit HIV; the presence of cuts or sores increases risk.

Sex with only one uninfected and totally faithful partner is without risk, but effective only if both partners are uninfected and completely monogamous.

Activities that don't involve the exchange of body fluids carry no risk: hugging, massage, closed-mouth kissing, masturbation, phone sex, and fantasy.

Abstinence is completely without risk. For many people, it can be an effective and reasonable method of avoiding HIV infection and other STDs during certain periods of life.

No Risk

FIGURE 13.4 **What's risky and what's not: The approximate relative risk of HIV transmission of various sexual activities.**

live in developing countries, where these treatments are unlikely to be available to anyone except the wealthiest few. Besides financial cost, receiving HIV treatment is challenging in many other ways. Common short-term side effects include nausea, vomiting, diarrhea, and fatigue. People on HIV drugs must take their medicines on time, every time, because drug resistance can develop if the medicines are taken inconsistently.

Patients who take antiretroviral medications for an extended period sometimes develop serious problems including abnormal blood lipids, heart disease, liver problems, bone loss, kidney disease, and cancers. Changes in body shape and facial appearance due to alterations in fat distribution is a common and troubling side effect of long-term antiretroviral drug use. Generally, people with HIV who have no symptoms and have relatively high CD4 counts may opt to delay treatment; however, immediate treatment is still recommended for anyone who is experiencing symptoms and for all pregnant women.

How Can You Protect Yourself? Although AIDS is currently incurable, it is preventable. You can protect yourself by avoiding behaviors that may bring you into contact with HIV.

In a sexual relationship, the current and past behaviors of you and your partner determine the amount of risk involved (Figure 13.4). If you are uninfected and in a mutually monogamous relationship with another uninfected person, you are not at risk for HIV. Having a series

6800 new HIV infections occurred daily in 2007.

—UNAIDS, 2007

of monogamous relationships is not a safe prevention strategy, however.

People who inject drugs should avoid sharing needles, syringes, or anything that might have blood on it. Any injectable drug, legal or illegal, can be associated with HIV transmission. Needles can be decontaminated with a solution of bleach and water, but it is not a foolproof procedure, and HIV can survive in a syringe for a month or longer. (Boiling needles and syringes does not necessarily destroy HIV either.) Fore more guidelines and tips, see the box "Preventing HIV Infection and Other STDs."

One-third of surveyed HIV-positive people said they did not reveal their infection to their sexual partners.

—CDC, 2006

Preventing HIV Infection and Other STDs

For those who aren't in a long-term monogamous relationship with an uninfected partner, abstinence is the only truly safe option for avoiding STDs.

Safer sexual activities that allow close person-to-person contact with almost no risk of contracting STDs or HIV include fantasy, hugging, massage, rubbing clothed bodies together, self-stimulation by both partners, and kissing with lips closed.

If you choose to be sexually active, talk with potential partners about HIV, safer sex, and the use of condoms before you begin a sexual relationship. The following behaviors will help lower your risk of exposure to STDs during sexual activities:

• Don't drink alcohol or use drugs in sexual situations. Mood-altering drugs can affect your judgment and make you more likely to take risks.

• Limit the number of partners. Avoid sexual contact with people who have HIV or an STD or who have engaged in risky behaviors.

• Use condoms during every act of intercourse and oral sex. Condoms do not provide perfect protection, but they provide a high level of protection against HIV and greatly reduce your risk of contracting most STDs.

• Use condoms properly to obtain maximum protection. Use a water-based lubricant; don't use oil-based lubricants such as petroleum jelly or baby oil or any vaginal product containing mineral or vegetable oil. Avoid using lubricants or condoms containing nonoxynol-9, particularly for anal intercourse.

• Use latex squares or dental dams during oral-genital or oral-anal contact.

• Avoid sexual contact that could cause cuts or tears in the skin or tissue.

• Get periodic screening tests for STDs and HIV. Young women need yearly pelvic exams and Pap tests.

• Get vaccinated for hepatitis B. Young women should consider getting vaccinated against HPV.

• Get prompt treatment for any STDs you contract.

If you inject drugs of any kind, don't share needles, syringes, or anything that might have blood on it. If your community has a syringe exchange program, use it. Seek treatment; stop using injectable drugs.

If you are at risk for HIV infection, don't donate blood, sperm, or body organs. Get tested for HIV soon, and get treated. HIV-infected people who get early treatment generally feel better and live longer than those who delay.

Chlamydia

Chlamydia trachomatis causes **chlamydia,** the most prevalent bacterial STD in the United States. The highest rates of infection occur in single people between ages 15 and 24. Both men and women are susceptible to chlamydia, but, as with most STDs, women bear the greater burden because of possible complications and consequences of the disease (see the box "Women Are Hit Hard by STDs" on p. 338). *C. trachomatis* can be transmitted by oral sex as well as by other forms of sexual intercourse. In most women, chlamydia produces no early symptoms. If left untreated, it can lead to pelvic inflammatory disease (PID), which is discussed later in this chapter. Chlamydia also greatly increases a woman's risk for infertility and ectopic (tubal) pregnancy. The U.S. Preventive Services Task Force currently recommends routine screening for all sexually active women age 25 or younger and for older women who are at increased risk (such as those who have multiple sex partners).

Chlamydia can also lead to infertility in men, although not as often as in women. In men under age 35, chlamydia is the most common cause of **epididymitis,** inflammation of the sperm-carrying ducts. And up to half of all cases of **urethritis,** inflammation of the urethra, in men are caused by chlamydia. Despite these statistics, many infected men have no symptoms.

Infants of infected mothers can acquire the infection through contact with the pathogen in the birth canal during delivery. Every year, over 150,000 newborns suffer from eye infections and pneumonia as a result of untreated maternal chlamydial infections.

Symptoms   In men, chlamydia symptoms include painful urination, a slight watery discharge from the penis, and sometimes pain around the testicles. Although most women with chlamydia are asymptomatic, some notice increased vaginal discharge, burning with urination, pain or bleeding with intercourse, and lower abdominal pain. Symptoms in both men and women can begin within 5 days of infection. However, most people experience few or no

chlamydia   An STD transmitted by the pathogenic bacterium *Chlamydia trachomatis.*

epididymitis   An inflammation of the small body of sperm-carrying ducts that rests on the testes.

urethritis   Inflammation of the tube that carries urine from the bladder to the outside opening.

TERMS

Women Are Hit Hard by STDs

Sexually transmitted diseases cause suffering for all who are infected, but in many ways, women and girls are the hardest hit, for both biological and social reasons. Among Americans, 62% of all cases of adverse health problems from STDs occur in women. Worldwide, as many women as men now die from AIDS each year.

Male-to-female transmission of many infections is more likely to occur than female-to-male transmission. This is particularly true of HIV: Studies show that it is three to eight times easier for an HIV-positive man to transmit the virus to a woman than it is for an HIV-positive woman to infect a man.

Teenagers have been hit especially hard, and 26% of American girls age 14–19 are infected with at least one of the most common STDs. Young women are more vulnerable to STDs than older women because the less-mature cervix is more susceptible to injury and infection. As a woman ages, the cells at the opening of the cervix become more resistant to infection. Young women are also more vulnerable for social and emotional reasons: Lack of control in relationships, fear of discussing condom use, and having an older sex partner are all linked to increased STD risk.

Once infected, women tend to suffer more consequences of STDs than men. For example, gonorrhea and chlamydia can cause PID and permanent damage to the oviducts in women, but these infections tend to have less serious effects in men. HPV infection causes nearly all cases of cervical cancer. HPV infection is also associated with penile cancer, which is much less common than cervical cancer. Women also have the added concern of the potential effects of STDs during pregnancy.

Between 1985 and 2005, the proportion of new U.S. AIDS cases in women increased from 5% to 27%. Women may become sicker at lower viral loads compared with men. Women and men with HIV do about equally well if they have similar access to treatment, but in many cases women are diagnosed later in the course of HIV infection, receive less treatment, and die sooner.

Worldwide, social and economic factors play a large role in the transmission and consequences of AIDS and other STDs for women. Sexual violence against women is spreading AIDS, as are such practices as very early marriage for women, often to much older men who have had many sexual partners. Cultural gender norms that promote premarital and extramarital relationships for men, combined with women's lack of power to negotiate safer sex, make HIV a risk even for women who are married and monogamous. In addition, lack of education and economic opportunities can force women into commercial sex work, placing them at high risk for all STDs.

SOURCES: Ebrahim, S. H., M. T. McKenna, and J. S. Marks. 2005. Sexual behaviour: Related adverse health burden in the United States. *Sexually Transmitted Infection* 81(1): 38–40; Dunkle, K. M., et al. 2004. Gender-based violence, relationship power, and risk of HIV infection in women attending antenatal clinics in South Africa. *Lancet* 363(9419): 1415–1421; Joint United Nations Programme on HIV/AIDS. 2004. *AIDS Epidemic Update, December 2004.* Geneva: UNAIDS; World Health Organization. 2003. *Gender and HIV/AIDS.* Geneva: World Health Organization.

symptoms, increasing the likelihood that they will inadvertently spread the infection to their partners.

Diagnosis and Treatment   Chlamydia is typically diagnosed through laboratory tests on a urine sample or a small amount of fluid from the urethra or cervix. Once chlamydia has been diagnosed, the infected person and his or her partner(s) are given antibiotics. Studies show that younger women were more likely than older women to be reinfected by an untreated, infected partner.

Gonorrhea

More than 350,000 cases of **gonorrhea** were reported to the CDC in 2007, an increase of 1% over 2006. The highest incidence is among 15–24-year-olds. Like chlamydia, untreated gonorrhea can cause PID in women and urethritis and epididymitis in men. It can also cause arthritis, rashes, and eye infections, and it occasionally involves internal organs. A woman who is infected during pregnancy is at risk for preterm delivery and for having a baby with life-threatening gonorrheal infection of the blood or joints. An infant passing through the birth canal of an infected mother may contract **gonococcal conjunctivitis,** an infection in the eyes that can cause blindness if not treated.

Symptoms   In males, the incubation period for gonorrhea is brief, generally 2–7 days. The first symptoms are due to urethritis, which causes urinary discomfort and a thick, yellowish white or yellowish green discharge from the penis. The lips of the urethral opening may become inflamed and swollen. In some cases, the lymph glands in the groin become enlarged and swollen. Up to half of males have very minor symptoms or none at all.

Most females with gonorrhea are asymptomatic. Those who do have symptoms often experience pain with urination, increased vaginal discharge, and severe menstrual cramps. Up to 40% of women with untreated gonorrhea develop PID. Gonorrhea can also infect the throat or rectum of people who engage in oral or anal sex.

Diagnosis and Treatment   Several tests—gram stain, detection of bacterial genes or DNA, or culture—may be

> After dropping **74%** between 1975 and 1997, gonorrhea rates are again rising in the United States.
>
> —CDC, 2007

performed; depending on the test, samples of urine or cervical, urethral, throat, or rectal fluids may be collected. Gonorrhea can be cured with antibiotics, but increasing drug resistance is a major concern. Today only one class of antibiotics, the cephalosporins, remains consistently effective against gonorrhea.

Pelvic Inflammatory Disease

Pelvic inflammatory disease (PID) is a major complication in 10–40% of women who have been infected with either gonorrhea or chlamydia and have not received adequate treatment. PID occurs when the initial infection with gonorrhea and/or chlamydia travels upward into the uterus, oviducts, ovaries, and pelvic cavity. PID is often serious enough to require hospitalization and sometimes surgery. Even if the disease is treated successfully, about 25% of affected women will have long-term problems such as a continuing susceptibility to infection, ectopic pregnancy, infertility, and chronic pelvic pain. PID is the leading cause of infertility in young women.

Women under age 25 are much more likely to develop PID than are older women. As with all STDs, the more sex partners a woman has had, the greater her risk of PID. Smokers have twice the risk of PID as nonsmokers. Using IUDs for contraception also increases the risk of PID.

Symptoms Some women, especially those with chlamydia, may be asymptomatic; others may feel very ill with abdominal pain, fever, chills, nausea, and vomiting. Early symptoms are essentially the same as those described earlier for chlamydia and gonorrhea. Symptoms often begin or worsen during or soon after a woman's menstrual period. Many women have abnormal vaginal bleeding—either bleeding between periods or heavy and painful menstrual bleeding.

Diagnosis and Treatment Diagnosis of PID is made on the basis of symptoms, physical examination, ultrasound, and laboratory tests. Laparoscopy may be used to confirm the diagnosis and obtain material for cultures. Antibiotics are usually started immediately; in severe cases, the woman may be hospitalized and antibiotics given intravenously. It is especially important that an infected woman's partners be treated. As many as 60% of the male contacts of women with PID are infected but asymptomatic.

Human Papillomavirus Infection

Human papillomavirus (HPV) infection is the most common STD in the United States. HPV infection causes a variety of human diseases, including common warts, **genital warts,** and genital cancers. HPV is the cause of virtually all cervical cancer, but HPV also causes penile cancer and some forms of anal and oropharyngeal cancers. Genital HPV is usually spread from one person to another through sexual activity, including oral sex. HPV is especially common in young people, with some of the highest rates of infection among college students. Many young women contract HPV infection within 3 months of becoming sexually active.

Genital HPV infection is quite contagious. Condoms and other barrier methods can help prevent the transmission of HPV, but HPV infection frequently occurs in areas where condoms are not fully protective. These areas are the labia in women, the base of the penis and the scrotum in men, and around the anus in both men and women.

In 2006, the FDA approved a vaccine for HPV (Gardasil), and additional vaccines are in development. Gardasil protects against four types of HPV virus that together account for 90% of genital warts and 70% of cervical cancers; the drug has also been shown to prevent cancers of the vagina and vulva. Vaccination is available for girls and women age 9–26. The CDC recommends the vaccine for all girls between the ages of 11 and 12 because the vaccine is most effective before the onset of sexual activity.

Symptoms HPV-infected tissue often appears normal; it may also look like anything from a small bump on the skin to a large, warty growth. Depending on location and size, genital warts are sometimes painful. Untreated warts can grow together to form a cauliflower-like mass. In males, they appear on the penis and often involve the urethra, appearing first at the opening and then spreading inside. The growths may cause irritation and bleeding, leading to painful urination and a urethral discharge. Warts may also appear around the anus or within the rectum. In women, warts may appear on the labia or vulva and may spread to the perineum, the area between the vagina and the rectum, and on the cervix.

The incubation period ranges from 1 month to 2 years from the time of contact. People can be infected with the

gonorrhea A sexually transmitted bacterial infection that usually affects mucous membranes.

gonococcal conjunctivitis An inflammation of the mucous membrane lining of the eyelids, caused by the gonococcus bacterium.

pelvic inflammatory disease (PID) An infection that progresses from the vagina and cervix to the uterus, oviducts, and pelvic cavity.

human papillomavirus (HPV) The pathogen that causes human warts, including genital warts.

genital warts A sexually transmitted viral infection characterized by growths on the genitals; also called *genital HPV infection* or *condyloma.*

virus and be capable of transmitting it to their sex partners without having any symptoms at all. The vast majority of people with HPV infection have no visible warts or symptoms of any kind.

Diagnosis and Treatment   Genital warts are usually diagnosed based on the appearance of the lesions. HPV infection of the cervix is often detected on routine Pap tests. Special tests are now available to detect the presence of HPV infection and to distinguish among the more common strains of HPV, including those that cause most cases of cervical cancer.

Treatment focuses on reducing the number and size of warts. The currently available treatments do not eradicate HPV infection. Warts may be removed by cryosurgery (freezing), electrocautery (burning), or laser surgery. Direct applications of podophyllin or other cytotoxic acids may be used, and there are treatments that patients can use at home. Warts are more likely to persist and become severe in people with an impaired immune system.

Even after treatment and the disappearance of visible warts, the individual may continue to carry HPV in healthy-looking tissue and can probably still infect others. Anyone who has ever had HPV infection should inform all partners and use condoms, even though they do not provide total protection. Because of the relationship between HPV and cervical cancer, women who have had genital warts should have Pap tests at least every 12 months.

Genital Herpes

About one in five adults in the United States has **genital herpes.** Worldwide, genital herpes is extremely common, and is a major factor in the transmission of HIV. Two types of herpes simplex viruses, HSV 1 and HSV 2, cause genital herpes and oral-labial herpes (cold sores). Genital herpes is usually caused by HSV 2, and oral-labial herpes is usually caused by HSV 1, although both virus types can cause either genital or oral-labial lesions. Many people wrongly assume that they are unlikely to pick up an STD if they limit their sexual activity to oral sex, but this is not true, particularly in the case of genital herpes. HSV can also cause rectal lesions, usually transmitted through anal sex. Infection with HSV is generally lifelong; after infection, the virus lies dormant in nerve cells and can reactivate at any time.

HSV 1 infection is so common that 50–80% of U.S. adults have antibodies to HSV 1 (indicating previous exposure to the virus); most were exposed to HSV 1 during childhood. HSV 2 infection usually occurs during adolescence and early adulthood, often between ages 18 and 25.

HSV 2 is almost always sexually transmitted. The infection is more easily transmitted when people have active sores, but HSV 2 can be transmitted to a sex partner even when no obvious lesions are present. Because HSV is asymptomatic in 80–90% of people, the infection is often acquired from a person who does not know that he or she is infected. If you have ever had an outbreak of genital herpes, you should consider yourself always contagious and inform your partners. Avoid intimate contact when any sores are present, and use condoms during all sexual contact.

Newborns can occasionally be infected with HSV, usually during passage through the birth canal of an infected mother or due to HSV infection acquired by the mother during the third trimester of pregnancy. Without treatment, 65% of newborns with HSV will die, and most who survive will have some degree of brain damage. The risk is low (less than 1%) in women with long-standing herpes infection.

Symptoms   Up to 90% of people who are infected with HSV have no symptoms. Those who do develop symptoms often first notice them within 2–20 days of having sex with an infected partner. (However, it is not unusual for the first outbreak to occur months or even years after initial exposure.) The first episode of genital herpes frequently causes flulike symptoms in addition to genital lesions. The lesions usually heal within 3 weeks, but the virus remains alive in an inactive state within nerve cells. A new outbreak of herpes can occur at any time. On average, newly diagnosed people will experience five to eight outbreaks per year, with a decrease in the frequency of outbreaks over time. Recurrent episodes are usually less severe than the initial one, with fewer and less painful sores that heal more quickly. Outbreaks can be triggered by stress, illness, fatigue, sun exposure, sexual intercourse, and menstruation (see the box "Stress and Genital Herpes").

Diagnosis and Treatment   Genital herpes is often diagnosed on the basis of symptoms; a sample of fluid from the lesions may also be sent to a laboratory for culture. There are also several blood tests can detect the presence of HSV antibodies.

There is no cure for herpes. Once infected, a person carries the virus for life. Antiviral drugs such as acyclovir can be taken at the beginning of an outbreak to shorten the severity and duration of symptoms. People who have frequent outbreaks can take acyclovir or similar drugs daily to suppress outbreaks and decrease viral shedding between outbreaks. A person on suppressive therapy can still transmit HSV to an uninfected partner, but the risk is probably reduced by about half. Using condoms consis-

TERMS

genital herpes   A sexually transmitted infection caused by the herpes simplex virus.

hepatitis   Inflammation of the liver, which can be caused by infection, drugs, or toxins; some forms of infectious hepatitis can be transmitted sexually.

syphilis   A sexually transmitted bacterial infection caused by the spirochete *Treponema pallidum*.

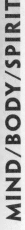
Stress and Genital Herpes

Patients and health care workers alike have long suspected that stress and genital herpes outbreaks are related. A recent study of women with genital herpes found that persistent stressors (those lasting more than a week) and persistent high levels of anxiety were associated with increased outbreaks. Short-term stress, mood changes, and brief negative life experiences did not influence the rate of herpes outbreaks.

Experts suspect that stress has a negative impact on the immune system.

Studies have shown that immune function and antibody levels may drop in response to psychological stress. Perhaps herpes viruses that are usually dormant in nervous system tissue become activated when immune function declines due to stress.

The next step is to investigate whether stress-reduction techniques such as meditation or exercise result in reduced rates of herpes outbreaks. Until such research becomes available, it makes sense for people who suffer recurrent genital

herpes outbreaks to do what they can to reduce stress, especially long-term stress and anxiety. If you have herpes, joining a support group may help reduce your stress and improve your ability to cope with this chronic disease. Keep in mind that regardless of stress level, genital herpes outbreaks naturally tend to become less and less frequent over time. Knowing that your outbreaks are likely to diminish can, in and of itself, help reduce your feelings of stress.

---

tently and taking suppressive medication is a reasonable way to reduce the risk of passing herpes to an uninfected sexual partner. It is always important to inform a sexual partner if you have genital herpes.

Hepatitis B

Hepatitis (inflammation of the liver) can cause serious and sometimes permanent damage to the liver. One of the many types of hepatitis is caused by hepatitis B virus (HBV). HBV is somewhat similar to HIV; it is found in most body fluids of an infected person, and it can be transmitted sexually, by injection drug use, and during pregnancy and delivery. However, HBV is much more contagious than HIV, and it can also be spread through nonsexual close contact. Hepatitis B is a potentially fatal disease with no cure, but fortunately there is an effective vaccine. Vaccination is recommended for everyone under age 19 and for all adults at increased risk for hepatitis B, including people who have more than one sex partner in 6 months, men who have sex with other men, those who inject illegal drugs, and health care workers who are exposed to blood and body fluids.

Other forms of viral hepatitis can also be sexually transmitted. Hepatitis A is of particular concern for people who engage in anal sex; a vaccine is available and is recommended for all people at risk. Less commonly, hepatitis C can be transmitted sexually. Experts believe that traumatic sexual activity that causes tissue damage is most likely to transmit HCV.

Transmission HBV is easily transmitted through any sexual activity that involves the exchange of body fluids, the use of contaminated needles, and any blood-to-blood contact, including the use of contaminated razor blades, toothbrushes, and eating utensils. The primary risk factors for acquiring HBV are sexual exposure and injection drug use; having multiple partners greatly increases risk. A pregnant woman can transmit HBV to her unborn child.

Symptoms Many people infected with HBV never develop symptoms; they have what are known as silent infections. Mild cases of hepatitis can cause flulike symptoms such as fever, body aches, chills, and loss of appetite. As the illness progresses, there may be nausea, vomiting, dark-colored urine, abdominal pain, and jaundice.

Most adults who have acute hepatitis B recover completely, but they can become chronic carriers of the virus, capable of infecting others for the rest of their life. Some chronic carriers remain asymptomatic, while others develop chronic liver disease. Chronic hepatitis can cause cirrhosis of the liver, liver failure, and a deadly form of liver cancer.

Diagnosis and Treatment Blood tests can diagnose hepatitis by analyzing liver function and detecting the infecting organism. There is no cure for hepatitis B and no specific treatment for acute infections; antiviral drugs and immune system modulators may be used for cases of chronic HBV infection.

Syphilis

Syphilis, a disease that once caused death and disability for millions, can now be effectively treated with antibiotics. The number of new cases in the United States hit an all-time low in 2000 but has been on the rise since then. Studies have found an association between syphilis infection and the use of the Internet as a means to meet sex partners among men who have sex with men. Another recent trend is an increase in the proportion of cases of syphilis from oral sex.

Syphilis is caused by a spirochete called *Treponema pallidum,* a thin, corkscrew-shaped bacterium. The disease is usually acquired through sexual contact, although infected pregnant women can transmit it to the fetus. The pathogen passes through any break or opening in the skin or mucous membranes and can be transmitted by kissing, vaginal or anal intercourse, or oral-genital contact.

Symptoms Syphilis progresses through several stages. *Primary syphilis* is characterized by an ulcer called a **chancre** that appears within 10–90 days after exposure. Chancres contain large numbers of bacteria and make the disease highly contagious when present; they are often painless and typically heal on their own within a few weeks. If the disease is not treated during the primary stage, about a third of infected individuals progress to chronic stages of infections.

Secondary syphilis is usually marked by mild, flulike symptoms and a skin rash that appears 3–6 weeks after the chancre. The rash may cover the entire body or only a few areas, but the palms of the hands and soles of the feet are usually involved. Areas of skin affected by the rash are highly contagious but usually heal within several weeks or months. If the disease remains untreated, the symptoms of secondary syphilis may recur over a period of several years; affected individuals may then lapse into an asymptomatic latent stage in which they experience no further consequences of infection. However, in about a third of cases of untreated secondary syphilis, the individual develops *late,* or *tertiary, syphilis.* Late syphilis can damage many organs of the body, possibly causing severe dementia, cardiovascular damage, blindness, and death.

In infected pregnant women who aren't treated, the probable result is stillbirth, prematurity, or congenital deformity. In many cases, the infant is also born infected (*congenital syphilis*) and requires treatment.

Diagnosis and Treatment Syphilis is diagnosed by examination of infected tissues and with blood tests. All stages can be treated with antibiotics, but damage from late syphilis can be permanent.

Other STDs

Trichomoniasis (often called *trich*) is the most common curable STD among young women. The single-celled organism that causes trich, *Trichomonas vaginalis,* thrives in warm, moist conditions, making women particularly susceptible to these infections in the vagina. Women who become symptomatic with trich develop a greenish, foul-smelling vaginal discharge and severe itching and pain in the vagina. Prompt treatment with metronidazole (Flagyl)

is important because studies suggest that trich may increase the risk of HIV transmission and, in pregnant women, premature delivery.

Bacterial vaginosis (BV) is the most common cause of abnormal vaginal discharge in women of reproductive age. BV occurs when healthy bacteria that normally inhabit the vagina become displaced by unhealthy species. BV is clearly associated with sexual activity and often occurs after a change in partners. Symptoms of BV include vaginal discharge with a fishy odor and sometimes vaginal irritation. BV is treated with topical and oral antibiotics.

Pubic lice (commonly known as *crabs*) and **scabies** are highly contagious parasitic infections. Treatment is generally easy, although lice infestation can require repeated applications of medications.

WHAT YOU CAN DO

You can take responsibility for your health and contribute to a general reduction in the incidence of STDs in three major areas: education, diagnosis and treatment, and prevention.

Education

Education efforts targeted at increasing public awareness about AIDS through the media have included public service announcements, dramatic presentations, and support from well-known public figures. Free pamphlets and other literature are available from public health departments, health clinics, physicians' offices, student health centers, and Planned Parenthood, and easy-to-understand books are available in libraries and bookstores. Several national hotlines have been set up to provide free, confidential information and referral services to callers anywhere in the country.

Learning about STDs is still up to every person individually. You must assume responsibility for learning about the causes and nature of STDs and their potential effects on you, those with whom you have sexual relationships, and the children you may have.

Diagnosis and Treatment

Early diagnosis and treatment of STDs can help you and your sex partner(s) avoid unnecessary complications and help prevent the spread of STDs.

TERMS

chancre The sore produced by syphilis in its earliest stage.

trichomoniasis A protozoal infection caused by *Trichomonas vaginalis,* transmitted sexually and externally.

bacterial vaginosis (BV) A condition linked to sexual activity; caused by an overgrowth of certain bacteria inhabiting the vagina.

pubic lice Parasites that infest the hair of the pubic region, commonly called *crabs.*

scabies A contagious skin disease caused by a type of burrowing parasitic mite.

Get Vaccinated   Every young, sexually active person should be vaccinated for hepatitis B; vaccines are available for all age groups. Men who have sex with men should be vaccinated for hepatitis A, and girls and women age 9–26 should be vaccinated for HPV.

Be Alert for Symptoms   If you are sexually active, be alert for any sign or symptom of disease, such as a rash, a discharge, sores, or unusual pain, and have a professional examination if you notice such a symptom.

Get Tested   Remember that almost all STDs—including HIV infection—can be completely asymptomatic for long periods of time. The CDC recommends that everyone between the ages of 13 and 64 be tested for HIV at least once during routine medical care. Sexually active young women should have pelvic exams and Pap tests at least once a year, with chlamydia and gonorrhea screening in most cases. Sexually active men, especially if they have had more than one partner, should have periodic STD screenings.

The CDC recommends that sexually active men who have sex with men be tested annually for HIV, chlamydia, syphilis, and gonorrhea. All sexually active gay and bisexual men should be vaccinated for hepatitis A and B.

Inform Your Partners   Telling a partner that you have exposed him or her to an STD isn't easy. Despite the awkwardness and difficulty, it is crucial that your sex partner or partners be informed and urged to seek testing and/or treatment as quickly as possible.

Get Treated   With the exception of AIDS treatments, treatments for STDs are safe and generally inexpensive. If you are being treated, follow instructions carefully and complete all the medication as prescribed. Don't stop taking the medication just because you feel better or your symptoms have disappeared. Above all, don't give any of your medication to anyone else, including your partner. Being cured of an STD does not mean that you will not

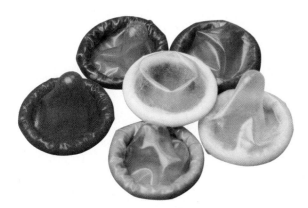

The use of condoms declined as more advanced methods of contraception, such as birth control pills and IUDs, became available. But condoms are once again gaining in popularity because of the protection they provide against STDs.

get it again, and exposure does not confer lasting immunity, nor does it prevent you from getting any other STD.

Prevention

If you choose to be sexually active, think about prevention *before* you have a sexual encounter, and plan accordingly. Remember that you are likely to be less cautious about sex when you have been drinking than you would be if you were sober. Being intoxicated leaves you vulnerable to sexual assault and greatly increases your risk of acquiring an STD.

Most people don't want to think, talk, or ask questions about STDs. There are many ways to bring up the subject of safer sex and condom use with your partner. Be honest about your concerns and stress that protection against STDs means that you care about yourself and your partner. Find out about your partner's sexual history and practices, but even if your partner's past seems low-risk, still insist on using a condom every time you have sex. You may find that your partner is just as concerned as you are. By thinking and talking about responsible sexual behavior, you are expressing a sense of caring for yourself, your potential partner, and your future children.

QUESTIONS FOR CRITICAL THINKING AND REFLECTION

If you are sexually active, have you talked seriously with your partner about STDs and safer sex practices? If not, why? How would you react if your partner started such a discussion?

TIPS FOR TODAY AND THE FUTURE

Your immune system is a remarkable germ-fighting network, but it needs your help to work at its best.

RIGHT NOW YOU CAN

- Move your bedtime up 15 minutes, starting tonight, to ensure that you're getting enough sleep.
- Make an appointment with your health care provider if you are worried about possible STD infection.
- Resolve to discuss condom use with your partner if you are sexually active and are not already using condoms.

IN THE FUTURE YOU CAN

- Learn how to communicate effectively with a partner who resists safer sex practices or is reluctant to discuss his or her sexual history. Support groups and educational classes can help.
- Make sure all your vaccinations are up-to-date; ask your doctor if you should be vaccinated against hepatitis B or any other STDs.

- The step-by-step process by which infections are transmitted from one person to another involves the pathogen, its reservoir, a portal of exit, a means of transmission, a portal of entry, and a new host.

- The immune response is carried out by white blood cells that are continuously produced in the bone marrow. It has four stages: recognition of the invading pathogen; rapid replication of killer T cells and B cells; attack by killer T cells and macrophages; and suppression of the immune response.

- Immunization is based on the body's ability to remember previously encountered organisms and retain its strength against them.

- Allergic reactions occur when the immune system responds to harmless substances as if they were dangerous antigens.

- Bacteria are single-celled organisms; some cause disease in humans. Bacterial infections include pneumonia, meningitis, strep throat, toxic shock syndrome, tuberculosis, Lyme disease, and ulcers.

- Viruses cannot grow or reproduce themselves; different viruses cause the common cold, influenza, measles, mumps, rubella, chicken pox, cold sores, mononucleosis, encephalitis, hepatitis, polio, and warts.

- Other diseases are caused by certain types of fungi, protozoa, parasitic worms, and prions.

- Autoimmune diseases occur when the body identifies its own cells as foreign.

- HIV affects the immune system, making an otherwise healthy person less able to resist a variety of infections.

- HIV is carried in blood and blood products, semen, vaginal and cervical secretions, and breast milk. HIV is transmitted through the exchange of these fluids.

- There is currently no cure or vaccine for HIV infection. Drugs have been developed to slow the course of the disease and to prevent or treat certain secondary infections.

- Chlamydia causes epididymitis and urethritis in men; in women, it can lead to PID and infertility if untreated.

- Pelvic inflammatory disease (PID), a complication of untreated gonorrhea or chlamydia, is an infection of the uterus and oviducts that may extend to the ovaries and pelvic cavity. It can lead to infertility, ectopic pregnancy, and chronic pelvic pain.

- Human papillomavirus (HPV) causes genital warts and cervical cancer. Treatment does not eradicate the virus, which can be passed on by asymptomatic people.

- Genital herpes is a common incurable infection that can be fatal to newborns. After an initial infection, outbreaks may recur at any time.

- Hepatitis B is a viral infection of the liver transmitted through sexual and nonsexual contact.

- Syphilis is a highly contagious bacterial infection that can be treated with antibiotics. If left untreated, it can lead to deterioration of the central nervous system and death.

- All STDs are preventable; the key is practicing responsible sexual behaviors. Those who are sexually active are safest with one mutually monogamous, uninfected partner. Using a condom properly with every act of sexual intercourse helps protect against STDs.

BOOKS

Engel, J. 2007. *The Epidemic: A Global History of AIDS.* New York: Collins. *A historical, social, and cultural perspective on the AIDS epidemic, from its beginning in 1981 to the present day, from a medical historian.*

Klausner, J. D., and E. W. Hook. 2007. *Current Diagnosis and Treatment of Sexually Transmitted Diseases.* New York: McGraw-Hill. *Written for the clinician; provides an easy-to-use reference of the latest diagnostic and treatment information available on STDs.*

McIlvenna, T. 2005. *The Complete Guide to Safer Sex.* Fort Lee, N.J.: Barricade Books. *Provides practical advice for STD prevention.*

Siegel, M. 2006. *Bird Flu: Everything You Need to Know About the Next Pandemic.* New York: Wiley. *A practicing physician and teacher examines the potential threat of an avian flu outbreak and explains the measures we can take to protect ourselves.*

Sompayrac, L. M. 2008. *How the Immune System Works.* 3rd ed. Malden, Mass.: Blackwell Science. *A highly readable overview of basic concepts of immunity.*

ORGANIZATIONS, HOTLINES, AND WEB SITES

American College Health Association. Offers free brochures on STDs, alcohol use, acquaintance rape, and other health issues.
http://www.acha.org

CDC National Center for Infectious Diseases. Provides extensive information on a wide variety of infectious diseases.
http://www.cdc.gov/ncidod

CDC National Immunization Program. Information and answers to frequently asked questions about immunizations.
http://www.cdc.gov/nip
http://www.cdc.gov/travel

CDC National Prevention Information Network. Provides extensive information and links on HIV/AIDS and other STDs.
http://www.cdcnpin.org

ASHA/CDC STD and AIDS Hotlines. Callers can obtain information, counseling, and referrals for testing and treatment. The hotlines offer information on more than 20 STDs and include Spanish and TTY service.
800-227-8922

HIV InSite: Gateway to AIDS Knowledge. Provides information about prevention, education, treatment, statistics, clinical trials, and new developments.

http://hivinsite.ucsf.edu

Joint United Nations Programme on HIV/AIDS (UNAIDS). Provides statistics and information on the international HIV/AIDS situation.

http://www.unaids.org

The NAMES Project Foundation AIDS Memorial Quilt. Includes the story behind the quilt, images of quilt panels, and information and links relating to HIV infection.

http://www.aidsquilt.org

National Institute of Allergies and Infectious Disease: Sexually Transmitted Infections. Provides up-to-date fact sheets and brochures.

http://www3.niaid.nih.gov/topics/sti

Planned Parenthood Federation of America. Provides information on STDs, family planning, and contraception.

http://www.plannedparenthood.org

World Health Organization: Infectious Diseases. Provides fact sheets about many emerging and tropical diseases as well as information about current outbreaks.

http://www.who.int/topics/infectious_diseases/en/

SELECTED BIBLIOGRAPHY

American Association of Blood Banks. 2007. *Blood Donation Frequently Asked Questions* (http://www.aabb.org/Content/Donate_Blood/Blood_Donation_FAQs/donatefaqs.htm; retrieved February 17, 2009).

American Social Health Association. 2008. *Frequently Asked Questions About Cervical Cancer/HPV Vaccine Access in the U.S.* (http://www.ashastd.org/hpv/hpv_vaccines.cfm; retrieved February 17, 2009).

Brown, D. R., et al. 2005. A longitudinal study of genital human papillomavirus infection in a cohort of closely followed adolescent women. *Journal of Infectious Diseases* 191(2): 182–192.

Centers for Disease Control and Prevention. 2006. Revised recommendations for HIV testing of adults, adolescents, and pregnant women in health-care settings. *Morbidity and Mortality Weekly Report* 55(RR-14): 1–17.

Centers for Disease Control and Prevention. 2007. *Healthcare-Associated Methicillin Resistant Staphylococcus Aureus (HA-MRSA)* (http://www.cdc.gov/ncidod/dhqp/ar-mrsa.html; retrieved February 16, 2009).

Centers for Disease Control and Prevention. 2007. *STD Surveillance 2006* (http://www.cdc.gov/std/stats06/toc2006.htm; retrieved February 17, 2009).

Centers for Disease Control and Prevention. 2008. *Asthma: General Information* (http://www.cdc.gov/asthma/basics.htm; retrieved February 16, 2009).

Centers for Disease Control and Prevention. 2008. *BSE (Bovine Spongiform Encephalopathy, or Mad Cow Disease)* (http://www.cdc.gov/ncidod/dvrd/bse; retrieved February 16, 2009).

Centers for Disease Control and Prevention. 2008. *Flu Activity and Surveillance* (http://www.cdc.gov/flu/weekly/fluactivity.htm; retrieved February 16, 2009).

Centers for Disease Control and Prevention. 2008. *Genital HPV Infection—CDC Fact Sheet* (http://www.cdc.gov/std/hpv/stdfact-hpv.htm; retrieved February 17, 2009).

Centers for Disease Control and Prevention. 2008. HIV prevalence estimates—United States, 2006. *Morbidity and Mortality Weekly Report* 57(39): 1073–1076.

Centers for Disease Control and Prevention. 2008. *New Estimates of U.S. HIV Prevalence, 2006.* (http://www.cdc.gov/hiv/topics/surveillance/resources/factsheets/pdf/prevalence.pdf; retrieved February 17, 2009).

Centers for Disease Control and Prevention. 2008. Trends in tuberculosis—United States, 2007. *Morbidity and Mortality Weekly Report* 57(11): 281–285.

Centers for Disease Control and Prevention. 2008. *West Nile Virus Basics* (http://www.cdc.gov/ncidod/dvbid/westnile/index.htm; retrieved February 16, 2009).

Centers for Disease Control and Prevention. 2009. Recommended immunization schedules for persons aged 0–18 years—United States, 2009. *Morbidity and Mortality Weekly Report* 57(51): Q1–Q4.

Cohen, Myron. 2004. HIV and sexually transmitted diseases: A lethal synergy. *Topics in HIV Medicine* 12(4):104–107.

Fairweather, D., and N. R. Rose. 2004. Women and autoimmune diseases. *Emerging Infectious Diseases* 10(11): 2005–2011.

Fauci, A. S. 2004. Emerging infectious diseases: A clear and present danger to humanity. *Journal of the American Medical Association* 292(15): 1887–1888.

Food and Drug Administration. 2004. *FDA Approves First Oral Fluid Based Rapid HIV Test Kit* (http://www.fda.gov/bbs/topics/news/2004/NEW01042.html; retrieved February 17, 2009).

Hightow, L. B., et al. 2005. The unexpected movement of the HIV epidemic in the southeastern United States: Transmission among college students. *Journal of Acquired Immune Deficiency Syndrome* 38(5): 531–537.

Joint United National Programme on HIV/AIDS (UNAIDS). 2008. *2008 Report on the Global AIDS Epidemic.* Geneva: UNAIDS.

Kimberlin, D., and D. Rouse. 2004. Genital herpes. *New England Journal of Medicine* 350(19): 1970–1977.

Levy, S. B., and B. Marshall. 2004. Antibacterial resistance worldwide: Causes, challenges, and responses. *Nature Medicine* 10(12 Suppl): S122–S129.

Mathers, C. D., and Loncar, D. 2006. Projections of global mortality and burden of disease from 2002 to 2030. Public Library of Science, *Medicine* 3(11):2011–2030.

Merson, M. 2006. The HIV-AIDS pandemic at 25—The global response. *New England Journal of Medicine* 354(23): 2414–2417.

Miller, W. C., et al. 2004. Prevalence of chlamydial and gonococcal infections among young adults in the United States. *Journal of the American Medical Association* 291(18): 2229–2236.

National Immunization Program. 2005. *Epidemiology and Prevention of Vaccine-Preventable Diseases,* 8th ed. Rev. Waldorf, Md.: Public Health Foundation.

Samandari, T., B. P. Bell, and G. L. Armstrong. 2004. Quantifying the impact of hepatitis A immunization in the United States, 1995–2001. *Vaccine* 22(31–32): 4342–4350.

World Health Organization. 2004. *WHO Guidelines for the Global Surveillance of Severe Acute Respiratory Syndrome (SARS), Updated Recommendations, October 2004.* Geneva: World Health Organization.

World Health Organization. 2007. *The World Health Report 2007.* Geneva: World Health Organization.

Xu, F., et al. 2006. Trends in herpes simplex virus type 1 and type 2 seroprevalence in the United States. *Journal of the American Medical Association* 296(8): 964–973.

Yeni, P. G., et al. 2004. Treatment for adult HIV infection. *Journal of the American Medical Association* 292(2): 251–265.

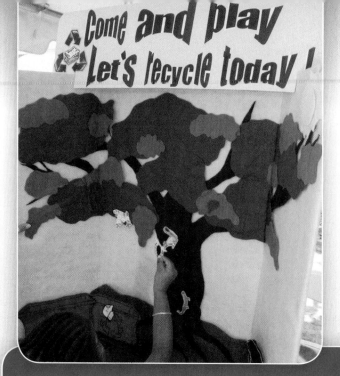

LOOKING AHEAD>>>>>

AFTER READING THIS CHAPTER, YOU
SHOULD BE ABLE TO:

- Explain how population growth affects the earth's environment and contributes to pollution and climate change

- Discuss the causes and effects of air and water pollution, and describe strategies that people can take to protect these resources

- Discuss the issue of solid waste disposal and the impact it has on the environment and human health

- Identify key sources of chemical and radiation pollution, and discuss methods for preventing such pollution

- Explain how energy use affects the environment, and describe steps everyone can take to use energy more efficiently

ENVIRONMENTAL HEALTH

14

We are constantly reminded of our intimate relationship with everything that surrounds us—our environment. Although the planet provides us with food, water, air, and everything else that sustains life, it also provides us with natural occurrences—earthquakes, tsunamis, hurricanes, drought, climate changes—that destroy life and disrupt society. In the past, humans frequently had to struggle against the environment to survive. Today, in addition to dealing with natural disasters, we also have to find ways to protect the environment from the by-products of our way of life.

ENVIRONMENTAL HEALTH DEFINED

The field of **environmental health** grew out of efforts to control communicable diseases. These efforts led to systematic garbage collection, sewage treatment, filtration and chlorination of drinking water, food inspection, and the establishment of public health enforcement agencies. Cleaning up the environment changed the health profile of the developed world, reducing or eliminating deaths from diseases like typhoid fever and cholera. Unfortunately, infectious diseases continue to take a huge toll worldwide.

In the United States, a complex public health system is constantly at work behind the scenes. Every time the system is disrupted, danger recurs. After any disaster situation that damages a community's public health system, prompt restoration of basic health services becomes crucial to human survival. And every time we venture beyond the boundaries of our everyday world, we are reminded of the importance of these basics: clean water, sanitary waste disposal, safe food, and insect and rodent control.

Over the last few decades, the focus of environmental health has expanded and become more complex. We now recognize that environmental pollutants contribute not only to infectious diseases but to many chronic diseases

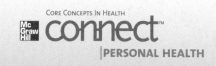

as well. Technological advances have increased our ability to affect and damage the environment. Rapid population growth, which has resulted partly from past environmental improvements, means that far more people are consuming and competing for resources than ever before.

Environmental health is therefore seen as encompassing all the interactions of humans with their environment and the health consequences of these interactions. Fundamental to this definition is a recognition that we hold the world in trust for future generations and for other forms of life. Our responsibility is to pass on a world no worse, and preferably better, than the one we enjoy today.

POPULATION GROWTH AND CONTROL

Throughout most of history, humans have been a minor pressure on the planet. About 300 million people were alive in the year A.D. 1; by the time Europeans were settling in the United States 1600 years later, the world population had increased gradually to a little over 500 mil-

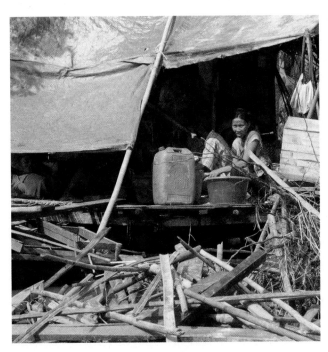

Natural events—such as the 2008 cyclone that struck Myanmar—can directly kill thousands of people while wiping out essential services, polluting water, and facilitating the spread of diseases.

QUESTIONS FOR CRITICAL THINKING AND REFLECTION
How often do you think about the environment's impact on your personal health? In what ways do your immediate surroundings (your home, neighborhood, school, workplace) affect your well-being? In what ways do you influence the health of your personal environment?

lion. But then it began rising exponentially—zooming to 1 billion by about 1800, more than doubling by 1930, and then doubling again in just 40 years (Figure 14.1).

The United Nations projects that world population will reach 9.1 billion by 2050 and will continue to increase until it levels off above 10 billion in 2200. Virtually all of this increase is taking place in less-developed regions. This rapid expansion of population, particularly in the past 50 years, is generally believed to be responsible for most of the stress humans put on the environment.

No one knows how many people the world can support, but most scientists agree that there is a limit. A 2006 report from the United Nation's Convention on Biological Diversity states that the population's demand for resources already exceed the earth's capacity by 20%. The primary factors that may eventually put a cap on human population are likely to be the limits of the earth's resources—food, land, water, and energy. The mass media have exposed the entire world to the American lifestyle and raised people's expectations of living at a comparable level. But such a lifestyle is

supported by levels of energy consumption that the earth cannot support worldwide. The United States has about 5% of the world's population but uses 25% of the world's energy.

Although it is apparent that population growth must be controlled, population trends are difficult to influence and manage. A variety of interconnecting factors fuel the current population explosion, including high fertility rates, lack of family planning resources, and lower death rates.

environmental health The collective interactions of humans with the environment and the short-term and long-term health consequences of those interactions.

FIGURE 14.1 World population growth.
The United Nations estimates that the world's population will continue to increase dramatically until it stabilizes above 10 billion people in 2200.

SOURCES: United Nations Population Division. 2007. *World Population Prospects: The 2006 Revision.* New York: United Nations; U.S. Bureau of the Census.

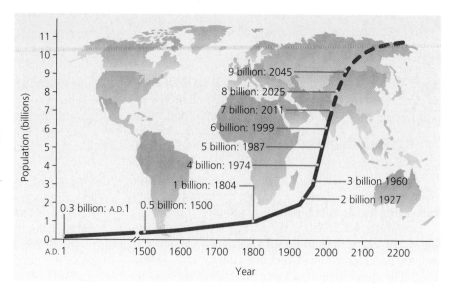

To be successful, population management must change the condition of people's lives, especially poverty, to remove the pressures for having large families. Research indicates that the combination of improved health, better education, and increased literacy and employment opportunities for women works together with family planning to decrease fertility rates. Unfortunately, in the fastest-growing countries, the needs of a rapidly increasing population use up financial resources that might otherwise be used to improve lives and ultimately slow population growth.

AIR QUALITY AND POLLUTION

Air pollution is not a human invention or even a new problem. The air is polluted naturally with every forest fire, pollen bloom, and dust storm, as well as with countless other natural pollutants. To these natural sources, humans have always contributed the by-products of their activities. Air pollution is linked to a wide range of health problems; the very young and the elderly are among those most susceptible to air pollution's effects.

Air Quality and Smog

The EPA uses a measure called the **Air Quality Index (AQI)** to indicate whether air pollution levels pose a health concern. The AQI is used for five major air pollutants: carbon monoxide (CO), sulfur dioxide (SO_2), nitrogen dioxide (NO_2), particulate matter (PM), and ground-level ozone. A major source of those pollutants is the burning of **fossil fuels** in vehicles and industrial processes. AQI values run from 0 to 500; the higher the AQI, the greater the level of pollution and associated health danger. Local AQI information is often available in newspapers, on television and radio, on the Internet, and from state and local telephone hotlines.

The term **smog** was first used in the early 1900s in London to describe the combination of smoke and fog. What we typically call smog today is a mixture of pollutants, with ground-level ozone being the key ingredient. Major smog occurrences are linked to the combination of several factors: Heavy motor vehicle traffic, high temperatures, and sunny weather can increase the production of ozone. Pollutants are also more likely to build up in areas with little wind and/or where a topographic feature such as a mountain range or valley prevents the wind from pushing out stagnant air.

> **113 million**
> Americans live in counties where the air is unhealthy at least some of the time.
>
> —Environmental Protection Agency, 2008

The Greenhouse Effect and Global Warming

The temperature of the earth's atmosphere depends on the balance between the amount of energy the planet absorbs from the sun (mainly as high-energy ultraviolet radiation) and the amount of energy radiated back into

QUESTIONS FOR CRITICAL THINKING AND REFLECTION

What is the population of your town or city? Does the sheer number of people in your town make living there difficult, or more enjoyable? In what ways? Do you believe your town has adequate infrastructure and resources to support its residents?

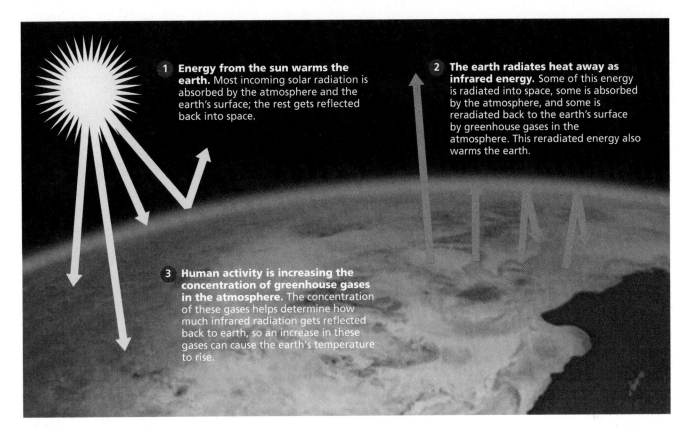

FIGURE 14.2 The greenhouse effect.

1. **Energy from the sun warms the earth.** Most incoming solar radiation is absorbed by the atmosphere and the earth's surface; the rest gets reflected back into space.

2. **The earth radiates heat away as infrared energy.** Some of this energy is radiated into space, some is absorbed by the atmosphere, and some is reradiated back to the earth's surface by greenhouse gases in the atmosphere. This reradiated energy also warms the earth.

3. **Human activity is increasing the concentration of greenhouse gases in the atmosphere.** The concentration of these gases helps determine how much infrared radiation gets reflected back to earth, so an increase in these gases can cause the earth's temperature to rise.

space as lower-energy infrared radiation. Key components of temperature regulation are carbon dioxide, water vapor, methane, and other **greenhouse gases**—so named because, like the glass panes in a greenhouse, they let through visible light from the sun but trap some of the resulting infrared radiation and reradiate it back to the earth's surface. This reradiation causes a buildup of heat that raises the temperature of the lower atmosphere, a natural process known as the **greenhouse effect** (Figure 14.2). Without it, the atmosphere would be far cooler and much more hostile to life.

There is growing consensus that human activity is causing **global warming** or *climate change*. The concentration of greenhouse gases is increasing because of human activity, especially the combustion of fossil fuels. Carbon dioxide levels in the atmosphere have increased rapidly in recent decades. The use of fossil fuels pumps more than 20 billion tons of carbon dioxide into the atmo-

sphere every year. Deforestation, often by burning, also sends carbon dioxide into the atmosphere and reduces the number of trees available to convert carbon dioxide into oxygen.

In 2006, the National Research Council reported that the overall global temperature had increased 0.6°C during the twentieth century (Figure 14.3). There is growing

Air Quality Index (AQI)   A measure of local air quality and what it means for health.

fossil fuels   Buried deposits of decayed animals and plants that are converted into carbon-rich fuels by exposure to heat and pressure over millions of years; oil, coal, and natural gas are fossil fuels.

smog   Hazy atmospheric conditions resulting from increased concentrations of ground-level ozone and other pollutants.

greenhouse gas   A gas (such as carbon dioxide) or vapor that traps infrared radiation instead of allowing it to escape through the atmosphere, resulting in a warming of the earth (the greenhouse effect).

greenhouse effect   A warming of the earth due to a buildup of carbon dioxide and certain other gases.

global warming   An increase in the earth's atmospheric temperature when averaged across seasons and geographical regions; also called *climate change*.

TERMS

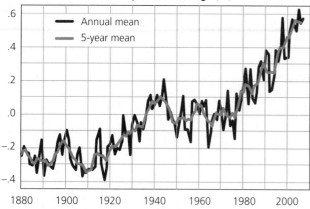

Global Temperature Change (°C)

- Annual mean
- 5-year mean

FIGURE 14.3   Trend in annual mean temperature. This graph traces the trend in the annual mean temperature relative to the 1951–1980 mean value. There has been a strong warming trend over the past 30 years.

SOURCE: Goddard Institute for Space Studies. 2009. *GISS Surface Temperature Analysis, Global Temperature Trends: 2009 Summation* (http://data.giss.nasa.gov/gistemp/2007; retrieved February 19, 2009).

agreement among scientists that temperatures will continue to rise, although estimates vary as to how much they will change. If global warming persists, experts say the impact may be devastating (see the box "Global Warming, Local Action"). Possible consequences include increased rainfall and flooding in some regions, increased drought in others; increased mortality from heat stress, urban air pollution, tropical diseases, and extreme weather events; a poleward shift of 50–350 miles in the location of vegetation zones, affecting crop yields, irrigation demands, and forest productivity; and increasingly rapid and drastic melting of the earth's polar ice caps.

According to estimates from the Environmental Protection Agency (EPA), the earth's average surface temperature is likely to increase 2.0–11.5°F (1.1–6.4°C) by the end of the twenty-first century.

Thinning of the Ozone Layer

Another air pollution problem is the thinning of the **ozone layer** of the atmosphere, a fragile, invisible layer about 10–30 miles above the earth's surface that shields the planet from the sun's hazardous ultraviolet (UV) rays.

TERMS

ozone layer   A layer of ozone molecules (O_3) in the upper atmosphere that screens out UV rays from the sun.

chlorofluorocarbons (CFCs)   Chemicals used as spray-can propellants, refrigerants, and industrial solvents, implicated in the destruction of the ozone layer.

Since the mid-1980s, scientists have observed the seasonal appearance and growth of a hole in the ozone layer over Antarctica. More recently, thinning over other areas—including Canada, Scandinavia, the northern United States, Russia, Australia, and New Zealand—has been noted.

The ozone layer is being destroyed primarily by **chlorofluorocarbons (CFCs)**, industrial chemicals that rise into the atmosphere and release chlorine atoms, which destroy ozone. In the Northern Hemisphere, ozone levels have declined by about 10% since 1980, and certain areas may be temporarily depleted in late winter and early spring by as much as 40%. Without the ozone layer to absorb the sun's UV radiation, life on Earth would be impossible. The potential effects of increased long-term exposure to UV light for humans include skin cancer, wrinkling and aging of the skin, cataracts and blindness, and reduced immune response. UV light may interfere with photosynthesis and cause lower crop yields; it may also kill phytoplankton and krill, the basis of the ocean food chain.

Worldwide production and use of CFCs have declined rapidly since the danger to the ozone layer was recognized. Ozone-depleting substances have very long lifetimes in the atmosphere, however, so despite these efforts, the ozone hole is not expected to recover until 2070. The gradual recovery is masked by annual variations caused by weather fluctuations over Antarctica.

Energy Use and Air Pollution

Americans are the biggest energy consumers in the world, leading China, Russia, Japan, India, and European countries. About 85% of the energy we use comes from fossil fuels—oil, coal, and natural gas. The remainder comes from nuclear power and renewable energy sources (such as hydroelectric, wind, and solar power). Energy consumption is at the root of many environmental problems, especially those relating to air pollution. Two key strategies for controlling energy use are conservation and the development of nonpolluting, renewable sources of energy. Although the use of renewable energy sources has increased in recent years, renewables still supply only a small proportion of our energy. Despite increases in U.S. consumer gas prices, more than 70% of commuters drive alone to work, and low-fuel-economy sport utility vehicles (SUVs) remain popular. Every gallon of gas burned puts about 20 pounds of carbon dioxide into the atmosphere, and the largest SUVs increase greenhouse gas emissions by 6 or more tons per year more than an average car.

Global Warming, Local Action

At current rates of consumption, we are using up the earth's resources so rapidly that they may run out sooner than anyone expects. Some experts say that humankind is already outstripping the planet's biological capacity by 20%. A 2006 report from the Worldwatch Institute says that if fast-growing nations like China and India start using the earth's stores at the same rate as the United States, we will need the resources of *a second earth* to keep everyone satisfied.

In addition, we use millions of tons of fossil fuel each year to power homes, cars, and factories. However unintentionally, we are also using them to destroy our planet.

Evidence of Global Warming

There is ample evidence that global warming is a reality. Here are just a few examples:

• Scientists have been measuring atmospheric carbon dioxide (CO_2) levels for years and say the amount of CO_2 is continually rising.

• Glaciers and other large ice formations are melting at a quickening pace and shrinking measurably. Such melting threatens to raise ocean levels around the world—possibly as much as 3 to 5 feet in the coming decades.

• The World Health Organization says that ecological damage caused by human activities (such as burning fossil fuels and destroying forests and wetlands) is threatening our health. WHO also predicts dramatic increases in disease during the next 50 years, along with food and water shortages.

Who Is Responsible?

To some degree, we are all responsible for climate change, just as we all stand to suffer because of it. Scientists can calculate just how much each person, house, car, appliance, and factory contributes to global warming; they call this measure an "environmental footprint." The footprint's size is determined by the amount of greenhouse gases the source generates, either directly (such as a car or factory) or indirectly (such as an electric appliance, which runs on electricity produced by a fossil-fuel-burning power plant). For example, for each gallon of gas your car burns, it releases about 20 pounds of CO_2 into the atmosphere; a typical refrigerator is responsible for more than 2000 pounds of CO_2 annually; and a typical American home generates 28,000 pounds of greenhouse gases each year, both directly and indirectly.

What Is Being Done?

At the global level, many governments are taking initiatives to slow the release of greenhouse gases. One result of these efforts is the Kyoto Protocol to the United Nations Convention on Climate Change, which took effect in 2005. Under terms of this agreement, participating countries must reduce greenhouse gas emissions to an average of 5% below 1990 levels by 2012. Under previous administrations, the United States did not participate in the Kyoto Protocol, as government leaders contended the accord placed too great a financial burden on industry. The United Nations has called on the United States to take a more ac-

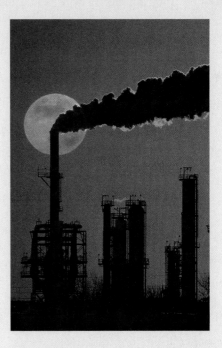

tive role in combating global warming under President Obama.

Industries are slowly getting on the bandwagon, too. Many companies are investing in cleaner fuel technology and "scrubbing" their emissions before they enter the environment. Automakers are improving existing hybrid automobiles and making more models available, while focusing on the development of all-electric cars and hydrogen fuel cell technologies that virtually eliminate automotive pollution.

Individuals are making a difference, too. You can learn more about global warming and what it means to our future by checking out the organizations and Web sites listed in the For More Information section at the end of the chapter.

Alternative Fuels The U.S. Department of Energy (DOE) is encouraging researchers and automobile manufacturers to produce vehicles that can handle alternative fuels such as ethanol. Ethanol, a form of alcohol, is a renewable and largely domestic transportation fuel produced from fermenting plant sugars such as corn, sugar cane, and other starchy agricultural products. Ethanol use reduces the amount of imported oil required to produce gasoline, reduces overall greenhouse gas emissions from automobiles, and supports the U.S. agricultural industry. Drawbacks of ethanol include the amount of energy required to produce it, which may exceed the amount of energy it

yields, and the diversion of corn crops from the food supply to the fuel industry, which is thought to contribute to high food prices and food shortages around the world.

Hybrid and Electric Vehicles A more positive trend has been the introduction of hybrid electric vehicles (HEVs). Hybrid vehicles use two or more distinct power sources to propel the vehicle, such as an on-board energy storage system (batteries, for example) and an internal combustion engine and electric motor. The hybrid vehicle typically realizes greater fuel economy than a conventional car does and produces fewer polluting emissions.

Another type of alternative vehicle is all-electric. In these vehicles, electricity is stored in battery packs and then converted into mechanical power that runs the vehicle. These vehicles do not produce tailpipe emissions, but generators that produce the electricity for the batteries do emit pollutants.

Indoor Air Pollution

Although most people associate air pollution with the outdoors, your home may also harbor potentially dangerous pollutants. Some of these compounds trigger allergic responses, and others have been linked to cancer. Common indoor pollutants include environmental tobacco smoke (ETS); carbon monoxide and other combustion by-products from woodstoves, fireplaces, kerosene heaters and lamps, and gas ranges; formaldehyde gas from certain construction materials, paints, floor finishes, permanent press clothing, and nail polish; biological pollutants, including bacteria, dust mites, mold, and animal dander; and indoor mold, which can cause health problems when inhaled, especially for people with asthma and other respiratory conditions.

Preventing Air Pollution and Conserving Energy

You can do a great deal to reduce air pollution and conserve energy. Here are a few ideas:

- Cut back on driving. Ride your bike, walk, use public transportation, or carpool in a fuel-efficient vehicle.

- Keep your car tuned up and well maintained, and keep your tires inflated at recommended pressures. To save energy when driving, avoid quick starts, stay within the speed limit, limit the use of air conditioning, and don't let your car idle unless absolutely necessary. Have your car's air conditioner checked and serviced by a station that uses environmentally friendly refrigerants (car air conditioners made before 1994 are a major source of CFCs).

- Buy energy-efficient appliances, and run the washing machine, dryer, and dishwasher only when you have full loads. Do laundry in warm or cold water

instead of hot. Clean refrigerator coils and clothes dryer lint screens frequently.

- Replace incandescent bulbs with compact fluorescent bulbs (CFLs). Although they cost more initially, they save you money over the long term because they use less electricity to produce light and last up to ten times longer than incandescent bulbs. Burned-out CFLs should be recycled rather than disposed of in the trash.

- Make sure your home is well-insulated, and use insulating shades and curtains. In cold weather, put on a sweater and turn down the thermostat. In hot weather, use a fan instead of an air conditioner to cool yourself.

- Plant and care for trees in your yard and neighborhood. Because they recycle carbon dioxide, trees work against global warming. They also provide shade and cool the air, so less air conditioning is needed.

- Before discarding a refrigerator, air conditioner, or humidifier, check with the waste hauler or your local government to ensure that ozone-depleting refrigerants will be removed prior to disposal. If you use a metered-dose inhaler, ask your physician if an ozone-safe inhaler is available for your medication.

- Keep paints, cleaning agents, and other chemical products tightly sealed in their original containers.

- Clean and inspect chimneys, furnaces, and other appliances regularly. Install carbon monoxide detectors.

WATER QUALITY AND POLLUTION

Few parts of the world have enough safe, clean drinking water, but few things are as important to human health.

Water Contamination and Treatment

Many cities rely at least in part on wells that tap local groundwater, but often it is necessary to tap lakes and rivers to supplement wells. Because such surface water is more likely to be contaminated with both organic matter and pathogenic microorganisms, it is purified in water-treatment plants before being piped into the community.

In most areas of the United States, water systems have adequate, dependable supplies, are able to control waterborne disease, and provide water without unacceptable color, odor, or taste. However, problems do occur. The Centers for Disease Control and Prevention (CDC) estimate that 1 million Americans become ill and 900–1000 die each year from microbial illnesses from drinking water.

? QUESTIONS FOR CRITICAL THINKING AND REFLECTION

What are your views on the issue of climate change? Do you believe it is a real problem, or that it has been overly hyped by the media and some politicians? How do you support your views?

Water Shortages

Water shortages are a growing concern in many regions of the world. Some parts of the United States are experiencing rapid population growth that outstrips the ability of local systems to provide adequate water to all. Groundwater pumping and the diversion of water from lakes and rivers for irrigation are further reducing the amount of water available to local communities.

Sewage

Most cities have sewage-treatment systems that separate fecal matter from water in huge tanks and ponds and stabilize it so that it cannot transmit infectious diseases. Once treated and biologically safe, the water is released back into the environment. The sludge that remains behind is often contaminated with **heavy metals** and is handled as hazardous waste; if not contaminated, sludge may be used as fertilizer.

Many cities have now begun expanded sewage-treatment measures to remove heavy metals and other hazardous chemicals. This action has resulted from many studies linking exposure to chemicals such as mercury, lead, and **polychlorinated biphenyls (PCBs)** with long-term health consequences, including cancer and damage to the central nervous system.

Protecting the Water Supply

By taking steps to keep the water supply clean, you reduce pollution overall and help protect the land, wildlife, and other people from illness.

- Take showers, not baths, to minimize your water consumption. Don't let water run when you're not actively using it while brushing your teeth, shaving, or hand-washing clothes.

- Install sink faucet aerators and water-efficient showerheads, which use two to five times less water with no noticeable decrease in performance. Purchase a water-saver toilet, or put a displacement device in your toilet tank to reduce the amount of water used with each flush.

- Fix any leaky faucets in your home. Leaks can waste thousands of gallons of water per year.

- Don't pour toxic materials such as cleaning solvents, bleach, or motor oil down the drain. Store them until you can take them to a hazardous waste collection center.

- Don't pour old medicines down the drain or flush them down the toilet. The best way to discard old medicines is to mix them with coffee grounds or cat litter, seal them in a container, and put them in the trash.

SOLID WASTE POLLUTION

Humans generate huge amounts of waste, which require proper handling to ensure environmental safety.

Solid Waste

The bulk of the organic food garbage produced in American kitchens is now dumped in the sewage system by way of the garbage disposal. The garbage that remains is not very hazardous from the standpoint of infectious disease because there is very little food waste in it, but it does represent an enormous disposal and contamination problem.

> The average American generates **4.6 pounds** of trash per day; about 1.5 pounds of this is recycled.
>
> —Environmental Protection Agency, 2008

QUICK STATS

What's In Our Garbage? The biggest single component of household trash by weight is paper products, including junk mail, glossy mail-order catalogs, and computer printouts (Figure 14.4). About 1% of the solid waste is toxic; a new source of toxic waste is the disposal of computer components in both household and commercial waste. Burning, as opposed to burial, reduces the bulk of solid waste, but it may release hazardous material into the air. Manufacturing, mining, and other industries all produce large amounts of potentially dangerous materials that cannot simply be dumped.

Disposing of Solid Waste Since the 1960s, billions of tons of solid waste have been buried in **sanitary landfill**

heavy metal A metal with a high specific gravity, such as lead, copper, or tin.

polychlorinated biphenyl (PCB) An industrial chemical used as an insulator in electrical transformers and linked to certain human cancers.

sanitary landfill A disposal site where solid wastes are buried.

TERMS

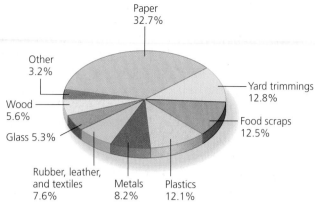

Paper
32.7%

Other
3.2%

Yard trimmings
12.8%

Wood
5.6%

Food scraps
12.5%

Glass 5.3%

Rubber, leather,
and textiles
7.6%

Metals
8.2%

Plastics
12.1%

Due to rounding, these numbers do not add up to 100%.

FIGURE 14.4 Components of municipal solid waste, by weight, before recycling.

SOURCE: Environmental Protection Agency, 2008. *Municipal Solid Waste Generation, Recycling and Disposal in the United States: Facts and Figures for 2007* (http://www.epa.gov./epa.waste/nonhaz/municipal/pubs/msw07-fs.pdf; retrieved February 19, 2009).

disposal sites. Sometimes protective liners are used around the site, and nearby monitoring wells are now required in most states. Layers of solid waste are regularly covered with thin layers of dirt until the site is filled. Some communities then plant grass and trees and convert the site into a park. Landfill is relatively stable; almost no decomposition occurs in the solidly packed waste. Much of this waste contains chemicals, ranging from leftover pesticides to paints and oils, which should not be released indiscriminately into the environment. Despite precautions, buried contaminants sometimes leak into the surrounding soil and groundwater. Burial is also expensive and requires huge amounts of space.

The term **biodegradable** means that certain products can break down naturally, safely, and quickly into the raw materials of nature, then disappear back into the environment. Table 14.1 shows the amount of time required for different types of material to biodegrade.

Recycling In **recycling**, many kinds of waste materials are collected and used as raw materials in the production of new products. Recycling is a good idea because it puts unwanted objects back to good use and it reduces the

biodegradable Refers to the ability of some materials to break down naturally and disappear back into the environment.

recycling The use of waste materials as raw materials in the production of new products.

asbestosis A lung condition caused by inhalation of microscopic asbestos fibers, which inflame the lung and can lead to lung cancer.

TERMS

Table 14.1	Biodegrading Times of Different Objects

Item	Time Required to Biodegrade
Banana peel	2–10 days
Paper	2–5 months
Rope	3–14 months
Orange peel	6 months
Wool sock	1–5 years
Cigarette butt	1–12 years
Plastic-coated milk carton	5 years
Aluminum can	80–100 years
Plastic six-pack holder ring	450 years
Glass bottle	1 million years
Plastic bottle	Forever

amount of solid waste sitting in landfills, some of which takes decades to decay naturally.

Discarded Technology Americans scrap about 400 million consumer electronic devices each year. This "e-waste" is the fastest-growing portion of our waste stream. Junked electronic devices are toxic, hazardous waste because they contain varying amounts of lead, mercury, and other heavy metals.

Reducing Solid Waste

By recycling more and throwing away less, you can conserve landfill space and put reusable items back into service.

- Buy products with the least amount of packaging you can, or buy products in bulk (see the box "How to Be a Green Consumer") or packaged in recyclable containers.

- Buy recycled or recyclable products. Avoid disposables; instead, use long-lasting or reusable products such as rechargeable batteries.

- Avoid using foam or paper cups and plastic stirrers by bringing your own coffee mug to work or wherever you drink coffee or tea. Pack your lunch in a reusable sack or box.

- To store food, use glass jars and reusable plastic containers rather than foil and plastic wrap.

- Recycle your newspapers, glass, cans, paper, and other recyclables. If you receive something packaged with foam pellets, take them to a commercial mailing center that accepts them for recycling.

- Do not throw electronic items, batteries, or fluorescent lights into the trash. Take all these to state-approved recycling centers.

- If you have a yard, start a compost pile for your organic garbage (non-animal food and yard waste).

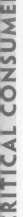
How to Be a Green Consumer

You can quickly and easily develop habits that direct your consumer dollar toward environmentally friendly products and companies.

- Remember the four Rs of green consumerism:

  Reduce the amount of trash and pollution you generate by consuming and throwing away less.

  Reuse as many products as possible—either yourself or by selling them or donating them to charity.

  Recycle all appropriate materials and buy recycled products whenever possible.

  Respond by educating others about reducing waste and recycling, by finding creative ways to reduce waste and toxicity, and by making your preferences known.

- Choose products packaged in refillable, recycled, reusable containers, such as paper, cardboard, aluminum, or glass. Don't buy products that are excessively packaged or wrapped.

- Look for products made with the highest possible content of recycled paper, metal, glass, plastic, and other materials.

- Choose simple products containing the lowest amounts of bleaches, dyes, and fragrances. Look for organic foods from local sources and clothes made from organically grown cotton or Fox Fibre or another naturally colored type of cotton.

- Buy high-quality appliances that have an Energy Star seal from the EPA or some other type of certification indicating that they are energy- and water-efficient.

- Get a reusable cloth shopping bag. If you forget your bag, it doesn't matter much whether you choose paper or plastic—what is important is that you reuse whatever bag you get.

- Look beyond the products to the companies that make them. Support those with good environmental records. If some of your favorite products are overpackaged or contain harmful ingredients, write to the manufacturer.

- Keep in mind that doing something is better than doing nothing. Even if you can't be a perfectly green consumer, doing your best on any purchase *will* make a difference.

SOURCES: U.S. Environmental Protection Agency. 2009. *Consumer Handbook for Reducing Solid Waste* (http://www.epa.gov/osw/wycd/catbook; retrieved February 19, 2009); Natural Resources Defense Council. 2009. *NRDC's Guide to Greener Living* (http:// www.nrdc.org/cities/living/gover. asp; retrieved February 19, 2009).

- Stop junk mail. To cancel junk mail, send a request to Mail Preference Service, Direct Marketing Association, 1120 Avenue of the Americas, New York, NY 10036-6700 (http://www.dmaconsumers.org).

QUESTIONS FOR CRITICAL THINKING AND REFLECTION

What are your own waste-disposal habits like? Do you recycle everything you possibly can? Do you get rid of items that are still usable? Even if you are conscientious about the way you deal with waste, how could you improve your habits?

CHEMICAL POLLUTION AND HAZARDOUS WASTE

New chemical substances are constantly being introduced into the environment—as pesticides, herbicides, solvents, and hundreds of other products. More people and wildlife are exposed and potentially exposed to them than ever before.

STATS

The Superfund national priorities list included 1255 sites as of May 2008.

—EPA, 2008

Asbestos

A mineral-based compound, asbestos was widely used for fire protection and insulation in buildings until the late 1960s. Microscopic asbestos fibers can be released into the air when this material is applied or when it later deteriorates or is damaged. These fibers can lodge in the lungs, causing **asbestosis**, lung cancer, and other serious lung diseases. Similar conditions expose workers to risk in the coal mining industry, from coal and silica dust (black lung disease), and in the textile industry, from cotton fibers (brown lung disease).

Lead

Thanks to better preventive efforts, lead poisoning is not as serious a problem today as it was a few years ago. Still, the CDC estimates that about 435,000 children under age 6 may have unsafe lead levels in their blood. Many of these children live in poor, inner-city areas (see the box "Poverty and Environmental Health" on p. 356). When lead is ingested or inhaled, it can damage the central nervous system, cause permanent mental impairment, hinder oxygen transport in the blood, create digestive problems, and cause coma or even death.

Young children can easily ingest lead from their environment by picking up dust and dirt on their hands and then putting their fingers in their mouth. Lead-based paints are the chief culprit in lead poisoning of children and were banned from residential use in 1978, but as

Residents of poor and minority communities are often exposed to more environmental toxins than residents of wealthier communities, and they are more likely to suffer from health problems caused or aggravated by pollutants.

Poor neighborhoods are often located near highways and industrial areas that have high levels of air and noise pollution; they are also common sites for hazardous waste production and disposal. Residents of substandard housing are more likely to come into contact with lead, asbestos, carbon monoxide, pesticides, and other hazardous pollutants associated with peeling paint, old plumbing, poorly maintained insulation and heating equipment, and attempts to control high levels of pests such as cockroaches and rodents.

Poor people are more likely to have jobs that expose them to asbestos, silica dust, and pesticides, and they are more likely to catch and consume fish contaminated with PCBs, mercury, and other toxins.

The most thoroughly researched and documented link among poverty, the environment, and health is lead poisoning in children. Many studies have shown that children of low-income black families are much more likely to have elevated levels of lead in their blood than white children. One survey found that two-thirds of urban African American children from families earning less than $6000 a year had elevated lead levels. The CDC and the American Academy of Pediatrics recommend annual testing of blood lead levels for all children under age 6, with more frequent testing for children at special risk.

Asthma is another health threat that appears to be linked with both environmental and socioeconomic factors. The number of Americans with asthma has grown dramatically in the past 20 years; most of the increase has occurred in children, with African Americans and the poor hardest hit. Researchers are not sure what accounts for this increase, but suspects include household pollutants, pesticides, air pollution, cigarette smoke, and allergens like cockroaches. These risk factors are likely to cluster in poor urban areas where inadequate health care may worsen asthma's effects.

---

many as 57 million American homes still contain lead paint. In 2006, the EPA proposed new guidelines requiring contractors to take special lead-containment measures when doing renovations, repairs, or painting in certain buildings. The use of lead in plumbing is now also banned, but some old pipes and faucets contain lead.

Pesticides

Pesticides are used to prevent the spread of insectborne diseases and to maximize food production by killing insects that eat crops. Both uses have risks as well as benefits. Most pesticide hazards to date have been a result of overuse, but there are concerns about the health effects of long-term exposure to small amounts of pesticide residues in foods, especially for children.

Mercury

A naturally occurring metal, mercury is a toxin that affects the nervous system and may damage the brain, kidneys, and gastrointestinal tract; increase blood pressure, heart rate, and heart attack risk; and cause cancer. Mercury slows fetal and child development and causes irreversible deficits in brain function. Coal-fired power plants are the largest producers of mercury; other sources include mining and smelting operations and the disposal of consumer products containing mercury. Mercury persists in the environment and, like pesticides, it is bioaccumulative. In particular, large, long-lived fish may carry high levels of mercury. See the box "Gender and Environmental Health" for more on issues affecting pregnant women.

Other Chemical Pollutants

Hazardous wastes are also found in the home and should be handled and disposed of properly. They include automotive supplies (motor oil, antifreeze, transmission fluid), paint supplies (turpentine, paint thinner, mineral spirits), art and hobby supplies (oil-based paint, solvents, acids and alkalis, aerosol sprays), insecticides, batteries, computer and electronic components, and household cleaners containing sodium hydroxide (lye) or ammonia. These chemicals are dangerous when

TERMS

pesticides Chemicals used to prevent the spread of diseases transmitted by insects and to maximize food production by killing insects that eat crops.

radiation Energy transmitted in the form of rays, waves, or particles.

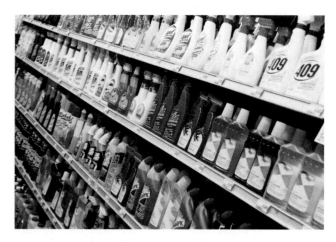

Hazardous chemicals accumulate in many homes, as well as in businesses and industrial sites.

Gender and Environmental Health

Although many environmental health risks are shared by all, some risks disproportionately affect women or men. Women and men often have different roles and responsibilities with respect to family, community, and the workforce.

In many societies, women are more often involved in day-to-day activities associated with the environment, including food preparation, agricultural work, and tasks around the home. These activities can expose women to greater levels of indoor air pollution, water pollution, foodborne pathogens, agricultural chemicals, and waste contamination. Indoor pollutants, especially soot from burning wood, charcoal, and other solid fuels used for home heating and cooking, are a particular risk for women. Exposure to this particulate pollution increases the risk of respiratory diseases, lung cancer, and reproductive problems.

All humans are exposed to chemicals in air, food, and drinking water, and we all carry a body load of chemicals. Some of these chemicals bioaccumulate in our bones, blood, or fatty tissues. Women are smaller than men, on average, and

have a higher percentage of body fat; so chemicals that accumulate in fatty tissue may pose a relatively greater risk for women. On the other hand, men may be more likely to work in industries that involve significant occupational exposures to disease-related toxins; for example, coal miners have an increased risk of lung cancer (black lung disease).

Although any chemical exposure can be a concern for health, women face the added risk of passing pollutants to a developing fetus during pregnancy or to an infant through breastfeeding. Even relatively low exposure to pollutants can result in a significant chemical body load in an infant or young child because of their small body size. And because infants and children are still developing, the effects of chemical exposure can be significant and devastating. It is not unusual for dangerous environmental toxin exposures to be first recognized through noticeable effects on infants or children.

Even in industrialized countries with strong environmental laws, infants and children are affected by such chemicals as lead and mercury. In 2005, scientists

announced that they had found elevated levels of the rocket fuel chemical perchlorate in human breast milk in amounts above the safe dose set by the National Academy of Sciences. Many other chemicals, including PCBs and pesticides, have already been found in breast milk.

Studies are ongoing to identify and reduce environmental hazards in the United States and throughout the world. However, many of the people most directly affected by environmental health problems—women, children, and people living in poor communities—have limited economic, social, and political power. It is important that everyone affected by environmental problems be given a voice in determining environmental policies.

SOURCES: Kirk, A. B., et al. 2005. Perchlorate and iodide in dairy and breast milk. *Environmental Science and Technology,* Web release, February 22; McCally, M., ed. 2002. *Life Support: The Environment and Human Health.* Cambridge, Mass.: MIT Press; Population Reference Bureau. 2002. *Women, Men, and Environmental Change: The Gender Dimensions of Environmental Policies and Programs.* Washington, D.C.: Population Reference Bureau.

inhaled or ingested, when they contact the skin or the eyes, or when they are burned or dumped. Many cities provide guidelines about approved disposal methods and have hazardous waste collection days. Look online or in the government pages of your phone book under Hazardous Waste or Waste Disposal.

Preventing Chemical Pollution

You can take steps to reduce the chemical pollution in your community.

- When buying products, read the labels, and try to buy the least toxic ones available. Choose nontoxic nonpetrochemical cleansers, disinfectants, polishes, and other personal and household products.

- Dispose of your household hazardous wastes properly. If you are not sure whether something is hazardous or don't know how to dispose of it, contact your local environmental health office or health department. Don't burn trash.

- Buy organic produce or produce that has been grown locally. Wash, scrub, and, if appropriate, peel fruits and vegetables. Consider eating less meat; animal products require more pesticides, fertilizer, water, and energy to produce.

- If you must use pesticides or toxic household products, store them in a locked place. Don't measure chemicals with food-preparation utensils, and wear gloves whenever handling them.

- If you have your house fumigated for pest control, be sure to hire a licensed exterminator. Keep everyone, including pets, out of the house while the crew works and, if possible, for a few days after.

RADIATION

Radiation can come in different forms and from different sources, such as the sun, uranium, and nuclear weapons. Of most concern to health are gamma rays produced by

QUESTIONS FOR CRITICAL THINKING AND REFLECTION
Are there any hazardous chemicals in your home, such as cleaning products, solvents, paint, or batteries? Would you know what to do if one of these chemicals spilled? How would you clean it up?

radioactive sources such as nuclear weapons, nuclear energy plants, and radon gas; these high-energy waves are powerful enough to penetrate objects and break molecular bonds. Although gamma radiation cannot be seen or felt, its effects at high doses can include **radiation sickness** and death; at lower doses, chromosome damage, sterility, tissue damage, cataracts, and cancer can occur. Other types of radiation can also affect health; for example, exposure to UV radiation from the sun or from tanning salons can increase the risk of skin cancer. The effects of some sources of radiation, such as cell phones, remain controversial.

Nuclear weapons pose a health risk of the most serious kind to all species. Reducing the stockpiles of nuclear weapons is a challenge and a goal for the twenty-first century. Power-generating plants that use nuclear fuel also pose health problems. When **nuclear power** was first developed as an alternative to oil and coal, it was promoted as clean, efficient, inexpensive, and safe. In general, this has proven to be the case. However, despite all the built-in safeguards and regulating agencies, accidents in nuclear power plants do happen, and the consequences of such accidents are far more serious than those of similar accidents in other types of power-generating plants. An additional, enormous problem is disposing of the radioactive wastes these plants generate. To date, no storage method has been devised that can provide infallible, infinitely durable shielding for nuclear waste.

Medical Uses of Radiation

Another area of concern is the use of radiation in medicine, primarily the X ray. Studies have revealed that X ray exposure is cumulative and that no exposure is absolutely

TERMS

radiation sickness An illness caused by excess radiation exposure, marked by low white blood cell counts and nausea; possibly fatal.

nuclear power The use of controlled nuclear reactions to produce steam, which in turn drives turbines to produce electricity.

radon A naturally occurring radioactive gas emitted from rocks and natural building materials that can become concentrated in insulated homes, causing lung cancer.

decibel A unit for expressing the relative intensity of sounds on a scale from 0 for the average least perceptible sound to about 120 for the average pain threshold.

safe. From a personal health point of view, no one should ever have a "routine" X ray examination; each such exam should have a definite purpose, and its benefits and risks should be carefully weighed.

Radiation in the Home and Workplace

Another area of concern is **radon**, a naturally occurring radioactive gas found in certain soils, rocks, and building materials. When the breakdown products of radon are inhaled, they cling to lungs and bombard sensitive tissue with radioactivity. Radon can enter a home by rising through the soil into the basement through dirt floors, cracks, and other openings. In 2005, the Surgeon General issued a national health advisory on radon, recommending that Americans test their homes for radon every 2 years, and retest any time they move, make structural changes to a home, or occupy a previously unused level of a residence. Problem levels can be dealt with through such measures as sealing cracks or installing basement ventilation systems. More information is available at the EPA Web site or by calling 1-800-SOS-RADON.

Avoiding Radiation

- Get X rays only when absolutely necessary, and keep a record of the date and location of every X ray you get.
- Follow the Surgeon General's recommendations for radon testing.
- Find out if there are radioactive sites in your area. If you live or work near such a site, form or join a community action group to get the site cleaned up.

NOISE POLLUTION

Loud noise in the environment can cause both hearing loss and stress. Prolonged exposure to sounds above 80–85 **decibels** (a measure of the intensity of a sound wave) can cause permanent hearing loss. Hearing damage can occur after 8 hours of exposure to sounds louder than 80 decibels. Regular exposure for longer than 1 minute to more than 100 decibels can cause permanent hearing loss. Children may suffer damage to their hearing at lower noise levels than adults.

Two common sources of excessive noise are the workplace and large gatherings of people at sporting events and rock concerts. The Occupational Safety and Health

Administration (OSHA) sets legal standards for noise in the workplace, but no laws exist regulating noise levels at rock concerts, which can be much louder than most workplaces. Here are some ways to avoid exposing yourself to excessive noise:

- Wear ear protectors when working around noisy machinery.

- When listening to music on a headset with a volume range of 1–10, keep the volume no louder than 6; your headset is too loud if you are unable to hear people around you speaking in a normal tone of voice. Earbuds should not be used more than 30 minutes a day unless the volume is set below 60% of maximum; headphones can be used up to 1 hour.

- Avoid loud music. Don't sit or stand near speakers or amplifiers at a rock concert, and don't play a car radio or stereo so high that you can't hear the traffic.

YOU AND THE ENVIRONMENT

Faced with a vast array of confusing and complex environmental issues, you may feel overwhelmed and conclude that there isn't anything you can do about global problems. But this is not true. If everyone made individual changes in his or her life, the impact would be tremendous. At the same time, it is important to recognize that large corporations and manufacturers are the ones primarily responsible for environmental degradation. Many of them have jumped on the environmental bandwagon with public relations and advertising campaigns designed to make them look good but haven't changed their practices. To influence them, people have to become educated, demand changes in production methods, and elect people to office who consider environmental concerns along with sound business practices (see the box "Making Your Letters Count" on page 360).

What you do every day *does* count. Following the suggestions throughout this chapter will help you make a difference in the environment. In addition, you can become a part of larger community actions by sharing what you learn about environmental issues with your friends and family, joining, supporting, or volunteering your time to organizations working on environmental causes that are important to you.

QUESTIONS FOR CRITICAL THINKING AND REFLECTION

How often do you listen to loud music? Do you ever use headphones? At what volume level do like to listen? Do you think your listening habits pose a threat to your hearing? Would you let a child listen at the same volume level?

TIPS FOR TODAY AND THE FUTURE

Environmental health involves protecting ourselves from environmental dangers and protecting the environment from the dangers created by humans.

RIGHT NOW YOU CAN

- Turn off the lights, televisions, and stereos in any unoccupied rooms.
- Turn down the heat a few degrees and put on a sweater, or turn off the air conditioner and change into cooler clothes.
- Check your trash for recyclable items and take them out for recycling. If your town does not provide curbside pickup for recyclable items, find out where the nearest community recycling center is.

IN THE FUTURE YOU CAN

- As your existing light bulbs burn out, replace them with compact fluorescent light bulbs.
- Have your car checked to make sure it runs as well as it can and puts out the lowest amount of polluting emissions possible.
- Go online and find one of the many calculators available that can help you estimate your environmental footprint. After calculating your footprint, figure out ways to reduce it.

SUMMARY

- Environmental health encompasses all the interactions of humans with their environment and the health consequences of those interactions.

- Factors that may eventually limit human population are food, availability of land and water, energy, and minimum acceptable standard of living.

- Increased amounts of air pollutants are especially dangerous for children, older adults, and people with chronic health problems.

- Heavy motor vehicle traffic, hot weather, and stagnant air contribute to the development of smog.

- Carbon dioxide and other natural gases act as a greenhouse around the earth, increasing the temperature of the atmosphere. Levels of these gases are rising through human activity; as a result, the world's climate could change.

- Environmental damage from energy use can be limited through energy conservation and the development of nonpolluting, renewable sources of energy.

- Indoor pollutants can trigger allergies and illness in the short term and cancer in the long term.

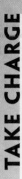

Making Your Letters Count

It takes only a few minutes to write to an elected official, but it can make a difference on an environmental issue you care about. When elected officials receive enough letters or e-mails on an issue, it does influence their vote—they want to be reelected, and your vote counts! To give your letter the greatest possible influence, use these guidelines:

•   Use your own words and your own stationery.

•   Be clear and concise. Keep your letter to one or two paragraphs, never more than one page.

•   Focus on only one subject in each letter, and identify it clearly. Refer to legislation by its name or number.

•   Request a specific action—vote a particular way on a piece of legislation, request hearings, cosponsor a bill—and state your reasons for your position.

•   If you live or work in the legislator's district, say so.

•   Courteous letters work best. Don't be insulting or unnecessarily critical.

You can send letters via regular mail; however, increased security screenings often delay delivery. You can e-mail the president or vice president at the following addresses:

president@whitehouse.gov

vice-president@whitehouse.gov

To locate the contact information for your United States senators and representatives, visit the following Web sites:

Senate: www.senate.gov

House of Representatives: www.house.gov/writerep

•   Concerns with water quality focus on pathogenic organisms and hazardous chemicals from industry and households, as well as on water shortages.

•   Sewage treatment prevents pathogens from contaminating drinking water; it often must also deal with heavy metals and hazardous chemicals.

•   The amount of garbage is growing all the time; paper is the biggest component. Recycling can help reduce solid waste disposal problems.

•   Potentially hazardous chemical pollutants include asbestos, lead, pesticides, mercury, and many household products. Proper handling and disposal are critical.

•   Radiation can cause radiation sickness, chromosome damage, and cancer, among other health problems.

•   Loud or persistent noise can lead to hearing loss and/or stress.

FOR MORE INFORMATION

BOOKS

Ausenda, F. 2009. *Green Volunteers: The World Guide to Voluntary Work in Nature Conservation,* 7th ed. New York: Universe. *Describes a variety of opportunities to volunteer for environmental causes, in many different parts of the world.*

Brown, M. J. 2007. *Building Powerful Community Organizations: A Personal Guide to Creating Groups That Can Solve Problems and Change the World.* Chicago: Long Haul Press. *Provides advice for facing environmental (and other) challenges through local organizing and recruiting.*

Cunningham, W. P., et al. 2007. *Environmental Science: A Global Concern,* 10th ed. New York: McGraw-Hill. *A nontechnical survey of basic environmental science and key concerns.*

Nadakavukaren, A. 2005. *Our Global Environment: A Health Perspective,* 6th ed. Prospect Heights, Ill.: Waveland Press. *A broad survey of major environmental issues and their effects on personal and community health.*

ORGANIZATIONS, HOTLINES, AND WEB SITES

CDC National Center for Environmental Health. Provides brochures and fact sheets on a variety of environmental issues.
    http://www.cdc.gov/nceh/default.htm

Ecological Footprint. Calculates your personal ecological footprint based on your diet, transportation patterns, and living arrangements.
    http://www.myfootprint.org

Energy Efficiency and Renewable Energy (EERE). U.S. Department of Energy. Provides information about alternative fuels and tips for saving energy at home and in your car.
    http://www.eere.doe.gov

Fuel Economy. Provides information on the fuel economy of cars made since 1985 and tips on improving gas mileage.
    http://www.fueleconomy.gov

Indoor Air Quality Information Hotline. Answers questions, provides publications, and makes referrals.
    800-438-4318

National Oceanic and Atmospheric Administration (NOAA): Climate. Provides information on a variety of issues related to climate, including global warming, drought, and El Niño and La Niña.
    http://www.noaa.gov/climate.html

National Safety Council Environmental Health Center. Provides information on lead, radon, indoor air quality, hazardous chemicals, and other environmental issues.
    http://www.nsc.org/ehc.aspx

Student Environmental Action Coalition (SEAC). A coalition of student and youth environmental groups; the Web site has contact information for local groups.
    http://www.seac.org

United Nations. Several U.N. programs are devoted to environmental problems on a global scale; the Web sites provide information on current and projected trends and on international treaties developed to deal with environmental issues.

http://www.un.org/popin (Population Division)

http://www.unep.org (Environment Programme)

U.S. Environmental Protection Agency (EPA). Provides information about EPA activities and many consumer-oriented materials. The Web site includes special sites devoted to global warming, ozone loss, pesticides, and other areas of concern.

http://www.epa.gov

Worldwatch Institute. A public policy research organization focusing on emerging global environmental problems and the links between the world economy and the environment.

http://www.worldwatch.org

There are many national and international organizations working on environmental health problems. A few of the largest and best known are listed below:

Greenpeace: 800-326-0959; http://www.greenpeace.org

National Audubon Society: 212-979-3000; http://www .audubon.org

National Wildlife Federation: 800-822-9919; http://www.nwf.org

Nature Conservancy: 800-628-6860; http://www.nature.org

Sierra Club: 415-977-5500; http://www.sierraclub.org

World Wildlife Fund—U.S.: 800-960-0993; http://www .worldwildlife.org

SELECTED BIBLIOGRAPHY

CDC National Center for Environmental Health. 2007. *Children's Blood Lead Levels in the United States* (http://www.cdc.gov/nceh/lead/research/kidsBLL.htm; retrieved February 19, 2009).

Delworth-Bart, J. E., and C. F. Moore. 2006. Mercy mercy me: Social injustice and the prevention of environmental pollutant exposures among ethnic minority and poor children. *Child Development* 77(2): 247–265.

Dominici, F., et al. 2006. Fine particulate air pollution and hospital admission for cardiovascular and respiratory diseases. *Journal of the American Medical Association* 295(10): 1127–1134.

Energy Information Agency. 2009. *Gasoline and Diesel Fuel Update* (http://tonto.eia.doe.gov/oog/info/gdu/gasdiesel.asp; retrieved February 19, 2009).

Environmental Protection Agency. 2008. *Municipal Solid Waste: Basic Facts* (http://www.epa.gov.epaoswer/non-hw/muncpl/facts.htm; retrieved February 19, 2009).

NASA Goddard Institute for Space Studies. 2008. *Global Temperature Trends: 2007 Summation* (http://www.giss.nasa.gov/gistemp/2008; retrieved February 19, 2009).

The National Academies. 2006. *Surface Temperature Reconstructions for the Last 2,000 Years.* Washington, D.C.: National Academies Press.

National Oceanic and Atmospheric Administration. 2008. *Billion Dollar U.S. Weather Disasters, 1980–2007* (http://www.ncdc.noaa.gov/oa/reports/billionz.html; retrieved February 19, 2009).

United Nations Population Division. 2007. *World Population Prospects: The 2006 Revision.* New York: United Nations.

U.S. Department of Health and Human Services. 2005. *Surgeon General Releases National Health Advisory on Radon* (http://www.surgeongeneral.gov/pressreleases/sg01132005.html; retrieved February 19, 2009).

U.S. Environmental Protection Agency. 2007. *Superfund National Accomplishments Summary Fiscal Year 2007* (http://www.epa.gov/superfund/accomp/numbers07.htm; retrieved February 19, 2009).

World Health Organization. 2005. *International Decade for Action: Water for Life 2005–2015* (http://www.who.int/water_sanitation_health/2005advocguide/en/index1.html; retrieved February 19, 2009).

World Health Organization. 2006. *Fuel for Life: Household Energy and Health.* Geneva: WHO Press.

Worldwatch Institute. 2007. *Vital Signs 2007–2008.* New York: Norton.

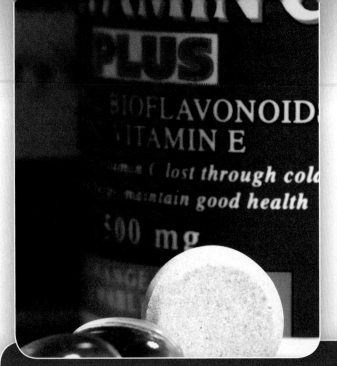

CONVENTIONAL AND COMPLEMENTARY MEDICINE

15

Today, people are becoming more empowered and confident in their ability to solve personal health problems on their own. People who manage their own health care gather information and learn skills from a variety of resources; they solicit opinions and advice, make decisions, and take action. They know how to practice safe, effective self-care, and they know how to make decisions about professional medical care, whether conventional Western medicine or complementary and alternative medicine.

This chapter will help you develop the skills both to identify and manage medical problems and to make the health care system work effectively for you.

SELF-CARE

Effectively managing medical problems involves developing several skills. First, you need to learn to be a good observer of your own body and assess your symptoms. You also must be able to decide when to seek professional advice and when you can safely deal with the problem on your own. You need to know how to safely and effectively self-treat common medical problems. Finally, you need to know how to develop a partnership with physicians and other health care providers and how to carry out treatment plans.

Self-Assessment

Symptoms are often an expression of the body's attempt to heal itself. A fever may be an attempt to make the body less hospitable to infectious agents. A cough can help clear the airways and protect the lungs. Carefully observing symptoms also lets you identify those signals that suggest you need professional assistance. Begin by noting when the symptom began, how often and when it occurs, what makes it worse, what makes it better, and whether you have any associated symptoms. You can also monitor your body's vital signs, such as temperature and heart rate. Medical self-tests for blood pressure, blood sugar,

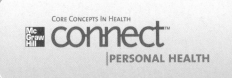

pregnancy detection, and urinary tract infections can also help you make a more informed decision about when to seek medical help and when to self-treat.

Knowing When to See a Physician

In general, you should see a physician for symptoms that you would describe as follows:

1. *Severe.* If the symptom is very severe or intense, medical assistance is advised. Examples include severe pains, major injuries, and other emergencies.

2. *Unusual.* If the symptom is peculiar and unfamiliar, it is wise to check it out with your physician. Examples include unexplained lumps, changes in a mole, problems with vision, difficulty swallowing, numbness, weakness, unexplained weight loss, and blood in sputum, urine, or stool.

3. *Persistent.* If the symptom lasts longer than expected, seek medical advice. Examples in adults include fever for more than 5 days, a cough lasting longer than 2 weeks, a sore that doesn't heal within a month, and hoarseness lasting longer than 3 weeks.

4. *Recurrent.* If a symptom tends to return again and again, medical evaluation is advised. Examples include recurrent headaches, stomach pains, and backache.

Sometimes a single symptom is not a cause for concern, but when the symptom is accompanied by other symptoms, the combination suggests a more serious problem. For example, a fever with a stiff neck suggests meningitis.

If you think that you need professional help, you must decide how urgent the problem is. If it is a true emergency, go (or call someone to take you) to the nearest emergency room (ER). Emergencies include the following:

- Major trauma or injury, such as head injury, suspected broken bone, deep wound, severe burn, eye injury, or animal bite
- Uncontrollable bleeding or internal bleeding, as indicated by blood in the sputum, vomit, or stool
- Intolerable and uncontrollable pain or severe chest pain
- Severe shortness of breath
- Persistent abdominal pain, especially if associated with nausea and vomiting
- Poisoning or drug overdose

- Loss of consciousness or seizure
- Stupor, drowsiness, or disorientation that cannot be explained
- Severe or worsening reaction to an insect bite or sting or to a medication, especially if breathing is difficult

If your problem is not an emergency but still requires medical attention, call your physician's office. Often you can be given medical advice over the phone without the inconvenience of a visit.

Self-Treatment

In most cases, your body itself can relieve your symptoms and heal the disorder. Patience and careful self-observation are often the best choices in self-treatment. Nondrug options can be easy, inexpensive, safe, and highly effective. For example, massage, ice packs, and neck exercises may at times be more helpful than drugs in relieving headaches and other pains. Getting adequate rest, increasing exercise, drinking more water, eating more or less of certain foods, using humidifiers, changes in ergonomics when working at a desk, and so on are just some of the hundreds of nondrug options for preventing or relieving many common health problems. For a variety of disorders caused or aggravated by stress, the treatment of choice may be relaxation or other stress-management strategies (see the box "Expressive Writing and Chronic Conditions" on page 364).

Self-Medication Self-treatment with nonprescription medications is an important part of health care. Nonprescription or **over-the-counter (OTC) medications** are medicines that the Food and Drug Administration (FDA) has determined are safe for use without a physician's prescription. There are more than 100,000 OTC drugs on the market; about 60% of all medications are sold over the counter. More than 600 products sold over the counter today use ingredients or dosage strengths available only by prescription 20 years ago. With this increased consumer choice, however, comes increased consumer responsibility for using OTC drugs safely.

Although many OTC products are effective, others are unnecessary or divert attention

over-the-counter (OTC) medication A medication or product that can be purchased by the consumer without a prescription.

TERMS

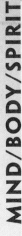

Expressive Writing and Chronic Conditions

The act of writing down feelings and thoughts about stressful life events has been shown to help people improve their health. Investigators remain unsure why writing about one's feelings has beneficial effects. It may be that expressing feelings about a traumatic event helps people work through the event and put it behind them. The resulting sense of release and control may reduce stress levels and have positive physical effects such as reduced heart rate and blood pressure and improved immune function. Alternatively, expressive writing may change the way people think about previous stressful events in their lives and

help them cope with new stressors. Whatever the cause, it's clear that expressive writing can be a safe, inexpensive, and effective supplement to standard treatment of certain chronic illnesses.

What about the effects of expressive writing on otherwise healthy individuals? Other studies have found a similar benefit: People who wrote about traumatic experiences reported fewer symptoms, fewer days off work, fewer visits to the doctor, improved mood, and a more positive outlook.

If you'd like to try expressive writing to help you deal with a traumatic event, set aside a special time—15 minutes a

day for 4 consecutive days, for example, or 1 day a week for 4 weeks. Write in a place where you won't be interrupted or distracted. Explore your very deepest thoughts and feelings and why you feel the way you do. Don't worry about grammar or coherence or about what someone else might think about what you're writing; you are writing just for yourself. You may find the writing exercise to be distressing in the short term—sadness and depression are common when dealing with feelings about a stressful event—but most people report relief and contentment soon after writing for several days.

---

from better ways of coping. Many ingredients in OTC drugs—perhaps 70%—have not been proven to be effective. And any drug may have risks and side effects. Follow these simple guidelines to self-medicate safely:

1. Always read labels and follow directions carefully. The information on most OTC drug labels now appears in a standard format developed by the FDA (Figure 14.1).

2. Do not exceed the recommended dosage or length of treatment unless you discuss this change with your physician.

3. Use caution if you are taking other medications or supplements, because OTC drugs and herbal supplements can interact with some prescription drugs. If you have questions about drug interactions, ask your pharmacist or another qualified health care provider *before* you mix medicines.

4. Try to select medications with one active ingredient rather than combination products. A product with multiple ingredients is likely to include drugs for symptoms you don't even have.

5. When choosing medications, try to buy **generic drugs**, which contain the same active ingredient as

the brand-name product but generally at a much lower cost.

6. Never take or give a drug from an unlabeled container or in the dark when you can't read the label.

7. If you are pregnant or nursing or have a chronic condition such as kidney or liver disease, consult your health care provider before self-medicating.

8. The expiration date marked on many medications is an estimate of how long the medication is likely to be safe and effective. However, an extensive study by the FDA found that 90% of all prescription and OTC medications are potent for several years after their stated expiration date. Exceptions include the antibiotic tetracycline, liquid antibiotics, nitroglycerine, and insulin. Expiration dates are very conservative. If you have any question about a medicine's expiration date, ask a pharmacist.

9. Store your medications in a cool, dry place that is out of the reach of children.

10. Use special caution with aspirin. Because of an association with a rare but serious problem known as Reye's syndrome, aspirin should not be used by children or adolescents who may have the flu, chicken pox, or any other viral illness. Outdated aspirin that has an acidic odor should be discarded.

QUESTIONS FOR CRITICAL THINKING AND REFLECTION

Do you often self-medicate for common medical problems, such as headaches or colds? If so, how careful are you about reading product labels and following directions? For example, would you know if you were taking two OTC medications that contained the same ingredient (such as ibuprofen) at the same time?

PROFESSIONAL CARE

When self-treatment is not appropriate or sufficient, you need to seek professional medical care. The health care system is a broad network of professionals and organizations, including independent practitioners, health care providers, hospitals, clinics, and public and private insurance programs.

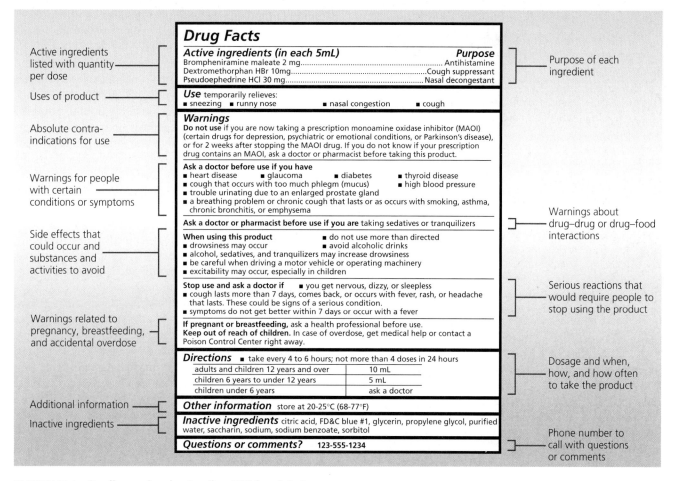

Active ingredients listed with quantity per dose

Uses of product

Absolute contra-indications for use

Warnings for people with certain conditions or symptoms

Side effects that could occur and substances and activities to avoid

Warnings related to pregnancy, breastfeeding, and accidental overdose

Additional information

Inactive ingredients

Drug Facts

Active ingredients (in each 5mL)   *Purpose*
Brompheniramine maleate 2 mg.. Antihistamine
Dextromethorphan HBr 10mg...Cough suppressant
Pseudoephedrine HCl 30 mg.. Nasal decongestant

Use temporarily relieves:
■ sneezing ■ runny nose   ■ nasal congestion   ■ cough

Warnings
Do not use if you are now taking a prescription monoamine oxidase inhibitor (MAOI) (certain drugs for depression, psychiatric or emotional conditions, or Parkinson's disease), or for 2 weeks after stopping the MAOI drug. If you do not know if your prescription drug contains an MAOI, ask a doctor or pharmacist before taking this product.

Ask a doctor before use if you have
■ heart disease   ■ glaucoma   ■ diabetes   ■ thyroid disease
■ cough that occurs with too much phlegm (mucus)   ■ high blood pressure
■ trouble urinating due to an enlarged prostate gland
■ a breathing problem or chronic cough that lasts or as occurs with smoking, asthma, chronic bronchitis, or emphysema

Ask a doctor or pharmacist before use if you are taking sedatives or tranquilizers

When using this product   ■ do not use more than directed
■ drowsiness may occur   ■ avoid alcoholic drinks
■ alcohol, sedatives, and tranquilizers may increase drowsiness
■ be careful when driving a motor vehicle or operating machinery
■ excitability may occur, especially in children

Stop use and ask a doctor if   ■ you get nervous, dizzy, or sleepless
■ cough lasts more than 7 days, comes back, or occurs with fever, rash, or headache that lasts. These could be signs of a serious condition.
■ symptoms do not get better within 7 days or occur with a fever

If pregnant or breastfeeding, ask a health professional before use.
Keep out of reach of children. In case of overdose, get medical help or contact a Poison Control Center right away.

Directions   ■ take every 4 to 6 hours; not more than 4 doses in 24 hours

adults and children 12 years and over	10 mL
children 6 years to under 12 years	5 mL
children under 6 years	ask a doctor

Other information   store at 20-25°C (68-77°F)

Inactive ingredients citric acid, FD&C blue #1, glycerin, propylene glycol, purified water, saccharin, sodium, sodium benzoate, sorbitol

Questions or comments?   123-555-1234

Purpose of each ingredient

Warnings about drug–drug or drug–food interactions

Serious reactions that would require people to stop using the product

Dosage and when, how, and how often to take the product

Phone number to call with questions or comments

FIGURE 15.1   **Reading and understanding OTC drug labels.**

SOURCE: Food and Drug Administration. 1999. Over-the-counter human drugs; labeling requirements; final rule. *Federal Register* 64(51), 17 March, 13254-13303.

In recent years, many Americans have also sought health care from practitioners of **complementary and alternative medicine (CAM)**, defined as those therapies and practices that do not form part of conventional, or mainstream, health care and medical practices as taught in most U.S. medical schools and offered in most U.S. hospitals. The most commonly used CAM therapies are relaxation techniques, herbal medicine, massage, and chiropractic (Table 15.1). People often use CAM therapies in addition to their conventional medical treatments, but many do not tell their physicians about it.

Consumers turn to CAM for a large variety of purposes related to health and well-being, such as boosting their immune system, lowering their cholesterol levels, losing weight, quitting smoking, or enhancing their memory. There are indications that people with chronic conditions, including cancer, asthma, autoimmune diseases, and HIV infection, are particularly likely to try CAM therapies. Despite their growing popularity, many CAM practices remain controversial, and individuals need to be critically aware of safety issues.

In the next sections of this chapter, we examine the principles and providers of both **conventional medicine**—the dominant medical system in the United States and Europe, also referred to as standard Western medicine or biomedicine—and complementary and alternative medicine, with particular attention to consumer issues.

generic drug   A drug that is not registered or protected by a trademark; a drug that does not have a brand name.

complementary and alternative medicine (CAM) Therapies or practices that are not part of conventional or mainstream health care and medical practice as taught in most U.S. medical schools and available at most U.S. health care facilities; examples of CAM practices include acupuncture and herbal remedies.

conventional medicine   A system of medicine based on the application of the scientific method; diseases are thought to be caused by identifiable physical factors and characterized by a representative set of symptoms; also called biomedicine or standard Western medicine.

Table 15.1	Use of Complementary and Alternative Therapies in the United States	
		Percent Who Ever Used Therapy
Prayer		55.3
Natural products (nonvitamin, nonmineral)		25.0
Chiropractic care		19.9
Deep breathing exercises		14.6
Meditation		10.2
Massage		9.3
Yoga		7.5
Diet-based therapies		6.8
Progressive relaxation		4.2
Acupuncture		4.0
Megavitamin therapy		3.9
Homeopathic treatment		3.6
Guided imagery		3.0
T'ai chi		2.5
Hypnosis		1.8
Energy healing therapy/Reiki		1.1
Biofeedback		1.0
Any therapy		**74.6**

SOURCE: Barnes, P. M., et al. 2004. Complementary and alternative medicine use among adults: United States, 2002. *Advance Data from Vital and Health Statistics* No. 343. Hyattsville, Md.: National Center for Health Statistics.

CONVENTIONAL MEDICINE

Referring to conventional medicine as standard Western medicine draws attention to the fact that it differs from the various medical systems that have developed in China, Japan, India, and other parts of the world. Calling it "biomedicine" reflects conventional medicine's foundation in the biological and physical sciences.

Premises and Assumptions of Conventional Medicine

One of the important characteristics of Western medicine is the belief that disease is caused by identifiable physical factors. Western medicine identifies the causes of disease as pathogens (such as bacteria and viruses), genetic factors, and unhealthy lifestyles that result in changes at the

QUESTIONS FOR CRITICAL THINKING AND REFLECTION

What are your views about the use of CAM treatments and therapies? What events or information have shaped those views? At this point in your life, would you consider using complementary or alternative medicine?

molecular and cellular levels. In most cases, the focus is primarily on the physical causes of illness rather than mental or spiritual imbalance.

Another feature that distinguishes Western biomedicine from other medical systems is the concept that every disease is defined by a certain set of symptoms and that these symptoms are similar in most patients suffering from this disease. Western medicine tends to treat illnesses as isolated biological disturbances that can occur in human beings, rather than as integral in some way to the individual with the illness.

Related to the idea of illness as the result of invasion by outside factors is the strong orientation toward methods of destroying pathogens or preventing them from causing serious infection. The public health measures of the nineteenth and twentieth centuries—chlorination of drinking water, sewage disposal, food safety regulations, vaccination programs, education about hygiene, and so on—are an outgrowth of this orientation.

The implementation of public health measures is one way to control pathogens; another is the use of drugs and surgery. The discovery and development of sulfa drugs, antibiotics, and steroids in the twentieth century, along with advances in chemistry that made it possible to identify the active ingredients in common plant-derived remedies, paved the way for the current close identification of Western medicine with **pharmaceuticals** (medical drugs, both prescription and over-the-counter). Western medicine also relies heavily on surgery and on advanced medical technology to discover the physical causes of disease and to correct, remove, or destroy them.

Further, Western medicine is based on the scientific method of obtaining knowledge and explaining health-related phenomena. Scientific explanations are:

- *Empirical*—they are based on the evidence of the senses and on objective and systematic observation, often carried out under carefully controlled conditions; they must be capable of verification by others.

- *Rational*—they follow the rules of logic and are consistent with known facts.

- *Testable*—either they are verifiable through direct observation or they lead to predictions about what should occur under conditions not yet observed.

- *Parsimonious*—they explain phenomena with the fewest number of causes.

- *General*—they have broad explanatory power.

- *Rigorously evaluated*—they are constantly evaluated for consistency with the evidence and known principles, for parsimony, and for generality.

- *Tentative*—scientists are willing to entertain the possibility that their explanations are faulty, based on new, better, or connected evidence.

Western medicine translates the scientific method into practice through the research process, a highly refined and well-established approach to exploring the causes of

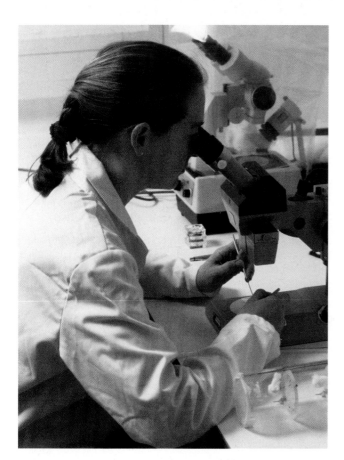

Conventional Western medicine is firmly grounded in scientific explanations resulting from the application of the scientific method to a question or problem.

of professionals are permitted to practice specific fields of medicine independently, including medical doctors, osteopaths, podiatrists, optometrists, and dentists.

• **Medical doctors** are practitioners who hold a doctor of medicine (M.D.) degree from an accredited medical school. In the United States, an education in medicine involves 7 to 11 years of study and residency beyond 4 years of undergraduate premedical education.

• **Doctors of osteopathic medicine** (D.O.) receive a medical education similar to that of medical doctors, but their training places special emphasis on musculoskeletal problems and manipulative therapy. M.D.s and D.O.s are the two types of "complete" physicians in the United States, meaning they are trained and licensed to perform surgery and prescribe medication.

• **Podiatrists** are practitioners who specialize in the medical and surgical care of the feet. They hold a doctor of podiatric medicine (D.P.M.) degree.

• **Optometrists** are practitioners trained to examine the eyes, detect eye diseases, and treat vision problems. They hold a doctor of optometry (O.D.) degree.

• **Dentists** specialize in the care of the teeth and mouth. They are graduates of 4-year dental schools and hold the doctor of dental surgery (D.D.S.) or doctor of medical dentistry (D.M.D.) degree.

In addition to these practitioners, there are millions of other trained health care

disease and ensuring the safety and efficacy of treatments. Research ranges from case studies—descriptions of a single patient's illness and treatment—to randomized controlled trials (RTCs) conducted on large populations. The process of drug development is equally rigorous. Drugs are developed and tested through an elaborate course that begins with preliminary research in the lab and continues through trials with human participants, review and approval by the FDA, and monitoring of the drug's effects even after it is on the market. The process may take 12 years or more, and only about 20% of drugs are eventually approved for marketing.

When results of research studies are published in medical journals, a community of scientists, physicians, researchers, and scholars has the opportunity to share the findings and enter a dialogue about the subject. Publication of research often prompts further research designed to replicate and confirm the findings, challenge the conclusions, or pursue a related line of thought or experiment. (See the box "Evaluating Health News.")

The Providers of Conventional Medicine

Conventional medicine is practiced by a wide range of health care professionals in the United States. Several kinds

TERMS

pharmaceuticals Medical drugs, both prescription and over-the-counter.

medical doctor An independent practitioner who holds a doctor of medicine degree from an accredited medical school.

doctor of osteopathic medicine A medical practitioner who has graduated from an osteopathic medical school; osteopathy incorporates the theories and practices of scientific medicine but focuses on musculoskeletal problems and manipulative therapy.

podiatrist A practitioner who holds a doctor of podiatric medicine degree and specializes in the medical and surgical care of the feet.

optometrist A practitioner who holds a doctor of optometry degree and is trained to examine the eyes, detect eye diseases, and prescribe corrective lenses.

dentist A practitioner who holds a doctor of medical dentistry or doctor of dental surgery degree and who specializes in the prevention and treatment of diseases and injuries of the teeth, mouth, and jaws.

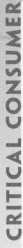

Evaluating Health News

Media reports of health-related research studies may oversimplify or exaggerate both the results and what those results mean to the average person. Researchers do not set out to mislead people, but they must often strike a balance between reporting promising preliminary findings to the public, thereby allowing people to act on them, and waiting 10–20 years until long-term studies confirm (or disprove) a particular finding.

The following questions can help you better assess the health advice that appears in the popular media:

1. *Is the report based on research or on an anecdote?* Information or advice based on one or more carefully designed research studies has more validity than one person's experiences.

2. *What is the source of the information?* A study published in a respected peer-reviewed journal has been examined by editors and other researchers in the field, people who are in a position to evaluate the merits of a study and its results. Many journal articles also include information on the authors and funders of research, alerting readers to any possible conflicts of interest. Research presented at medical meetings should be considered very preliminary because the results have not yet undergone a thorough prepublication review; many such studies are never published. It is also wise to ask who funded a study to determine whether there is any potential for bias. Information from government agencies and national research organizations is usually considered fairly reliable.

3. *How big was the study?* A study involving many subjects is more likely to yield reliable results than a study involving only a few subjects. Another important indication that a finding is meaningful is if several studies yield the same results.

4. *Who were the participants involved in the study?* Research findings are more likely to apply to you if you share important characteristics with the participants in the study. For example, the results of a study on men over age 50 who smoke may not be particularly meaningful for a 30-year-old nonsmoking woman.

5. *What kind of study was it?* Epidemiological studies involve observation or interviews in order to trace the relationships among lifestyle, physical characteristics, and diseases. While epidemiological studies can suggest links, they cannot establish cause-and-effect relationships. Clinical or interventional studies or trials involve testing the effects of different treatments on groups of people who have similar lifestyles and characteristics. They are more likely to provide conclusive evidence of a cause-and-effect relationship. The best interventional studies share the following characteristics:

   - *Controlled.* A group of people who receive the treatment is compared with a matched group of people (called a *control group*) who do not receive the treatment. The matched control group may receive an inert placebo or an established active treatment.

   - *Randomized.* The treatment and control groups are selected randomly.

   - *Double-blind.* Researchers and participants are unaware of who is receiving the treatment.

   - *Multicenter.* The experiment is performed at more than one institution.

   A third type of study, meta-analysis, involves combining the results of individual studies to get an overall view of the effectiveness of a treatment.

6. *What do the statistics really say?* If a study is large and well designed, its results can be deemed statistically significant, meaning there is less than a 5% chance that the findings resulted from chance.

7. *Is new health advice being offered?* If the media report new guidelines for health behavior or medical treatment, examine the source. Government agencies and national research foundations usually consider a great deal of evidence before offering health advice. Above all, use common sense, and check with your physician before making a major change in your health habits based on news reports.

SOURCES: Stevens, L. M. 2006. Medical journals. *Journal of the American Medical Association* 295(15); 1860; Nemours Foundation. 2006. *Figuring Out Health News* (http://www.kidshealth.org/teen/safety/safebasics/healthnews.html; retrieved September 17, 2006); Tufts University. 2006. Studying research studies: 10 questions you need to ask. *Tufts University Health and Nutrition Letter*, June, 4–5; Patient Inform. 2005. *Understanding Medical Research: What to Look for When Reading Medical Research* (http://www.patientinform.org/understanding-medical-research/; retrieved September 17, 2006).

professionals, known as **allied health care providers,** working in the United States. They include registered nurses (R.N.s), licensed vocational nurses (L.V.N.s), physical therapists, social workers, registered dietitians (R.D.s), physician assistants (P.A.s), nurse practitioners, and certified nurse midwives.

Choosing a Primary Care Physician

Most experts believe it is best to have a primary care physician, someone who gets to know you, who coordinates your medical care, and who refers you to specialists when you need them. Primary care physicians include those certified in family practice, internal medicine, pediatrics, and gynecology. These physicians are able to diagnose and treat the vast majority of common health problems; they also provide many preventive health services. The best time to look for a physician is before you are sick.

To select a physician, begin by making a list of possible choices. If your insurance limits the health care providers you can see, check the plan's list first. Ask for recommendations from family, friends, coworkers, local medical societies, and the physician referral service at a local clinic or hospital. Once you have the names of a few physicians you might want to try, call their offices to find out information such as the following:

- Is the physician covered by your health plan and accepting new patients?
- What are the office hours, and when is the physician or office staff available? What do patients do if they need urgent care or have an emergency?
- Which hospitals does the physician use?
- How many other physicians are available to cover when he or she isn't available, and who are they?
- How long does it usually take to get a routine appointment?
- Does the physician (or a nurse or physician assistant) give advice over the phone for common problems?

Schedule a visit with the physician you think you would most like to use. During that first visit, you'll get a sense of how well matched you are and how well he or she might meet your medical needs.

Getting the Most Out of Your Medical Care

The key to making the health care system work for you lies in good communication with your physician and other members of the health care team.

The Physician-Patient Partnership The physician-patient relationship is undergoing an important transformation. The image of the all-knowing physician and the passive patient is fading. What is emerging is a physician-patient *partnership,* in which the physician acts more like a consultant and the patient participates more actively. You should expect your physician to be attentive, caring, and able to listen and clearly explain things to you. You also must do your part. You need to be assertive in a firm but nonaggressive manner. You need to express your feelings and concerns, ask questions and, if necessary, be persistent. If your physician is unable to communicate clearly with you despite your best efforts, you probably need to change physicians.

Your Appointment with Your Physician Prepare for your visit ahead of time by making a list of your key concerns and questions, along with notes about your symptoms. Present your concerns at the beginning of the visit, to set the agenda. Be specific and concise about your symptoms, and be open and honest about your concerns. Let your physician know if you are taking any drugs, are allergic to any medications, are breast-feeding, or may be pregnant. At the end of the visit, briefly repeat the physician's diagnosis, prognosis, and instructions. Make sure you understand your next steps.

The Diagnostic Process The first step in the diagnostic process is the medical history, including the primary rea-

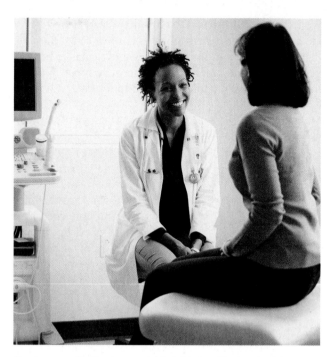

Good communication is a crucial factor in an effective physician-patient partnership.

son for your visit, your current symptoms, your past medical history, and your social history (job, family life, major stressors, living conditions, and health habits). Keeping up-to-date records of your medical history can help you provide your physician with key facts about your health.

The next step is the physical exam, which usually begins with a review of vital signs: blood pressure, heart rate (pulse), breathing rate, and temperature. Depending on your primary complaint, your physician may give you a complete physical, or the exam may be directed to specific areas, such as your ears, nose, and throat.

Additionally, your physician may order medical tests to complete the diagnosis. Physicians can order X rays, biopsies, blood and urine tests, scans, and **endoscopies** to view, probe, or analyze almost any part of the body. If your physician orders a test for you, be sure you know why you need it, what the risks and benefits of the test are for you, how you should prepare for it, and what the test will involve. Also ask what the test results mean, because no test is 100% accurate—**false positives** and **false negatives** do occur—and interpretation of some tests is subjective.

allied health care providers Health care professionals who typically provide services under the supervision or control of independent practitioners.

endoscopy A medical procedure in which a viewing instrument is inserted into a body cavity or opening.

false positive A test result that incorrectly detects a disease or condition in a healthy person.

false negative A test result that fails to correctly detect a disease or condition.

TERMS

Medical and Surgical Treatments Many conditions can be treated in a variety of ways; in some cases, lifestyle changes are enough. In other cases, physicians prescribe a medication. Thousands of lives are saved each year by antibiotics, insulin, and other prescription drugs, but we pay a price for having such powerful tools. A 2006 report from the Institute of Medicine (IOM) estimates that 1.5 million prescription drug-related errors—called *adverse drug events,* or ADEs—occur each year in the United States. ADEs happen for several reasons:

• *Medication errors:* Physicians may overprescribe drugs, prescribe the wrong drug, or prescribe a dangerous combination of drugs; such problems are especially prevalent for older adults, who typically take multiple medications (see the box "Medical Errors, Adverse Events, and Their Prevention"). At the pharmacy, patients may receive the wrong drug or may not be given complete information about drug risks, side effects, and interactions.

• *Off-label drug use:* Once a drug is approved by the FDA for one purpose, it can legally be prescribed (although not marketed) for purposes not listed on the label. Many off-label uses are safe and supported by some research, but both consumers and health care providers need to take special care with off-label use.

• *Online pharmacies:* Some online pharmacies may sell products that are adulterated, expired, ineffective, or counterfeit drugs. The FDA recommends that consumers avoid sites that prescribe drugs without a physical exam, sell prescription drugs without a prescription, or sell medications not approved by the FDA. You should also avoid sites that do not provide access to a registered pharmacist to answer questions or that do not provide a U.S. address and phone number to contact in case of a problem. The National Association of Boards of Pharmacy sponsors a voluntary certification program for Internet pharmacies. To be certified, a pharmacy must have a state license and allow regular inspections.

• *Costs:* Spending on prescription drugs is now the fastest-growing portion of U.S. health care spending. Consumers may be able to lower their drug costs by using generic versions of medications; by joining a drug discount program sponsored by a company, organization, or local pharmacy; and by investigating mail-order or Internet pharmacies.

Patients also share some responsibility for problems with prescription drugs. Many people don't take their medications properly, skip doses, take incorrect doses, stop too soon, or do not take the medication at all. An estimated 30–50% of the more than 3 billion prescriptions dispensed annually in the United States are not taken correctly and thus do not produce the desired results. Consumers can increase the safety and effectiveness of their treatment by carefully reading any prescription's label and fact sheets or brochures and by asking the following questions:

• Are there nondrug alternatives?
• What is the name of the medication, and what is it supposed to do, within what period of time?
• How and when do I take the medication, how much do I take, and for how long? What should I do if I miss a dose?
• What other medications, foods, drinks, or activities should I avoid?
• What are the side effects, and what do I do if they occur?
• Can I take a generic drug rather than a brand-name one?
• Is there written information about the medication?

Surgery is another staple of Western medical treatment. Each year, more than 70 million operations and related procedures are performed in the U.S. If a health care provider suggests surgery for any reason, ask the following questions:

• Why do I need surgery at this time?
• Are any nonsurgical options available, such as medicine or physical therapy?
• What are the risks and complications of the surgery?
• Can the operation be performed on an outpatient basis?
• What can I expect before, during, and after surgery?

COMPLEMENTARY AND ALTERNATIVE MEDICINE

Where conventional Western medicine tends to focus on the body, on the physical causes of disease, and on ways to eradicate pathogens in order to restore health, CAM tends to focus on an integration of mind, body, and spirit in seeking ways to restore the whole person to harmony so that he or she can regain health. Where conventional medicine is based primarily on science, CAM tends to be based on healing traditions and accumulated experience. Caution is in order when choosing any mode of treat-

Medical Errors, Adverse Events, and Their Prevention

The Institute of Medicine (IOM) estimates that 44,000 to 98,000 deaths occur each year in hospitals due to medical errors. Even at the lower estimate, medical errors could rank as one of the ten leading causes of death in the United States.

The IOM defines a *medical error* as "the failure to complete a planned action as intended or the use of a wrong plan to achieve an aim." An *adverse event* is "an injury caused by medical management rather than by the underlying disease or condition of the patient."

Medical errors may involve surgical mismanagement, misdiagnosis leading to incorrect therapy, misinterpretation of or failure to order diagnostic tests, failure to act on abnormal test results, equipment failure, blood transfusion injuries, misinterpretation of physician orders leading to use of the wrong drug or an incorrect dosage, and hospital-acquired infections.

Medication Errors

Errors involving medication are fairly common in the United States. Nationally, about 7000 patients die each year from medication errors.

The FDA defines a *medication error* as "any preventable event that may cause or lead to inappropriate medication use or patient harm while the medication is in the control of the health care professional, patient, or consumer." Such events may include prescribing, order communication, and product labeling, packaging, dispensing, administration, and use.

Hospital Errors

Approximately 10 percent of all hospitalized patients acquire a significant infec-

tion. Most are caused by common bacteria that normally inhabit the skin and mucous membranes. Proper handling of equipment and frequent hand washing by providers are the major ways to avoid such infections.

Prevention Within the System

Fortunately, most errors are preventable. Major system improvements proposed in an IOM report include the application of standardized procedure and equipment guidelines, medical rounds that include a pharmacist on the team, and the use of computer technology and barcodes.

Studies show that most medical errors are system-related and not attributable to negligence or misconduct by individual providers. Public awareness of these issues can be used to encourage patient participation.

Prevention Through Patient Involvement

According to the United States Agency for Healthcare Research and Quality (AHRQ), physicians often do not sufficiently help patients make informed health care decisions. Health-conscious patients inform themselves as much as possible about their condition, inquire about their health care options, and partner with their physicians, using them as information resources and health facilitators. The AHRQ says the most effective way a patient can help prevent medical errors is by taking an active role in the health care team.

As a patient, you can take the following steps to prevent medical errors:

- Take all medications exactly as prescribed, for as long as prescribed. If you don't understand why you are being given a medication, ask your physician or pharmacist to explain.

- If you require hospitalization, select your hospital carefully. If possible, choose a hospital with extensive experience treating patients with your type of condition.

- When being discharged from a hospital, ask about any special care, precautions, medications, and other procedures that will be required upon returning home.

- Recruit a patient advocate, someone who can give support and speak on your behalf in order to protect your rights, promote your interests, and assist you in making decisions.

- Rely on a hospitalist, a physician who specializes in the care of hospitalized patients. Hospitalists focus on advocacy and safety, and help remedy the lack of continuity that occurs among hospital providers. They manage a patient's course through the hospital, coordinate the various providers and consultants, and stay in touch with the patient's family and primary care physician. Hospitalists help remedy many of the problems that lead to medical errors. Hospitalist medicine is today's fastest-growing specialty.

---

ment—conventional or unconventional—that has not been scientifically evaluated for safety and effectiveness (see the box "Avoiding Health Fraud and Quackery" on p. 372).

The National Center for Complementary and Alternative Medicine (NCCAM), a branch of the National Institutes of Health (NIH), was established in the 1990s to apply rigorous scientific standards for proving or disproving the safety and effectiveness of CAM. NCCAM groups CAM practices into five domains: alternative medical systems, mind-body interventions, biological-based therapies, manipulative and body-based methods, and energy

therapies. What follows is a general introduction to the types of CAM available and a brief description of some of the more widely used ones.

QUESTIONS FOR CRITICAL THINKING AND REFLECTION

What sort of relationship do you have with your primary physician? Do you think he or she really understands your needs and is familiar enough with your history? What could you do to improve this relationship?

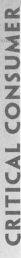
Alternative Medical Systems

Many cultures elaborated complete systems of medical philosophy, theory, and practice long before the current biomedical approach was developed. The complete systems that are best known in the United States are probably traditional Chinese medicine (TCM), also known as traditional Oriental medicine, and homeopathy. Traditional medical systems have also been developed in many other regions of the world, including North, Central, and South America; the Middle East; India; Tibet; and Australia. In many countries, these medical approaches continue to be used today—frequently alongside Western medicine and quite often by physicians trained in Western medicine.

Alternative medical systems tend to have concepts in common. For example, the concept of life force or energy exists in many cultures. In traditional Chinese medicine, the life force contained in all living things is called *qi* (sometimes spelled chi). Most traditional medical systems think of disease as a disturbance or imbalance not just of physical processes but also of forces and energies within the body, the mind, and the spirit. Treatment aims at reestablishing equilibrium, balance, and harmony. Because the whole patient, rather than an isolated set of symptoms, is treated in most comprehensive alternative medical systems, it is rare that only a single treatment approach is used. Most commonly, multiple techniques and methods are employed and are continually adjusted according to the changes in the patient's health status that occur naturally or are brought about by the treatment.

Traditional Chinese Medicine In **traditional Chinese medicine (TCM)**, the free and harmonious flow of qi produces health—a positive feeling of well-being and vitality in body, mind, and spirit. Illness occurs when the flow of qi is blocked or disturbed. TCM works to restore and balance the flow of blocked qi; the goal is not only to treat illnesses but also to increase energy, prevent disease, and support the immune system.

Two of the primary treatment methods in TCM are herbal remedies and **acupuncture.** Chinese herbal remedies number about 5800 and include plant products, animal parts, and minerals. The use of a single medicinal botanical is rare in Chinese herbal medicine; rather, several different plants are combined in very precise proportions, often to make a tea or soup.

Acupuncture works to correct disturbances in the flow of qi through the insertion of thin needles at appropriate points in the skin. Qi is believed to flow through the body along several *meridians*, or pathways, and there are at least 2000 acupuncture points located along these meridians. The points chosen for acupuncture are highly individualized for each patient, and they change over the course of treatment as the patient's health status changes.

The World Health Organization has compiled a list of over 40 conditions in which acupuncture may be beneficial. At a conference called by the National Institutes of Health (NIH), a panel of experts found evidence that acupuncture was effective in relieving nausea and vom-

QUICK STATS

More than **8 million** Americans have had acupuncture at least once.

—CDC, 2005

Several forms of alternative medicine, such as traditional Chinese medicine, rely heavily on remedies made from plant and animal parts. Although millions of people claim that these remedies are beneficial, their production now threatens the very existence of several species. Here are some examples:

- Today there are fewer than 10,000 tigers living in the wild (and about 5000 being raised on farms). Despite their dwindling numbers and status as an endangered species, hundreds of tigers are poached every year. The carcasses are sold to purveyors of traditional medicine, who use tiger body parts in some of their remedies.

- Only a few thousand rhinoceros live in the wild today, but they continue to be poached for their horns, which are prized by traditional healers. Rhinos are classified as "critically endangered" and will disappear within a few years unless they are protected.

- Other species, such as seahorses, musk deer, and bears, are being harvested at a rate that may put them at risk of extinction soon.

  For more than a decade, environmentalists and wildlife protection officials worldwide have been calling for practitioners of traditional medicine to either stop using endangered plants and animals in their remedies, or to support farming of these species as an alternative to harvesting them from the environment. Progress is slow, but according to organizations like the International Fund for Animal Welfare, practitioners have started responding positively.

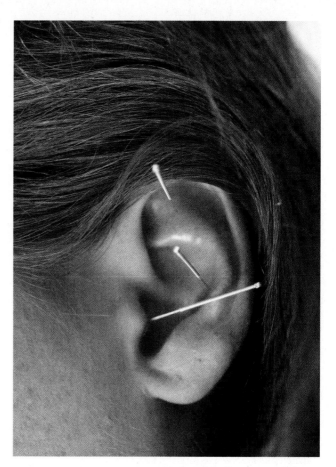

Acupuncture involves the insertion of needles at appropriate points in the skin to restore balance to the flow of qi.

iting after chemotherapy and pain after surgery, including dental surgery. Newer studies show that acupuncture may help relieve the painful symptoms of fibromyalgia and reduce the joint pain and stiffness of osteoarthritis. There is not yet enough evidence to show conclusively that acupuncture is effective for menstrual cramps, tennis elbow, carpal tunnel syndrome, asthma, or certain other conditions. Western researchers typically use a different framework for understanding the effects of acupuncture. For example, they might explain pain relief not in terms of qi but in terms of altering nervous system pathways and the release of hormones and neurotransmitters.

Very few negative side effects have been reported in conjunction with acupuncture. Nonetheless, problems can occur from the improper insertion and manipulation of needles and from the use of unsterile needles. The FDA regulates acupuncture needles like other standard medical devices and requires that they be sterile. Most states require licensing for acupuncture practitioners, but requirements vary widely.

Homeopathy An alternative medical system of Western origin, **homeopathy** is based on two main principles: "Like cures like," and remedies become more effective with greater dilution. "Like cures like" summarizes the concept that a substance that produces the symptoms of an illness in a healthy person can cure the illness when given in very minute quantities. Remedies containing very small quantities of a particular substance are obtained by repeatedly diluting the original solution. The extent of dilution varies, but the final extract is often so dilute that few, if any, of the original molecules are left in it.

Over 1000 different substances (plant and animal parts, minerals, and chemicals) are used to prepare homeopathic

traditional Chinese medicine (TCM) The traditional medical system of China, which views illness as the result of a disturbance in the flow of qi, the life force; therapies include acupuncture, herbal medicine, and massage.

acupuncture Insertion of thin needles into the skin at points along meridians, pathways through which qi is believed to flow.

homeopathy An alternative medical system that treats illnesses by giving very small doses of drugs that in larger doses would produce symptoms like those of the illness.

The Power of Belief: The Placebo Effect

connect™

A placebo is a chemically inactive substance or ineffective procedure that a patient believes is an effective therapy for his or her condition. Researchers frequently give placebos to the control group in an experiment testing the efficacy of a particular drug or other treatment. By comparing the effects of the actual treatment with the effects of the placebo, researchers can judge whether the treatment is effective.

The *placebo effect* occurs when a patient improves after receiving a placebo. In such cases, the effect of the placebo on the patient cannot be attributed to the specific actions or properties of the drug or procedure.

Researchers have consistently found that 30–40% of all patients given a pla-

cebo show improvement. This result has been observed for a wide variety of conditions or symptoms, including coughing, seasickness, depression, migraines, and angina. For some conditions, placebos have been effective in up to 70% of patients. In some cases, people given a placebo even report having the side effects associated with an actual drug. Placebos are particularly effective when they are administered by a practitioner whom the patient trusts.

Studies on patients with depression and people with Parkinson's disease have found that treatment with an inactive placebo results in changes in brain function. Such changes in the electrical or chemical activity of the brain may help explain the placebo effect. Other possi-

ble explanations for the placebo effect involve relaxation and stress reduction.

The placebo effect can be exploited by unscrupulous people who sell worthless medical treatments to the scientifically unsophisticated public. But placebo power can also be harnessed for its beneficial effects. When a skilled and compassionate medical practitioner provides a patient with a sense of confidence and hope, the positive aspects of placebo power can boost the benefits of standard medical treatment. Getting well, like getting sick, is a complex process. Anatomy, physiology, mind, emotions, and the environment are all inextricably intertwined. But the placebo effect does show that belief can have both psychological and physical effects.

remedies, and each of these substances is thought to have different effects at different dilutions. That means a homeopath must not only choose the correct remedy for a particular patient but also decide on the specific dilution of that remedy in order to achieve the desired effect.

In order to assess a patient's condition, homeopaths generally spend quite a bit of time talking with a patient and assessing his or her physical, psychological, and emotional health before deciding on the correct remedy at the proper dilution. This intensive interaction between the practitioner and the patient might play an important role in the success of the therapy. Indeed, critics of homeopathy often attribute its reported effectiveness to this nonspecific placebo effect (see the box "The Power of Belief: The Placebo Effect"). However, when the results of 185 homeo-

pathic trials were analyzed recently, it was concluded that the clinical effects of homeopathy could not be completely explained by the placebo effect. Homeopathy remains one of the most controversial forms of CAM.

To date, the FDA has not found any serious adverse events associated with the use of homeopathy, with the possible exception of situations in which a patient might have been successfully treated with standard medical approaches but chose to rely solely on homeopathy. The FDA regulates some homeopathic remedies, but they are subject to many fewer restrictions than prescription or over-the-counter drugs. A few states require practitioners to have special licenses, but most providers practice homeopathy as a specialty under another medical license, such as medical doctor or nurse practitioner.

Mind-Body Interventions

Mind-body interventions make use of the integral connection between mind and body and the effect each can have on the other. They include many of the stress-management techniques discussed in Chapter 2, including meditation, yoga, visualization, taijiquan, and biofeedback. Psychotherapy, support groups, prayer, and music, art, and dance therapy can also be thought of as mind-body interventions. The placebo effect is one of the most widely known examples of mind-body interdependence.

Some forms of **hypnosis** are considered to be CAM therapies, although the use of hypnotherapy for certain conditions was accepted more than 40 years ago by the American Medical Association. Hypnosis involves the induction of a state of deep relaxation during which the patient is more suggestible (more easily influenced). While

TERMS

hypnosis The process by which a practitioner induces a state of deep relaxation in which an individual is more suggestible; commonly used in cases of pain, phobia, and addiction.

biological-based therapies CAM therapies that include biologically based interventions and products; examples include herbal remedies, extracts from animal tissues, and dietary supplements.

pharmacopoeia A collection of descriptions and formulas for drugs and medicinal preparations.

chiropractic A system of manual healing most frequently used to treat musculoskeletal problems; the primary treatment is manipulation of the spine and other joints.

energy therapies Forms of CAM treatment that use energy fields originating either within the body or from outside sources to promote health and healing.

the patient is in such a hypnotic trance, the practitioner tries to help him or her change unwanted behavior or deal with pain and other symptoms. Hypnosis is sometimes used in smoking cessation programs and as a nondrug approach to anxiety disorders such as phobias and chronic conditions such as irritable bowel syndrome.

Hypnosis can be used by medical professionals (M.D.s, D.O.s, D.D.S.s) but is also offered by hypnotherapists. Physicians are certified by their own associations; many states require hypnotherapists to be licensed, but the requirements for licensing vary substantially.

Biological-Based Therapies

Biological-based therapies consist primarily of herbal therapies or remedies, botanicals, extracts from animal tissues (such as shark cartilage), and dietary supplements. Herbal remedies are a major component of all indigenous forms of medicine; prior to the development of pharmaceuticals at the end of the nineteenth century, people everywhere in the world relied on materials from nature for pain relief, wound healing, and treatment of a variety of ailments. Herbal remedies are also a common element in most systems of traditional medicine. Much of the **pharmacopoeia** of modern scientific medicine originated in the folk medicine of native peoples, and many drugs used today are derived from plants.

A majority of botanical products are sold as dietary supplements, that is, in the form of tablets, pills, capsules, liquid extracts, or teas. Like foods, dietary supplements must carry ingredient labels. As with food products, it is the responsibility of the manufacturers to ensure that their dietary supplements are safe and properly labeled prior to marketing. The FDA is responsible for monitoring the labeling and accompanying literature of dietary supplements and for overseeing their safety once they are on the market.

Well-designed clinical studies have been conducted on only a small number of biologically-based therapies. A few commonly used botanicals, their uses, and the evidence supporting their efficacy are presented in Table 15.2. Participants in clinical trials with St. John's wort, ginkgo, and echinacea experienced only minor adverse events. However, most clinical trials of this type last for only a few weeks, so the tests did not indicate whether it is safe to take these botanicals for longer periods of time. They also didn't examine the effects of different dosages or how these therapies interact with conventional drugs.

Although most drug-herb interactions are relatively minor compared to conventional drug–drug interactions, some can be potentially serious. An example is the use of herbs that have anticoagulant (anticlotting) properties, such as ginkgo biloba, when used concurrently with the commonly prescribed anticoagulant Coumadin.

Studies have shown that most people do not reveal their use of CAM therapies to their conventional health care providers, an oversight that can have severe health consequences. Any herbs or drugs used in combination should be evaluated for safety by a knowledgeable health care provider such as a pharmacist. See the box "Herbal Remedies: Are They Safe?" on p. 377.

Manipulative and Body-Based Methods

Touch and body manipulation are long-standing forms of health care. Manual healing techniques are based on the idea that misalignment or dysfunction in one part of the body can cause pain or dysfunction in that or another part; correcting these misalignments can bring the body back to optimal health.

Manual healing methods are an integral part of physical therapy and osteopathic medicine, now considered a form of conventional medicine. Other physical healing methods include massage, acupressure, Feldenkrais, Rolfing, and numerous other techniques. The most commonly used CAM manual healing method is **chiropractic,** a method that focuses on the relationship between structure, primarily of joints and muscles, and function, primarily of the nervous system, to maintain or restore health. An important therapeutic procedure is the manipulation of joints, particularly those of the spinal column. However, chiropractors also use a variety of other techniques, including exercise, patient education and lifestyle modification, nutritional supplements, and orthotics (mechanical supports and braces) to treat patients.

Chiropractors, or doctors of chiropractic, are trained for a minimum of four full-time academic years at accredited chiropractic colleges and can go on to postgraduate training in many countries. Chiropractic is accepted by many health care and health insurance providers to a far greater extent than the other types of CAM therapies. Chiropractic is effective in controlling back pain, and promising results have been reported with the use of chiropractic techniques in neck pain and headaches.

20% of American adults have received chiropractic care.

—NCCAM, 2007

Spinal manipulation performed by a person without proper chiropractic training can be extremely dangerous. The American Chiropractic Association can help you find a licensed chiropractor near you.

Energy Therapies

Energy therapies are forms of treatment that use energy originating either within the body (biofields) or from other sources (electromagnetic fields). Biofield therapies are based on the idea that energy fields surround and penetrate the body and can be influenced by movement, touch, pressure, or the placement of hands in or through the fields.

Table 15.2 — Commonly Used Botanicals, Their Uses, Evidence for Their Effectiveness, and Contraindications

Botanical	Use	Evidence	Examples of Adverse Effects and Interactions
Cranberry (*Vaccinium macrocarpon*)	Prevention or treatment of urinary tract disorders	May eliminate and prevent bacteria from infecting the urinary tract	None known
Dandelion (*Taraxacum officinale*)	As a "tonic" against liver or kidney ailments	None yet	May cause diarrhea in some users; people with gallbladder or bile duct problems should not take dandelion
Echinacea (*Echinacea purpurea, E. angustifolia, E. pallida*)	Stimulation of immune functions; to prevent colds and flulike diseases; to lessen symptoms of colds and flus	Some trials showed that it prevents colds and flus and helps patients recover from colds faster	Might cause liver damage if taken over long periods of time (more than 8 weeks); since it is an immune stimulant, it is not advisable to take it with immune suppressants (e.g., corticosteroids) or during chemotherapy
Evening primrose oil (*Oenothera biennis L.*)	Reduction of inflammation	Long-term supplementation effective in reducing symptoms of rheumatoid arthritis	None known
Feverfew (*Tanacetum parthenium*)	Prevention of headaches and migraines	The majority of trials indicate that it is more effective than placebo	Should not be used by people allergic to other members of the aster family; has the potential to increase the effects of warfarin and other anticoagulants
Garlic (*Allium sativum*)	Reduction of cholesterol	Short-term studies have found a modest effect	May interact with some medications, including anticoagulants, cyclosporine, and oral contraceptives
Ginkgo (*Ginkgo biloba*)	Improvement of circulation and memory	Improves cerebral insufficiency and slows progression of Alzheimer's disease and other types of senile dementia in some patients; improves blood flow in legs	Could increase bleeding time; should not be taken with nonsteroidal anti-inflammatory drugs or anticoagulants; gastrointestinal disturbance
Ginseng (*Panax ginseng*)	Improvement of physical performance, memory, immune function, and glycemic control in diabetes; treatment of herpes simplex 2	No conclusive evidence exists for any of these uses	Interacts with warfarin and alcohol in mice and rats, hence should probably not be used with these drugs; may cause liver damage
St. John's wort (*Hypericum perforatum*)	Treatment of depression	There is strong evidence that it is significantly more effective than placebo, is as effective as some standard antidepressants for mild to moderate depression, and causes fewer adverse effects	Known to interact with a variety of pharmaceuticals and should not be taken together with digoxin, theophylline, cyclosporine, indinavir, and serotonin-reuptake inhibitors
Saw palmetto (*Serenoa repens*)	Improvement of prostate health	Early studies showed that saw palmetto may reduce mild prostate enlargement	Has no known interactions with drugs, but should probably not be taken with hormonal therapies
Valerian (*Valeriana officinalis*)	Treatment of insomnia	Appears to help with sleep disorders	Interacts with thiopental and pentobarbital and should not be used with these drugs

Qigong, a component of traditional Chinese medicine, combines movement, meditation, and regulation of breathing to enhance the flow of qi, improve blood circulation, and enhance immune function. **Therapeutic touch** is derived from the ancient technique of laying-on of hands; it is based on the premise that healers can identify and correct energy imbalances by passing their hands over the patient's body. **Reiki** is one form of therapeutic touch; it is intended to correct disturbances in the flow of life energy (ki is the Japanese form of the Chinese qi) and enhance the body's healing powers through the use of 13 specific hand positions on the patient.

Bioelectromagnetics is the study of the interaction between living organisms and electromagnetic fields, both those produced by the organism itself and those produced by outside sources. The recognition that the body produces electromagnetic fields has led to the development of many diagnostic procedures in Western medicine, including electroencephalography (EEG), electrocardiography (ECG), and nuclear magnetic resonance (NMR) scans.

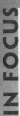

IN FOCUS

Herbal Remedies: Are They Safe?

Consider the following research findings and FDA advisories:

• St. John's wort interacts with drugs used to treat HIV infection and heart disease; the herb may also reduce the effectiveness of oral contraceptives, antirejection drugs used with organ transplants, and some medications used to treat infections, depression, asthma, and seizure disorders.

• Supplements containing kava kava have been linked to severe liver damage, and anyone who has liver problems or takes medications that can affect the liver are advised to consult a physician before using kava kava–containing supplements.

• In a sample of ayurvedic herbal medicine products, 20% were found to contain potentially harmful levels of lead, mercury, and/or arsenic.

These findings highlight growing safety concerns about dietary supplements, which now represent annual sales of more than $15 billion in the United States.

Drug Interactions

Botanicals may decrease the effects of drugs, making them ineffective, or increase their effects, in some cases making them toxic. Most patients fail to tell their physicians about their use of herbal substances. Botanicals can also interact

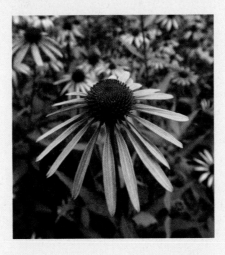

with alcohol, usually heightening alcohol's effects. Many manufacturers are offering new combinations of botanical preparations without empirical or scientific information about the interactions of the individual products.

Lack of Standardization

The Dietary Supplement Health and Education Act of 1994 requires that dietary supplement labels list the name and quantity of each ingredient. However, confusion can result because different plant species—with distinct chemical compositions and effects—may have the same common name. The content of

herbal preparations is also variable. Botanicals are naturally grown products. Herb producers do not have complete control over natural processes any more than farmers have control over the vitamin content of fruit.

As an attempt toward standardization, herb producers have identified one or two substances that indicate quality; these substances should be listed on a product's label with their corresponding concentrations, lot numbers, and purity analysis data. Avoid any herbal product whose label is missing this information. Reputable retailers sell only products with this identifying information, and some send qualified inspectors to the site of production to verify the label information.

The Role of Government in Safety Issues

In the United States, because herbs are considered supplements rather than food or drug products, they do not have to meet FDA food and drug standards for safety or effectiveness, nor do they currently have to meet any manufacturing standards. The manufacturer is responsible for ensuring that a supplement is safe before it is marketed; the FDA has the power to restrict a substance if it is found to pose a health risk after it is on the market.

Bioelectromagnetic-based therapies involve the use of electromagnetic fields to manage pain and to treat conditions such as asthma. Although promising, the available research is still very limited and does not allow firm conclusions about the efficacy of these therapies.

Evaluating Complementary and Alternative Therapies

Because there is less information available about complementary and alternative therapies, as well as less regulation of associated products and providers, consumers need to take an active role when they are thinking about using them.

Working with Your Physician The NCCAM advises consumers not to seek complementary therapies without first visiting a conventional health care provider for an evaluation and diagnosis of their symptoms. It's usually best to discuss and try conventional treatments that have

been shown to be beneficial for your condition. If you are thinking of trying any alternative therapies, it is critically important to tell your physician in order to avoid any dangerous interactions with conventional treatments you are receiving. Areas to discuss with your physician or

TERMS

qigong A component of traditional Chinese medicine that combines movement, meditation, and regulation of breathing to enhance the flow of qi, improve blood circulation, and enhance immune function.

therapeutic touch A CAM practice based on the premise that healers can identify and correct energy imbalances by passing their hands over the patient's body.

Reiki A CAM practice intended to correct disturbances in the flow of life energy and enhance the body's healing powers through the use of 13 hand positions on the patient.

bioelectromagnetic-based therapies CAM therapies based on the notion that electromagnetic fields can be used to promote healing and manage pain.

pharmacist include the *safety* of the complementary tretment; evidence for its effectiveness, if any; issues of timing; and likely cost.

If appropriate, schedule a follow-up visit with your physician to assess your condition and your progress after a certain amount of time using a complementary therapy. Keep a symptom diary to more accurately track your symptoms and gauge your progress. (Symptoms such as pain and fatigue are very difficult to recall with accuracy, so an ongoing symptom diary is an important tool.) If you plan to pursue a therapy against your physician's advice, you need to tell him or her.

Questioning the CAM Practitioner   You can also get information from individual practitioners and from schools, professional organizations, and state licensing boards. Ask about education, training, licensing, and certification. If appropriate, check with local or state regulatory agencies or the consumer affairs department to determine if any complaints have been lodged against the practitioner. Some guidelines for talking with a CAM practitioner include the following:

- Ask the practitioner why he or she thinks the therapy will be beneficial for your condition. Ask for a full description of the therapy and any potential side effects. In all cases, demand an evidence-based approach.

- Describe in detail any conventional treatments you are receiving or plan to receive.

- Ask how long the therapy should continue before it can be determined if it is beneficial.

- Ask about the expected cost of the treatment. Does it seem reasonable? Will your health insurance pay some or all of the costs?

If anything an alternative practitioner says or recommends directly conflicts with advice from your physician, discuss it with your physician before making any major changes in any current treatment regimen or in your lifestyle.

Doing Your Own Research   You can investigate CAM therapies on your own by going to the library or doing research online, although caution is in order when using Web sites for the various forms of CAM. A good place to start is the Web sites of government agencies like the FDA or NCCAM and of universities and similar organizations that conduct government-sponsored research on CAM ap-

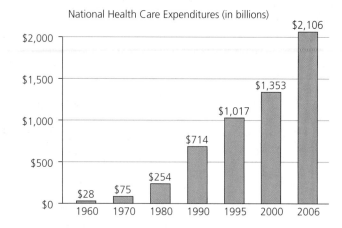

National Health Care Expenditures (in billions)

FIGURE 15.2   National health care expenditures (public and private) 1960–2006.

SOURCE: National Center for Health Statistics. 2009. *Health, United States: 2008.* Hyattsville, Md.: National Center for Health Statistics.

proaches. Perhaps more so than for any other consumer products and services, the use of CAM calls for consumer skills, critical thinking, and caution.

PAYING FOR HEALTH CARE

The American health care system is one of the most advanced and comprehensive in the world, but it is also the most expensive (Figure 15.2). In 2006, the United States spent $2.1 trillion on health care, or more than $7000 per person. Many factors contribute to the high cost of health care in the United States, including the cost of advanced equipment and new technology, expensive treatments for some illnesses, the aging of the population, high earnings by some people in the health care industry, and the demand for profits by investors.

Health Insurance

Health insurance enables people to receive health care they might not otherwise be able to afford. Health insurance plans are either fee-for-service (indemnity) or managed

care. With both types the individual or the employer pays a basic premium, usually on a monthly basis; there are often other payments as well (see the box "Who Are the Uninsured?").

Traditional Fee-for-Service (Indemnity) Plans   In a fee-for-service, or indemnity, plan, you can use any medical provider (such as a physician or a hospital) you choose.

QUESTIONS FOR CRITICAL THINKING AND REFLECTION

Have you ever considered using a complementary or alternative treatment? If so, was it in addition to conventional treatment, or instead of it? What kind of research did you do before having the treatment? What advice did your primary health care provider give you about it?

Who Are the Uninsured?

connect™

Despite high national levels of spending on health care, many Americans under age 65—17%, or nearly 1 in 5, according to the National Center for Health Statistics—did not have health insurance in 2006. (Americans age 65 and over are often covered by government programs.) This overall statistic about the uninsured hides some important differences among groups (see table).

- *Low income:* The factor most closely associated with lack of health insurance is low income.
- *Age:* Young adults may not be regularly employed and so may not be covered by an insurance plan through work.
- *Ethnicity:* Many of the ethnic disparities are explained by socioeconomic status. However, other factors may also contribute, including language barriers, differing cultural attitudes toward medical care, living in medically underserved communities, and citizenship status.

People without health insurance receive less health care and lower quality of care. They have fewer physician visits and less preventive care. To help overcome the health gap between ethnic minorities and the general population, the U.S. Department of Health and Human Services sponsors "Take a Loved One for a Checkup Day." Held on the third Tuesday in September, this event is designed to encourage people to obtain preventive care. People are encouraged to make an appointment for themselves or for a friend or family member who hasn't seen a health care provider recently.

People who don't have a regular health care provider or who don't have health insurance can contact a local health department or local community center to find out more about free or low-cost care. For more information, visit the Closing the Health Gap Web site (http://www.omhrc.gov/healthgap/).

Uninsured Americans Under Age 65 (Percent), 2006	
Total	**17.0**
Income (percent of poverty level)	
Below 100%	35.7
100–149%	37.5
150–199%	34.3
200% or more	13.7
Age (years)	
Under 18	13.2
18–24	36.4
25–34	33.8
35–44	22.6
45–54	17.9
55–64	12.9
Ethnicity	
White	16.6
Asian American	18.0
African American	22.1
Latino	38.8

SOURCES: Centers for Disease Control and Prevention. 2009. *Health, United States, 2008.* Hyattsville, Md.: National Center for Health Statistics.

You or the provider sends the bill to your insurance company, which pays part of it. Usually you have to pay a deductible amount each year, and then the plan will pay a percentage—often 80%—of what they consider the "usual and customary" charge for covered services.

Managed-Care Plans Managed-care plans have agreements with a network of specified physicians, hospitals, and health care providers to offer a range of services to plan members at reduced cost. In general, you have lower out-of-pocket costs and less paperwork with a managed-care plan than with an indemnity plan, but you also have less freedom in choosing health care providers. Managed-care plans may follow several different models:

- **Health maintenance organizations (HMOs)** offer members a range of services for a set monthly fee. You choose a primary care physician who manages your care and refers you to specialists if you need them.
- **Preferred provider organizations (PPOs)** have arrangements with physicians and other providers who have agreed to accept lower fees.
- **Point-of-service (POS) plans** are options offered by many HMOs in which you can see a physician outside the plan and still be partially covered.

Many managed-care plans try to reduce costs over the long term by paying for routine preventive care, such as regular checkups, screening tests, and prenatal care; they may also encourage prevention by offering health education and lifestyle modification programs for members. Other cost-cutting measures are less consumer-oriented. Consumers' choice of physicians is limited, and they may have to wait longer for appointments and travel farther to see participating doctors.

Health Savings Accounts Health savings accounts (HSAs) include two parts: a health plan with a high

TERMS

managed-care plan A health care program that integrates the financing and delivery of services by using designated providers, utilization review, and incentives for following the plan's policies; HMOs, PPOs, and POS plans are managed-care plans.

health maintenance organization (HMO) A prepaid health insurance plan that offers health care from designated providers.

preferred provider organization (PPO) A prepaid health insurance plan in which providers agree to deliver services for discounted fees; patients can go to any provider, but using nonparticipating providers results in higher costs to the patient.

point-of-service (POS) plan A managed-care plan that covers treatment by an HMO physician but permits patients to seek treatment elsewhere with a higher copayment.

health savings account (HSA) Health insurance coverage that includes a health plan with a high deductible and a tax-exempt personal savings account that is used for qualified medical expenses.

deductible and a tax-exempt personal savings account that is used for qualified medical expenses. The individual makes pre-tax contributions to the savings account and later uses these funds or other cash payments to cover medical expenses until the plan's deductible is met. Once the deductible is met, the plan pays remaining medical costs according to the type of policy. An HSA may give the consumer more control over health care spending; it can also potentially lower premiums for some people because health plans with high deductibles tend to have lower premiums.

Government Programs Americans who are 65 or older and younger people with certain disabilities can be covered by **Medicare**, a federal health insurance program that helps pay for hospitalization, physician services, and prescription drugs. **Medicaid** is a joint federal-state health insurance program that covers some low-income people, especially children, pregnant women, and people with certain disabilities.

Choosing a Policy

Choosing health insurance can be complicated; it's important to evaluate the coverage provided by different plans and decide which one is best for you. Colleges typically provide medical services through a student health center; some require students to purchase additional insurance if they are not covered by family policies. It's usually economical to remain on a family policy as long as possible. After college, most people secure group coverage through their place of employment or through membership in an organization. If you are choosing insurance, consider a number of different plans and use your critical thinking skills to find the one that best suits your needs.

TERMS

Medicare A federal health insurance program for people 65 or older and for younger people with certain disabilities.

Medicaid A federally subsidized state-run plan of health care for people with low income.

TIPS FOR TODAY AND THE FUTURE
Most of the time, you can take care of yourself without consulting a health care provider. When you need professional care, you can still take responsibility for yourself by making informed decisions.

RIGHT NOW YOU CAN
- Make sure you have enough of your prescription medications on hand, and that your prescriptions are up-to-date.
- If you take any supplements (dietary or herbal), ask your pharmacist if they can interact with any prescription drugs you are taking.

IN THE FUTURE YOU CAN
- Thoroughly research any form of complementary or alternative medical treatments you are using or considering; make sure it is considered safe and effective.
- Review your medical insurance policy and make sure you are familiar with your coverage and the policy's terms. If you have any questions about your policy, contact your insurance agent. If you don't have any medical insurance, start investigating your options.

SUMMARY

- Informed self-care requires knowing how to evaluate symptoms. It's necessary to see a physician if symptoms are severe, unusual, persistent, or recurrent.

- Self-treatment doesn't necessarily require medication, but OTC drugs can be a helpful part of self-care.

- Conventional medicine is characterized by a focus on the external, physical causes of disease; the identification of a set of symptoms for different diseases; the development of public health measures to prevent disease and of drugs and surgery to treat them; the use of rational, scientific thinking to understand phenomena; and a well-established research methodology.

- Conventional practitioners include medical doctors, doctors of osteopathic medicine, podiatrists, optometrists, and dentists, as well as allied health care providers.

- The diagnostic process involves a medical history, a physical exam, and medical tests. Patients should ask questions about medical tests and treatments recommended by their physicians.

- Safe use of prescription drugs requires knowledge of what the medication is supposed to do, how and when to take it, and what the side effects are.

- Complementary and alternative medicine (CAM) is defined as those therapies and practices that do not form part of conventional health care and medical practice as taught in most U.S. medical schools and offered in most U.S. hospitals.

- CAM is characterized by a view of health as a balance and integration of body, mind, and spirit; and a body of knowledge based on accumulated experience and observations of patient reactions.

- Alternative medical systems such as traditional Chinese medicine and homeopathy are complete systems of medical philosophy, theory, and practice.

- Mind-body interventions include meditation, biofeedback, group support, hypnosis, and prayer.

- Biological-based therapies consist of herbal remedies, botanicals, animal-tissue products, and dietary supplements.

- Manipulative and body-based methods include massage and other physical healing techniques; the most frequently used is chiropractic.

- Energy therapies are designed to influence the flow of energy in and around the body; they include qigong, therapeutic touch therapies, and Reiki.

- Because there is less information available about CAM and less regulation of its practices and providers, consumers must be proactive in researching and choosing treatments, using critical thinking skills and exercising caution.

- Health insurance plans are usually described as either fee-for-service (indemnity) or managed-care plans. Indemnity plans allow consumers more choice in medical providers, but managed-care plans are less expensive.

FOR MORE INFORMATION

BOOKS

Committee on the Use of Complementary and Alternative Medicine by the American Public. 2005. *Complementary and Alternative Medicine in the United States.* Washington, D.C.: National Academy Press. *Outlines ways of integrating conventional and complementary therapies, and proposes changes to dietary supplement laws.*

Mayo Clinic. 2007. *The Mayo Clinic Book of Alternative Medicine.* New York: Time-Life. *A concise review of currently popular CAM therapies and treatments.*

Thompson, W. G. 2005. *The Placebo Effect and Health: Combining Science and Compassionate Care.* New York: Prometheus Books. *Describes the placebo effect and how it may be used to benefit health.*

PDR. 2007. *PDR for Nonprescription Drugs, Dietary Supplements, and Herbs, 2008,* 29th ed. Montvale, N.J.: Thomson Healthcare. *A reference covering the safety and efficacy of over-the-counter medications.*

ORGANIZATIONS, HOTLINES, AND WEB SITES

American Board of Medical Specialties. Provides information on board certification, including information on specific physicians.
    http://www.abms.org

American Chiropractic Association. Provides information on chiropractic care, consumer tips, and a searchable directory of certified chiropractors.
    http://www.amerchiro.org

American Medical Association (AMA). Provides information about physicians, including their training, licensure, and board certification.
    http://www.ama-assn.org

American Osteopathic Association. Provides information on osteopathic physicians, including board certification.
    http://www.osteopathic.org

Food and Drug Administration: Information for Consumers. Provides materials on dietary supplements, foods, prescription and OTC drugs, and other FDA-regulated products.
    http://www.fda.gov/consumer/default.htm

National Center for Complementary and Alternative Medicine (NCCAM). Provides general information packets, answers to frequently asked questions about CAM, consumer advice for safer use of CAM, research abstracts, and bibliographies.
    http://nccam.nih.gov

National Council Against Health Fraud. Provides news and information about health fraud and quackery and links to related sites.
    http://www.ncahf.org

Quackwatch. Provides information on health fraud, quackery, and health decision making.
    http://www.quackwatch.org

U.S. Treasury Department: Health Savings Accounts. Provides information about HSAs and links to relevant IRS forms.
    http://www.treas.gov/offices/public-affairs/hsa/

SELECTED BIBLIOGRAPHY

American Medical Association. 2004. *Health Savings Accounts at a Glance.* Chicago: American Medical Association.

Babones, S. J. 2008. Income inequality and population health: Correlation and causality. *Social Science and Medicine* 66(7): 1614–1626.

Burke, A., et al. 2006. Acupuncture use in the United States: Findings from the national health interview survey. *Journal of Alternative and Complementary Medicine* 12(7): 639–648.

Centers for Disease Control and Prevention. 2004. Complementary and alternative medicine use among adults: United States, 2002. *Advance Data from Vital and Health Statistics* No. 343. Hyattsville, Md.: National Center for Health Statistics.

Cyna, A. M., et al. 2006. Antenatal self-hypnosis for labour and childbirth: A pilot study. *Anaesthesia and Intensive Care* 34(4): 464–469.

Ernst, E. 2004. Prescribing herbal medications appropriately. *Journal of Family Practice* 53(12): 985–988.

Frazier, S. C. 2005. Health outcomes and polypharmacy in elderly individuals: An integrated literature review. *Journal of Gerontological Nursing* 31(9): 4–11.

Grzywacz, J. G., et al. 2008. Age-related differences in the conventional health care–complementary and alternative medicine link. *American Journal of Health Behavior* 32(6): 650–663.

Kaiser Family Foundation. 2005. *Trends and Indicators in the Changing Health Care Marketplace.* Menlo Park, Calif.: Kaiser Family Foundation.

Miller, F. G., et al. 2004. Ethical issues concerning research in complementary and alternative medicine. *Journal of the American Medical Association* 291(5): 599–604.

National Academy of Sciences, Institute of Medicine. 2006. *Preventing Medication Errors.* Washington, D.C.: National Academies Press.

National Center for Health Statistics. 2005. Trends in health insurance and access to medical care for children under age 19 years. *Advance Data from Vital Health Statistics* No. 355.

National Center for Health Statistics. 2008. *Early Release of Selected Estimates Based on Data from the 2007 National Health Interview Survey.* Hyattsville, Md.: National Center for Health Statistics.

National Center for Health Statistics. 2009. *Health, United States, 2008.* Hyattsville, Md.: National Center for Health Statistics.

Radley, D. C., et al. 2006. Off-label prescribing among office-based physicians. *Archives of Internal Medicine* 166(9): 1021–1026.

Rados, C. 2004. FDA reiterates warning against online drug buying. *FDA Consumer,* September/October.

Remler, D. K., and S. A. Glied. 2006. How much more cost sharing will health savings accounts bring? *Health Affairs* 25(4): 1070–1078.

Saha, S., et al. 2008. Racial and ethnic disparities in the VA health care system: A systematic review. *Journal of General Internal Medicine* 23(5): 654–671.

Schoen, C., et al. 2008. How many are underinsured? Trends among U.S. adults, 2003 and 2007. *Health Affairs,* 10 June [epub].

U.S. Department of the Treasury. 2008. *Health Savings Accounts (HSAs)* (http://www.ustreas.gov/offices/public-affairs/hsa; retrieved February 20, 2009).

Wahbeh, H., S. M. Elsas, and B. S. Oken. 2008. Mind-body interventions: Applications in neurology. *Neurology* 70(24): 2321–2328.

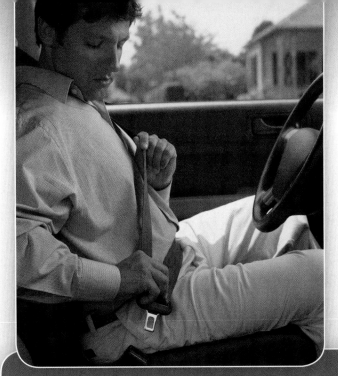

LOOKING AHEAD>>>>>

AFTER READING THIS CHAPTER, YOU SHOULD BE ABLE TO:

- Identify factors that contribute to unintentional injuries
- List the most common types of unintentional injuries and strategies for preventing them
- Describe factors that contribute to violence and intentional injuries
- Discuss different forms of violence and how to protect yourself from intentional injuries
- List strategies for helping others in an emergency situation

PERSONAL SAFETY

16

Each year, nearly 120,000 Americans die from injuries, and many more are temporarily or permanently disabled. The economic cost of injuries is high, with more than $650 billion spent each year for medical care and rehabilitation of injured people. Injuries also cause emotional suffering for injured people and their families, friends, and colleagues.

Engineering strategies such as safety belts can help lower injury rates, as can the passage and enforcement of safety-related laws, such as those requiring tamper-proof containers for OTC medications. Public education campaigns about risky behaviors such as driving under the influence of alcohol or smoking in bed can also help prevent injuries. Ultimately, though, it is up to each person to take responsibility for his or her actions and make wise choices about safety behaviors.

DIFFERENTIATING INJURIES

An **intentional injury** is one that is purposely inflicted, by oneself or by another person. If an injury occurs when no harm is intended, it is considered an **unintentional injury.** Motor vehicle crashes, falls, and fires often result in unintentional injuries. (Public health officials prefer not to use the word *accidents* to describe unintentional injuries because it suggests events beyond human control. *Injuries* are predictable outcomes of factors that can be controlled or prevented.) Although Americans tend to express more concern about intentional injuries, unintentional injuries are actually far more common. For example, the National Safety Council (NSC) estimates that in 2006, 329 Americans died each day from unintentional injuries, whereas 89 died of suicide and 50 died from

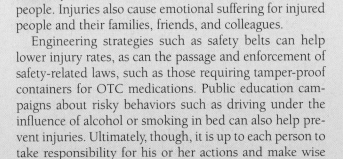

http://www.mcgrawhillconnect.com/personalhealth

homicide. Unintentional injuries are the fifth leading cause of death among all Americans and the leading cause of death for Americans under age 35.

UNINTENTIONAL INJURIES

Injury situations are generally categorized into four general classes, based on where they occur: motor vehicle injuries, home injuries, public injuries, and work injuries. The greatest number of deaths occur in motor vehicle crashes, but the greatest number of disabling injuries occur in the home (Table 16.1).

What Causes an Injury?

Most injuries are caused by a combination of human and environmental factors. Human factors are inner conditions or attitudes that lead to an unsafe state, whether physical, emotional, or psychological. Environmental factors are external conditions and circumstances, such as poor road conditions, a slippery surface, or the undertow of the ocean at the beach. A common human factor that leads to injuries is risk-taking behavior. Young men are especially prone to taking risks (see the box "Injuries Among Young Men"). Alcohol and drug use is another common risk factor that leads to many injuries and deaths.

Psychological and emotional factors can also play a role in injuries. People sometimes act on the basis of inadequate or inaccurate beliefs about what is safe or unsafe. However, many people who have accurate information still decide to engage in risky behavior. Young people often have unsafe attitudes, such as "I won't get hurt" or "It won't happen to me." Attitudes like this can lead to risk taking and ultimately to injuries.

Environmental factors leading to injury may be natural (weather conditions), social (a drunk driver), work-related (defective equipment), or home-related (faulty wiring). Making the environment safer is an important aspect of safety. Laws are often passed to try to make our environment safer; examples include speed limits on highways and workplace safety requirements.

Table 16.1 Unintentional Injuries in the United States

	Deaths	Disabling Injuries
Motor vehicle	44,700	2,400,000
Home	42,600	10,200,000
Public	30,000	10,000,000
Work	4,988	3,700,000
All classes*	120,000	26,200,000

*Deaths and injuries for the four separate classes total more than the "All classes" figures because of rounding and because some deaths and injuries are included in more than one class.

SOURCE: National Safety Council. 2008. *Injury Facts, 2008 Edition.* Itasca, Ill.: National Safety Council.

Motor Vehicle Injuries

According to the Centers for Disease Control and Prevention (CDC), nearly 45,000 Americans were killed and 3 million injured in motor vehicle crashes in 2006. Worldwide, motor vehicle crashes kill 1.2 million and injure up to 50 million people each year, making motor vehicle injuries the eleventh leading cause of death overall. **Motor vehicle injuries** also result in the majority of cases of paralysis due to spinal injuries, and they are the leading cause of severe brain injury in the United States.

> **QUICK STATS**
> Motor vehicle injuries cost Americans **$258 billion** in 2006.
> —NSC, 2008

Factors Contributing to Motor Vehicle Injuries
Common causes of motor vehicle injuries are speeding, aggressive driving, fatigue, inexperience, cell phones and other distractions, the use of alcohol and other drugs, and the incorrect use of safety belts and other safety devices.

SPEEDING Nearly 63% of all motor vehicle crashes are caused by bad driving, especially speeding. As speed increases, momentum and the force of impact increase, and the time allowed for the driver to react (reaction time) decreases. Speed limits are posted to establish the safest maximum speed limit for a given area under ideal conditions; if visibility is limited or the road is wet, the safe maximum speed may be considerably lower.

AGGRESSIVE DRIVING Aggressive driving includes frequent, erratic, and abrupt lane changes; tailgating; running red lights or stop signs; passing on the shoulder; and blocking other cars trying to change lanes or pass. Aggressive drivers increase the risk of crashes for themselves and others. Injuries may also occur if aggressive drivers stop their vehicles and confront each other following an incident.

Injuries Among Young Men

connect™

Males   Females

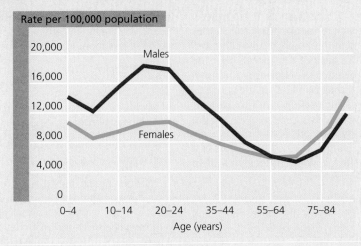

Figure 1   Nonfatal injury rate by age and sex.

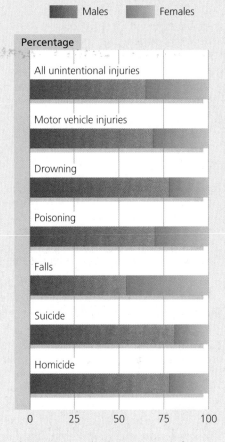

Figure 2   Injury deaths: Percentage of victims by sex.

Overall, rates of injury are highest among young adults and seniors over age 85. Except among the oldest group of adults, the nonfatal injury rate is substantially higher in males than in females—and it peaks among young adult males (Figure 1). Males also significantly outnumber females in injury deaths—whether unintentional or intentional (Figure 2).

Why do men, especially young men, have such high rates of injury? Gender roles may play a key role: Traditional gender roles for males may associate masculinity with risk-taking behavior and a disregard for pain and injury, and risk-taking behavior may be particularly common among young men. Men are more likely to drive dangerously, drink and drive, binge-drink, and use aggressive behavior to control situations—all of which can lead to higher rates of fatal and nonfatal injury. Men may also have a lower perception of risk of dangerous behaviors compared with women.

Traditional gender roles may also make it more difficult for men to admit to injury or emotional vulnerability. Physical injuries may worsen or become chronic if

care is not sought promptly. Untreated depression can lead to suicide.

In addition, men may have greater exposure to some injury situations. Compared with women, men may drive more miles, have greater access to firearms, and be more likely to ride motorcycles, operate machinery, and have jobs associated with high rates of workplace injuries. They may be more likely to engage in sports and other recreational activities associated with high rates of injuries. Greater access and use of firearms plays a role in higher rates of deaths among men from assault and suicide; as described in Chapter 3, women are more likely than men to attempt suicide, but men are much more likely to succeed, primarily because they are more likely to use firearms.

Some researchers suggest that the male hormone testosterone may play a role in risky and aggressive behavior. Differences in brain structure and activity may also influence how men and women respond to stressors and how quickly and to what degree they become verbally or physically aggressive in response to anger.

Further studies are needed to identify all the factors underlying excessive risk-taking among men and how these risk behaviors can be changed to lower the rates of fatal and nonfatal injury among men.

SOURCES: Centers for Disease Control and Prevention. 2004. Surveillance for fatal and nonfatal injuries—United States, 2001. *MMWR Surveillance Summaries* 53(SS7): 1–57; World Health Organization. 2002. *Gender and Road Traffic Injuries.* Geneva: World Health Organization; Courtenay, W. 1998. College men's health: An overview and a call to action. *Journal of American College Health* 46(6): 279–290.

FATIGUE AND SLEEPINESS   Driving requires mental alertness and attentiveness. Studies have shown that sleepiness causes slower reaction time, reduced coordination and vigilance, and delayed information processing. Research shows that even mild sleep deprivation causes a deterioration in driving ability comparable to that caused by a 0.05% blood alcohol concentration—a level considered hazardous when driving.

CELL PHONES AND OTHER DISTRACTIONS   Anything that distracts a driver can increase the risk of a motor vehicle injury. Several common causes of crashes, such as disregarding stop signs, have been linked to driver distraction. Distraction is a contributing factor in 25–50% of all crashes. A 2006 study showed that drivers who use cell phones are nearly six times as likely to be involved in a crash as drivers who don't. The same study showed that

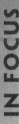

Cell Phones and Distracted Driving

connect™

At any given moment, about 5% of drivers are talking on a cell phone. In 2001, New York became the first state to ban the use of handheld cellular phones while driving; drivers there must use hand-free equipment or face fines of up to $100. Since then, four other states and the District of Columbia passed similar bans, and many other states have bans under consideration. Around the world, many countries have laws against the use of handheld cell phones while driving.

Available evidence indicates that use of a cell phone while driving can increase the risk of motor vehicle crashes. In a study using a driver-training simulator, cell phone users were about 20% slower to respond to sudden hazards than were other drivers, and they were about twice as likely to rear-end a braking car in front of them. Among young adult drivers who used a cell phone, reaction time was reduced to the level of a 70-year-old driver who was not using a phone. It is unclear,

however, if bans such as those in New York will help reduce the risk: Studies have not found much, if any, benefit in the use of headsets. It appears that the mental distraction of talking is a factor in crashes rather than holding the phone.

The safest strategy is not to use your phone while driving. For people who live in areas where cell phone use is legal while driving and who choose to use a phone, the following strategies may help increase safety:

• Be familiar with your phone and its functions, especially speed dial and redial.

• Store frequently called numbers on speed dial so you can place calls without looking at the phone.

• If your phone has voice-activated dialing, use it.

• Use a hands-free device so you can keep both hands on the steering wheel.

• Let the person you are speaking to know you are driving and be prepared to end the call at any time.

• Don't place or answer calls in heavy traffic or hazardous weather conditions.

• Don't take notes or look up phone numbers while driving.

• Time calls so that you can place them when you are at a stop.

• Never engage in stressful or emotional conversations while on the road. If you are discussing a complicated or emotional matter, pull off the road to complete your conversation.

Text messaging and e-mail are potentially even more distracting than talking on a cell phone. Washington, Minnesota, Alaska, California, Connecticut, Louisiana, New Jersey, and the District of Columbia prohibit text messaging while driving.

---

sober drivers using cell phones can perform worse than drivers who are inebriated. Five states (New York, New Jersey, California, Washington, and Connecticut) and the District of Columbia have banned the use of handheld phones while driving (see the box "Cell Phones and Distracted Driving").

ALCOHOL AND OTHER DRUGS Alcohol is involved in about 40% of all fatal crashes. Alcohol-impaired driving is illegal in all states; the legal limit for blood alcohol concentration (BAC) is 0.08%, but people can be impaired at much lower BACs. The combination of fatigue and alcohol use increases the risk even further. Because alcohol affects reason and judgment as well as the ability to make fast, accurate, and coordinated movements, a person who has been drinking will be less likely to recognize that he or she is impaired. Use of many over-the-counter and all psychoactive drugs is potentially dangerous if you drive.

SAFETY BELTS, AIR BAGS, AND CHILD SAFETY SEATS Although some type of mandatory safety belt law is in effect in 49 states (excluding New Hampshire) and the District of Columbia, only about 82% of motor vehicle occupants use safety belts even though they are the single most effective way to reduce the risk of crash-related death. If you wear a combination lap and shoulder belt, your chance of surviving a crash is three to four times better than that of a person who doesn't wear one.

Some people think that if they are involved in a crash they are better off being thrown free of their vehicle. In fact, the chances of being killed are 25 times greater if you are thrown from a vehicle. Safety belts also provide protection from the second collision: If a car is traveling at 65 mph and hits another vehicle, the car stops first; then the occupants stop because they, too, are traveling at 65 mph. The second collision occurs when occupants hit something inside the car, such as the dashboard or windshield. The safety belt stops the second collision from occurring and spreads the collision's force over the body.

Since 1998, all new cars and light trucks have been equipped with dual air bags—one for the driver and one for the front passenger. Many vehicles also offer optional side air bags, which further reduce the risk of injury. Although air bags provide supplementary protection in the event of a collision, most are useful only in head-on collisions. They also deflate immediately after inflating and therefore do not provide protection in collisions involving multiple impacts. Air bags are not a replacement for safety belts; everyone in a vehicle should buckle up.

Air bags deploy forcefully and can injure a child or short adult who is improperly restrained or sitting too close to the dashboard, although second-generation air bags are somewhat safer for children than the older devices. To ensure that air bags work safely, always follow these basic guidelines: Place infants in rear-facing infant seats in the back seat, transport children age 12 and under in the back seat, always use safety belts or appropriate safety seats, and keep 10 inches between the air bag cover and the breastbone of the driver or passenger. If necessary, adjust the steering wheel or use seat cushions to ensure that an inflating air bag will hit a person in the chest and not in the face. Children who have outgrown child safety seats but are still too small for adult safety belts alone (usually age 4–8) should be secured using booster seats that ensure that the safety belt is positioned low across the waist.

Preventing Motor Vehicle Injuries About 75% of all motor vehicle collisions occur within 25 miles of home and at speeds lower than 40 mph. Strategies for preventing motor vehicle injuries include the following:

- Obey the speed limit.
- Always wear a safety belt.
- Never drive under the influence of alcohol or other drugs, or ride with a driver who is.
- Keep your car in good working order.
- Always allow enough following distance. Use the 3-second rule: When the vehicle ahead passes a reference point, count out 3 seconds. If you pass the reference point before you finish counting, drop back and allow more following distance.
- Always increase your following distance and slow down if weather or road conditions are poor.
- Choose interstate highways rather than rural roads. Highways are much safer because of better visibility, wider lanes, fewer surprises, and other factors.
- Always signal when turning or changing lanes.
- Stop completely at stop signs. Follow all traffic laws.
- Take special care at intersections. Look left, right, and then left again. Make sure you have time to complete your maneuver in the intersection.
- Don't pass on two-lane roads unless you're in a designated passing area and have a clear view ahead.

Motorcycles and Mopeds About one out of every ten traffic fatalities among people age 15–34 involves someone riding a motorcycle. Injuries from motorcycle collisions are generally more severe than those involving automobiles because motorcycles provide little, if any, protection. Moped riders face additional challenges. Mopeds usually have a maximum speed of 30–35 mph and have

less power for maneuverability, especially in an emergency. Strategies for preventing motorcycle and moped injuries include the following:

- Wear light-colored clothing, drive with your headlights on, and correctly position yourself in traffic.
- Develop the necessary skills. Lack of skill is a major factor in motorcycle and moped injuries. Skidding from improper braking is the most common cause of loss of control.
- Wear a helmet. Helmets should be marked with the DOT symbol, certifying that they conform to federal safety standards established by the Department of Transportation. Helmet use is required by law in nearly half of the states.
- Protect your eyes with goggles, a face shield, or a windshield.
- Drive defensively, particularly when changing lanes and at intersections, and never assume that other drivers can see you.

Bicycles According to a 2006 estimate, bicycle crashes send more than 500,000 people to emergency rooms each year and result in about 1000 fatalities. Bicycle injuries result primarily from riders not knowing or understanding the rules of the road, failing to follow traffic laws, not having sufficient skill or experience to handle traffic conditions, or being intoxicated. Bicycles are considered vehicles; bicyclists must obey all traffic laws that apply to automobile drivers, including stopping at traffic lights and stop signs.

Head injuries are involved in about two-thirds of all bicycle-related deaths. Wearing a helmet reduces the risk of head injury by 85%, but only 50% of cyclists wear helmets (see the box "Choosing a Bicycle Helmet" on page 388). Safe cycling strategies include the following:

- Wear safety equipment, including a helmet, eye protection, gloves, and proper footwear. Secure the bottom of your pant legs with clips, so they don't get tangled in the chain.
- Wear light-colored, reflective clothing. Equip your bike with reflectors, and use lights, especially at night or when riding in wooded or other dark areas.
- Ride with the flow of traffic, not against it, and follow all traffic laws. Use bike paths when they are available.
- Ride defensively; never assume that drivers have seen you. Be especially careful when turning or crossing at corners and intersections. Watch for cars turning right.
- Stop at all traffic lights and stop signs. Know and use hand signals.
- Continue pedaling at all times when moving (no coasting) to help keep the bike stable and to maintain your balance.

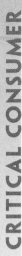

Choosing a Bicycle Helmet

Wearing a bicycle helmet can help you avoid serious head injury, brain damage, or even death in the event of a collision or fall. Helmets have a layer of stiff foam, which absorbs shock and cushions a blow to your head, covered by a thin plastic shell that will skid along the ground. For maximum protection, it's important to select a correctly fitting helmet. When you go shopping, remember the four S's: size, strap, straight, and sticker.

• *Size:* Try on several different sizes before making your selection; it may take several tries before you find the most comfortable fit. The helmet should be very snug but not overly tight on your head. Pads are usually provided to help adjust the fit. A good salesperson can also help you get the right fit. When

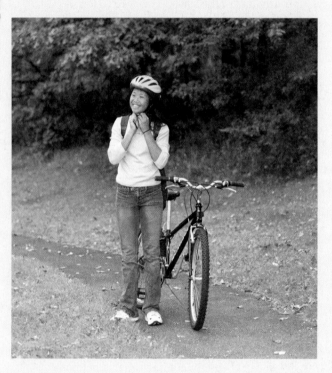

the helmet is strapped onto your head, it should not move more than an inch in any direction, and you should not be able to pull or twist it off no matter how hard you try.

• *Strap:* Be sure that the chin strap fits snugly under your chin and that the V in the strap meets under your ear. Avoid thin straps, which can be uncomfortable. Check to be sure that the buckle is strong and won't pop open and that the straps are sturdy.

• *Straight:* The helmet should sit straight on your head, not tilted back or forward. A rule of thumb is that the rim should be about two finger widths above your eyebrows (depending on the height of your forehead).

• *Sticker:* Since March 1999, helmets sold in the United States must meet uniform safety standards established by the U.S. Consumer Product Safety Commission (CPSC). Look for a sticker or label that says the helmet meets the CPSC standard. If a helmet does not have one, it does not meet federal safety standards and should not be used.

You are more likely to wear your helmet if it is comfortable, so be sure that vents on the helmet provide airflow to promote cooling and sweat control. You will be safer with a brightly colored helmet that makes you more visible to drivers, especially in rainy, foggy, or dark conditions. Reflective tape will also increase your visibility. Finally, a helmet is a good place to put emergency information (your name, address, and phone number, plus any emergency medical conditions and an emergency contact).

If you are involved in a crash, replace your helmet. Even if the helmet doesn't have any visible signs of damage, its ability to protect your head may be compromised.

SOURCES: Bicycle Helmet Safety Institute. 2009. *A Consumer's Guide to Bicycle Helmets* (http://www.helmets.org/guide.htm; retrieved February 21, 2009); Bicycle Helmet Safety Institute. 2007. *How to Fit a Bicycle Helmet* (http://www.helmets.org/fit.htm; retrieved February 21, 2009).

Home Injuries

The most common fatal **home injuries** are the result of falls, fires, poisoning, suffocation, and unintentional shootings.

Falls   Most deaths occurring from falls involve falling on stairs or steps or from one level to another. Falls also occur on the same level, from tripping, slipping, or stumbling. Alcohol is a contributing factor in many falls. Strategies for preventing falls include the following:

• Install handrails and nonslip surfaces in the shower and bathtub.

• Keep floors, stairs, and outside areas clear of objects or conditions that could cause slipping or tripping, such as ice, snow, electrical cords, and toys.

• Put a light switch by the door of every room so no one has to walk across a room to turn on a light.

Use night lights in bedrooms, halls, stairs, and bathrooms.

• When climbing a ladder, use both hands. Never stand higher than the third step from the top. When using a stepladder, make sure the spreader brace is in the locked position. With straight ladders, set the base out 1 foot for every 4 feet of height. Don't use chairs to reach things.

• If there are small children in the home, place gates at the top and bottom of stairs. Never leave a baby unattended on a bed or table. Install window guards to prevent children from falling out of windows.

Fires   A death caused by a residential fire occurs every 143 minutes. Cooking is the leading cause of home fire injuries; careless smoking is the leading cause of fire deaths, followed by problems with heating equipment and arson. To prevent fires, it's important to dispose of all cigarettes in ashtrays and to never smoke in bed. Other strategies include proper maintenance of fireplaces, furnaces, heaters, chimneys, and electrical outlets, cords, and appliances. If you use a portable heater, keep it at least 3 feet away from curtains, bedding, or anything else that might catch fire. Never leave heaters on unattended.

It's important to be adequately prepared to handle fire-related situations. Plan at least two escape routes out of each room, and designate a location outside the home as a meeting place. For practice, stage a home fire drill; do it at night, as that's when most deadly fires occur.

Install smoke detectors on every level of your home. Your risk of dying in a fire is almost twice as high if you do not use them. Clean the detectors and check the batteries once a month, and replace the batteries at least once a year. These strategies can help prevent injuries in a fire:

- Get out as quickly as possible, and go to the designated meeting place. Don't stop for a keepsake or a pet. Never hide in a closet or under a bed. Once outside, count heads to see if everyone is out. If you think someone is still inside the burning building, tell the firefighters. Never go back inside a burning building.

- If you're trapped in a room, feel the door. If it is hot or if smoke is coming in through the cracks, don't open it; use the alternative escape route. If you can't get out, go to the window and shout for help.

- Smoke inhalation is the largest cause of death and injury in fires. To avoid inhaling smoke, crawl along the floor away from the heat and smoke. Cover your mouth and nose, ideally with a wet cloth, and take short, shallow breaths.

- If your clothes catch fire, don't run. Drop to the ground, cover your face, and roll back and forth to smother the flames. Remember: stop-drop-roll.

Poisoning More than 2.4 million poisonings and over 19,000 poison-related deaths occur every year in the United States. Poisons come in many forms, some of which are not typically considered poisons. For example, even honey can be poisonous to children less than a year old. Medications are safe when used as prescribed, but overdosing or incorrectly combining medications with another substance may result in poisoning. Other poisonous substances include cleaning agents, petroleum-based products, insecticides and herbicides, cosmetics, nail polish and remover, and many houseplants. All potentially poisonous substances should be used only as directed and stored out of the reach of children.

The most common type of poisoning by gases is carbon monoxide poisoning. Carbon monoxide gas is emitted by motor vehicle exhaust and some types of heating equipment. The effects of exposure to this colorless, odorless gas include headache, blurred vision, and shortness of breath,

followed by dizziness, vomiting, and unconsciousness. Carbon monoxide detectors (similar to smoke detectors) are available for home use. To prevent poisoning by gases, never operate a vehicle in an enclosed space, have your furnace inspected yearly, and use caution with any substance or device that produces potentially toxic fumes.

Keep the national poison control hotline number (800-222-1222) in a convenient location. A call to the national hotline will be routed to a local Poison Control Center, which provides expert emergency advice 24 hours a day. If a poisoning does occur, it's important that you act quickly. Remove the poison from contact with the victim's eyes, skin, or mouth, or move the victim away from contact with poisonous gases. Call the Poison Control Center immediately for instructions; do not follow the emergency instructions on product labels because they may be incorrect. Do not induce vomiting. If you are advised to go to an emergency room, take the poisonous substance or container with you.

Suffocation and Choking Suffocation and choking account for about 3000 deaths annually. Children can suffocate if they put small items in their mouth, get tangled in their crib bedding, or get trapped in airtight appliances like old refrigerators. Keep small objects out of reach of children under age 3, and don't give them raw carrots, hot dogs, popcorn, gum, or hard candy. Examine toys carefully for small parts that could come loose; don't give plastic bags or balloons to small children.

Many choking victims can be saved with the **Heimlich maneuver.** The American Red Cross recommends abdominal thrusts as the easiest and safest thing to do when an adult is choking. Back blows in conjunction with abdominal thrusts are an acceptable procedure for dislodging an object from the throat of an infant.

Firearms About 40% of all unintended firearm deaths occur among people age 5–29. People who use firearms should remember the following:

- Always treat a gun as though it were loaded, even if you know it isn't.

- Never point a gun—loaded or unloaded—at anything you do not intend to shoot.

- Always unload a gun before storing it. Store unloaded firearms under lock and key, in a place separate from the ammunition.

home injuries Unintentional injuries and deaths that occur in the home and on home premises to occupants, guests, domestic servants, and trespassers; falls, burns, poisonings, suffocations, unintentional shootings, drownings, and electrical shocks are examples.

Heimlich maneuver A maneuver developed by Henry J. Heimlich, M.D., to help force an obstruction from the airway.

- Always inspect firearms carefully before handling.
- If you ever plan to handle a gun, take a firearms safety course first.
- If you own a gun, buy and use a gun lock designed specifically for that weapon.

Proper storage is critical. Do not assume that young children cannot fire a gun. Every year, about 120 Americans are unintentionally shot to death by children under 6. If you plan to handle a gun, avoid alcohol and drugs, which affect judgment and coordination.

Leisure Injuries

Leisure activities encompass a large part of our free time, so it is not surprising that **leisure injuries** are a significant health-related problem in the United States. Specific safety strategies for activities associated with leisure injuries include the following:

- Don't swim alone, in unsupervised places, under the influence of alcohol, or for an unusual length of time. Use caution when swimming in unfamiliar surroundings or in water colder than 70°F. Check the depth of water before diving. Make sure that residential pools are fenced and that children are never allowed to swim unsupervised.
- Always use a **personal flotation device** (also known as a life jacket) when on a boat.
- For all sports and recreational activities, make sure facilities are safe, follow the rules, and practice good sportsmanship. Develop adequate skill in the activity, and use proper safety equipment, including, where appropriate, a helmet, eye protection, correct footwear, and knee, elbow, and wrist pads.

- If using equipment such as skateboards, snowboards, mountain bikes, or all-terrain vehicles, wear a helmet and other safety equipment, and avoid excessive speeds and unsafe stunts. Playground equipment should be used only for those activities for which it is designed.
- If you are active in excessively hot and humid weather, drink plenty of fluids, rest frequently in the shade, and slow down or stop if you feel uncomfortable. Danger signals of heat stress include excessive perspiration, dizziness, headache, muscle cramps, nausea, weakness, rapid pulse, and disorientation.
- Do not use alcohol or other drugs during recreational activities—such activities require coordination and sound judgment.

Work Injuries

According to the Bureau of Labor Statistics, 4.1 million Americans suffered injuries on the job in 2006. Certain types of **work injuries**, including skin disorders and repetitive strain injuries, are increasing. Although laborers make up less than half of the workforce, they account for more than 75% of all work-related injuries and illnesses. Most fatal occupational injuries involve crushing injuries, severe lacerations, burns, and electrocutions; among women, the leading cause of workplace injury deaths is homicide.

Back problems accounted for about 280,000 work injuries in 2004; many of these could be prevented through proper lifting technique (Figure 16.1).

26 million Americans age 20–64 suffer frequent back pain.

—American Pain Foundation, 2007

QUICK STATS

- Avoid bending at the waist. Remain in an upright position and crouch down if you need to lower yourself to grasp the object. Bend at the knees and hips.
- Place feet securely about shoulder-width apart; grip the object firmly.
- Lift gradually, with straight arms. Avoid quick, jerky motions. Lift by standing up or pushing with your leg muscles. Keep the object close to your body.
- If you have to turn, change the position of your feet. Twisting is a common and dangerous cause of injury. Plan ahead so that your pathway is clear and turning can be minimized.
- Put the object down gently, reversing the steps for lifting.

Musculoskeletal injuries and disorders in the workplace include **repetitive strain injuries (RSIs)**. RSIs are caused

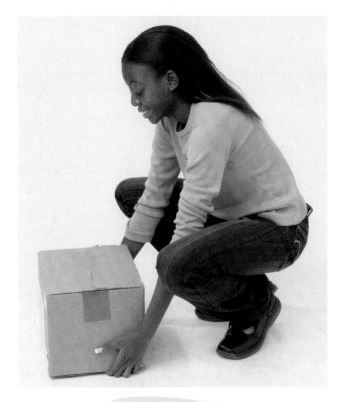

FIGURE 16.1 Correct lifting technique. Stay upright, bending at the knees and hips.

by repeated strain on a particular part of the body. Twisting, vibrations, awkward postures, and other stressors may contribute to RSIs. **Carpal tunnel syndrome** is one type of RSI that has increased in recent years due to increased use of computers (see the box "Carpal Tunnel Syndrome" on page 392).

(see the box "Carpal Tunnel Syndrome" on page 392)

THINKING ABOUT THE ENVIRONMENT

Every year, thousands of people are killed and injured by weather-related events such as floods and hurricanes. Earthquakes and tsunamis can cause massive destruction and loss of life, while leaving thousands or even millions of people homeless and injured.

In May 2008, a cyclone struck Myanmar (formerly Burma), leaving nearly 135,000 people dead or missing. That same month, an earthquake measuring 7.9 on the Richter scale struck Sichuan Province in China, killing 12,000 and injuring countless others.

Weather emergencies usually are not on such a vast scale. For example, about 60 Americans die each year after being struck by lightning, almost always in isolated incidents. According to the National Weather Service, 1159 tornadoes strike in the United States each year, causing an average of 62 deaths annually.

VIOLENCE AND INTENTIONAL INJURIES

Violence—the use of physical force with the intent to inflict harm, injury, or death upon oneself or another—is a major public health concern in the United States. According to the Federal Bureau of Investigation (FBI), over 1.4 million violent crimes occurred in the United States in 2007. Worldwide, interpersonal violence is the third leading cause of death among people age 15–44. In comparison to other industrialized countries, U.S. rates of violence are unusually high in only two areas—homicide and firearm-related deaths. The U.S. homicide death rate is four to ten times that of similar countries, and the firearm death rate is eight times that of other developed countries.

Factors Contributing to Violence

Most intentional injuries and deaths are associated with an argument or the committing of another crime. However, there are a great many forms of violence, and no single factor can explain all of them.

Social Factors Rates of violence vary by geographic region, neighborhood, socioeconomic level, and many other factors. According to the FBI, violence was highest in the South in 2007, followed closely by the West. Neighborhoods that are disadvantaged in status, power, and economic resources are typically the ones with the most violence. Rates of violence are highest among young people and minorities, groups that have relatively little power. In 2007, people under age 25 accounted for 45% of the arrests for violent crime in the United States and 50% of the arrests for homicide.

People who feel a part of society (have strong family and social ties), who are economically integrated (have a reasonable chance at getting a decent job), and who grow up in areas where there is a feeling of community (good schools, parks, and neighborhoods) are significantly less likely to engage in violence.

Studies have shown that the environment on college campuses can contribute to violence. The nature of college campuses—transitory communities rather than permanent places where people work and live together over

Carpal Tunnel Syndrome

Carpal tunnel syndrome (CTS) is a repetitive strain injury characterized by pressure on the median nerve in the wrist. It is the most commonly reported work-related medical problem, accounting for about half of all work-related injuries. Women are about twice as likely as men to be affected by CTS.

The median nerve travels from the forearm to the hand through a tunnel in the wrist formed by the carpal (wrist) bones and associated tendons and cov-ered by a ligament (see the figure). The median nerve can become compressed for a variety of reasons, including swelling of the surrounding tendons caused by pregnancy, diabetes, arthritis, or repetitive wrist motions during activities such as typing, cutting, or carpentry work. Symptoms of CTS include numbness, tingling, burning, and/or aching in the hand, particularly in the thumb and the first three fingers. The pain may worsen at night and may shoot up from the hand as far as the shoulder.

Many cases of carpal tunnel syndrome clear up on their own or with minimal treatment. Modification of the movement that is causing the problem is critically important. For example, adjusting the height of a computer keyboard so that the wrists can be held straight during typing can help relieve pressure on the wrists. CTS is often first treated by immobilizing the wrist with a splint during the night. People may also be given anti-inflammatory drugs or injections of cortisone in the wrist to reduce swelling. In a small percentage of severe cases, surgery to cut the ligament and reduce the pressure on the nerve may be recommended.

If you engage in activities like typing or cutting that involve repetitive motions, there are some strategies you can try to reduce your risk of developing carpal tunnel syndrome. Begin by modifying your work environment to reduce the stress on your wrists. Alternate activities to avoid spending long stretches of time engaged in the same motion. Warm up your wrists before you begin any repetitive motion activity, and take frequent breaks to stretch and flex your wrists and hands:

• Extend your arms out in front of you and stretch your wrists by pointing your fingers to the ceiling; hold for a count of five. Then straighten your wrists and relax your fingers for a count of five.

• With arms extended, make a tight fist with both hands and then bend your wrists so your knuckles are pointed toward the floor; hold for a count of five. Then straighten your wrists and relax your fingers for a count of five.

Repeat these stretches several times, and finish by letting your arms hang loosely at your sides and shaking them gently for several seconds.

SOURCES: Ly-Pen, D., et al. 2005. Surgical decompression versus local steroid injection in carpal tunnel syndrome: A one-year, prospective, randomized, open, controlled clinical trial. *Arthritis and Rheumatism* 52(2): 612–619; Carpal tunnel syndrome. 2002. *Journal of the American Medical Association* 288(10): 1310; American Academy of Orthopaedic Surgeons. 2007. *Ask an Orthopaedic Surgeon about Carpal Tunnel Syndrome* (http://orthoinfo.aaos.org/topic.cfm?topic=A00009; retrieved February 21, 2009).

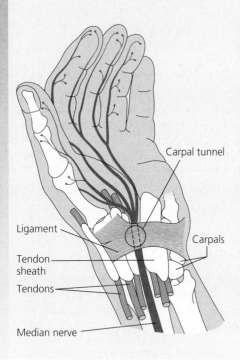

Carpal tunnel

Ligament

Carpals

Tendon sheath

Tendons

Median nerve

---

the long term—means that there is less incentive for people to cooperate and coexist amicably.

Violence in the Media The mass media play a major role in exposing audiences of all ages to violence as an acceptable and effective means of solving problems. Children may view as many as 10,000 violent acts on television and in movies each year. Computer and video games also include many violent acts, leading to concern that children's exposure to violence will make them more accepting or tolerant of it. The consequences of violence are depicted much less frequently.

Researchers have found that exposure to media violence at least temporarily increases aggressive feelings in children, making them more likely to engage in violent or fearful behavior; the direct, short-term effects on teens and adults are less clear. Parents should monitor the TV shows, movies, video games, music, and other forms of media to which children are exposed. Watching programs with children gives parents the opportunity to talk to children about violence and its consequences, to explain that violence is not the best way to resolve conflicts or solve problems, and to point out examples of positive behaviors such as kindness and cooperation.

Gender In most cases, violence is committed by men (Figure 16.2). Males are nine times more likely than females to commit murder and three times more likely than females to be murdered. Male college students are twice as likely to be the victim of violence as female students.

Women do commit acts of violence, including a small but substantial proportion of murders of spouses. This fact has been used to argue that women have the same capacity to commit violence as men, but most researchers note substantial differences. Men often kill their wives as the culmination of years of violence or after stalking them; they may kill their entire family and themselves at the same time. Women virtually never kill in such circum-

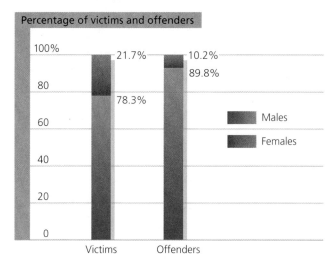

Percentage of victims and offenders

100%
21.7%   10.2%
80   89.8%
78.3%

60
Males
Females

40

20

0
Victims   Offenders

(a) Homicide victims and offenders by sex, 2007

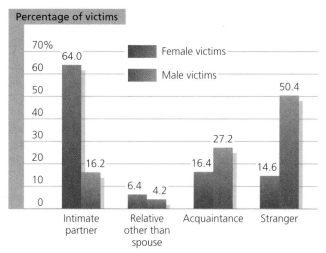

Percentage of victims

70%
64.0   Female victims
60   Male victims
50   50.4
40
30   27.2
20   16.2   16.4
14.6
10   6.4 4.2
0
Intimate   Relative   Acquaintance   Stranger
partner   other than
spouse

(b) Adult victims of violence by victim-offender relationship and sex
of victim

FIGURE 16.2   Facts about violence in the United States.

SOURCES: Federal Bureau of Investigation. 2008. *Crime in the United States 2007*. Washington, D.C.: U.S. Department of Justice; Tjaden, P., and N. Thoennes. 2000. *Full Report of the Prevalence, Incidence, and Consequences of Violence Against Women*. Washington, D.C.: U.S. Department of Justice.

stances; rather, they kill their husbands after repeated victimization or while being beaten.

Interpersonal Factors   Although most people fear attack from strangers, the majority of victims are acquainted with their attacker. Approximately 60% of murders of women and 80% of sexual assaults are committed by someone the woman knows. Crime victims and violent criminals tend to share many characteristics—that is, they are likely to be young, male, in a minority, and poor.

Alcohol and Other Drugs   Substance abuse and dependence are consistently associated with interpersonal violence and suicide. Intoxication affects judgment and may increase aggression in some people, causing a small

argument to escalate into a serious physical confrontation. On college campuses, alcohol is involved in about 95% of all violent crimes.

Firearms   Many criminologists feel that the high rate of homicide in the United States is directly related to the fact that we are the only industrialized country in which handguns are widespread and easily available. The use of a handgun can change a suicide attempt to a completed suicide and a violent assault to a murder.

Over 100,000 deaths and injuries occur in the United States

each year as a result of the use of firearms. Firearms are used in more than two-thirds of homicides, and studies reveal a strong correlation between the incidence of gun ownership and homicide rates for a given area of the country. Over half of all suicides involve a firearm, and people living in households in which guns are kept have a risk of suicide that is five or more times greater than that of people living in households without guns.

Assault

Assault is the use of physical force by a person or persons to inflict injury or death on another; homicide, aggravated assault, and robbery are examples of assault. The victims of assaultive injuries and their perpetrators tend to resemble one another in terms of ethnicity, educational

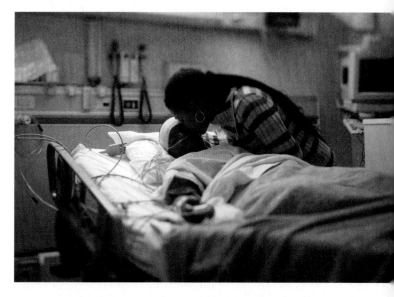

The victims of most types of violence are statistically likely to be young (under age 25), poor, in a minority, urban, and—except for rape and domestic violence—male.

background, psychological profile, and reliance on weapons. In many cases, the victim actually magnifies the confrontation through the use of a weapon.

Homicide

The FBI estimates that nearly 17,000 Americans were murdered in 2007. Men, teenagers, young adults, and members of minority groups, particularly African Americans and Latinos, are most likely to be murder victims. The murder rate for black males is about six times higher than the rate for the U.S. population as a whole. Poverty and unemployment have been identified as key factors in homicide, and this may account for the high rates of homicide among blacks and other minority groups. Most homicides are committed with a firearm, occur during an argument, and occur among people who know one another. Intrafamilial homicide, where the perpetrator and victim are related, accounts for about one out of every eight homicides. About 40% of family homicides are committed by spouses, usually following a history of physical and emotional abuse directed at the woman.

Gang-Related Violence

Gangs are most frequently associated with large cities, but gang activity also extends to the suburbs and even to rural areas. It is estimated that more than 1 million Americans belong to gangs; the average age for joining a gang is 14. Gang members are more likely than non–gang members to possess weapons, and violence may result from conflicts over territory or illegal activities. Gangs are more common in areas that are poor and suffer from high unemployment, population density, and crime. In these areas, an individual may feel that his or her hope of legitimate success in life is out of reach and know that involvement in the drug market makes some gang members rich. Often, gangs serve as a mechanism for companionship, self-esteem, support, and security; indeed, in some areas gang membership may be viewed as the only possible means of survival.

Hate Crimes

When bias against another person's race or ethnicity, national origin, religion, sexual orientation, or disability motivates a criminal act, the offense is classified as a hate crime. Hate crimes may be committed against people or property. Those against people may include intimidation, assault, and even rape or murder. Crimes against property most frequently involve graffiti, the desecration of churches or synagogues, cross burnings, and other acts of vandalism or property damage.

About 7700 hate crimes were reported in 2006; many more go unreported. Crimes against people made up about 60% of all incidents; intimidation and assault are the most common offenses. Racial or ethnic bias was cited as a motivation in 52% of the hate crimes reported in 2006. National origin or ethnicity was cited in 13% of cases, religion in 19%, and sexual orientation in 16%. But research indicates that a substantial number of hate crimes are committed by males under age 20. Hate crimes are frequently, but not always, associated with fringe groups that have extremist ideologies, such as the Ku Klux Klan and neo-Nazi groups. The rapid growth of hate sites on the Internet is another area of concern.

School Violence

Tragedies like the shootings at Columbine High School in Colorado and Red Lake Senior High School in Minnesota have brought national attention to the problem of violence in the schools. According to the National School Safety Center, about 450 school-associated violent deaths of students, faculty, and administrators have occurred since 1992. Most of these deaths occurred in urban areas, at high schools, and involved use of a firearm. As with other types of violence, both victims and offenders were predominantly young men. Homicide and suicide are the most serious but least common types of violence in schools; an estimated 400,000 less serious incidents of violence and crime occur each year, including theft, vandalism, and fights not involving weapons.

Children are actually much safer at school than away from it. Less than 1% of all homicides among youths age 5–19 occur at school, and 90% of schools report no incidents of serious violence. Children and adolescents are more likely to be killed by an adult in their own home or away from school than they are to die as a result of school-associated violence. According to the CDC, the overall number of violent incidents has decreased steadily since 1992, but the number of multiple-victim events may have increased.

Schools are basically safe places overall, but there are ways to identify at-risk youths and improve safety for all students. Characteristics associated with youths who have caused school-associated violent deaths include uncontrollable angry outbursts, violent and abusive language and behavior, isolation from peers, depression and irritability, access to and preoccupation with weapons, and lack of support and supervision from adults. Being a victim of teasing, bullying, or social exclusion (rejection) may lead to aggressive behavior and violence. Recommendations for reducing school violence include offering classroom training in anger management, social skills, and improved self-control; providing mental health and social services for students in need; developing after-school programs that help students build self-esteem and make friends; and keeping guns out of the hands of children and out of schools.

Workplace Violence

Each year U.S. workers experience an average of 1.5 million minor assaults, 400,000 serious assaults, 85,000 robberies, 50,000 sexual assaults, and 700 homicides. Most of the perpetrators of workplace violence are white males over

DIMENSIONS OF DIVERSITY

In 2002, the World Health Organization (WHO) issued its *World Report on Violence and Health,* which examines the magnitude and impact of violence throughout the world. Each year, more than 1.6 million people die from violent acts: Suicide claims a life every 40 seconds, homicide every minute, and armed conflict every 2 minutes. Violence is among the leading causes of death for people age 15–44, accounting for 14% of deaths among males and 7% of deaths among females. Millions more victims of violence survive but are left with physical, psychological, and reproductive problems. Beyond individual misery, violence has devastating social and economic consequences.

Interpersonal Violence

WHO defines *interpersonal violence* as the intentional use of physical force or power, threatened or actual, against another person that is likely to result in injury, death, psychological harm, or deprivation. Each year, more than 500,000 people die from interpersonal violence, and more than 60 million children and elderly adults are maltreated. It's estimated that 10–70% of women experience physical violence at the hands of an intimate partner during their lifetime; in addition, forced prostitution, child marriage, sexual trafficking, and female genital mutilation are prevalent in some areas of the world.

Worldwide, adolescents and young adults are the primary victims and perpetrators of interpersonal violence. Individual risk factors for violence highlighted in the WHO report include being young,

male, and poor; being intoxicated; and having easy access to firearms. At the community and social levels, risk factors include low social capital (norms and networks that promote coordination and cooperation), high crime rates, rapid social change, poverty, poor rule of law and corruption, gender inequality, firearm availability, and armed conflict.

Collective Violence

WHO applies the term *collective violence* to violence inflicted by one group against another group to achieve political, economic, or social objectives. Collective violence includes armed conflict within or between states; genocide, repression, and other human rights abuses; terrorism; and organized violent crime. Characteristics of countries with increased risk of violent conflict include long-standing tensions between groups, a lack of democratic processes, unequal access to power, unequal distribution and control of resources, and rapid demographic changes.

In the twentieth century, an estimated 191 million people—well over half of them civilians—lost their lives directly or indirectly as a result of armed conflict, and many more were injured. In addition to directly causing deaths and injuries, collective violence destroys infrastructure and disrupts trade, food production, and vital services, thus setting the stage for famine, increased rates of infectious diseases, and mass movements of refugees. The resulting social turmoil also increases rates of interpersonal violence.

What Can Be Done?

The WHO report emphasizes that violence is neither an inevitable part of the human condition nor an intractable social problem. Rather, the wide variation in violence within and among nations over time suggests that violence is the product of a complex but modifiable set of social and environmental factors. Potential strategies to reduce violence include the following:

• Individual and relationship approaches to encourage healthy attitudes and behaviors, such as training in social, parenting, and relationship skills and conflict resolution.

• Community-based efforts to raise public awareness and address local social and material causes of violence, such as creating safe places for children to play and adopting community policing

• Societal approaches to change underlying cultural, social, and economic factors, such as new laws and international treaties, policy changes to reduce poverty and inequality, efforts to change harmful social and cultural norms (for example, ethnic discrimination or gender inequality), and disarmament and demobilization programs in countries emerging from conflict

SOURCES: World Health Organization. 2002. *The World Health Report 2002: Reducing Risks, Promoting Healthy Life.* Geneva: World Health Organization; World Health Organization. 2002. *World Report on Violence and Health.* Geneva: World Health Organization.

age 21. Firearms are used in more than 80% of workplace homicides, and the majority of these homicides occur during the commission of a robbery or other crime. Police and corrections officers have the most dangerous jobs, followed by taxi drivers, security guards, bartenders, mental health professionals, and workers at gas stations and convenience and liquor stores. General crime prevention strategies, including use of surveillance cameras and silent alarms and limiting the amount of cash on hand, can help reduce workplace violence related to robberies. Clear guidelines about acceptable behavior and prompt action after any threats or incidents of violence can help control workplace violence.

Terrorism

In 2001, more Americans died as a result of terrorism than in any prior year; the attacks on September 11 killed more than 3000 people, including citizens of 78 countries. The FBI defines terrorism as the unlawful use of force or violence against persons or property to intimidate or coerce a government, the civilian population, or any segment thereof in furtherance of political or social objectives (see the box "Violence and Health: A Global View").

72 U.S. police officers were killed in the September 11, 2001, terrorist attacks.

—FBI, 2007

The fear of potential threats such as terrorist strikes or an outbreak of widespread violence—underscore the need for everyone to be prepared for an emergency. Two key elements of emergency preparedness are a well-stocked emergency supply kit and a well-reasoned emergency plan.

Emergency Supplies

An emergency supply kit should include everything you'll need to make it on your own for at least 3 days. You'll need nonperishable food, water, first aid supplies, essential medications, a battery-powered radio, toiletries, clothing, a flashlight or candles and matches, cash, keys, copies of important documents, and supplies for sleeping outdoors in any season/weather (blankets, sleeping bags, tent, and so on). Don't forget about special-needs items for infants, seniors, and pets.

In the case of certain types of terrorist attacks or industrial disasters, you may need supplies to "shelter in place"—to create a barrier between yourself and any dangerous airborne materials. These supplies might include filter masks or folded cotton towels that can be placed over the mouth and nose. Plastic sheeting and duct tape can be used to seal windows and doors.

You may want to create several kits of emergency supplies. The primary one would contain supplies for home use. Put together a smaller, lightweight version that you can take with you if you are forced to evacuate your residence and kits for your car and office.

A Family or Household Plan

You and the members of your household may not be together when a disaster strikes. You should have a plan about where to meet and how to communicate. Choose at least two potential meeting places—one in your neighborhood and one or more in other areas. Your community may also have set locations for community shelters.

Where you go may depend on the circumstances of the emergency situation. Use your common sense, and listen to the radio or television for instructions from emergency officials about whether to evacuate or stay in place. In addition, know all the transportation options in the vicinity of your home, school, and workplace; roadways and public transit may be affected, so keep walking shoes in your emergency kit.

Everyone in the household should also have the same emergency contact person to call, preferably someone who lives outside the immediate area. Local phone service may be significantly disrupted, so long-distance calls may be more likely to go through. Everyone should carry the relevant phone numbers and addresses at all times.

Check the emergency plans at any location where you or family members spend time, including schools and workplaces. For each location, know the safest place to be for different types of emergencies—for example, near load-bearing interior walls during an earthquake, the basement during a tornado, or a safe location miles away from a hurricane. Also know how to turn off water, gas, and electricity in case of damaged utility lines; keep the needed tools next to the shutoff valves.

Other steps you can take to help prepare for emergencies include taking a first aid class and setting up an emergency response group in your neighborhood or building. More complete information about emergency preparedness is available from the following sources:

American Red Cross (www.redcross.org)

Federal Emergency Management Agency (www.fema.gov)

U.S. Department of Homeland Security (www.ready.gov)

Terrorism can be either domestic, carried out by groups based in the United States, or international. It comes in many forms, including biological, chemical, nuclear, and cyber. Its intent is to promote helplessness by instilling fear of harm or destruction.

Terrorism-prevention activities occur at all levels of government. U.S. government efforts include close work with the diplomatic, law-enforcement, intelligence, economic, and military communities. The mission of the Department of Homeland Security is to help prevent, protect against, and respond to acts of terrorism on U.S. soil. It is coordinating efforts to protect electric and water supply systems, transportation, gas and oil, emergency services, the computer infrastructure, and other systems.

One step you can take is to put together an emergency plan and kit for your family or household that can serve for any type of emergency or disaster (see the box "Emergency Preparedness").

Family and Intimate Violence

Family violence generally refers to any rough and illegitimate use of physical force, aggression, or verbal abuse by one family member toward another. Such abuse may be physical and/or psychological in nature. Based on reported cases, an estimated 5–7 million women and children are abused each year in the United States.

Battering Studies reveal that 95% of domestic violence victims are women. Violence against wives or intimate

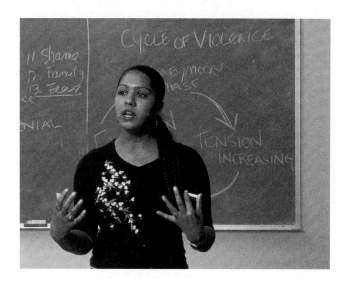

Education, counseling, and support can help the victims of family violence.

partners, or battering, occurs at every level of society but is more common at lower socioeconomic levels. It occurs more frequently in relationships with a high degree of conflict—an apparent inability to resolve arguments through negotiation and compromise. About 25% of women report having been physically assaulted or raped by an intimate partner. In more than 10% of cases, the domestic violence continues for 20 years or longer. The problem of intimate violence is even apparent among young people; each year, 1.5 million high school students are victims of physical violence while on a date.

At the root of much of this abusive behavior is the need to control another person. Abusive partners are controlling partners. They not only want to have power over another person, but also believe they are entitled to it, no matter what the cost to the other person. Abuse includes behavior that physically harms, arouses fear, prevents a person from doing what she wants, or compels her to behave in ways she does not freely choose.

In abusive relationships, the abuser (in most cases a man) usually has a history of violent behavior, traditional beliefs about gender roles, and problems with alcohol abuse. He has low self-esteem and seeks to raise it by dominating and imposing his will on another person. Research has revealed a three-phase cycle of battering, consisting of a period of increasing tension, a violent explosion and loss of control, and a period of contriteness in which the man begs forgiveness and promises it will never happen again. The batterer is drawn back to this cycle over and over again, but he never succeeds in changing his feelings about himself.

Battered women often stay in violent relationships for years. They may be economically dependent on their partners, feel trapped or fear retaliation if they leave, believe their children need a father, or have low self-esteem themselves. They may love or pity their husband, or they may believe they'll eventually be able to stop the violence.

They usually leave the relationship only when they become determined that the violence must end. Battered women's shelters offer physical protection, counseling, support, and other assistance.

Stalking and Cyberstalking Battering is closely associated with **stalking**, characterized by harassing behaviors such as following or spying on a person and making verbal, written, or implied threats. In the United States, it is estimated that 1 million women and 400,000 men are stalked each year; about 87% of stalkers are men. About half of female victims are stalked by current or former intimate partners; of these, 80% had been physically or sexually assaulted by that partner during the relationship. Stalking among female college students may be greater than that experienced by the general population. A stalker's goal may be to control or scare the victim or to keep her or him in a relationship. Most stalking episodes last a year or less.

The use of the Internet, e-mail, chat rooms, and other electronic communications devices to stalk another person is known as **cyberstalking.** As with offline stalking, the majority of cyberstalkers are men, and the majority of victims are women, although there have been same-sex cyberstalking incidents. Cyberstalkers may send harassing or threatening e-mails or chat room messages to the victim, or they may encourage others to harass the victim—for example, by impersonating the victim and posting inflammatory messages and personal information on bulletin boards or in chat rooms. Guidelines for staying safe online include the following:

- Never use your real name as an e-mail username or chat room nickname. Select an age- and gender-neutral identity.

- Avoid filling out profiles for accounts related to e-mail use or chat room activities with information that could be used to identify you.

- Do not share personal information in public spaces anywhere online or give it to strangers.

- Learn how to filter unwanted e-mail messages.

- If you experience harassment online, do not respond to the harasser. Log off or surf elsewhere.

If you receive unwanted online contact, make it clear to that person that you want all contact to stop. If harassment continues, contact the harasser's Internet service provider (ISP) by identifying the domain of the stalker's account (after the "@" sign); most ISPs have an e-mail address for complaints. Often, an ISP can try to stop the conduct by direct contact with the harasser or by closing his or her account. Save all communications for evidence, and contact your ISP and your local police department.

Violence Against Children Every year, at least 1 million American children are physically abused by their parents, and another 1 to 2 million are victims of neglect.

Parents who abuse children tend to have low self-esteem, to believe in physical punishment, to have a poor marital relationship, and to have been abused themselves (although many people who were abused as children do not grow up to abuse their own children). Poverty, unemployment, and social isolation are characteristics of families in which children are abused. External stressors related to socioeconomic and environmental factors are most closely associated with neglect, whereas stressors related to interpersonal issues are more closely associated with physical abuse. Single parents, both men and women, are at especially high risk for abusing their children.

Elder Abuse   Each year, 1–2 million older adults are abused, exploited, or mistreated by someone who is supposed to be giving them care and protection; only one in six incidents is reported. Most abusers are family members who are serving as caregivers. Elder abuse can take different forms: physical, sexual, or emotional abuse; financial exploitation; neglect; or abandonment. Neglect accounts for about 55% of reported cases. Physical abuse accounts for about 15% of reported cases, and financial exploitation for about 13%. Abuse often occurs when caring for a dependent adult becomes too stressful for the caregiver, especially if the elder is incontinent, has suffered mental deterioration, or is violent. Abuse may become an outlet for frustration. Many believe that the solution to elder abuse is support in the form of greater social and financial assistance, such as adult day-care centers and education and public care programs.

Sexual Violence

The use of force and coercion in sexual relationships is one of the most serious problems in human interactions. The most extreme manifestation of sexual coercion is rape, but sexual coercion occurs in many subtler forms, including sexual harassment.

Sexual Assault: Rape   Sexual coercion that relies on the threat and use of physical force or takes advantage of circumstances that render a person incapable of giving consent (such as when drunk) constitutes **sexual assault** or **rape.** When the victim is younger than the legally defined age of consent, the act constitutes **statutory rape,** whether or not coercion is involved. Coerced sexual activity in which the victim knows or is dating the rapist is often referred to as **date rape,** or *acquaintance rape.* Most victims know their assailant, but less than one-third of all sexual crimes are reported.

Any woman—or man—can be a rape victim. Between 100,000 and 130,000 cases of rape are reported each year. It is estimated that nearly 700,000 women are raped each year and that 1 in 6 women and 1 in 33 men has experienced an attempted or completed rape at some point in their lives. A study of college students found that between 1 in 4 and 1 in 5 college women experience a completed or attempted rape during their college years. Most male-on-male rapes do not occur in prison.

WHO COMMITS RAPE?   Men who commit rape may be any age and come from any socioeconomic group. Some rapists are exploiters in the sense that they rape on the spur of the moment and mainly want immediate gratification. Some attempt to compensate for feelings of sexual inadequacy and an inability to obtain satisfaction otherwise. Others are more hostile and sadistic and are primarily interested in hurting and humiliating a particular woman or women in general. Often, the rapist is more interested in dominance, control, and power than in sexual satisfaction.

Most women are in much less danger of being raped by a stranger than of being sexually assaulted by a man they know or date. Surveys suggest that as many as 25% of women have had experiences in which the men they were dating persisted in trying to force sex despite pleading, crying, screaming, or resisting. Surveys have also found that more than 60% of all rape victims were raped by a current or former spouse, boyfriend, or date.

Most cases of date rape are never reported to the police, partly because of the subtlety of the crime. Usually no weapons are involved, and direct verbal threats may not have been made. Victims of date rape tend to shoulder much of the responsibility for the incident, questioning their own judgment and behavior rather than blaming the aggressor.

FACTORS CONTRIBUTING TO DATE RAPE   Although the general status of women in society has improved, it is still a commonly held cultural belief that nice women don't say yes to sex (even when they want to) and that real men don't take no for an answer.

Men and women also differ in their perception of romantic encounters and signals. In one study, researchers found that men interpreted women's actions on dates, such as smiling or talking in a low voice, as indicating an interest in having sex, whereas the women interpreted the same actions as just being friendly. Men's thinking about forceful sex also tends to be unclear. One psychologist

TERMS

sexual assault or **rape**   The use of force to have sex with someone against that person's will.

statutory rape   Sexual interaction with someone under the legal age of consent.

date rape   Sexual assault by someone the victim knows or is dating; also called *acquaintance rape.*

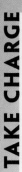

Preventing Date Rape

Guidelines for Women

• Believe in your right to control what you do. Set limits, and communicate these limits clearly, firmly, and early. Say no when you mean no.

• Be assertive with someone who is sexually pressuring you. Men often interpret passivity as permission.

• If you are unsure of a new acquaintance, go on a group date or double date. If possible, provide your own transportation.

• Remember that some men assume sexy dress and a flirtatious manner mean a desire for sex.

• Remember that alcohol and drugs interfere with clear communication about sex.

• Use the statement that has proven most effective in stopping date rape: "This is rape, and I'm calling the police."

Guidelines for Men

• Be aware of social pressure. It's OK to not score.

• Understand that no means no. Don't continue making advances when your date resists or tells you she wants to stop. Remember that she has the right to refuse sex.

• Don't assume sexy dress and a flirtatious manner are invitations to sex, that previous permission for sex applies to the current situation, or that your date's relationships with other men constitute sexual permission for you.

• Remember that alcohol and drugs interfere with clear communication about sex.

---

reports that men find "forcing a woman to have sex against her will" more acceptable than "raping a woman," even though the former description is the definition of rape.

DATE-RAPE DRUGS A 2006 study showed that drugs are a factor in more than 60% of sexual assaults and about 5% of victims are given date-rape drugs. The drugs used in date rapes include flunitrazepam (Rohypnol), gamma hydroxybutyrate (GHB), and ketamine hydrochloride ("Special K"). These drugs have a variety of effects, including sedation; if slipped surreptitiously into a drink, they can incapacitate a person within about 20 minutes and make her or him more vulnerable to assault. Rohypnol, GHB, and other drugs also often cause anterograde amnesia, meaning victims have little memory of what happened while they were under the influence of the drug. The Drug-Induced Rape Prevention and Punishment Act of 1996 adds up to 20 years to the prison sentence of any rapist who uses a drug to incapacitate a victim. Strategies such as the following can help ensure that your drink is not tampered with at a bar or party:

• Check with campus or local police to find out if drug-facilitated sexual assault has occurred in your area and, if so, where.

• Drink moderately and responsibly. Avoid group drinking and drinking games.

• Be wary of opened beverages—alcoholic or non-alcoholic—offered by strangers. When at an unfamiliar bar, watch the bartender pour your drink.

• If an opened beverage tastes, looks, or smells strange, do not drink it. If you leave your drink unattended, obtain a fresh drink when you return to your table.

• If you go to a party, club, or bar, go with friends. Have a prearranged plan for checking on each other visually and verbally. If you feel giddy or light-headed, get assistance.

Both males and females can take actions that will reduce the incidence of acquaintance rape; see the box "Preventing Date Rape" for specific suggestions.

DEALING WITH A SEXUAL ASSAULT Each situation is unique, and a woman should respond to the threat of rape in whatever way she thinks best. If a woman chooses not to resist, it does not mean that she has not been raped. If you are threatened by a rapist and decide to fight back, here is what Women Organized Against Rape (WOAR) recommends:

• Trust your gut feeling. If you feel you are in danger, don't hesitate to run and scream. It is better to feel foolish than to be raped.

• Yell—and keep yelling. It will clear your head and start your adrenaline going; it may scare your attacker and also bring help. Don't forget that a rapist is also afraid of pain and afraid of getting caught.

• If an attacker grabs you from behind, use your elbows for striking his neck, his sides, or his stomach.

• Try kicking. Your legs are the strongest part of your body, and your kick is longer than his reach. Kick with your rear foot and with the toe of your shoe. Aim low to avoid losing your balance.

• His most vulnerable spot is his knee; it's low, difficult to protect, and easily knocked out of place. Don't try to kick a rapist in the crotch; he has been protecting this area all his life and will have better protective reflexes there than at his knees.

- Once you start fighting, keep it up. Your objective is to get away as soon as you can.
- Remember that ordinary rules of behavior don't apply. It's OK to vomit, act crazy, or claim to have a sexually transmitted disease.

If you are raped, tell what happened to the first friendly person you meet. Call the police, tell them you were raped, and give your location. Try to remember as many facts as you can about your attacker; write down a description as soon as possible. Don't wash or change your clothes, or you may destroy important evidence. The police will take you to a hospital for a complete exam; show the physician any injuries. Tell the police simply, but exactly, what happened. Be honest, and stick to your story.

If you decide that you don't want to report the rape to the police, be sure to see a physician as soon as possible. You need to be checked for pregnancy and STDs.

THE EFFECTS OF RAPE Rape victims suffer both physical and psychological injury. For most, physical wounds heal within a few weeks. Psychological pain may endure and be substantial. Even the most physically and mentally strong are likely to experience shock, anxiety, depression, shame, and a host of psychosomatic symptoms after being victimized. Some victims experience rape trauma syndrome, a form of PTSD, characterized by fear, nightmares, fatigue, crying spells, and digestive upset. Self-blame is very likely; society has contributed to this tendency by perpetuating the myths that women can actually defend themselves and that no one can be raped if she doesn't want to be. Fortunately, these false beliefs are dissolving in the face of evidence to the contrary.

Many organizations offer counseling and support to rape victims. Look online or in the telephone directory under Rape or Rape Crisis Center for a hotline number to call. Your campus may have counseling services or a support group.

Child Sexual Abuse Child sexual abuse is any sexual contact between an adult and a child who is below the legal age of consent. Adults and older adolescents are able to coerce children into sexual activity because of their authority and power over them. Threats, force, or the promise of friendship or material rewards may be used to manipulate a child. Sexual contacts are typically brief and consist of genital manipulation; genital intercourse is much less common. Sexual abusers are usually male, heterosexual, and known to the victim. The

15% of rape and sexual assault victims are less than 12 years old.

—Rape, Abuse, & Incest National Network, 2008

abuser may be a relative, a friend, a neighbor, or another trusted adult acquaintance. Child abusers are often pedophiles, people who are sexually attracted to children. They may have poor interpersonal and sexual relationships with other adults and feel socially inadequate and inferior. One highly traumatic form of sexual abuse is **incest**, sexual activity between people too closely related to legally marry.

Child sexual abuse is often unreported. Surveys suggest that as many as 27% of women and 16% of men were sexually abused as children. An estimated 150,000–200,000 new cases of child sexual abuse occur each year. It can leave lasting scars; victims are more likely to suffer as adults from low self-esteem, depression, anxiety, eating disorders, self-destructive tendencies, sexual problems, and difficulties in intimate relationships.

If you were a victim of sexual abuse as a child and feel it may be interfering with your functioning today, you may want to address the problem. A variety of approaches can help, such as joining a support group of people who have had similar experiences, confiding in a partner or friend, or seeking professional help.

Sexual Harassment Unwelcome sexual advances, requests for sexual favors, and other verbal, visual, or physical conduct of a sexual nature constitute **sexual harassment** if such conduct explicitly or implicitly affects academic or employment decisions or evaluations; interferes with an individual's academic or work performance; or creates an intimidating, hostile, or offensive academic, work, or student living environment.

Extreme cases of sexual harassment occur when a manager, professor, or other person in authority uses his or her ability to control or influence jobs or grades to coerce people into having sex or to punish them if they refuse. A hostile environment can be created by conduct such as sexual gestures, displaying of sexually suggestive objects or pictures, derogatory comments and jokes, sexual remarks about clothing or appearance, obscene letters, and unnecessary touching or pinching.

12,510 sexual harassment charges were filed with the EEOC in 2007.

—U.S. Equal Employment Opportunity Commission, 2008

If you have been the victim of sexual harassment, you can take action to stop it. Be assertive with anyone who uses language or actions you find inappropriate. If possible, confront your harasser either in writing, over the telephone, or in person, informing him or her that the situation is unacceptable to you and you want the harassment to stop. If assertive communication doesn't work, assemble a file or log documenting the harassment, noting the details of each incident and information about any witnesses. You may

QUICK STATS

STATS

Staying Safe on Campus

College campuses can be the site of criminal activity and violence just as any other environment or living situation can be—and so they require the same level of caution and awareness that you would use in other situations. Two key points to remember: 80% of campus crimes are committed by a student against a fellow student, and alcohol or drug use is involved in 90% of campus felonies. Drinking or drug use can affect judgment and lower inhibitions, so be aware if you or another person is under the influence. Here are some suggestions for keeping yourself safe on campus:

• Don't travel alone after dark. Many campuses have shuttle buses that run from spots on campus such as the library and the dining hall to residence halls and other locations. Escorts are often available to walk with you at night.

• Be familiar with well-lit and frequently traveled routes around campus if you do need to walk alone.

• If you have a car, follow the usual precautions about parking in well-lit areas, keeping the doors locked while you are driving, and never picking up hitchhikers.

• Always have your keys ready as you approach your residence hall, room, and car. Don't lend your keys to others.

• Let friends and family members know your schedule of classes and activities to create a sort of buddy system.

• Be sure the doors and windows of your dorm room have sturdy locks, and use them.

• Don't prop open doors or hold doors open for nonstudents or nonresidents trying to enter your dorm. Be aware of non-residents around your dorm. If someone says that he or she is meeting a friend inside, that person should be able to call the friend from outside the building.

• Keep valuables and anything containing personal information—credit cards, wallets, jewelry, and so on—hidden. Secure expensive computer and stereo equipment with cables so that it can't be easily stolen. Use a quality U-shaped lock whenever you leave a bicycle unattended.

• Be alert when using an ATM, and don't display large amounts of cash.

• Stay alert and trust your instincts. Don't hesitate to call the police or campus security if something doesn't seem or feel right.

The Jeanne Clery Disclosure of Campus Security Policy and Campus Crime Statistics Act, named for a Lehigh University student who was murdered in her residence hall in 1986, requires colleges and universities to collect and report campus crime statistics. You can now review this information online at the Crime Statistics Web site of the U.S. Department of Education's Office of Postsecondary Education (http://ope.ed.gov/security/Search.asp).

discover others who have been harassed by the same person, which will strengthen your case. Then file a grievance with the harasser's supervisor or employer.

If your attempts to deal with the harassment internally are not successful, you can file an official complaint with your city or state Human Rights Commission or Fair Employment Practices Agency, or with the federal Equal Employment Opportunity Commission. You may also wish to pursue legal action under the Civil Rights Act or under local laws prohibiting employment discrimination. Very often, the threat of a lawsuit or other legal action is enough to stop the harasser.

What You Can Do About Violence

Violence in our society is a serious threat to our collective health and well-being. This is especially true on college campuses (see the box "Staying Safe on Campus"). Schools are now providing training for conflict resolution and are educating people about the diverse nature of our society, thereby encouraging tolerance and understanding.

Reducing gun-related injuries may require changes in the availability, possession, and lethality of the 8–12 million firearms sold in the United States each year. As part of the Brady gun control law, computerized instant background checks are performed for most gun sales to prevent purchases by convicted felons, people with a history of mental instability, and certain other groups. In some states, waiting periods are required in addition to the background checks. Some groups advocate a complete and universal federal ban on the sale of all handguns.

Safety experts also advocate the adoption of consumer safety standards for guns, including features such as child-proofing and indicators to show if a gun is loaded. Technologies are now available to personalize handguns to help prevent unauthorized use. Education about proper storage is also important.

incest Sexual activity between close relatives, such as siblings or parents and their children.

sexual harassment Unwelcome sexual advances, requests for sexual favors, and other conduct of a sexual nature that affects academic or employment decisions or evaluations; interferes with an individual's academic or work performance; or creates an intimidating, hostile, or offensive academic, work, or student living environment.

TERMS

PROVIDING EMERGENCY CARE

A course in **first aid** can help you respond appropriately when someone is injured. One important benefit of first aid training is learning what *not* to do in certain situations. For example, a person with a suspected neck or back injury should not be moved unless other life-threatening conditions exist. A trained person can assess emergency situations accurately before acting.

Emergency rescue techniques can save the lives of people who are choking, who have stopped breathing, or whose hearts have stopped beating. As described earlier, the Heimlich maneuver is used when a victim is choking. Pulmonary resuscitation (also known as rescue breathing, artificial respiration, or mouth-to-mouth resuscitation) is used when a person is not breathing. Cardiopulmonary resuscitation (CPR) is used when a pulse cannot be found. Training is required before a person can perform CPR; courses are offered by the American Red Cross and the American Heart Association (see the inside back cover).

A new feature of some of these courses is training in the use of automatic external defibrillators (AEDs), which monitor the heart's rhythm and, if appropriate, deliver an electrical shock to restart the heart. Because of the importance of early use of defibrillators in saving heart attack victims, these devices are being installed in public places, including casinos, airports, and many office buildings.

As a person providing assistance, you are the first link in the **emergency medical services (EMS) system.** Your responsibility may be to render first aid, provide emotional support for the victim, or just call for help. The basic pattern for providing emergency care is check-call-care:

- *Check the situation:* Make sure the scene is safe for both you and the injured person.
- *Check the victim:* Conduct a quick head-to-toe examination. Assess the victim's signs and symptoms, such as level of responsiveness, pulse, and breathing rate. Look for bleeding and any indications of broken bones or paralysis.
- *Call for help:* Call 9-1-1 or a local emergency number. Identify yourself and give as much information as you can about the condition of the victim and what happened.
- *Care for the victim:* If the situation requires immediate action (no pulse, shock, etc.), provide first aid if you are trained to do so.

TIPS FOR TODAY AND THE FUTURE

Protecting yourself from injuries means taking sensible safety precautions every day, and preparing yourself to deal with an emergency.

RIGHT NOW YOU CAN

- Check your home for any object or situation that could cause an injury, such as a tripping hazard, top-heavy shelves, and so on.
- Test the batteries in your home's smoke detectors, and change them if necessary. Test the detectors to make sure they work properly.
- If you ride a bike, check your helmet to ensure that it still fits properly and will protect you in a crash. If you have any doubts, throw it away and buy a new one.

IN THE FUTURE YOU CAN

- Get trained in CPR, rescue breathing, and the use of an automatic external defibrillator. If you have already had such training, take a refresher course.
- Be watchful for hazardous situations at your school and workplace. If you notice anything suspicious, report it to an appropriate person right away.

TERMS

first aid   Emergency care given to an ill or injured person until medical care can be obtained.

emergency medical services (EMS) system   A system designed to network community resources for providing emergency care.

Adopting Safer Habits

For the next 7–10 days, keep track of any mishaps you are involved in or injuries you receive, recording them on a daily behavior record like the one shown in Chapter 1. Count each time you cut, burn, or injure yourself, fall down, run into someone, or have any other potentially injury-causing mishap, no matter how trivial. Also record any risk-taking behaviors, such as failing to wear your safety belt or bicycle helmet, drinking and driving, exceeding the speed limit, putting off home or bicycle repairs, and so on. For each entry (injury or incidence of unsafe behavior), record the date, the time, what you were doing, who else was there and how you were influenced by him or her, what your motivations were, and what you were thinking and feeling at the time.

At the end of the monitoring period, examine your data. For each incident, determine both the human factors and the environmental factors that contributed to the injury or unsafe behavior. Were you tired? Distracted? Did you not realize this situation was dangerous? Did you take a chance? Did you think this incident couldn't happen to you? Was visibility poor? Were you using defective equipment? Then consider each contributing factor carefully, determining why it existed and how it could have been avoided or changed. Finally, consider what preventive actions you could take to avoid such incidents or to change your behaviors in the future.

As an example, let's say that you usually don't use a safety belt when you run local errands in your car and that several factors contribute to this behavior: You don't really think you could be involved in a crash so close to home, you only go on short trips, you just never think to use it, and so on. One of the contributing factors to your unsafe behavior is inadequate knowledge. You can change this factor by obtaining accurate information about auto crashes (and their usual proximity to a victim's home) from this chapter and from library or Internet research. Just acquiring information about auto crashes and safety belt use may lead you to examine your beliefs and attitudes about safety belts and motivate you to change your behavior.

Once you're committed, you can use behavior change techniques described in Chapter 1, such as completing a contract, asking family and friends for support, and so on, to build a new habit. Put a note or picture reminding you to buckle up in your car where you can see it clearly. Recruit a friend to run errands with you and to remind you about using your safety belt. Once your habit is established, you may influence other people—especially people who ride in your car—to use safety belts all the time. By changing this behavior, you have reduced the chances that you or your passengers will suffer a serious injury or even die in a vehicle crash.

SUMMARY

• Key factors in motor vehicle injuries include aggressive driving, speeding, a failure to wear safety belts, alcohol and drug intoxication, fatigue, and distraction.

• Motorcycle, moped, and bicycle injuries can be prevented by developing appropriate skills, driving or riding defensively, and wearing proper safety equipment.

• Most fall-related injuries are a result of falls at floor level, but stairs, chairs, and ladders are also involved in a significant number of falls.

• Careless smoking and problems with cooking or heating equipment are common causes of home fires. Being prepared for fire emergencies means planning escape routes and installing smoke detectors.

• The home can contain many poisonous substances, including medications, cleaning agents, plants, and fumes from cars and appliances.

• Performing the Heimlich maneuver can prevent someone from dying from choking.

• The proper storage and handling of firearms can help prevent injuries; assume that any gun is loaded.

• Many injuries during leisure activities result from the misuse of equipment, lack of experience, use of alcohol, and a failure to wear proper safety equipment.

• Most work-related injuries involve extensive manual labor; back problems and repetitive strain injuries are most common.

• Factors contributing to violence include poverty, the absence of strong social ties, the influence of the mass media, cultural attitudes about gender roles, problems in interpersonal relationships, alcohol and drug abuse, and the availability of firearms.

• Types of violence include assault, homicide, gang-related violence, hate crimes, school violence, workplace violence, and terrorism.

• Battering and child abuse occur at every socioeconomic level. The core issue is the abuser's need to control other people.

• Most rape victims are women, and most know their attackers. Factors in date rape include different standards of appropriate sexual behavior for men and women and different perceptions of actions.

- Sexual harassment is unwelcome sexual advances or other conduct of a sexual nature that affects academic or employment performance or evaluations or that creates an intimidating, hostile, or offensive academic, work, or student living environment.

- Steps in giving emergency care include making sure the scene is safe for you and the injured person, conducting a quick examination of the victim, calling for help, and providing emergency first aid.

BOOKS

Dacey, J. S., and L. B. Fiore. 2006. *The Safe Child Handbook.* San Francisco: Jossey-Bass. *A practical handbook for keeping your family safe and coping with the stress and fear associated with many real-world dangers.*

Henry, J., H. Larson, and J. Rubin. 2007. *Home Emergency Pocket Guide.* Tigard, OR.: Informed Publishing. *A small, spiral-bound guide that provides critical information to help in dealing with a variety of emergencies.*

MacPherson, J. 2003. *AAA Auto Guide: Driving Survival. How to Stay Safe on the Road.* Heathrow, Fl: AAA Publishing. *Provides helpful strategies for choosing and maintaining a safe vehicle and for handling a variety of driving situations.*

National Safety Council. 2007. *Standard First Aid, CPR, and AED.* Itasca, Ill.: National Safety Council. *An everyday guide to the most current first aid and emergency resuscitation techniques, with instructions for using automatic defibrillators.*

ORGANIZATIONS, HOTLINES, AND WEB SITES

American Bar Association: Domestic Violence. Provides information on statistics, research, and laws relating to domestic violence.
http://www.abanet.org/domviol/home.html

Consumer Product Safety Commission. Provides information and advice about safety issues relating to consumer products.
http://www.cpsc.gov

Insurance Institute for Highway Safety. Provides information about crashes on the nation's highways, as well as reports on topics such as speeding and crashworthiness of vehicles.
http://www.iihs.org

National Center for Injury Prevention and Control. Provides consumer-oriented information about unintentional injuries and violence.
http://www.cdc.gov/injury

National Center for Victims of Crime. An advocacy group for crime victims; provides statistics, news, safety strategies, tips on finding local assistance, and links to related sites.
http://www.ncvc.org

National Highway Traffic Safety Administration. Supplies materials about reducing deaths, injuries, and economic losses from motor vehicle crashes.
http://www.nhtsa.dot.gov

National Safety Council. Provides information and statistics about preventing unintentional injuries.
http://www.nsc.org

National Violence Hotlines. Provide information, referral services, and crisis intervention.
800-799-SAFE (domestic violence)
800-422-4453 (child abuse)
800-656-HOPE (sexual assault)

National Youth Violence Prevention Resource Center. Provides information about violence related to college students.
http://www.safeyouth.org/scripts/topics/college.asp

Occupational Safety and Health Administration. Provides information about topics related to health and safety issues in the workplace.
http://www.osha.gov

Prevent Child Abuse America. Provides statistics, information, and publications relating to child abuse, including parenting tips.
http://www.preventchildabuse.org

Rape, Abuse, and Incest National Network (RAINN). Provides guidelines for preventing and dealing with sexual assault and abuse.
http://www.rainn.org

Tolerance.Org: 10 Ways to Fight Hate on Campus. Offers suggestions for fighting hate and promoting tolerance; sponsored by the Southern Poverty Law Center.
http://www.tolerance.org/campus/index.jsp

World Health Organization: Violence and Injury Prevention. Provides statistics and information about the consequences of intentional and unintentional injuries worldwide.
http://www.who.int/violence_injury_prevention

The following sites provide statistics and background information on violence and crime in the United States:

Bureau of Justice Statistics: http://www.ojp.usdoj.gov/bjs
Federal Bureau of Investigation: http://www.fbi.gov
Justice Information Center: http://www.ncjrs.org

SELECTED BIBLIOGRAPHY

Browne, K. D., and C. Hamilton-Giachritsis. 2005. The influence of violent media on children and adolescents: A public-health approach. *Lancet* 365(9460): 702–710.

Carr, J. L. 2005. *American College Health Association Campus Violence White Paper.* Baltimore, Md.: American College Health Association.

Centers for Disease Control and Prevention. 2005. Increase in poisoning deaths caused by nonillicit drugs. *Morbidity and Mortality Weekly Report* 54(2): 33–36.

Centers for Disease Control and Prevention. 2006. Nonfatal injuries and restraint use among child passengers—United States, 2004. *Morbidity and Mortality Weekly Report* 55(22): 624–627.

Centers for Disease Control and Prevention. 2006. Notice to Readers: Buckle Up America Week—May 22–29, 2006. *Morbidity and Mortality Weekly Report* 55(19): 535–536.

Centers for Disease Control and Prevention. 2006. Physical dating violence among high school students—United States, 2003. *Morbidity and Mortality Weekly Report* 55(19): 532–535.

Commission for Global Road Safety. 2008. *Global Road Safety Fact File* (http://www.fiafoundation.com/commissionforglobalroadsafety/factfile/index.html; retrieved February 21, 2009).

Cummings, P., et al. 2006. Changes in traffic crash mortality rates attributed to use of alcohol, or lack of a seat belt, air bag, motorcycle helmet, or bicycle helmet, United States, 1982–2001. *Injury Prevention* 12(3): 148–154.

Federal Bureau of Investigation. 2007. *Hate Crime Statistics, 2006.* Washington, D.C.: U.S. Department of Justice.

Federal Bureau of Investigation. 2008. *Crime in the United States. Uniform Crime Reports, 2007.* Washington, D.C.: U.S. Department of Justice.

Graffunder, C. M., et al. 2004. Through a public health lens. Preventing violence against women: An update from the U.S. Centers for Disease Control and Prevention. *Journal of Women's Health* 13(1): 5–15.

Grossman, D. C., et al. 2005. Gun storage practices and risk of youth suicide and unintentional firearm injuries. *Journal of the American Medical Association* 293(6): 707–714.

Iudice, A., et al. 2005. Effects of prolonged wakefulness combined with alcohol and hands-free cell phone divided attention tasks on simulated driving. *Human Psychopharmacology* 20(2): 125–132.

National Center for Health Statistics. 2008. Deaths: Preliminary data for 2006. *National Vital Statistics Reports* 56(16).

National Center for Injury Prevention and Control. 2006. *Intimate Partner Violence Fact Sheet* (http://www.cdc.gov/ncipc/factsheets/ipvfacts.htm; retrieved September 21, 2006).

National Safety Council. 2008. *Injury Facts 2008.* Itasca, Ill.: National Safety Council.

National School Safety Center. 2008. *Report on School Associated Violent Deaths* (http://www.schoolsafety.us/pubfiles/savd.pdf; retrieved February 21, 2009).

National Traffic Safety Administration. 2007. *Traffic Safety Facts Research Note: Driver Cell Phone Use in 2006—Overall Results.* Washington, D.C.: National Traffic Safety Administration.

World Health Organization. 2004. *World Report on Road Traffic Injury Prevention.* Geneva: World Health Organization.

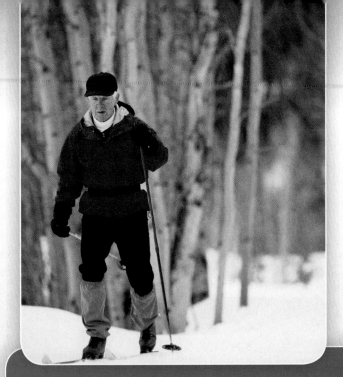

LOOKING AHEAD>>>>>

**AFTER READING THIS CHAPTER,
YOU SHOULD BE ABLE TO:**

- List strategies for healthful aging
- Explain the physical, social, and mental changes that may accompany aging and discuss how people can best confront these changes
- Describe practical considerations of older adults and caregivers, including housing, finances, health care, communication, and transportation
- Understand personal considerations in preparing for death, including making a will, assessing choices for end-of-life care, and making arrangements for a funeral or memorial service
- Describe the experience of living with a life-threatening illness and list ways to support a person who is dying
- Explain the grieving process and how support can be offered to adults and children who have experienced a loss

THE CHALLENGE OF AGING

17

Aging does not begin at some specific point in life, and there is no precise age at which a person becomes "old." Rather, aging is a normal process of development that occurs throughout life. If you optimize wellness during young adulthood, you can exert great control over the physical and mental aspects of aging, and you can better handle your response to events that might be out of your control. This chapter discusses the aging process, and it also addresses the process of dying and issues that arise around death.

GENERATING VITALITY AS YOU AGE

Biological aging includes all the normal, progressive, irreversible changes to one's body that begin at birth and continue until death. Psychological aging and social aging usually involve more abrupt changes in circumstance and emotion: relocating, changing homes, losing a spouse and friends, retiring, having a lower income, and changing roles and social status. These changes represent opportunities for growth throughout life.

Successful aging requires preparation. People need to establish good health habits in their teens and twenties. During their twenties and thirties, they usually develop important relationships and settle into a particular lifestyle. By their mid-forties, they generally know how much money they need to support the lifestyle they've chosen. At this point, they must assess their financial status and perhaps adjust their savings in order to continue enjoying that lifestyle after retirement. In their mid-fifties, they need to reevaluate their health insurance plans and may want to think about retirement housing. In their seventies and beyond, they need to consider ways of sharing their legacy with the next generation.

What Happens as You Age?

A significant number of older Americans describe themselves as being in poor health. Many of the characteristics

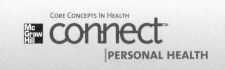

CORE CONCEPTS IN HEALTH

McGraw Hill connect™

|PERSONAL HEALTH

http://www.mcgrawhillconnect.com/personalhealth

Stem Cells

Nearly all the cells in the body are differentiated, meaning they are committed to specific functions. We have heart cells, skin cells, nerve cells—more than 260 kinds in all. Stem cells, on the other hand, are undifferentiated; they can renew themselves by continuing to divide in their undifferentiated state for long periods, or they can develop into specialized cells. Theoretically, stem cells can be used to create replacement cells for many diseased or injured tissues—for example, insulin-producing cells to treat diabetes, cardiac muscle cells to repair a damaged heart, or healthy brain cells for people with Parkinson's disease.

Embryonic Stem Cells

As their name suggests, embryonic stem cells are derived from embryos. About 4–5 days after fertilization, an embryo is a microscopic ball of cells, called a *blastocyst*. At this stage, the embryo contains about 30 stem cells; scientists can remove these cells and grow them, producing millions of embryonic stem cells. This method kills the embryo, however, and gives rise to the ethical debate that swirls around stem cell research. Most embryonic stem cells used in research are derived from eggs that have been fertilized in vitro, then donated to research; they are not taken from embryos fertilized in the womb.

Adult Stem Cells

Researchers believe that cellular repair is carried out by adult stem cells that lie dormant in tissues until they are needed. Adult stem cells seem to have some *plasticity* (the ability to differentiate), but there is only limited evidence to suggest that adult stem cells from one tissue can turn into functional cells of another type of tissue.

Another avenue of stem cell research is *somatic cell nuclear transfer*. In this technique, the nucleus from a somatic (body) cell is placed in an egg whose nucleus has been removed. The egg is allowed to grow into a blastocyst, and then the resulting stem cells are removed. This process, also called *therapeutic cloning*, produces a line of stem cells that are genetically matched to the original cell's donor; using these stem cells for transplant should eliminate problems with rejection. (This technique is distinct from reproductive cloning, in which an embryo is created through somatic cell transfer, then implanted into a woman's uterus and allowed to develop. This process results in an offspring who is genetically identical to the donor of the original somatic cell.)

The Stem Cell Controversy

Many experts believe that research into both embryonic and adult stem cells is needed to advance the therapeutic potential of stem cell research. However, the use of human embryos for such research is controversial. Some people advocate a complete ban; others would permit the use of existing stem cell lines, the use of extra embryos produced through in vitro fertilization, or the use of embryos created from eggs and sperm donated specifically for research.

Federal guidelines put in place under the Bush administration put severe restrictions on funding for stem cell research and limited researchers' access to stem cells. The result was a confusing patchwork of state laws regarding stem cells. President Obama promised to lift the federal ban on funding stem cell research.

In 2007, scientists at Wake Forest University found a new type of stem cell in amniotic fluid. This discovery could provide an alternative to embryonic stem cells. Additional research is being conducted, and preliminary tests show opportunities for future cell development and transplantation. Clinical trials have shown promise in treating heart failure, lupus, and other blood and bone diseases.

---

associated with aging are due not to aging but to neglect and abuse of our bodies and minds. These assaults lay the foundation for later psychological problems and chronic conditions like arthritis, heart disease, diabetes, hearing loss, and hypertension. But even with the healthiest behavior and environment, aging inevitably occurs as a result of biochemical processes we don't yet fully understand. Studies of healthy people indicate that functioning remains essentially constant until after age 70. Further research may help pinpoint the causes of aging and aid in the development of therapies to repair damage to aging organs (see the box "Stem Cells").

Life-Enhancing Measures: Age-Proofing

You can prevent, delay, lessen, or even reverse some of the changes associated with aging through good habits. Simple things you can do daily will make a vast difference to your level of energy and vitality—your overall wellness.

Challenge Your Mind Numerous studies show that older adults who stay mentally active have a lower risk of developing dementia. Reading, doing puzzles, learning language, and studying music are good ways to stimulate the brain. The more complex the activity, the more protective it may be.

Develop Physical Fitness Exercise significantly enhances both psychological and physical health. A 2006 study showed that elderly people who burned extra calories through daily activity had a much lower mortality rate than their peers who did not exercise. The positive effects of exercise include lower blood pressure and healthier cholesterol levels; better protection against heart attacks and an increased chance of survival should one occur; sustained or increased lung capacity; weight control through less accumulation of fat; maintenance of strength, flexibility, and balance; protection against osteoporosis and type 2 diabetes; increased effectiveness of the immune

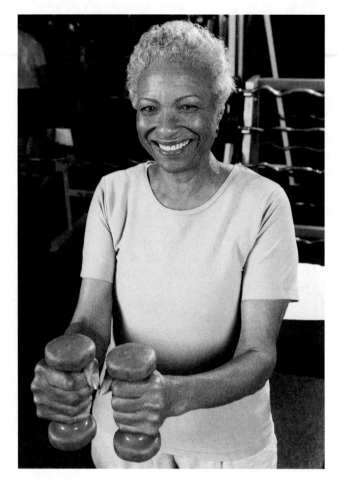

Regular exercise is a key to successful, healthy aging.

Table 17.1 — Exercise Recommendations for Older Adults

Type of Exercise	Days per Week	Duration
Moderate-intensity aerobic exercise	At least 5	At least 30 minutes
or		
Vigorous-intensity aerobic exercise	At least 3	At least 20 minutes
Strength training	At least 2	8–10 exercises, 10–15 repetitions each
Flexibility training	At least 2	At least 10 minutes

SOURCE: Nelson M. E., et al. 2007. Physical activity and public health in older adults: Recommendation from the American College of Sports Medicine and the American Heart Association. *Medical Science in Sports and Exercise* 39(8): 1435–1445.

system; and maintenance of mental agility and flexibility, response time, memory, and hand-eye coordination.

The stimulation that exercise provides also seems to protect against the loss of **fluid intelligence,** the ability to find solutions to new problems. Fluid intelligence depends on rapidity of responsiveness, memory, and alertness. Individuals who exercise regularly are also less susceptible to depression and dementia.

Regular physical activity is essential for healthy aging. Table 17.1 shows specific exercise recommendations for healthy adults age 65 or older and for adults age 50–64 with chronic conditions such as arthritis. Older individuals who have been sedentary should be encouraged to become more active. It's never too late to start exercising. Even in people over 80, endurance and strength training can improve balance, flexibility, and physical functioning and reduce the potential for dangerous falls.

Eat Wisely Good health at any age is enhanced by eating a varied diet full of nutrient-rich foods. Follow the recommendations in the 2005 Dietary Guidelines for Americans to get enough essential nutrients while maintaining a healthy weight.

- Get enough vitamin B-12 and extra vitamin D from fortified foods or supplements.

- To help control blood pressure, limit sodium intake to 1500 mg per day and get enough potassium (4700 mg per day).

- Consume foods rich in dietary fiber and drink plenty of water to help prevent constipation, which may occur in up to 20% of older adults. A diet rich in whole grains, vegetables, and fruits can meet the recommended goals for fiber.

- Pay special attention to food safety; older adults tend to be more susceptible to foodborne illness.

Maintain a Healthy Weight Weight management is especially difficult if you have been overweight most of your life. A sensible program of expending more calories through exercise, cutting calorie intake, or a combination of both will work for most people who want to lose weight, but there is no magic formula. Obesity is not physically healthy, and it leads to premature aging.

Control Drinking and Overdependence on Medications Alcohol abuse ranks with depression as a common hidden mental health problem, affecting about 10% of older adults. (The ability to metabolize alcohol decreases with age.) The problem is often not identified because the effects of alcohol or drug dependence can mimic disease, such as Alzheimer's disease. Signs of potential alcohol or drug dependence include unexplained falls or frequent injuries, forgetfulness, depression, and malnutrition. Problems can be avoided by not using alcohol to relieve anxiety or emotional pain and not taking medication when safer forms of treatment are available.

Don't Smoke The average pack-a-day smoker can expect to live about 13–14 years less than a nonsmoker. Furthermore, smokers suffer more illnesses that last longer, and they are subject to respiratory disabilities that limit their total vigor for many years before their death.

Premature balding, skin wrinkling, and osteoporosis have been linked to cigarette smoking.

Schedule Physical Examinations to Detect Treatable Diseases

When detected early, many diseases, including hypertension, diabetes, and many types of cancer, can be successfully controlled by medication and lifestyle changes. Regular testing for **glaucoma** after age 40 can prevent blindness from this eye disease. Recommended immunizations, including those for influenza and pneumococcus, can protect you from preventable infectious diseases.

Recognize and Reduce Stress

Stress-induced physiological changes increase wear and tear on your body. Cut down on the stresses in your life. Don't wear yourself out through lack of sleep, substance abuse or misuse, or overwork. Practice relaxation, using the techniques described in Chapter 2.

DEALING WITH THE CHANGES OF AGING

Just as you can act now to prevent or limit the physical changes of aging, you can also begin preparing yourself psychologically, socially, and financially for changes that may occur later in life.

Planning for Social Changes

Retirement marks a major change in the second half of life. As Americans' longevity has increased, people spend a larger proportion of their lives in retirement.

Changing Roles and Relationships

Changes in social roles are a major feature of middle age. Children become young adults and leave home, putting an end to daily parenting. Parents experiencing this empty-nest syndrome must adapt to changes in their customary responsibilities and personal identities. And although retirement may be a desirable milestone for most people, it may also be viewed as a threat to prestige, purpose, and self-respect—the loss of a valued or customary role—and will probably require some adjustment.

Retirement and the end of child rearing also bring about changes in the relationship between marriage partners. The amount of time a couple spends together will increase and activities will change. Couples may need a period of adjustment, in which they get to know each other as individuals again. Discussing what types of activities each partner enjoys can help couples set up a mutually satisfying routine of shared and independent activities.

Increased Leisure Time

Although retirement confers the advantages of leisure time and freedom from deadlines, competition, and stress, many people do not know how to enjoy their free time. If you have developed diverse interests, retirement can be a joyful and fulfilling period of your life. It can provide opportunities for expanding your horizons by giving you the chance to try new activities, take classes, and meet new people. Volunteering in your community can enhance self-esteem and allow you to be a contributing member of society.

The Economics of Retirement

Financial planning for retirement should begin early in life. People in their twenties and thirties should estimate how much money they need to support their standard of living, calculate their projected income,

and begin a savings program. The earlier people begin such a program, the more money they will have at retirement.

Financial planning for retirement is especially critical for women. American women are much less likely than men to be covered by pension plans, reflecting the fact that many women have lower-paying jobs or work part-time during their childbearing years. They tend to have less money vested in other types of retirement plans as well. Although the gap is narrowing, women currently outlive men by about 5–6 years, and they are more likely to develop chronic conditions that impair their daily activities later in life. The net result of these factors is that older women are almost twice as likely as older men to live in poverty. Women should investigate their retirement

fluid intelligence The ability to develop a solution when confronted with a new problem.

glaucoma A disease in which fluid inside the eye is under abnormally high pressure; can lead to the loss of peripheral vision and blindness.

plans and take charge of their finances to be sure they will be provided for as they get older.

Adapting to Physical Changes

Some changes in physical functioning are inevitable, and successful aging involves anticipating and accommodating these changes. Decreased energy and changes in health mean that older people have to develop priorities for how to use their energy. Rather than curtailing activities to conserve energy, they need to learn how to generate energy. This usually involves saying yes to enjoyable activities and paying close attention to the need for rest and sleep. Adapting, rather than giving up, favorite activities may be the best strategy for dealing with physical limitations. For example, if **arthritis** interferes with playing an instrument, a person can continue to enjoy music by taking up a different instrument or attending concerts.

Hearing Loss   The loss of hearing is a common physical change that can have a particularly strong effect on the lives of older adults. Hearing loss affects a person's ability to interact with others and can lead to a sense of isolation and depression. Hearing loss should be assessed and treated by a health care professional; in some cases, hearing can be completely restored by dealing with the underlying cause of hearing loss. In other cases, hearing aids may be prescribed.

Vision Changes   Vision usually declines with age. For some individuals this can be traced to conditions such as glaucoma or **age-related macular degeneration (AMD)**

that can be treated medically. Glaucoma is caused by increased pressure within the eye due to built-up fluid. The optic nerve can be damaged by this increased pressure, resulting in a loss of side vision and, if untreated, blindness. Medication can relieve the pressure by decreasing the amount of fluid produced or by helping it drain more efficiently. Laser and conventional surgery are other options. People over 60, African Americans over 40, and anyone with a family history of glaucoma are at risk.

AMD is a slow disintegration of the *macula,* the tissue at the center of the retina where fine, straight-ahead detail is distinguished. AMD affects more than 1.5 million Americans over 40 and is the leading cause of blindness in people over age 75. Losing this vision makes it difficult to read, drive, or perform other close-up activities. Risk factors for AMD are age, gender (women may be at higher risk than men), smoking, elevated cholesterol levels, and

family history. Some cases of AMD can be treated with laser surgery. Both glaucoma and AMD can be detected with regular screening.

By the time they reach their forties, many people have developed **presbyopia,** a gradual decline in the ability to focus on objects close to them. **Cataracts,** a clouding of the lens caused by lifelong oxidation damage (a by-product of normal body chemistry), may dim vision by the sixties.

Arthritis   More than 46 million American adults are estimated to have some form of arthritis. This degenerative disease causes joint inflammation leading to chronic pain, swelling, and loss of mobility. There are more than 100 different types of arthritis; osteoarthritis (OA) is by far the most common. In a person with OA, the cartilage that caps the bones in joints wears away, forming sharp spurs. It most often affects the hands and weight-bearing joints of the body—knees, ankles, and hips.

Strategies for reducing the risk of arthritis and, for those who already have OA, for managing it include exercise, weight management, and avoidance of heavy or repetitive muscle use. Exercise lubricates joints and strengthens the muscles around them, protecting them from further damage. Swimming, walking, and t'ai chi are good low-impact exercises. Maintaining an appropriate weight is important to avoid placing stress on the hips, knees, and ankles.

Many people with OA take medication to relieve inflammation and reduce pain. Nonsteroidal anti-inflammatory drugs like ibuprofen can help but can irritate the digestive tract; prescription drugs that relieve pain without damaging the stomach have been found to have other dangerous side effects. Acetaminophen can also reduce pain without upsetting the stomach, but exceeding the recommended dosage can cause liver damage.

Menopause   The natural process of menopause usually occurs during a woman's forties or fifties. The ovaries gradually stop functioning, estrogen levels drop, and eventually menstruation ceases. Several years before a woman stops menstruating, her periods usually become irregular, and she may experience hot flashes, vaginal dryness, sleep disturbances, and mood swings. This period, called *perimenopause,* can be troublesome for many women, some more than others. A 5-year study that concluded in 2006 showed that African American women are 60% more likely than white women to suffer aggravating or painful symptoms.

During the 1990s, about one-third of menopausal women used hormone replacement therapy (HT) to alleviate the symptoms of menopause and possibly prevent chronic diseases such as CVD and osteoporosis. The benefits of HT came into serious question, however, when a large-scale government-funded HT study (part of the Women's Health Initiative) was halted in 2002, after a significant number of participants suffered cardiovascular problems. This decision led many physicians to stop recommending HT for menopausal women. Newer data, however, are reopening the debate about HT. For example, a 2006 study published in the *Journal of Women's Health* reported that women who started HT near the beginning of menopause had a significantly lower risk of heart disease than women who did not take hormones. No benefit was found for women who started HT at older ages. Thus, age and the number of years a woman has been in menopause before starting therapy may be key considerations.

HT is effective for controlling severe menopausal symptoms, and it has been shown to reduce the risk of bone fractures and colon cancer. Decisions about HT should be made by individual women in consultation with their physicians, taking into account their overall health.

Osteoporosis As described in Chapter 9, **osteoporosis** is a condition in which bones become dangerously thin and fragile over time. Fractures are the most serious consequence of osteoporosis. Other problems associated with osteoporosis are loss of height and a stooped posture due to vertebral fractures, severe back and hip pain, and breathing problems.

Osteoporosis affects about 10 million Americans, 80% of whom are women. Women are at greater risk than men for osteoporosis because they have 10–25% less bone in their skeleton, and bone loss accelerates in women during the first 5–10 years after the onset of menopause because of the drop in estrogen production. Black women have higher bone density and fewer fractures than white or Asian women but may be at increased risk of osteoporosis due to lack of vitamin D (a condition caused by high levels of melatonin). Other risk factors include a family history of osteoporosis, early menopause (before age 45), abnormal or irregular menstruation, a history of anorexia, and a thin, small frame. Thyroid medication, corticosteroid drugs for arthritis or asthma, and long-term use of certain contraceptives can also have a negative effect on bone mass.

Preventing osteoporosis requires building as much bone as possible during your young years and then maintaining it as you age. Diet and exercise play key roles. Weight-bearing aerobic activities must be performed regularly throughout life to have lasting effects. Strength train-

ing improves bone density, muscle mass, strength, and balance, protecting against both bone loss and falls, a major cause of fractures. Even for people in their seventies, low-intensity strength training has been shown to improve bone density. Two other lifelong strategies for reducing the effects of osteoporosis are avoiding tobacco use and managing depression and stress. Bone mineral density testing can be used to gauge an individual's risk of fracture and help determine if any treatment is needed.

Handling Psychological and Mental Changes

Most older adults in good health remain mentally alert and retain their full capacity to learn and remember new information. Many people become smarter as they become older and more experienced.

Dementia Severe and significant brain deterioration in elderly individuals, termed **dementia**, affects about 7% of people under age 80 (the incidence rises sharply for people in their eighties and nineties). Early symptoms include slight disturbances in a person's ability to grasp the situation he or she is in. As dementia progresses, memory failure becomes apparent, and the person may forget conversations, the events of the day, or how to perform simple tasks. It is important to have any symptoms evaluated by a health care professional because some of the over 50 known causes of dementia are treatable.

The two most common forms of dementia among older people—**Alzheimer's disease** and multi-infarct dementia—are irreversible. Alzheimer's disease is characterized by changes in brain nerve cells. Multi-infarct dementia results from a series of small strokes or changes in the

arthritis Inflammation of a joint or joints, causing pain and swelling.

age-related macular degeneration (AMD) A deterioration of the macula (the central area of the retina) leading to blurred vision and sensitivity to glare; some cases can lead to blindness.

presbyopia The inability of the eyes to focus sharply on nearby objects, caused by a loss of elasticity of the lens that occurs with advancing age.

cataracts Opacity of the lens of the eye that impairs vision and can cause blindness.

osteoporosis The loss of bone density, causing bones to become weak, porous, and more prone to fractures.

dementia Deterioration of mental functioning (including memory, concentration, and judgment) resulting from a brain disorder; often accompanied by emotional disturbances and personality changes.

Alzheimer's disease A disease characterized by a progressive loss of mental functioning (dementia), caused by a degeneration of brain cells.

TERMS

Alzheimer's Disease

connect™

Alzheimer's disease (AD) is a fatal brain disorder that causes physical and chemical changes in the brain. As the brain's nerve cells are destroyed, the system that produces the neurotransmitter acetylcholine breaks down, and communication among parts of the brain deteriorates. Autopsies reveal that the interiors of the affected neurons are filled with clusters of proteins known as *tangles:* the spaces between the neurons are filled with protein deposits called *amyloid plaques.*

Almost 5 million Americans have Alzheimer's disease, and that number is expected to quadruple in the next 50 years, as more people live into their eighties and nineties. AD usually occurs in people over 60 but can occur in people as young as 40.

Symptoms

The first symptoms of AD are forgetfulness and inability to concentrate. A person may have difficulty performing familiar tasks at home and work and have problems with abstract thinking. As the disease progresses, people experience severe memory loss, especially for recent events. They may vividly remember events from their childhood but be unable to remember the time of day or their location. Depression and anxiety are also common.

In the later stages, people with AD are disoriented and may even hallucinate; some experience personality changes—becoming very aggressive or very docile. Eventually, they lose control of physical functioning and are completely dependent on caregivers. On average, a person will survive 8 years after the development of the first symptoms.

Causes

Scientists do not yet know what causes Alzheimer's disease. Age is the main risk factor, although about 10% of cases seem tied to inherited gene mutations. Inherited familial AD generally strikes people before age 65, while the more common late-onset AD occurs in people 65 and older. Some evidence suggests that many of the same factors that affect heart disease risk also apply to AD. In women, low levels of estrogen in the brain may contribute to AD.

People who regularly take nonsteroidal anti-inflammatory drugs (NSAIDs) like ibuprofen (often to control arthritis) and people who regularly consume fish rich in omega-3 fatty acids appear to have lower rates of AD, indicating a possible protective effect of substances that reduce inflammation. Some studies indicate that vitamin E and other antioxidants may reduce risk for AD or slow the progress of the disease, suggesting that

oxidative stress caused by free radicals may also play a role.

Diagnosis and Treatment

Currently, the only certain way to diagnose AD is to examine brain tissue during an autopsy. In most cases, physicians use a combination of medical history, neurological and psychological tests, physical exams, blood and urine tests, and a brain-imaging scan. Good early results have also been seen using a test that measures levels of a specific protein in spinal fluid, and less invasive blood tests to measure the same proteins are under development.

For people with mild to moderate AD, there are several drugs that provide modest improvements in memory. Several medications help maintain cognitive function by inhibiting the breakdown of the neurotransmitter acetylcholine but do not alter the course of the disease. These so-called cholinesterase inhibitors include Aricept (donepezil), Cognex (tacrine), Exelon (rivastigmine), and Reminyl (galantamine). Other medicines now under investigation may stop Alzheimer's progress before it can cause too much damage. People with AD may also be prescribed antidepressant or antianxiety medications.

---

brain's blood supply that destroy brain tissue (see the box "Alzheimer's Disease").

There is evidence that some cases of dementia are hereditary, but experts say genetics are not always a sure sign that a person will develop the disease. You can also take lifestyle steps to help ward off dementia, such as controlling weight and blood pressure, eating a balanced diet (including adequate B vitamins and omega-3 fatty acids), exercising, practicing stress reduction techniques, maintaining social contacts, and cultivating a variety of

mental pursuits, such as doing crossword puzzles. Strong evidence links the Mediterranean diet with reduced risk of Alzheimer's disease.

Grief Another psychological and emotional challenge of aging is dealing with grief and mourning. Aging is associated with loss—the loss of friends, peers, physical appearance, possessions, and health. Grief is the process of getting through the pain of loss, and it can be one of the loneliest and most intense times in a person's life. It can take a year or two or more to completely come to terms with the loss of a loved one. Unresolved grief can have serious physical and psychological or emotional health consequences and may require professional help.

Depression Unresolved grief can lead to depression, a common problem in older adults. If you notice the signs of depression in yourself or someone you know, consult a mental health professional. A marked loss of interest in usually pleasurable activities, decreased appetite, insom-

QUESTIONS FOR CRITICAL THINKING AND REFLECTION

Have you watched someone you know grow old? How did the aging process affect that person? In what ways did the person's physical and mental health change? In what ways were you affected, as you watched him or her age?

Why Do Women Live Longer?

Women live longer than men in most countries around the world, even in places where maternal mortality rates are high. In the United States, women on average can expect to live about 5 years longer than men. Worldwide, among people over age 100, women outnumber men about 9 to 1.

The reason for the gender gap in life expectancy is not entirely understood but may be influenced by biological, social, and lifestyle factors. Estrogen production and other factors during a woman's younger years may protect her from early heart disease and from age-related declines in the pumping power of the heart. Women may have lower rates of stress-related illnesses because they cope more positively with stress by seeking social support.

The news for women is not all good, however, because not all their extra years are likely to be healthy years. They are more likely than men to suffer from chronic conditions like arthritis and osteoporosis. Women's longer life spans, combined with the facts that men tend to marry younger women and that widowed men remarry more often than widowed women, means there are many more single older women than men. Older men are more likely to live in family settings, whereas older women are more likely to live alone. Older women are also less likely to be covered by a pension or to have retirement savings, so they are more likely to be poor.

Increased male mortality can be traced in part to higher rates of behaviors such as smoking and alcohol and drug abuse. Testosterone production may be partly responsible in that it is linked to aggressive and risky behavior and to unhealthy cholesterol levels. Men have much higher rates of death from car crashes and other unintentional injuries, firearm-related deaths, homicide, suicide, AIDS, and early heart attack. Gender roles that promote risky behavior among young men are a factor in many of these causes of death. Indeed, among people who have made it to age 65, the gender longevity gap is smaller.

Social and behavioral factors may be more important than physiological causes in explaining the gender gap; for example, among the Amish, a religious sect that has strict rules against smoking and drinking, men usually live as long as women. This suggests that the longevity gap could be substantially narrowed through lifestyle changes.

SOURCES: U.S. Census Bureau. 2005. *We the People: Women and Men in the United States.* Washington, D.C.: U.S. Census Bureau; National Center for Health Statistics. 2007. *Health, United States, 2007.* Hyattsville, Md.: National Center for Health Statistics; World Health Organization. 2003. *Gender, Health, and Aging.* Geneva: World Health Organization.

---

nia, fatigue, and feelings of worthlessness are signs of depression. Listen carefully when an older friend or relative complains about being depressed; it may be a request for help. Suicide rates are relatively high among the elderly, and depression should be taken seriously.

AGING AND LIFE EXPECTANCY

Life expectancy is the average length of time we can expect to live. In 2006, life expectancy for the total population was 78.1 years, but those who reach age 65 can expect to live even longer—18 more years or longer—because they have already survived hazards to life in the younger years. Women have a longer life expectancy than men (see the box "Why Do Women Live Longer?"). As life expectancy increases, a larger proportion of the population will be in their later years. This change will necessitate new govern-

ment policies and changes in our general attitudes toward older adults.

America's Aging Minority

People over 65 are a large minority in the American population—over 37.3 million people, about 12% of the total population in 2006. That number is expected to nearly double by the year 2030 (Figure 17.1). The enormous increase in the over-55 population is markedly affecting our stereotypes of what it means to grow old. The misfortunes associated with aging—frailty, forgetfulness, poor health, isolation—occur in fewer people in their sixties and seventies and are shifting instead to burden the very old, those over 85.

life expectancy   The average length of time a person is expected to live.

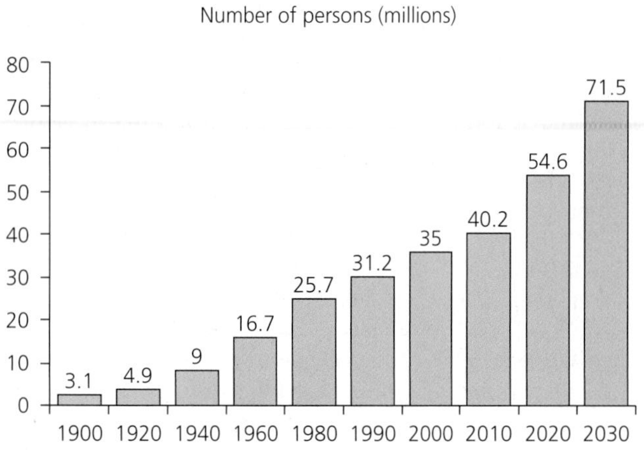

Number of persons (millions)

FIGURE 17.1   Increase in Americans over age 65, 1900–2030.

SOURCE: U.S. Department of Health and Human Services, Administration on Aging. 2008. *A Statistical Profile of Older Americans Aged 65+* (http://www.aoa.gov/press/prodsmats/fact/pdf/ss_stat_profile.pdf; retrieved February 22, 2009).

About 81% of older Americans own their homes. Their living expenses are lower after retirement because they no longer support children and have fewer work-related expenses; they consume and buy less food. They are more likely to continue practicing their expertise for years after retirement: Thousands of retired consultants, teachers, technicians, and craftspeople work until their middle and late seventies. They receive greater amounts of assistance, such as Medicare, pay proportionately lower taxes, and have greater net worth from lifetime savings. As the aging population increases proportionately, however, the number of older people who are ill and dependent rises. Health care remains the largest expense for older adults. Most older Americans have at least one chronic condition; many have more than one.

Retirement finds many older people with their incomes reduced to subsistence levels. The majority of older Americans live with fixed sources of income, such as pensions, that are eroded by inflation. **Social Security** benefits constitute 90% of the total income for one-third of Americans over age 65. Social Security was intended to serve as a supplement to personal savings and private pensions, not as a sole source of income. It is vital to plan for an adequate retirement income.

Family and Community Resources for Older Adults

With help from friends, family members, and community services, people in their later years can remain active and independent. About 66% of noninstitutionalized older Americans live with a spouse or other family member; the other 30% live alone. Only 4% live in institutional settings, but among those over age 85, about 15% live in a nursing home. In about three out of four cases, a spouse, a grown daughter, or a daughter-in-law assumes a caregiving role for elderly relatives. Recent surveys indicate

that the average woman will spend about 17 years raising children and 18 years caring for an aging relative.

Caregiving can be rewarding, but it is also hard work. If the experience is stressful and long-term, family members may become emotionally exhausted. Corporations are increasingly responsive to the needs of their employees who are family caregivers by providing services such as referrals, flexible schedules and leaves, and on-site adult care. Professional health care advice is another critical part of successful home care.

The best thing a family can do is talk honestly about the obligations, time, and commitment required by caregiving. Families should also explore the community resources and professional assistance that may be available to reduce the stress in this difficult job.

Government Aid and Policies

The federal government helps older Americans through several programs, such as food stamps, housing subsidies, Social Security, Medicare, and Medicaid. Medicare is a major health insurance program for the elderly and the disabled, paying about 30% of the medical costs of older Americans. It provides basic health care coverage for acute episodes of illness that require skilled professional care, and it pays for some preventive services. Medicare pays less than 2% of nursing home costs, and private insurers pay less than 1%, creating a tremendous financial burden for nursing home residents and their families. As of 2006, Medicare subscribers could enroll in privately managed prescription drug coverage plans, known as Medicare Part D, but the program is controversial for several reasons. The plans are complex and confusing, they leave gaps that enrollees must fill, and, according to some studies, they may actually drive up the cost of drugs for many people. When their financial resources are exhausted, people may apply for Medicaid, which provides medical insurance to low-income people of any age.

Health care policy planners hope that rising medical costs for older adults will shrink dramatically through education and prevention. Health care professionals, including **gerontologists** and **geriatricians,** are beginning to practice preventive medicine, just as pediatricians do. They advise older people about how to avoid and, if necessary, how to manage disabilities.

There can be benefits to aging, but they don't come automatically. They require planning and wise choices earlier

> In 2005, Social Security benefits accounted for **37%** of the aggregate income of the older population.
>
> —AOA, 2008

QUESTIONS FOR CRITICAL THINKING AND REFLECTION

What do you want your life to be like when you are old? Do you hope to retire, or keep working indefinitely? Where would you like to live? How much time do you spend thinking about these questions? Have you done any planning yet for old age?

in life. One octogenarian, Russell Lee, founder of a medical clinic in California, perceived the advantages of aging as growth: "The limitations imposed by time are compensated by the improved taste, sharper discretion, sounder mental and esthetic judgment, increased sensitivity and compassion, clearer focus—which all contribute to a more certain direction in living. . . . The later years can be the best of life for which the earlier ones were preparation."

WHAT IS DEATH?

Whether it is a powerful hurricane devastating New Orleans, a man in a crowded restaurant having a heart attack, or an elderly woman dying peacefully with her family close by, images of death are easy to envision. Nevertheless, very rarely do we think about the inevitability of death in our

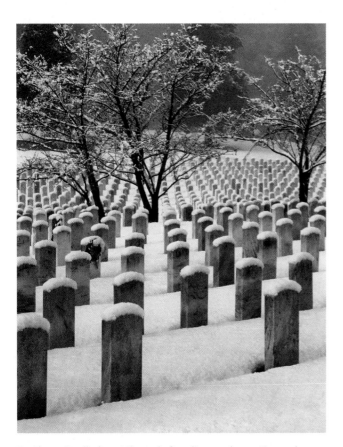

Death awaits all of us at the end of our lives, and accepting and dealing with death are difficult but important tasks.

own lives. Accepting and dealing with death are important tasks that present unique challenges to our sense of self, our relationships with others, and our understanding of the meaning of life itself. Although times of pain and distress may accompany the dying process, facing death also presents an opportunity for growth as well as affirmation of the preciousness of simple aspects of our daily lives.

Questions about the meaning of death and what happens when we die are central concerns of the great religions and philosophies. Some promise a better life after death. Others teach that everyone is evolving toward perfection or divinity, a goal reached after successive rounds of death and rebirth. There are also those who suggest that it is not possible to know what happens—if anything—after death and that any judgment about life's worth must be made on the basis of satisfactions or rewards that we create for ourselves in our lifetime.

Defining Death

Traditionally, death has been defined as cessation of the flow of vital body fluids. This occurs when the heart stops beating and breathing ceases. These traditional signs are adequate for determining death in most cases. However, the use of respirators and other **life-support systems** in modern medicine allows some body functions to be artificially sustained. The concept of **brain death** was developed to determine whether a person is alive or dead when the traditional signs are inadequate because of supportive medical technology.

According to the standards published by a Harvard Medical School committee, brain death involves four characteristics: (1) lack of receptivity and response to external stimuli, (2) absence of spontaneous muscular movement and spontaneous breathing, (3) absence of observable reflexes, and (4) absence of brain activity, as signified by a flat **electroencephalogram (EEG)**. The Harvard criteria require a second set of tests to be performed after 24 hours

TERMS

Social Security   A government program that provides financial assistance to people who are unemployed, disabled, or retired (and over a certain age); financed through taxes on business and workers.

gerontologist   One who studies the biological, psychological, and social phenomena associated with aging and old age.

geriatrician   A physician specializing in the diseases, disabilities, and care of older adults.

life-support systems   Medical technologies, such as the respirator, that allow vital body functions to be artificially sustained.

brain death   A medical determination of death as the cessation of brain activity indicated by various diagnostic criteria, including a flat EEG reading.

electroencephalogram (EEG)   A record of the electrical activity of the brain (brain waves).

have elapsed, and they exclude cases of hypothermia (body temperature below 90°F) and situations involving central nervous system depressants, such as barbiturates.

In contrast to **clinical death,** which is determined by either the cessation of heartbeat and breathing or the criteria for establishing brain death, **cellular death** refers to a gradual process that occurs when heartbeat, respiration, and brain activity have stopped. It encompasses the breakdown of metabolic processes and results in complete nonfunctionality at the cellular level.

The way in which death is defined has potential legal and social consequences in a variety of areas, including criminal prosecution, inheritance, taxation, treatment of the corpse, and even mourning. It also affects the practice of organ transplantation, because some organs—hearts, most obviously—must be harvested from a human being who is legally determined to be dead.

Learning About Death

Our understanding of death changes as we grow and mature, as do our attitudes toward it. A child's understanding of death evolves greatly from about age 5 to age 9. During this period, most children come to understand that death is final, universal, and inevitable. A child who consciously recognizes these facts is said to possess a **mature understanding of death.** This understanding of death is further refined during the years of adolescence and young adulthood by considering the impact of death on close relationships and contemplating the value of religious or philosophical answers to the enigma of death.

It is important to add, however, that individuals who possess a mature understanding of death commonly hold nonempirical ideas about it as well. Such nonempirical ideas—that is, ideas not subject to scientific proof—deal mainly with the notion that human beings survive in some form beyond the death of the physical body. What happens to an individual's personality after he or she dies? Does the self or soul continue to exist after the death of the physical body? If so, what is the nature of this afterlife? Developing personally satisfying answers to such questions is also part of the process of acquiring a mature understanding of death.

Denying Versus Welcoming Death

Our ability to find meaning and comfort in the face of mortality depends not only on our having an understanding of the facts of death, but also on our attitudes toward it. Many people seek to avoid any thought or mention of death. The sick and old are often isolated in hospitals and nursing homes. Relatively few Americans have been present at the death of a loved one. Instead of facing death directly, we tend to amuse ourselves with unrealistic portrayals on television and movie screens.

Although some commentators characterize the predominant attitude toward death in the United States as "death denying," others are reluctant to paint society as a whole with such a broad brush. Individuals often maintain conflicting or ambivalent attitudes toward death. Those who come to view death as a relief or release from insufferable pain may have at least a partial sense of welcoming death, but few people wholly avoid or wholly welcome death. Problems can arise, however, when avoidance or denial fosters the notion that death happens to others but not to you or me. (For another perspective, see the box "El Día de los Muertos: The Day of the Dead.")

PLANNING FOR DEATH

Acknowledging the inevitability of death allows us to plan for it. Adequate planning can help ensure that a sudden, unexpected death is not made even more difficult for survivors. Even when death is not sudden, many decisions can be anticipated, considered, and discussed with close relatives and friends.

Making a Will

Surveys indicate that about seven out of ten Americans die without leaving a will. A **will** is a legal instrument expressing a person's intentions and wishes for the disposition of his or her property after death. It is a declaration of how one's **estate**—that is, money, property, and other possessions—will be distributed after death. During the life of the **testator** (the person making the will), a will can be changed, replaced, or revoked. Upon the testator's death, it becomes a legal instrument governing the distribution of the testator's estate.

When a person dies **intestate**—that is, without having left a valid will—property is distributed according to rules set up by the state. If you haven't yet made a will, start thinking about how you'd like your property distributed in the case of your death. If you have a will, consider whether it needs to be updated in response to a key life

El Día de los Muertos: The Day of the Dead

In contrast to the solemn attitude toward death so prevalent in the United States, a familiar and even ironic attitude is more common among Mexicans and Mexican Americans. In the Mexican worldview, death is another phase of life, and those who have passed into it remain accessible. Ancestors are not forever lost, nor is the past dead. This sense of continuity has its roots in the culture of the Aztecs, for whom regeneration was a central theme. When the Spanish came to Mexico in the sixteenth century, their beliefs about death, along with symbols such as skulls and skeletons, were absorbed into the native culture.

Mexican artists and writers confront death with humor and even sarcasm, depicting it as the inevitable fate that all—even the wealthiest—must face. At no time is this attitude toward death livelier than at the beginning of each November on the holiday known as Día de los Muertos, "the Day of the Dead." This holiday coincides with All Souls' Day, the Catholic commemoration of the dead, and represents a unique blending of indigenous ritual and religious dogma.

The celebration in honor of the dead typically spans two days—one day devoted to dead children, one to adults. It reflects the belief that the dead return to Earth in spirit once a year to rejoin their families and partake of holiday foods prepared especially for them. The fiesta usually begins at midday on October 31, with flowers and food—candies, cookies, honey, milk—set out on altars in each house for the family's dead. The next day, family groups stream to the graveyards, where they have cleaned and decorated the graves of their loved ones, to celebrate and commune with the dead. They bring games, music, and special food; they sit on the graves, eat, sing, and talk with the departed ones. Tears may be shed as the dead are remembered, but mourning is tempered by the festive mood of the occasion.

During the season of the dead, graveyards and family altars are decorated with yellow candles and yellow marigolds—the "flower of death." In some Mexican villages, yellow flower petals are strewn along the ground, connecting the graveyard with all the houses visited by death during the year. Wherever Mexican Americans have settled in the United States, Día de los Muertos celebrations keep the traditions alive.

Keeping death in the forefront of consciousness may provide solace to the living, reminding them of their loved ones and assuring them that they themselves will not be forgotten when they die. Yearly celebrations and remembrances may help people keep in touch with their past, their ancestry, and their roots. The festive atmosphere may help dispel the fear of death, allowing people to look at it more directly. Although it is possible to deny the reality of death even when surrounded by images of it, such practices as Día de los Muertos may help people face death with more equanimity.

SOURCES: Adapted from DeSpelder, L., and A. Strickland. 2007. *The Last Dance*, 8th ed. New York: McGraw-Hill; Azcentral. 2000. *Día de los Muertos* (http://www.azcentral.com/rep/dead; retrieved September 14, 2006); Puente, T. 1991. Día de los Muertos. *Hispanic*, October; Milne, J. 1965. *Fiesta Time in Latin America*. Los Angeles: Ward Ritchie Press.

event such as marriage, the birth of a child, or the purchase of a home.

You can also help your family members by completing a *testamentary letter;* this document includes information about your personal affairs, such as bank accounts, credit cards, the location of documents and keys, the names of your professional advisers, the names of people who should be notified of your death, and so on.

Considering Options for End-of-Life Care

An appropriate balance in end-of-life care may involve a combination of home care, hospital stays, and hospice or palliative care.

? QUESTIONS FOR CRITICAL THINKING AND REFLECTION

What situations or events make you think seriously about your own mortality? Is this something you consider often, or do you avoid thinking about death? What has influenced your willingness or reluctance to think about death?

Home Care Many people express a preference to be cared for at home during the end stage of a terminal illness. An obvious advantage of home care is the fact that the dying person is in a familiar setting, ideally in the

clinical death A determination of death made according to accepted medical criteria. cellular death The breakdown of metabolic processes at the level of the cell.

cellular death The breakdown of metabolic processes at the level of the cell.

mature understanding of death The recognition that death is universal and irreversible, that it involves the cessation of all physiological functioning, and that there are biological reasons for its occurrence.

will A legal instrument expressing a person's intentions and wishes for the disposition of his or her property after death.

estate The money, property, and other possessions belonging to a person.

testator The person who makes a will.

intestate Referring to the situation in which a person dies without having made a legal will.

company of family and friends. For home care to be an option, however, support generally must be provided not only by family and friends, but also by skilled, professional caregivers.

Hospital-Based Palliative Care   Although hospitals are primarily organized to provide short-term intensive treatment for acute injury and illness, they are also adopting the principles of **palliative care** for patients who require comprehensive care at the end of life. Unlike acute care, which involves taking active measures to sustain life, palliative care focuses on controlling pain and relieving suffering by caring for the physical, psychological, spiritual, and existential needs of the patient. Although the emphasis is generally placed on comfort care, palliative therapies can be combined with cure-oriented treatment approaches in some cases. In all cases, the goal of palliative care is to achieve the best possible quality of life for patients and their families.

Hospice Programs   As a comprehensive program of care offering a set of services designed to support terminally ill patients and their families, **hospice** is a well-known form of palliative care. Although the term *hospice* sometimes refers to a freestanding medical facility to which terminally ill patients are admitted, most hospice care takes place in patients' homes with family members as primary caregivers.

Hospice care allows many people to choose where they die, a comforting fact for patients and families. A 2006 study revealed that nursing home residents who chose hospice care were 50% less likely to spend their final 30 days of life in a hospital. Hospitalization can negatively impact a dying person's quality of life.

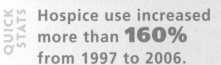

Deciding to Prolong Life or Hasten Death

Modern medicine can keep the human organism alive despite the cessation of normal heart, brain, respiratory, or kidney function. But should a patient without any hope of recovery be kept alive by means of artificial life support? What if a patient has fallen into a **persistent vegetative state,** a state of profound unconsciousness, lacking any sign of normal reflexes and unresponsive to external stimuli, with no reasonable hope of improvement?

Ethical questions about a person's right to die have become prominent since the landmark case of Karen Ann Quinlan in 1975. At age 22, she was admitted in a coma-

tose state to an intensive care unit, where her breathing was sustained by a respirator. When she remained unresponsive, her parents asked that the respirator be disconnected. The request to withdraw treatment eventually reached the New Jersey Supreme Court, which ruled that artificial respiration could be discontinued.

Since then, courts have ruled on removing other types of life-sustaining treatment, including artificial feeding mechanisms that provide nutrition and hydration to permanently comatose patients who are able to breathe on their own. Most notable was the case of Nancy Beth Cruzan, heard before the U.S. Supreme Court in 1990. As a result of injuries she received in 1983, Cruzan was in a persistent vegetative state. To provide nourishment, Nancy's physicians implanted a feeding tube, the only form of life support she was receiving. Nancy's parents asked that the tube be removed, but the hospital refused. In this case, the U.S. Supreme Court upheld the right to refuse treatment, even if it sustains life. However, the court said states can require that such refusal come from the patient; because Nancy had not expressed her wishes, the state did not have to honor the family's request. Later testimony from Nancy's friends convinced a state court that she would have refused life support, so permission was granted to remove her feeding tube.

In 2003, the Terri Schiavo case presented a similar dilemma. Terri had been diagnosed as being in a persistent vegetative state. Contending that she would not want to continue living on life support, Terri's husband requested that her feeding tube be removed. Terri's parents contested the request, and a series of legal actions ensued. Finally, in 2005, after intervention by the U.S. Supreme Court, doctors were allowed to remove the tube. Cases like those of Nancy Cruzan and Terri Schiavo highlight the importance of expressing one's wishes about life-sustaining treatment, in writing, before the need arises.

Withholding or Withdrawing Treatment   The right of a competent patient to refuse unwanted treatment is now generally established in both law and medical practice. The consensus is that there is no medical or ethical distinction between withholding (not starting) a treatment and withdrawing (stopping) a treatment once it has been started. The choice to forgo life-sustaining treatment involves refusing treatments that would be expected to extend life. The right to refuse treatment remains constitutionally protected even when a patient is unable to communicate. Although specific requirements vary, all states authorize some type of written advance directive to honor the decisions of individuals unable to speak for themselves but who have previously recorded their wishes in an appropriate legal document.

The practice of withholding or withdrawing a treatment that could potentially sustain life is sometimes termed **passive euthanasia,** although many people consider this term a misnomer because it tends to confuse the widely accepted practice of withholding or withdrawing treatment with the generally unacceptable and unlawful practice of taking active steps to cause death.

Assisted Suicide and Active Euthanasia In contrast to withdrawing or withholding treatment, assisted suicide and active euthanasia refer to practices that intentionally hasten a person's death. In **physician-assisted suicide (PAS),** a physician provides lethal drugs or other interventions—at the patient's request—with the understanding that the patient plans to use them to end his or her life. The patient administers the fatal dose.

In 1997, the Supreme Court reviewed two cases relating to physician-assisted suicide. The decisions in these cases (*Washington v. Glucksberg* and *Vacco v. Quill*) are important for several reasons. First, the Court upheld the distinction between, on the one hand, withholding or withdrawing treatment and, on the other hand, physician-assisted suicide. Second, the Court affirmed the rights of states to craft policy concerning physician-assisted suicide, either prohibiting it, as most states now do, or permitting it under a regulatory system.

Oregon is currently the only state where PAS is permitted. The Death with Dignity Act, a ballot initiative, was passed by Oregon voters in 1994 and, after surviving judicial challenges, was reaffirmed in 1997. During its first 9 years of implementation, 292 people were reported to have legally committed suicide with the assistance of their physicians. These patients exhibited strong beliefs in personal autonomy and a determination to control the end of their lives. The Death with Dignity Act withstood Supreme Court scrutiny in 2006, when the court ruled that the federal government could not block Oregon physicians from prescribing lethal drugs to patients who qualified for PAS under the act's provisions.

A third finding of importance in the Supreme Court's 1997 rulings about PAS relates to the concept of **double effect** in the medical management of pain. The doctrine of double effect states that a harmful effect of treatment, even if it results in death, is permissible if the harm is not intended and occurs as a side effect of a beneficial action. Sometimes the dosages of medication needed to relieve a patient's pain must be increased to levels that can cause respiratory depression, resulting in the patient's death. Such medication for pain, even if it hastens death, is not physician-assisted suicide if the intent is to relieve pain.

Unlike physician-assisted suicide, **active euthanasia** is the intentional act of killing someone who would otherwise suffer from an incurable and painful disease. *Voluntary euthanasia* (also known as voluntary active euthanasia, or VAE) is the intentional termination of life at the patient's request. In practice, this generally means that a competent patient requests direct assistance to die, and he or she receives assistance from a qualified medical practitioner. Voluntary active euthanasia is legal in Belgium and the Netherlands, but is currently unlawful in the United States. Taking active steps to end someone's life is a crime—even if the motive is mercy.

Completing an Advance Directive

To make your preferences known about medical treatment, you need to document them through a written **advance directive.** Two forms of advance directives are legally important. First is the **living will,** which enables

palliative care A form of medical care aimed at reducing the intensity or severity of a disease by controlling pain and other discomforting symptoms.

hospice A program of care for dying patients and their families.

persistent vegetative state A condition of profound unconsciousness in which a person lacks normal reflexes and is unresponsive to external stimuli, lasting for an extended period with no reasonable hope of improvement.

passive euthanasia The practice of withholding (not starting) or withdrawing (stopping) treatment that could potentially sustain a person's life, with the recognition that, without such treatment, death is likely to occur.

physician-assisted suicide (PAS) The practice of a physician intentionally providing, at the patient's request, lethal drugs or other means for a patient to hasten death with the understanding that the patient plans to use them to end his or her life.

double effect A situation in which a harmful effect occurs as an unintended side effect of a beneficial action, such as when medication intended to control a patient's pain has the unintended result of causing the patient's death.

active euthanasia A deliberate act intended to end another person's life; voluntary active euthanasia involves the practice of a physician administering—at the request of a patient—medication or some other intervention that causes death.

advance directive Any statement made by a competent person about his or her choices for medical treatment should he or she become unable to make such decisions or communicate them in the future.

living will A type of advance directive that allows individuals to provide instructions about the kind of medical care they wish to receive if they become unable to participate in treatment decisions.

individuals to provide instructions about the kind of medical care they wish to receive if they become incapacitated or otherwise unable to participate in treatment decisions. The second important form of advance directive is the **health care proxy,** which is also known as a *durable power of attorney for health care.* This document makes it possible to appoint another person to make decisions about medical treatment if you become unable to do so. This decision maker, also known as a **surrogate,** may be a family member, close friend, or attorney with whom you have discussed your treatment preferences. The proxy is expected to act in accordance with your wishes as stated in an advance directive or as otherwise made known.

For advance directives to be of value, you must do more than merely complete the paperwork. Discuss your wishes ahead of time with caregivers and family members as well as with your physician.

Becoming an Organ Donor

Each day about 77 people receive an organ transplant while another 19 people on the waiting list die because not enough organs are available. There are currently more than 98,000 Americans waiting for organ transplants, including more than 13,000 people under age 35.

If you decide to become a donor, the first step is to indicate your wish by completing a **Uniform Donor Card** (Figure 17.2); alternatively, you can indicate your wish on your driver's license. Be sure to discuss your decision with your family.

Planning a Funeral or Memorial Service

Funerals and memorial services are rites of passage that commemorate a person's life and acknowledge his or her passing from the community. Funerals and memorials allow survivors to support one another as they cope with their loss and express their grief. The presence of death rites in every human culture suggests that they serve innate human needs.

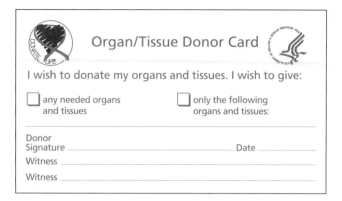

FIGURE 17.2 A sample organ/tissue donor card.

SOURCE: U.S. Department of Health and Human Services (http://www.organdonor .gov/donor/index.htm; retrieved June 17, 2008).

Disposition of the Body   People generally have a preference about the final disposition of their body. For most Americans, the choice is either burial or cremation. *Burial* usually involves a grave dug into the soil or entombment in a mausoleum. *Cremation* involves subjecting a body to intense heat. Cremated remains can be buried, placed in a columbarium niche, put into an urn kept by the family or interred in an urn garden, or scattered at sea or on land. If the body is to be viewed during a wake or will be present at the funeral, **embalming** is generally done.

> **31%** of corpse dispositions were done via cremation in 2005.
>
> —National Funeral Directors Association, 2008

Arranging a Service   Although it is becoming more common for individuals and families to express a preference for no services, bereaved relatives and friends can derive important benefits from having an opportunity to honor the deceased and express their grief through ceremony. Decisions about your last rites are ideally made with a view to the needs and wishes of your survivors. Religious and cultural or ethnic traditions play a major role in shaping the way people honor their dead. The diversity of life and death in the United States calls for a diversity of rites. A meaningful funeral or memorial service can be designed in many ways. Making at least some plans ahead of time and discussing the options with family members can help reduce the burden on survivors who find themselves facing a number of tasks and decisions once death occurs.

COPING WITH DYING

There is no one right way to live with or die of a life-threatening illness. Every disease has its own set of problems and challenges, and each person copes with these

TERMS

health care proxy   A type of advance directive that allows an individual to appoint another person as an agent in making health care decisions in the event he or she becomes unable to participate in treatment decisions; also known as a *durable power of attorney for health care.*

surrogate   The agent or substitute decision maker appointed by a person to act on his or her behalf by means of a health care proxy.

Uniform Donor Card   A consent form authorizing the use of the signer's body parts for transplantation or medical research upon his or her death.

embalming   The process of removing blood and other fluids and replacing them with chemicals to disinfect and temporarily retard deterioration of a corpse.

problems and challenges in his or her own way. Living with an illness that is life-threatening and incurable can be described as a living-dying experience. Hope and honesty are often delicately balanced—honesty to face reality as it is, hope for a positive outcome. The object of hope changes. The early hope that the symptoms are not really serious gives way to hope that a cure is possible. When the illness is deemed incurable, there is hope for more time. As time begins to run out, one hopes for a pain-free death, a "good death" (see the box "In Search of a Good Death" on page 422).

The Tasks of Coping

In her 1969 book *On Death and Dying,* Elisabeth Kübler-Ross suggested that the response to an awareness of imminent death involves five psychological stages: denial, anger, bargaining, depression, and acceptance. Individuals go back and forth among the stages during the course of an illness, and different stages can occur simultaneously. More recently, the notion of stages has been deemphasized in favor of highlighting the tasks that deserve attention in

coping with a life-threatening illness. Charles Corr, for example, distinguishes four primary dimensions in coping with dying:

1. *Physical:* Satisfying bodily needs and minimizing physical distress
2. *Psychological:* Maximizing a sense of security, self-worth, autonomy, and richness in living
3. *Social:* Sustaining significant relationships and addressing the social implications of dying
4. *Spiritual:* Identifying, developing, or reaffirming sources of meaning and fostering hope

People who apparently cope best with life-threatening illness often exhibit a fighting spirit that views the illness not only as a threat but also as a challenge. These people strive to inform themselves about their illness and take an active part in treatment decisions. They are optimistic and have a capacity to discover positive meaning in ordinary events. Holding to a positive outlook despite distressing circumstances involves creating a sense of meaning that is bigger than the threat. In the context of life-threatening illness, this encompasses a person's ability to comprehend the implications an illness has for the future, as well as for his or her ability to accomplish goals, maintain relationships, and sustain a sense of personal vitality, competence, and power.

Supporting a Dying Person

People often feel uncomfortable in the presence of a person who is close to dying. What can we say? How should we act? It may seem that any attempt to be comforting could result only in words that are little more than stale platitudes. Yet we want to express concern and establish meaningful contact with the person who is facing death. In such circumstances, the most important gift we can bring is that of listening. Offering the dying person opportunities to speak openly and honestly about his or her experience can be crucial, even when such conversation is initially painful.

We tend to place dying people in a special category, but the reality is that their needs are not fundamentally different from anyone else's, although their situation is perhaps more urgent. Dying people need to know that they are valued, that they are not alone, that they are not being unfairly judged, and that those closest to them are also striving to come to terms with a difficult situation. As with any relationship, there are opportunities for growth on both sides.

COPING WITH LOSS

Even if we have not experienced the death of someone close, we are all survivors of losses that occur in our lives because of changes and endings. The loss of a job, the ending of a relationship, transitions from one school or neighborhood

In Search of a Good Death

Participants in a recent study were asked to discuss the deaths of family members, friends, or patients and reflect on what made their deaths good or bad. From these discussions, six major themes emerged as components of a good death.

The first component was pain and symptom management. Many people fear dying in pain, and portrayals of bad deaths usually included inadequate pain management. Every health care provider in the study told regret-filled stories of patients who died in pain. Patients were concerned with pain control; when reassured that pain could be managed, they were less anxious.

The second component of a good death was clear decision making. Both providers and families feared entering a medical crisis without knowing the patient's preferences. Patients and families who had good communication with health care providers and had discussed treatment decisions ahead of time felt empowered, and providers felt they were giving good care. Although all uncertainty about end-of-life decisions cannot be eliminated, tolerance for uncertainty may increase if values and preferences are clarified.

The third component was preparation for death. Patients expressed satisfaction when they had time to prepare their wills and help plan their funeral arrangements. Many times, providers avoided end-of-life discussions to prevent their patients from losing hope, thus depriving them of

the opportunity to plan ahead. Patients and families also wanted to know what to expect during the course of the illness and what physical and psychosocial changes would take place as death approached.

The fourth component was completion, the opportunity to review one's life, to resolve conflicts, to spend time with loved ones, and to say good-bye. Participants confirmed the deep importance of spirituality or meaningfulness at the end of life. Many times, patients were able to view their experience of dying as part of a broader life trajectory and thus continue to grow emotionally and spiritually in their last days. Issues of faith were often mentioned as important to healing.

The fifth component was contributing to others. Patients wanted to know that they still had something to offer to others, whether it was making someone laugh or lightening the load of someone closer to death. Many patients found that as they reflected on their lives, what they valued most was their personal relationships with family and friends, and they were anxious to impart this wisdom to others.

The sixth component of a good death was affirmation of the whole person. Patients appreciated empathic health care providers, and family members were comforted by those who treated their loved ones as unique and whole people, rather than as a disease. The quality of dying is related to the acknowledgment that

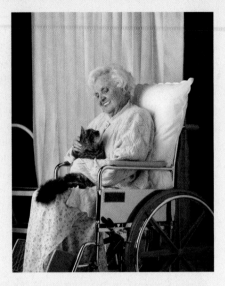

people die in character, that is, as an extension of who they have been in their lives.

The study affirmed that most people think of death as a natural part of life, not as a failure of technology. Although the biomedical aspects of end-of-life care are crucial, they merely provide a point of departure toward a good death. When pain is properly managed and the practical aspects of dying are taken care of, patients and their families have the opportunity to address the important emotional, psychological, and spiritual issues that all human beings face at the end of life.

---

to another—these are examples of the kinds of losses that occur in all our lives. Such losses are sometimes called little deaths and, in varying degrees, they all involve grief.

Experiencing Grief

Grief is the reaction to loss. It encompasses thoughts and feelings, as well as physical and behavioral responses. Mental distress may involve disbelief, confusion, anxiety,

disorganization, and depression. The emotions that can be present in normal grief include not only sorrow and sadness, but also relief, anger, and self-pity, among others. Common behaviors associated with grief include crying, searching for the deceased, and talking incessantly about the deceased and the circumstances of the death. Bereaved

QUESTIONS FOR CRITICAL THINKING AND REFLECTION

What is your notion of a "good death"? In what setting does it take place, and who is there? In the last days of your life, what do you think you'll need to say, and to whom will you want to say it? If you were terminally ill, what would be the most supportive things others could do for you?

people may be restless, as if not knowing what to do with themselves. Physically, grief may involve frequent sighing, insomnia, and loss of appetite. Grief may also evoke a re-examination of religious or spiritual beliefs as a person struggles to make meaning of the loss. All such manifestations of grief can be present as part of one's total response to **bereavement**—that is, the event of loss.

Mourning is closely related to grief and is often used as a synonym for it. However, mourning refers not so much to the *reaction* to loss but to the *process* by which a bereaved person adjusts to loss and incorporates it into his or her life. How this process is managed is determined, at least partly, by cultural and gender norms for the expression of grief.

Tasks of Mourning　Experiencing grief is part of the process by which a bereaved person integrates a significant loss into his or her life. Psychologist William Worden has identified four tasks that must be attended to:

1. *Accepting the reality* of the loss
2. *Working through the pain* of grief
3. *Adjusting to a changed environment* in which the deceased is absent
4. *Emotionally relocating the deceased and moving on with life*

Accomplishing the fourth task does not mean dishonoring the deceased's memory or denying normal feelings of connection that persist beyond death. Making the journey of grief and attending to the various tasks along the way, we come to a place where we learn how to keep a special place for the deceased in our hearts and memories while moving forward with our lives.

The Course of Grief　Grieving, like dying, is highly individual. In the first hours or days following a death, a bereaved person is likely to experience overwhelming shock and numbness, as well as a sense of disbelief. The cause or mode of death—natural, accidental, homicide, or suicide—has an influence on how grief is experienced (see the box "Profound Trauma and Loss" on page 424). Even when a death is anticipated, grief is not necessarily diminished when the loss becomes real.

The sense of disorganization experienced by survivors during the early period of grief is set against the need to attend to decisions and actions surrounding the disposition of the deceased's body. As family and friends gather to offer mutual support, funeral ceremonies are held. Engaging in such activities promotes accepting the reality of the death and moving beyond the initial shock and numbness.

In its middle phase, the course of grief is characterized by anxiety, apathy, and pining for the deceased. The pangs of grief are felt as the bereaved person deeply experiences the pain of separation. There is often a sense of despair as a person repeatedly goes over the events surrounding the

loss, perhaps fantasizing that somehow everything could be undone and be as it was before.

In moving toward the restoration of one's well-being, the last phase of active grief involves resolution. The acute pain and emotional turmoil of grief subside. Physical and mental balance is reestablished. The bereaved becomes increasingly reintegrated into his or her social world. Sadness doesn't go away completely, but it recedes into the background.

Some people, however, have more trouble resolving their grief than others. Such people may get stuck in the grieving process for months or even years, sometimes becoming so burdened with loss that they lose the ability to cope with daily living. Experts call this long-term, unresolved grief *complicated grief* and describe it as truly debilitating. Complicated grief is most likely to occur when a person has lost a loved one in a sudden, violent manner (such as homicide) or experienced an untimely death (such as the loss of a child). Grief counseling or therapy can help people work through complicated grief.

Supporting a Grieving Person

In experiencing a significant loss, a person initially may feel and behave much like a frightened, helpless child. He or she may respond best to the kind of loving support that is given by a parent. A hug may be more comforting than any words. Also, because talking about a loss is an important way that survivors cope with the changed reality, simply listening can be very helpful. The key to being a good listener is to refrain from making judgments about whether the feelings expressed by a survivor are right or wrong, good or bad.

Funerals and other ceremonies generally help survivors gain a sense of closure and begin to integrate a loss into their lives. Social support for the bereaved is as critical during the later course of grief as it is during the first days after a loss. In offering support, we can reassure them that grief is normal, permissible, and appropriate. They may also need permission to occasionally give themselves a break from grieving. An extended need for support often continues through the first year or two of mourning. Bereaved people also may want to share their stories and concerns through organized support groups, such as those for widows and widowers. Many support groups are organized around some specific type of bereavement.

Children tend to cope with loss in a healthier fashion when they are included as part of their family's experience

QUESTIONS FOR CRITICAL THINKING AND REFLECTION

Have you ever been in the position of being supportive to a bereaved person? What kind of support did he or she seem to appreciate most? Why do you think that was the case? How did the experience affect you?

Profound Trauma and Loss

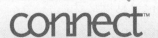
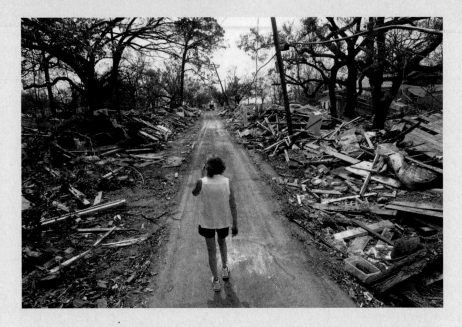

Profoundly traumatic events—Hurricane Katrina, the terrorist attacks of September 11, 2001, the deaths and destruction resulting from the wars in Iraq and Afghanistan—all represent a category of loss far beyond normal comprehension. Experiencing traumatic loss in such extraordinary circumstances can cause severe and disruptive reactions in emotion and behavior.

Many World War I veterans developed psychological symptoms that collectively were described as shell shock. However, it was not until after the Vietnam War that the medical community became fully aware of how disruptive and enduring the psychological effects could be for those experiencing profound traumatic loss.

It is now widely recognized that significant psychological symptoms can follow the experiencing of loss in traumatic circumstances. Elements commonly seen in a customary reaction to grief, such as sadness, disbelief, crying, insomnia, and loss of appetite, are frequently exaggerated in the aftermath of profoundly traumatic events and will often include more pronounced symptoms, such as overwhelming distress, numbness, doubt, despair, guilt, and disabling depression and anxiety.

Depending on the severity of exposure and a person's underlying vulnerability, the symptoms can persist long after the original trauma. Memories and images of the event may suddenly pop into the victim's mind, causing anxiety, depression, and anger. Insomnia and nightmares can disrupt the sleep-wake cycle. The person may start avoiding everything that serves as a reminder of the event and, as a kind of self-protection, may begin to become numb, to lose all feelings. Such people may startle easily and have difficulty concentrating. Their work life, social life, and intimate relationships may become markedly impaired. People experiencing these severe symptoms most likely have PTSD, which can persist for months or years.

The events of September 11, 2001, are an example of a profound trauma that caused PTSD in affected people. As described in Chapter 3, PTSD symptoms occurred among survivors, rescue workers, passersby, residents of Manhattan, and some people exposed to the events through repeated television images. Researchers who interviewed residents of Manhattan found that about 7.5% reported symptoms consistent with a diagnosis of PTSD and 9.7% reported symptoms consistent with new onset of depression; these numbers are about twice as high as the expected rates in surveys of this type. Among people who lived closest to the World Trade Center, the prevalence of PTSD was as high as 20%.

Many people experience disabling depression or anxiety but do not meet the full criteria for PTSD. More persistent and severe grief reactions, unexplained physical symptoms, and the increased use of alcohol and drugs are frequent occurrences for people who have undergone such trauma. In addition, family and interpersonal conflict and financial strain are commonly seen. All too frequently, in war or natural disasters, the primary wage earner of the family dies or the family's house and belongings are destroyed.

How long will an individual's symptoms last after experiencing an event like September 11 or witnessing a friend killed by a roadside bomb in Iraq? Factors such as the severity of the trauma, the individual's proximity to the event, and his or her emotional closeness to those who have died can all play important roles in the magnitude and duration of the reaction to traumatic loss. In general, though, symptoms will diminish with time, especially in the absence of new threats and traumatic losses. Studies of those who have developed full-blown PTSD suggest that approximately half of the cases resolve within 2 years but that nearly a third never fully recover.

Psychological support and treatment can greatly help many of those who suffer from disabling emotional symptoms in reaction to traumatic loss. Building on research and work done with Vietnam veterans in the 1970s and 1980s, clinicians have developed multiple therapeutic strategies involving group therapy, individual psychological support, and pharmacologic intervention to treat persistent symptoms.

SOURCES: Coker, A. L., et al. 2006. Social and mental health needs assessment of Katrina evacuees. *Disaster Management and Response* 4(3): 88-94; Watanabe, T., et al. 2006. Acute stress syndrome in a victim of the Indian Ocean Tsunami. *Psychiatry and Clinical Neurosciences* 60(5): 644; Galea, S., and H. Resnick. 2005. Posttraumatic stress disorder in the general population after mass terrorist incidents: Considerations about the nature of exposure. *CNS Spectrums* 10(2): 107–115; Galea, S., et al. 2002. Psychological sequelae of the September 11 terrorist attacks in New York City. *New England Journal of Medicine* 346(13): 982–987; Shuster, M., et al. 2001. A national survey of stress reactions after the September 11, 2001, terrorist attacks. *New England Journal of Medicine* 345(20): 1507–1512; Ornstein, R. D., and R. K. Pitman, section eds. 2000. Trauma and post-traumatic stress disorder. In *Massachusetts General Hospital Psychiatry Update and Board Preparation*, 2nd ed., eds. T. A. Stern and J. B. Herman. New York: McGraw-Hill.

of grief and mourning. In talking about death with children, the most important guideline is to be honest. Set the explanation you are offering at the child's level of understanding. In general, it's advisable to keep the explanation simple, stick to basics, and verify what the child has understood from your explanation. A child's readiness for more details can usually be assessed by paying attention to his or her questions.

COMING TO TERMS WITH DEATH

We may wish we could keep death out of view and not make a place for it in our lives. But this wish cannot be fulfilled. With the death of a beloved friend or relative, we are confronted with emotions and thoughts that relate not only to the immediate loss but also to our own mortality. Our encounters with dying and death teach us that relationships are more important than things and that life offers no guarantees. In discovering the meaning of death in our own lives, we find that life is both precious and precarious. Allowing ourselves to make room for death, we discover that it touches not only the dying or bereaved person and his or her family and friends but also the wider community of which we are all part. We recognize that dying and death offer opportunities for extraordinary growth in the midst of loss.

TIPS FOR TODAY AND THE FUTURE
The best way to ensure a high-quality life in later years is by cultivating healthy habits in your younger years.

RIGHT NOW YOU CAN
- Think about any unhealthy habits you have and resolve to change them. Set a timetable and start developing a plan.
- Think about how you want your body to be disposed of when you die.
- Think about how you would want your worldly goods to be distributed if you were to die soon.
- Think about organ donation. If you want to be an organ donor, start making the appropriate arrangements now, as described in this chapter.

IN THE FUTURE YOU CAN
- Learn a new skill, such as a language or a game of strategy.
- Talk to your parents or grandparents about their wishes for end-of-life care and funeral arrangements, and discuss ways you can be involved.

SUMMARY

- People who take charge of their health during their youth have greater control over the physical and mental aspects of aging.

- A lifetime of interests and hobbies helps maintain creativity and intelligence. Exercise and a healthy diet throughout life enhances physical and psychological health.

- Retirement can be a fulfilling and enjoyable time of life for those who adjust to their new roles, enjoy participating in a variety of activities, and have planned ahead for financial stability.

- Slight confusion and forgetfulness are not signs of a serious illness; however, severe symptoms may indicate Alzheimer's disease or another form of dementia.

- Resolving grief and mourning and dealing with depression are important tasks for older adults.

- People over 65 form a large minority in the United States, and their status is improving.

- Family and community resources can help older adults stay active and independent.

- Government aid to the elderly includes food stamps, housing subsidies, Social Security, Medicare, and Medicaid.

- Dying and death are more than biological events; they have social and spiritual dimensions.

- The traditional criteria for determining death focus on vital signs such as breathing and heartbeat. Brain death is characterized by a lack of physical responses other than breathing and heartbeat.

- A will is a legal instrument that governs the distribution of a person's estate after death.

- End-of-life care may involve a combination of home care, hospital stays, and hospice or palliative care.

- The practice of withholding or withdrawing potentially life-sustaining treatment is sometimes termed passive euthanasia.

- Physician-assisted suicide occurs when a physician provides lethal drugs or other interventions, at a patient's request, with the understanding that the patient plans to use them to end his or her life.

- Advance directives, such as living wills and health care proxies, are used to express one's wishes about the use of life-sustaining treatment.

- People can donate their bodies or specific organs for transplantation and other medical uses after death.

- Bereaved people usually benefit from participating in a funeral or memorial service to commemorate a loved one's death.

- Coping with dying involves physical, psychological, social, and spiritual dimensions.

- In offering support to a dying person, the gift of listening can be especially important.

- Grief encompasses thoughts and feelings, as well as physical and behavioral responses.

- Mourning, the process by which a person integrates a loss into his or her life, is determined partly by social and cultural norms for expressing grief.

FOR MORE INFORMATION

BOOKS

Batuello, J. T. 2003. *End of Life Decisions: A Practical Guide.* College Station, Tx.: Virtualbookworm. *A guide to end-of-life decisions, including those related to pain relief and palliative and hospice care.*

DeSpelder, L. A., and A. L. Strickland. 2009. *The Last Dance: Encountering Death and Dying,* 8th ed. New York: McGraw-Hill. *A comprehensive and readable text highlighting a broad range of topics related to dying and death.*

Johns Hopkins Medical Center. 2007. *The Johns Hopkins Medical Guide to Health After 50.* New York: Black Dog & Leventhal. *A practical guide to healthy aging for all wellness dimensions.*

National Institute on Aging. 2006. *Fitness Over Fifty: An Exercise Guide from the National Institute on Aging,* book and DVD ed. New York: Hatherleigh Press. *A practical guide to physical activity and exercise, with specific guidelines for safe exercise for older adults.*

Weil, A. 2007. *Healthy Aging: A Lifelong Guide to Your Physical and Spiritual Well-Being.* New York: Anchor. *One of America's best-known complementary care physicians discusses the aging process and explains methods for maintaining health during the latter years of life.*

ORGANIZATIONS AND WEB SITES

AARP. Provides information on all aspects of aging, including health promotion, health care, and retirement planning.
>   http://www.aarp.org

Alzheimer's Association. Offers tips for caregivers and patients and information on the causes and treatment of Alzheimer's disease.
>   http://www.alz.org

Association for Death Education and Counseling (ADEC). Provides resources for education, bereavement counseling, and care of the dying.
>   http://www.adec.org

Dying Well. A Web site focused on wellness through the end of life.
>   http://www.dyingwell.org

FirstGov.gov: Senior Citizens' Resources. A gateway to government resources on the Internet for older Americans.
>   http://www.usa.gov/Topics/Seniors.shtml

Hospice Foundation of America. Promotes the hospice concept of care through education and leadership.
>   http://www.hospicefoundation.org

Medicare. Provides information about Medicare.
>   http://www.medicare.gov

National Council on Aging. Provides helpful information on retirement planning, health promotion, and lifelong learning.
>   http://www.ncoa.org

National Funeral Directors Association (NFDA). Provides resources related to funerals and funeral costs, body disposition, and bereavement support.
>   http://www.nfda.org

National Institute on Aging. Provides fact sheets and brochures on aging-related topics.
>   http://www.nih.gov/nia
>   http://nihseniorhealth.gov

Nolo Press: Wills and Estate Planning. Provides answers to questions about planning for death, from writing a basic will to organ donation.
>   http://www.nolo.com

On Our Own Terms: Public Broadcasting System. A companion Web site to the Bill Moyers PBS series on improving end-of-life care.
>   http://www.pbs.org/wnet/onourownterms

Oregon Department of Health and Human Services. Provides information about Oregon's Death with Dignity Act.
>   http://egov.oregon.gov/DHS/ph/pas

SELECTED BIBLIOGRAPHY

Annas, G. J. 2005. "Culture of life" politics at the bedside—the case of Terri Schiavo. *New England Journal of Medicine,* 23 March [epub].

Anderson, K., et al. 2005. Depression and the risk of Alzheimer's disease. *Epidemiology* 16(2): 233–238.

Beyond menopause: Life after estrogen. 2005. *Mayo Clinic Health Letter Supplement,* February.

Centers for Disease Control and Prevention. 2006. Prevalence of doctor-diagnosed arthritis and arthritis-attributable activity limitation—United States, 2003–2005. *Morbidity and Mortality Weekly Report* 55(40): 1089–1092.

Chochinov, H. M. 2006. Dying, dignity, and new horizons in palliative end-of-life care. *CA: A Cancer Journal for Clinicians* 56(2): 84–103.

Christ, G. H., and A. E. Christ. 2006. Current approaches to helping children cope with a parent's terminal illness. *CA: A Cancer Journal for Clinicians* 56(4): 197–212.

Curtis, L. H., et al. 2004. Inappropriate prescribing for elderly Americans in a large outpatient population. *Archives of Internal Medicine* 164(15): 1621–1625.

Donatelli, L. A., et al. 2006. Ethical issues in critical care and cardiac arrest: Clinical research, brain death, and organ donation. *Seminars in neurology* 26(4): 452–459.

DuBois, J. M., and E. E. Anderson. 2006. Attitudes toward death criteria and organ donation among healthcare personnel and the general public. *Progress in Transplantation* 16(1): 65–73.

Field, N. P. 2006. Unresolved grief and continuing bonds: An attachment perspective. *Death Studies* 30(8): 739–756.

Harvard Medical School. 2006. Minding your mind: 12 ways to keep your brain young with proper care and feeding. *Harvard Men's Health Watch* 10(10): 1–4.

Heyn, P. C., et al. 2008. Endurance and strength training outcomes on cognitively impaired and cognitively intact older adults: A meta-analysis. *Journal of Nutrition, Health & Aging* 12(6): 401–409.

Jager, R. D., et al. 2008. Age-related macular degeneration. *New England Journal of Medicine* 258(24): 2606–2617.

Lipkin, K. M. 2006. Identifying a proxy for health care as part of routine medical inquiry. *Journal of General Internal Medicine,* 17 July [online early ed.].

Mayo Clinic. 2006. Osteoporosis: Treatments for men and women. *Mayo Clinic Health Letter* 24(6): 4–5.

Mudge, A. M., et al. 2008. Exercising body and mind: An integrated approach to functional independence in hospitalized older people. *Journal of the American Geriatrics Society* 56(4): 630–635.

Oregon Department of Health and Human Services, Public Health Division. 2008. *"Death With Dignity Act" Annual Report: Year 9—2006 Summary* (http://www.oregon.gov/dhs/ph/pas/index.shtml; retrieved June 16, 2008).

Rietjens, J. A., et al. 2006. Terminal sedation and euthanasia: A comparison of clinical practices. *Archives of Internal Medicine* 166(7): 749–753.

Rosengren, A., et al. 2005. Body mass index, other cardiovascular risk factors, and hospitalization for dementia. *Archives of Internal Medicine* 165(3): 321–326.

Satel, S. 2006. Death's waiting list. *New York Times,* 15 May.

Scarmeas, N., et al. 2006. Mediterranean diet, Alzheimer disease, and vascular mediation. *Archives of Neurology* 63: December [early online release].

Schulz, R., et al. 2006. Predictors of complicated grief among dementia caregivers: A prospective study of bereavement. *American Journal of Geriatric Psychiatry* 14(8): 650–658.

Siminoff, L. A., et al. 2006. Racial disparities in preferences and perceptions regarding organ donation. *Journal of General Internal Medicine* 21(9): 995–1000.

Sorrell, J. M. 2008. As good as it gets? Rethinking old age. *Journal of Psychosocial Nursing and Mental Health Services* 46(5): 21–24.

Tufts University. 2006. Pendulum swings on estrogen and women's heart health risk. *Tufts University Health & Nutrition Letter* 24(3): 1–2.

U.S. Department of Health and Human Services. 2008. *Organ Donor Card* (http://www.organdonor.gov/donor/index.htm; retrieved February 23, 2009).

Ward, E. M. 2006. A weekly to-do list to help delay or prevent dementia. *Environmental Nutrition* 29(5): 2.

Wolfe, M. S. 2006. Shutting down Alzheimer's. *Scientific American* 294(5): 72–79.

Arby's

	Serving size	Calories	Protein	Total fat	Saturated fat	Trans fat	Total carbohydrate	Sugars	Fiber	Cholesterol	Sodium	Vitamin A	Vitamin C	Calcium	Iron	% calories from fat
	g		g	g	g	g	g	g	g	mg	mg		% Daily Value			
Regular roast beef	154	320	21	14	5	.5	34	5	2	44	953	0	0	6	20	39
Super roast beef	198	398	21	19	6	.5	40	10	2	44	1060	7	10	7	21	43
Junior roast beef	125	272	16	10	4	0	34	5	2	29	740	0	0	6	17	33
Market Fresh® Ultimate BLT	294	779	23	45	11	0.5	75	18	6	51	1571	16	28	17	26	52
Market Fresh® Roast Turkey & Swiss	345	708	41	30	8	0.5	74	17	5	83	1677	13	17	36	29	37
Market Fresh® Southwest chicken wrap	246	581	32	31	10	1	45	4	7	77	1719	12	10	37	28	48
Chicken fillet sandwich (grilled)	244	395	32	17	3	0	38	8	2	60	1002	10	17	8	17	39
Chopped turkey club salad (w/o dressing)	293	233	22	11	6	0.5	10	0	3	54	6	81	50	25	14	34
Balsamic vinaigrette dressing	43	130	0	12	2	0	5	4	0	0	460	-	-	-	-	83
Curly fries (medium)	156	496	7	29	5	0.5	55	0	6	0	1160	11	12	6	14	53
Jalapeno Bites®, regular (5)	110	305	5	21	9	1	29	3	2	28	526	14	1	3	5	63
Apple turnover	128	380	4	14	7	0.5	58	37	3	0	287	1	3	1	7	33
Chocolate shake, regular	397	507	13	13	8	0	83	81	0	34	357	8	9	51	3	23

SOURCE: Arby's © 2008, Arby's, Inc. (http://www.arbysrestaurant.com). Used with permission of Arby's, Inc.

Burger King

	Serving size	Calories	Protein	Total fat	Saturated fat	Trans fat	Total carbohydrate	Sugars	Fiber	Cholesterol	Sodium	Vitamin A	Vitamin C	Calcium	Iron	% calories from fat
	g		g	g	g	g	g	g	g	mg	mg		% Daily Value			
Original Whopper®	290	680	29	40	11	1.5	51	11	3	75	1020	10	15	15	30	53
Original Double Whopper® w/cheese	398	1010	53	66	24	2.5	52	11	3	160	1530	15	15	30	45	59
Original Whopper Jr.®	158	370	16	21	6	1	31	6	2	40	570	4	6	8	20	51
Whopper® Junior w/o mayonnaise	147	290	16	12	4.5	0.5	31	6	2	35	500	4	6	8	20	38
Original Chicken Sandwich	219	660	24	40	8	2.5	52	5	4	65	1430	2	2	10	20	55
Chicken Tenders® (8 pieces)	123	370	24	23	6	3.5	18	<1	<1	55	870	2	0	2	6	57
French fries (medium, salted)	116	360	4	20	4.5	4.5	41	1	4	0	590	0	15	2	4	45
Onion rings (medium)	91	310	4	15	3.5	2.5	37	4	3	0	440	0	0	6	6	45
Tendergrill™ Chicken Garden Salad	292	240	33	9	3.5	0	8	3	4	80	720	200	60	15	15	33
Croissan'wich® w/bacon, egg & cheese	122	340	15	20	7	2	27	15	5	155	890	10	0	15	15	53
Hershey®'s sundae pie	79	300	3	18	12	1.5	31	23	1	10	190	2	0	4	6	53
Vanilla shake (value)	228	310	6	11	7	0	44	43	0	45	180	8	4	30	0	32

SOURCE: BURGER KING® trademarks and nutritional information used with permission from Burger King Brands, Inc.

Jack in the Box

	Serving size	Calories	Protein	Total fat	Saturated fat	Trans fat	Total carbohydrate	Sugars	Fiber	Cholesterol	Sodium	Vitamin A	Vitamin C	Calcium	Iron	% calories from fat
	g		g	g	g	g	g	g	g	mg	mg	% Daily Value				
Breakfast Jack®	125	290	17	12	4.5	0	29	4	1	220	760	N/A	N/A	N/A	N/A	38
Supreme croissant	151	450	18	25	9	3.5	36	5	1	235	860	N/A	N/A	N/A	N/A	51
Hamburger	109	280	14	12	4.5	0.5	30	6	1	30	580	N/A	N/A	N/A	N/A	39
Jumbo Jack® w/cheese	286	690	25	42	16	1.5	54	12	3	70	1310	N/A	N/A	N/A	N/A	54
Sourdough Jack®	245	710	17	51	18	3	36	7	3	75	1230	N/A	N/A	N/A	N/A	65
Chicken fajita pita w/ whole grain, no salsa	193	300	23	9	3.5	0	33	4	4	60	1090	N/A	N/A	N/A	N/A	27
Sourdough grilled chicken club	266	530	36	28	7	2	34	5	2	85	1430	N/A	N/A	N/A	N/A	47
Deli Trio Pannido™	271	645	30	34	8.5	0	53	4	2	95	2530	N/A	N/A	N/A	N/A	47
Jack's Spicy Chicken®	270	620	25	31	6	3	61	8	4	50	1100	N/A	N/A	N/A	N/A	46
Monster taco	112	240	8	14	5	2	20	4	3	20	390	N/A	N/A	N/A	N/A	54
Egg rolls (3)	170	400	14	19	6	3	44	4	6	15	920	N/A	N/A	N/A	N/A	43
Chicken strips, crispy (4)	201	500	35	25	6	6	36	1	3	80	1260	N/A	N/A	N/A	N/A	44
Stuffed jalapeños (7)	168	530	15	30	13	4.5	51	5	4	45	1600	N/A	N/A	N/A	N/A	51
Barbeque dipping sauce	28	45	0	0	0	0	11	4	0	0	330	N/A	N/A	N/A	N/A	0
Seasoned curly fries (medium)	125	400	6	23	5	7	45	1	5	0	890	N/A	N/A	N/A	N/A	52
Onion rings	119	500	6	30	6	10	51	3	3	0	420	N/A	N/A	N/A	N/A	54
Side salad	123	50	3	3	1.5	0	5	2	2	10	60	N/A	N/A	N/A	N/A	50
Ranch dressing	57	310	1	33	5	1	3	2	0	20	470	N/A	N/A	N/A	N/A	96
Oreo® cookie ice-cream shake (small)	339	770	12	40	26	1.5	88	69	1	115	240	N/A	N/A	N/A	N/A	47

SOURCE: Jack in the Box, Inc. 2008 (http://www.jackinthebox.com). The following trademarks are owned by Jack in the Box, Inc.: Breakfast Jack,® Jumbo Jack,® Sourdough Jack,® Jack in the Box.® Reproduced with permission from Jack in the Box, Inc.

KFC

	Serving size	Calories	Protein	Total fat	Saturated fat	Trans fat	Total carbohydrate	Sugars	Fiber	Cholesterol	Sodium	Vitamin A	Vitamin C	Calcium	Iron	% calories from fat
	g		g	g	g	g	g	g	g	mg	mg	% Daily Value				
Original Recipe® Chicken breast	161	360	37	21	5	0	7	0	0	115	1020	2	2	8	6	53
Original Recipe® Chicken thigh	126	330	20	24	6	0	8	0	0	110	870	4	2	4	8	67
Extra Crispy™ Chicken breast	162	440	34	27	6	0	15	0	0	105	970	2	2	6	6	57
Extra Crispy™ thigh	114	370	18	28	6	0	12	0	0	85	850	2	0	2	6	68
Tender Roast® sandwich w/ sauce	236	380	37	13	3	0	29	4	2	80	1180	6	15	8	15	32
Tender Roast® sandwich w/o sauce	217	300	37	4.5	1.5	0	28	3	2	70	1060	6	15	8	15	13
Hot Wings™ (5 pieces)	112	350	20	24	5	0	14	0	2	105	740	4	0	4	8	63
Popcorn chicken (large)	160	550	29	35	6	0	30	0	3	80	1600	4	2	4	10	58
Chicken pot pie	423	770	33	40	15	14	70	2	5	115	1680	200	0	0	20	47
Roasted Caesar Salad w/o dressing and croutons	301	220	30	8	4.5	0	6	3	3	70	830	45	35	25	10	36
KFC® creamy parmesan caesar dressing	57	260	2	26	5	0	4	2	0	15	540	2	0	6	2	88
Corn on the cob (5.5")	162	150	6	3	1	0	26	10	7	0	10	0	10	6	6	17
Mashed potatoes w/gravy	151	140	1	5	1	0.5	20	1	1	0	560	2	2	4	8	32
Baked beans	136	220	20	1	0	0	45	20	7	0	730	6	2	10	15	5
Cole slaw	130	180	4	10	1.5	0	22	18	3	5	270	10	20	4	4	50
Biscuit (1)	57	220	2	11	2.5	3.5	24	2	1	0	640	2	0	4	10	45
Potato salad	128	180	6	9	1.5	0	22	6	2	5	470	2	10	0	2	45

SOURCE: KFC Corporation, 2008. Nutritional information provided by KFC Corporation from its web site (www.kfc.com) as of July 30, 2008 and subject to the conditions listed therein. KFC and related marks are registered trademarks of KFC Corporation. Reproduced with permission from KFC Corporation.

McDonald's

	Serving size (g)	Calories	Protein (g)	Total fat (g)	Saturated fat (g)	Trans fat (g)	Total carbohydrate (g)	Sugars (g)	Fiber (g)	Cholesterol (mg)	Sodium (mg)	Vitamin A (% DV)	Vitamin C (% DV)	Calcium (% DV)	Iron (% DV)	% calories from fat
Hamburger	100	250	12	9	3.5	0.5	31	6	2	25	528	0	2	10	15	40
Quarter Pounder®	169	410	24	19	7	1	37	8	3	65	730	2	4	15	20	41
Quarter Pounder® w/cheese	198	510	29	26	12	1.5	40	9	3	90	1190	10	4	30	25	45
Big Mac®	214	540	25	29	10	1.5	45	9	3	75	1040	6	2	25	25	48
Big N' Tasty®	206	460	24	24	8	1.5	37	8	3	70	720	6	8	15	25	47
Filet-O-Fish®	142	380	15	18	3.5	0	38	5	2	40	640	2	0	15	10	45
McChicken®	143	360	14	16	3	0	40	5	2	35	830	0	2	10	15	42
Medium French Fries	117	380	4	19	2.5	0	48	0	5	0	270	0	10	2	6	45
Chicken McNuggets® (6 pieces)	95	280	14	17	3	0	16	0	0	40	600	2	2	2	4	57
Chicken Select® Premium Breast Strips (5 pieces)	219	660	38	40	6	0	39	0	0	85	1680	0	6	4	8	55
Tangy Honey Mustard Sauce	43	70	1	2.5	0	0	13	9	0	5	170	0	0	0	1	29
Bacon Ranch Salad w/Grilled Chicken (w/o dressing)	321	260	33	9	4	0	12	5	3	90	1010	130	50	15	10	35
Caesar Salad w/Crispy Chicken (w/o dressing)	314	330	130	17	4.5	0	20	6	3	60	840	130	50	20	10	46
Newman's Own® Ranch Dressing (2 oz)	59	170	1	15	2.5	0	9	4	0	20	530	0	0	4	0	76
Egg McMuffin®	139	300	18	12	5	0	30	3	2	260	820	10	2	30	20	37
Sausage Biscuit w/ Egg	163	510	18	33	14	0	36	2	2	250	1170	6	0	8	20	57
Hotcakes (w/o syrup & margarine)	151	350	8	9	2	0	60	14	3	20	590	2	0	15	15	23
Fruit 'n Yogurt Parfait	149	160	4	2	1	0	31	21	1	5	85	0	15	15	4	13
Chocolate Triple Thick® Shake (16 oz)	444	580	13	14	8	1	102	84	1	50	250	20	0	45	10	21

SOURCE: McDonald's Corporation, 2008. (http://www.mcdonalds.com). Used with permission from McDonald's Corporation. For the most current information, visit the McDonald's Web site.

Subway

Based on standard formulas with 6-inch subs on Italian or wheat bread

	Serving size (g)	Calories	Protein (g)	Total fat (g)	Saturated fat (g)	Trans fat (g)	Total carbohydrate (g)	Sugars (g)	Fiber (g)	Cholesterol (mg)	Sodium (mg)	Vitamin A (% DV)	Vitamin C (% DV)	Calcium (% DV)	Iron (% DV)	% calories from fat
6" Italian BMT®	242	450	23	21	8	0	47	8	5	55	1770	10	35	15	25	42
6" Meatball marinara	377	560	24	24	11	1	63	13	8	45	1590	15	60	20	40	39
6" Prime rib	278	400	29	12	6	0.5	48	9	6	60	1110	10	40	15	40	27
Subway Melt®	254	380	26	12	5	0	48	8	5	45	1600	10	35	15	25	29
Tuna	250	530	22	31	7	0.5	44	7	4	45	1010	10	35	15	30	53
Sweet onion chicken teriyaki wrap	304	480	26	90	10	3.5	70	14	2	50	1450	8	40	8	25	19
Roast beef wrap	248	400	19	10	4	0	15	3	2	15	1150	8	30	5	35	23
Turkey breast wrap	248	380	18	80	9	3	37	2	2	20	1250	8	35	6	25	21
Veggie Delite® wrap	192	330	9	8	2.5	0	55	2	2	0	750	8	35	6	25	20
Turkey Breast salad (w/o dressing)	378	110	12	2.5	0.5	0	13	6	4	20	580	60	50	6	10	20
New England style clam chowder	310	150	6	5	1	0	20	2	4	10	990	0	-	4	6	30
Chili con carne	310	290	19	8	3.5	0	35	13	12	25	990	15	20	8	20	25
Chocolate chip cookie	45	210	2	10	6	0	30	18	1	15	150	6	0	0	6	43

SOURCE: Subway U.S. Nutrition Info as found on http://www.subway.com, 7/30/2008. Reprinted by permission of Doctor's Associates, Inc.

Taco Bell

	Serving size	Calories	Protein	Total fat	Saturated fat	Trans fat	Total carbohydrate	Sugars	Fiber	Cholesterol	Sodium	Vitamin A	Vitamin C	Calcium	Iron	% calories from fat
	g		g	g	g	g	g	g	g	mg	mg	% Daily Value				
Crunchy Taco	92	150	7	8	2.5	0	13	1	3	20	370	4	2	8	6	47
Crunchy Taco Supreme®	113	210	9	13	6	.5	15	2	3	40	370	10	6	10	6	57
Soft taco, beef	113	180	8	70	7	3	21	2	3	20	650	4	2	10	10	39
Gordita Supreme®, steak	153	290	15	13	5	0	28	6	2	40	530	6	6	10	15	41
Grilled steak soft taco	128	160	10	4.5	1.5	0	20	3	2	20	550	4	10	8	10	25
Gordita Baja®, chicken	153	320	17	16	3.5	0	28	6	3	40	800	8	6	10	10	44
Chalupa Supreme, beef	153	380	14	23	7	0.5	30	4	3	40	620	8	6	15	15	55
Chalupa Supreme, chicken	153	360	17	20	5	0	29	4	2	45	650	6	8	10	15	49
1/2 lb. Beef combo burrito	241	440	21	18	7	1	51	4	8	45	1630	15	6	20	30	36
Bean burrito	198	350	13	9	3.5	0.5	54	4	8	5	1190	10	8	20	25	23
Burrito Supreme®, chicken	248	400	20	13	6	0.5	49	5	6	45	1360	15	15	20	25	30
Grilled stuffed burrito, beef	325	680	27	30	10	1	76	6	9	55	2120	15	4	30	40	40
Tostada	170	240	11	10	3.5	0.5	27	2	7	15	730	10	8	20	10	39
Zesty Chicken Border Bowl™ w/dressing	418	640	22	35	6	1	60	4	10	30	1800	15	15	15	25	37
Express taco salad	475	610	25	32	10	1.5	56	8	14	65	1420	20	20	30	25	48
Steak quesadilla	184	520	26	28	13	1	39	4	3	70	1300	10	0	45	20	50
Nachos Supreme	191	440	12	26	6	1	40	3	7	30	790	8	8	10	10	52
Nachos BellGrande®	305	770	19	44	8	1	77	5	12	30	1270	8	8	20	20	51
Pintos 'n cheese	128	160	9	6	3	0.5	19	1	7	15	670	10	6	15	8	31
Mexican rice	85	110	2	3	0	0	19	0	1	0	460	15	6	10	8	23

SOURCE: Taco Bell Corporation, 2008. (http://www.tacobell.com). Reproduced courtesy of Taco Bell Corporation.

Wendy's

	Serving size	Calories	Protein	Total fat	Saturated fat	Trans fat	Total carbohydrate	Sugars	Fiber	Cholesterol	Sodium	Vitamin A	Vitamin C	Calcium	Iron	% calories from fat
	g		g	g	g	g	g	g	g	mg	mg	% Daily Value				
Classic Single® w/everything	226	430	25	20	7	1	39	9	2	75	870	8	8	4	25	42
Jr. Hamburger	98	230	13	8	3	0	27	5	1	30	490	0	0	2	20	30
Jr. Bacon Cheeseburger	136	320	17	16	6	0.5	26	5	1	50	670	10	6	10	20	44
Ultimate Chicken Grill Sandwich	211	320	28	7	1.5	0	36	8	2	70	950	6	10	4	20	19
Spicy Chicken Sandwich	223	440	28	16	2.5	0	46	6	3	60	1300	6	8	4	15	34
Homestyle Chicken Fillet Sandwich	226	430	25	16	2.5	0	48	6	2	45	1120	6	8	4	15	33
10 Piece Chicken Nuggets	150	460	24	30	6	0	24	0	0	70	1040	0	0	2	6	59
Caesar Side Salad (no toppings or dressing)	142	260	8	19	4	0	14	2	2	490	270	100	35	10	6	57
Mandarin Chicken® Salad w/grilled chicken fillet	402	540	31	25	3	0.5	50	31	5	65	1260	70	50	6	10	43
Southwest Taco Salad (no toppings or dressing	520	640	30	39	16	1	44	12	9	110	1570	80	35	45	20	55
Creamy ranch dressing	64	200	1	20	3.5	0	4	2	0	15	400	0	0	4	2	87
Reduced fat creamy ranch dressing	64	90	1	7	1.5	0	6	3	1	10	400	0	0	6	2	70
Large French Fries	184	550	7	26	4	0	73	0	7	0	480	4	15	2	10	42
Sour Cream & Chive Baked Potato	308	320	8	4	2	0	63	4	7	10	50	4	60	8	15	11
Strawberry Frosty™ shake, small	325	390	7	11	7	0.5	67	58	0	35	170	2	2	22	6	26
Chili, small, plain	227	190	14	6	2.5	0	19	6	5	40	830	4	4	8	15	32
Crispy Chicken Nuggets™ (5)	75	230	12	15	3	0	12	0	0	35	520	0	0	0	2	59
Barbecue sauce (1 packet)	28	45	1	0	0	0	10	8	0	0	170	0	0	0	4	0
Vanilla Frosty™, medium	298	410	11	10	6	0.5	68	57	0	45	240	20	0	40	20	22

SOURCE: Wendy's International, Inc., 2008. (http://www.wendys.com). Reproduced with permission from Wendy's International, Inc. The information contained in Wendy's International Information is effective as of July 30, 2008. Wendy's International, Inc., its subsidiaries, affiliates, franchises, and employees do not assume responsibility for a particular sensitivity or allergy (including peanuts, nuts or other allergies) to any food product provided in our restaurants. We encourage anyone with food sensitivities, allergies, or special dietary needs to check on a regular basis with Wendy's Consumer Relations Department to obtain the most up-to-date information.

Information on additional foods and restaurants is available online; see the Web sites listed in this appendix and the following additional sites: **Hardees:** http://www.hardees.com; **White Castle:** http://www.whitecastle.com

PHOTO CREDITS

INDEX

Boldface numbers indicate pages on which glossary definitions appear.

AA (Alcoholics Anonymous), 168, 169
AAP (American Academy of Pediatrics), 262
ABCD test, melanoma, 307
abortion, 114–115, 125, **140**, 140–147. *See also* miscarriage
abstinence, **134**, 134–135
abuse. *See* alcohol abuse; psychoactive drugs; substance abuse; violence
academic stress, 32
Acceptable Macronutrient Distribution Ranges (AMDRs), 208
ACOG (American College of Obstetricians and Gynecologists), 212
acquired immune deficiency syndrome (AIDS), **331**. *See also* HIV/AIDS; human immuno-deficiency virus
    sexual orientation and, 11
    women and, 338
acquired immunity, **320**
ACS (American Cancer Society), 301, 303, 310, 312
ACSM (American College of Sports Medicine), 248, 255
active euthanasia, **419**
acupuncture, 372–373, **373**
addiction, **151**. *See also* psychoactive drugs; substance dependence
addictive behavior, 149–152, **151**
Adequate Intake (AI), 218
ADHD (attention-deficit/hyperactivity disorder), 164
adolescence, 66
adoption, 144
adrenal androgens, 253
adrenal glands, **93**
adulthood, **66**, 66–67
adults, dietary challenges and, 226
advance directive, **419**, 419–420
advertising. *See* media
AEDs (automated external defibrillators), 402
AFP (alpha-fetoprotein), 216
African Americans
    alcohol use by, 186, 187
    cardiovascular disease among, 286, 292
    diabetes in, 267
    drug use/dependence among, 168
    genetic diseases in, 112
    health concerns of, 7, 11
    hypertension in, 286
    life expectancy of, 413
    sodium consumption and, 286
age, contraception use according to, 138
age-related macular degeneration (AMD), 410, **411**
aggressive driving, 384
aging, 96, 290, 406–415
    adapting to physical changes, 410–411
    age-proofing measures, 407–409
    diet and, 408
    elder abuse, 398
    exercise and, 408
    government aid/policies and, 414–415
    psychological/mental changes with, 411–413
    social changes with, 409–410
    successful, 406
agoraphobia, **57**

AI (Adequate Intake), 218
AIDS. *See* acquired immune deficiency syndrome
air bags, 386–387
air pollution, 348–352. *See also* chemical pollution; pollution
    energy use and, 350–352
    global warming/greenhouse effect, 13, 348–350, **349**
    indoor, 352
    ozone layer thinning and, **350**
    prevention of, 352
Air Quality Index (AQI), 348, **349**
alarm reaction, 28
Alaska Natives
    alcohol use by, 168, 188
    cardiovascular disease among, 292
    diabetes in, 267
    drug use by, 168
    health concerns of, 11
alcohol, 175–189, **176**, 310
    absorption of, 176
    dose-response function from, 180
    intake, 177
    metabolism/excretion of, 176, 178
    poisoning, 178
alcohol abuse, 154, 177, 180–188, **183**
alcohol use, 113, 123, 162, 271–296
    aggression and, 179
    body fat and, 176
    cancer and, 181–182
    cardiovascular disease and, 298
    cardiovascular system effects of, 181
    CVD and, **284**, 290, 298
    deaths from, 4, 5, 276, 280, 281
    by demographics, 186
    digestive system and, 180–181
    drugs with, 179
    employment and, 168
    ethnicity and, 177, 186
    gender differences in, 9, 177, 186–187
    health benefits of, possible, 182–183
    injuries and, 386
    in lifestyle assessment, 16
    moderation in, 290–291
    motor-vehicle injuries and, 386
    pregnancy and, 113, 182, 281–282
    stress and, 42
    violence and, 179, 277, 393
alcoholic beverages, 176
Alcoholics Anonymous (AA), 168, 169
alcoholism, **183**, 184–186
alcohol-related neurodevelopmental disorder (ARND), **182**, 183
allergic response, 322
allergies, 40, **232**, 233, 322–323, **323**
allied health care providers, **369**
allostatic load, 29–30, **30**
alpha-fetoprotein (AFP), 216
altered states of consciousness, **166**
alternative medicine, 62, 372–374
Alzheimer's disease, 352, **411**, 411–412
AMD (age-related macular degeneration), **410**
AMDRs. *See* Acceptable Macronutrient Distribution Ranges
amenorrhoea, **269**
American Cancer Society (ACS), 301, 303, 310, 312

American College of Sports Medicine (ACSM), 248, 255
American Indians
    alcohol use by, 188
    cardiovascular disease among, 292
    diabetes in, 267
    drug use/dependence among, 168
    health concerns of, 9–10
American Psychiatric Association (APA), 58
amino acids, **206**, 253
amniocentesis, **111**
amniotic fluid, **215**
amniotic sac, 108
amphetamines, 162–163
anabolic steroids, **253**
anal intercourse, 101
anaphylaxis, **322**, 323
anatomy, sexual, 90–92
androgens, **93**
andropause, 96
anemia, **215**
aneurysm, 296, **297**
anger, 54, 289
angina pectoris, 293–294, **294**
angiogram, **294**
anorexia nervosa, 276–277, **277**
antibiotics, **324**, 325
    resistance to, 326, 329
antibody, **320**, 334
anticarcinogens, **310**
antidepressants, 63, 221
antigens, **320**
antioxidants, **212**, 216–217
anti-tobacco legislation, 197, 198
antiviral medications, 328, 334
anxiety, **55**, 289. *See also* stress
    test, 27, 44
anxiety disorders, 55–58, 60
    panic disorder, 74
    post-traumatic stress disorder, 40, 45, **76**, 76–77
aorta, **284**
APA (American Psychiatric Association), 58, 240
Apgar score, **118**, 119
AQI (Air Quality Index), 348, **349**
ARND (alcohol-related neurodevelopmental disorder), **182**, 183
arousal. *See* female sexual arousal disorder; sexual functioning
arrhythmias, **294**
ART (assisted reproductive technology), 106
arteries, **284**
arteriosclerosis, 293
arthritis, 246, 320, 330, 376, 410, **411**
artificial insemination, **106**
asbestosis, **354**, 355
Asian Americans, 7
    cardiovascular disease among, 292
    diabetes in, 267
    drug use and, 168
    family life/education values of, 168
aspirin, 94–95, 364
assault, 393–395. *See also* sexual assault
assertiveness, **53**
assisted reproductive technology (ART), **106**
asthma, 7, 10, 246
asymptomatic diseases, **331**, 343

atherosclerosis, **192**, **193**, **286**. *See also* peripheral arterial disease
athletes, 226, 252, 253
atria, **204**
attachment, **70**, 119
attention-deficit/hyperactivity disorder (ADHD), 164
AUDIT (Alcohol Use Disorders Test), 291
auditory hallucinations, 64, 67
authenticity, **49**
authoritarian parent, 85
authoritative parent, 85–86
autoeroticism, 100–101, **101**
autoimmune diseases, **320**, 330
automated external defibrillators (AEDs), 402
autonomic nervous system, **25**, 33
autonomy, **48**, 49

BAC (blood alcohol concentration), **176**, 176–178, 180
bacterial vaginosis (BV), **342**
bacterium/bacteria, **323**, 323–326
    foodborne illness types of, 228, 231
balloon angioplasty, **294**, 295
barrier method, 122, **123**
basal cell carcinoma, **307**
battering, 396–397
BDD (body dysmorphic disorder), 276
beans, 224
beer, 176
behavior. *See* addictive behavior; sexual behavior
behavior change, **14**
    cycle of, 21
    goal-setting for, 22–23
    maintenance of, 21, 25–26
    motivation for, 15–17, 25
    personal contract for, 20
    personalized plans for, 18–20
    readiness for, 20–21
    relapse in, 18
    rewards for, 24
    self-efficacy in, **15**
    social influences in, 25
    stages of change model, 17–18
    stress barrier to, 25
    target behavior, **15**, 19
    techniques/effort in, 25
behavior change strategies
    beverages and, 234
    dietary, 315
    drug use, 172
    injury prevention, 403
    social anxiety, 67
    test anxiety, 44
    tobacco use/smoking, 202
    weight management, 280
benign tumors, **299–300**
Benson-Henry Institute for Mind Body Medicine, 58
bereavement, **422**, 423
beverages, 273
bicycles, 387
bidis, clove cigarettes and, 195–196
binge drinking, **183**, 183–184
binge-eating disorder, **278**
bioelectromagnetic-based therapies, **377**
biofeedback, **54**
biological model, 83–85
biological-based therapies, **374**, 375
biopsy, **300**
bioterrorism, 330
bipolar disorder, **61**, 61–62
birth control, **122**, **123**. *See also* childbirth; contraception
    pills, 124–125
birth defects, 111

blastocyst, **108**, 109
blood. *See also* cholesterol
    cardiovascular system, 284
    glucose levels in, **211**
blood alcohol concentration (BAC), **176**, 176–178, 180
blood pressure, 286, 299. *See also* high blood pressure
blood tests
    prenatal care and, 113
    prostate-specific antigen, 304
BMI (body mass index), **264**, 264–265
Bod Pod, 265
body composition, **242**, 262–263, 264–265
analysis, 418
body dysmorphic disorder (BDD), 276
body fat
    body composition and, **242**, 262–263, 264–265
    distribution and, 266–267
    excess, 265–266, 268–270
    percent, **263**
    wellness and, 265–267, 419–420, 422
body image, 268, **269**, 272, 276, 277
body mass index (BMI), 264–265, **265**
body weight. *See* body fat
bone marrow, **300**
bones
    nutrition and, 216
    osteoporosis, 213, **215**, 216
botanicals. *See* herbal remedies
brain
    alcohol effects on, 182
    psychoactive drug influence on, 157
    stress and, 41
brain death, **415**
breakfast cereals, 213
breast cancer, 302–303
breast self exams (BSE), 304
breastfeeding, 118–119
breathing, 40–41, 54
BSE (breast self-exams), 304
bulimia nervosa, 278, **278**
Bupropion (zyban/Wellbutrin), 200
burnout, **33**
BV (bacterial vaginosis), **342**

CAD. *See* coronary artery disease
caffeine, 164
    beverage content of, 164
    pregnancy and, 114, 220
calcium, 216, 298
calories, 270–271, 407
    cardiovascular disease and, 298
    discretionary calorie allowance, 225
    energy and, 263
    food labels and, 229
    nutrient classes and, 218
    weight management and, 270–271
CAM. *See* complementary/alternative medicine
cancer, 245, **299**, 299–316, 330
    alcohol use and, 181–182, 310
    breast, 302–303
    carcinomas, **300**
    causes of, 309–312
    cervical, 305–306
    colon/rectal, 302
    diagnosis of, 302, 312–313
    diet and, 310
    DNA role in, 309
    early detection of, 312
    endometrial, 306
    female reproductive tract, 305–306
    incidence of, 301
    leukemia, **300**
    lung, 301–302, 309
    lymphomas and, **300**, 301

melanoma and, 306, **307**
metastasis and, **300**
myths about, 311
obesity and, 310, 311
oral, 307, 309
ovarian, 306
prevention of, 307, 314
prostate, 303–305
quackery, 313
sarcomas and, **300**
skin, 306–307
testicular, 309
tobacco use and, 306, 309–310, 313, 314
treatment of, 302, 312–313
tumors and, **299**, 299–300
types of, 300
uterine, 306
viruses and, 165
cannabis products, marijuana/other, 164–165
capacity for intimacy, 48
capillaries, **284**
carbohydrates, **208**, 209–212, 299
    AMDRs for protein/fat and, 208
    cardiovascular disease and, 299
    diet planning with, 219–220
    diets with low, 274
    energy from, 209–212
    glycemic index for, **211**, 211–212
    recommended intake of, 212
    simple/complex, 209–210
    whole grains v. refined, 210–211
carbon dioxide (CO_2), 349, 352
carbon monoxide (CO), 348
carcinogens, **191**, 310
    anti-, **310**
    environmental tobacco smoke, 315
carcinoma, **300**, 307
cardiac arrest, 295. *See also* sudden cardiac death
cardiac myopathy, **181**
cardiopulmonary resuscitation (CPR), **294**, 402
cardiorespiratory endurance exercise and, 240–241, **241**, 243–244, 250, 254
cardiovascular disease (CVD), **40**, 283–299, **284**, 314. *See also* atherosclerosis; heart attack; stroke
    aging and, 290
    alcohol use and, 284, 290, 298
    cholesterol and, 287, 299
    congenital heart defects, **297**
    diet and, 286, 292, 298–299
    drug use and, 290
    ethnicity and, 286, 291, 292
    exercise and, 245, 299
    gender differences in, 290
    heredity and, 290
    high blood pressure and, 286–287
    homocysteine and, 292
    inflammation/C-Reactive protein and, 291
    insulin resistance and, 291–292
    LDL and, 286, 287, 298–299
    major forms of, 292–299
    metabolic syndrome and, 291–292
    obesity and, 287–288
    prevention of, 298–299, 314
    psychological/social factors in, 288–290
    risk assessment for, 291–292
    sodium intake and, 298
    stress and, 30–31, 289
    tobacco use and, 192–193, 285, 299
    triglyceride levels and, 288
cardiovascular system, 283–284, **284**
    alcohol effects on, 181
    blood vessels, 284
caregiving, 417–418
carpal tunnel syndrome, **390**, 391, 392
cataracts, 410, **411**

Caucasians
  alcohol use by, 186
  cardiovascular disease among, 292
  diabetes in, 267
  drug use/dependence among, 168
  genetic diseases in, 112
  life expectancy of, 413
CD4 T cell, **331**, 334
CDC. *See* Center for Disease Control
CDC (Center for Disease Control), 252
celibacy, **100**
cell phones, 385–386
cellular death, **417**
Center for Disease Control (CDC), 252
central nervous system (CNS), **160**. *See also* depressants, CNS; stimulants, CNS
cerebral cortex, **192**, **193**
cerebrovascular accident. *See* stroke
cervical cancer, 305–306
cervix, **91**
cesarean section, **118**, **119**
CFCs (chlorofluorocarbons), **350**
chain of infection, 318–319
chancre, **342**
CHD. *See* coronary heart disease
chemical pollution, 355–357
chemicals, ingested, 310–311
chemotherapy, **303**
chicken pox, 326
child safety seats, 386
child sexual abuse, 400
childbirth, 114, 116–119, 231. *See also* birth control
children
  adoption of, 144
  aspirin and, 364
  congenital heart defects in, **297**
  death in, causes of, 328
  depression and, 86
  diabetes in, 267
  dietary challenges with, 226
  divorce and, 84
  lead poisoning in, 355–356
  mercury poisoning in, 356
  school violence and, 394
  sexual abuse of, 400
  television violence and, 392
  violence against, 397–398
chiropractic, **374**, 375
chlamydia, 337–338
chlorofluorocarbons (CFCs), **350**
choking, 389
cholera, 347
cholesterol, **208**, 287, 298, 299
  good v. bad, 287
  guidelines, 287
  smoking and, 310
chorionic villi, 109
chorionic villus sampling (CVS), **111**
chromium picolinate, 253
chronic disease, **4**, 364
chronic obstructive pulmonary disease (COPD), 193
cigar smoking, 195, 314
cigarette tar, **191**
cigarette tax, 198
cigarettes. *See also* smoking; tobacco/tobacco use
  clove/bidis, 195–196
  light/low-tar, 191
  menthol, 191–192
circumcision, **93**
cirrhosis, **181**
civil unions, same-sex marriage and, 82
clinical death, **417**
clitoris, **91**
clove cigarettes, 195–196

club drugs, 161, 252
cluster headaches, 32
CMV (cytomegalovirus), 326
CNS. *See* central nervous system
CO_2 (carbon dioxide), 349, 352
cocaine, 162
cocarcinogens, **191**
codependency, **170**
coercion, sexual, **103**
coffee, caffeine content in, 164
cognitive distortion, **51**, 52
cognitive techniques, stress management through, 38–39
cohabitation, **78**, 78–81
cold sores, 326
collective violence, 395
college students, 49
  binge drinking by, 185
  dietary challenges with, 226
  drug use by, 154
  eating disorders among, 276
  eating strategies for, 227
  sexual behavior and, 102
  stress and, 32–33
  test anxiety of, 27, 44
  violence on campus and, 391–392, 401
  wellness concerns of, 13
colon/rectal cancer, 302
colostrum, **119**
combination pill, 124
commercial sex, 103–104
commitment
  family life success and, 87
  love and, 83, 87, 98
  marriage and, 83
  unequal/premature, 73
common cold, 326
communication
  contraception and, 139
  family life and, 118–119
  gender differences in, 75, 77
  guidelines for effective, 105
  "I" statements, 105
  intimate relationships, 75–78, 103–107
  psychological health and, 53
  sexual behavior and, 104, 105
  skills, 75
competitiveness, 73
complementary/alternative medicine (CAM), **365**, 370–378
  biological-based therapies, **374**, 375
  energy therapies, 375–377
  evaluation of, 377–378
  manipulative/body-based methods, 375
  mind-body interventions, 374–375
compulsion, **58**, **59**, 151–152
computed tomography (CT) scanning, **297**
conception, **123**. *See also* prenatal care
condoms
  female, 130, 131
  male, **129**, 129–131
  STDs and, 129, 343
  trends in use of, 129
confidants, statistics on, 97–98
conflict/conflict resolution, 75–78
congenital heart defect, **297**
congenital malformations, **113**
congestive heart failure, **297**
consciousness. *See* altered states of consciousness
constructive thinking, 50
contagion, 321
contemplation, 17
continuation rate, **123**
contraception, 104, 122–148, **123**, 187
  abstinence, **134**, 134–135
  age of use by type of, 138

barrier method, 122, **123**
choosing right, 139–140
combining methods of, 135
communicating about, 139
condom, **129**, 129–131
continuation rate, **154**, 155–156
contraceptive failure rate, **123**
deaths from abortion and, 125
diaphragm, **131**, 131–133
effectiveness, 126, 127, 129, 136
emergency, **127**, 128, 130
ethnicity and, 138
female condoms, 130, 131
FemCap, **132**, 133
fertility awareness method (FAM), **134**, 134–135
health risks and, 139
hormonal method, 122, **123**
hysterectomy, **139**
implants, 126
injectable, 126–127
intrauterine device, **127**, 127–129, 176, 180
IUD, 180
laparoscopy, **137**
Lea's Shield, 132–133
male condoms, **129**, 129–131
men's involvement in, 140
natural method, **123**
oral, **123**, 156–158
over-the-counter contraceptives, 130
partner communication about, 139
permanent/sterilization, **136**, 136–139, **137**
Plan B, 127, 128, 130
reversible, 123–136
risk statistics on, 125
sexually transmitted diseases and, 136, 139
skin patch, 125
socioeconomic status and, 138
spermicide, **129**, 130
sponge, 130, **132**, 133
STDs and, 122, 124, 129, 131, 136
surgical method, **123**
trends in use of, 129, 138
vaginal contraceptive ring, 125–126
vaginal spermicides, **129**, 129–130, 166, 170–171
withdrawal, **134**, 134–135
contraceptive failure rate, **123**
contractions, labor, **116**, **117**
conventional medicine, **365**, 366–370
COPD (chronic obstructive pulmonary disease), 193
coronary arteries, **284**
coronary artery disease (CAD), 290, 293, 294
coronary bypass surgery, **294**, 295
coronary heart disease (CHD), 192, **193**, 287, 289, **293**
  plaques and, **193**, **293**
  tobacco use and, 192–193
corpus luteum, **94**, **95**
cortisol, **25**
costs
  cancer, 300
  cardiovascular disease, 292
  drug abuse, 167
  health care, 378–380
  injuries, 383
  psychoactive drug use, 153
  smoking, 194
  tobacco use, 197
Cowper's glands, **93**
CPR (cardiopulmonary resuscitation), **294**, 402
C-reactive protein (CRP), 291
cream, prostaglandin, 137
Creatine Monohydrate, 253
creativity, self-actualization and, **48**
crime, hate, 394

cross-training, **258**
CRP (C-reactive protein), 291
cruciferous vegetables, **217**
Cruzan, Nancy, 418
culture
    death/dying and, 417
    drug use and, 168
    ethnicity and, 9
    gender identity/gender roles and, 138
    lifestyle and, 10–11
    stress and, 28
cunnilingus, **101**
CVA. *See* stroke
CVD. *See* cardiovascular disease
CVS (chorionic villus sampling), **111**
cybersex, 103–104, **104**
cyberstalking, **396**, 397
cycle of behavior change, 21
cystic fibrosis, 8, 14–15, 112
cytokines, **320**, 321

D & C (dilation and curettage), **144**
D & E (dilation and evacuation), **145**
Daily Values, **219**
DASH diet, 218, 286, 299
date rape, **398**, 398–399
date rape drugs, 161, 399
dating, 78
Day of the Dead, 417
death, causes of. *See also* suicide
    alcohol use, 4, 5, 276, 280, 281
    among Americans, statistics on, 5–6
    cancer, 301, 311, 313
    cardiovascular disease, 288
    childhood, nutrition-related, 207
    in children, 328, 389
    chronic liver disease, 280
    contraception/abortion, 125
    diabetes, 420
    ethnicity and, 11
    firearms, 390
    heart disease, 292
    indoor fires, 388–389
    infant mortality among ethnic groups and, 11
    injuries, 383
    lifestyle choices and, 4, 5
    lung cancer, 301, 315
    natural disasters, 391
    obesity, 5, 268
    physical inactivity, 382
    teens, 4
    terrorism, 395
    tobacco use, 4, 5, 300, 309–310
    in U.S., 4
Death with Dignity Act, 418
death/dying, 415–425
    advance directives, **419**, 419–420
    coming to terms with, 425
    coping with dying, 420–421
    defining death, 415–416
    denying v. welcoming, 416
    end-of-life care, 417–418
    funeral/memorial service planning, 420
    grief and, 412, 422–425
    prolonging/hastening death, 418–419
    wills, 416–417, 419
decibels, **358**
deep breathing, 40–41
defense mechanisms, 51–52, 53, **53**
Defense of Marriage Act (DOMA), 82
dementia, **411**
dendritic cells, 320, 321
dentists, **367**
deoxyribonucleic acid (DNA), 309, 331
Department of Homeland Security, 396
dependence. *See* substance dependence

depersonalization, marijuana and, 165
Depo-Provera, 160–161
depressants, CNS, **160**, 160–162
depression, 58–62, **59**, 412–413
    cardiovascular disease and, 289
    childhood, 86
    gender differences in, 9
    herbal remedies/alternative medical systems for, 62
    postpartum, **119**
    suicide and, 60
development
    embryonic, early, 109
    fetal, 108–111
development stages, 66, 67
diabetes
    ethnicity and, 267
    exercise and, 246
    gestational, **115**, 267
    mellitus, 265–266
    prevention/treatment of, 267
    statistics on, 389
    symptoms of, 420
    Type 1, 266
    Type 2, 245–246, 266
    types of, 267
diagnostic process, 369–370
diaphragm, contraceptive, **131**, 131–133
diastole, **284**
diet(s). *See also* dietary supplements; food(s)
    aging and, 408
    aids, 272–273
    cancer and, 310, 315
    carbohydrates in, 219–220
    cardiovascular disease and, 286, 292, 298–299
    cholesterol and, 287
    DASH, 218, 286, 299
    death statistics and, 5
    eating habits and, 56, 332
    exercise and, 255–256
    grains in, 210–211, 222, 352–353
    incorporating fruits/vegetables into, 217, 222, 315
    low-carbohydrate, 274
    Mediterranean, 221–222
    MyPyramid, **217**, 218, 221–225, 270, 273
    nutritional guidelines for planning, 217–227
    personal plan for, 228–233
    PMS, 95
    pregnancy, 113
    special population groups, 226–227
    unhealthy eating habits, **56**
    weight management/eating habits and, 218, 269, 270–271, 274, 280
diet sodas, 270
dietary fat, 208–209, 350, 355–356. *See also* body fat; fat(s)
    AMDRs for carbohydrate/protein and, 208
    cancer and, 310, 350, 355–356
    cholesterol and, 218–219, **334**
    low-density lipoprotein, **208**, **286**, 287, 298, 299
    recommended intake of, 208–209
dietary fiber, **212**, 213
Dietary Guidelines for Americans, **217**, 218–221
Dietary Reference Intakes (DRIs), **217**, 217–218, 237–239
dietary reference intakes (DRIs), 237
Dietary Supplement Health and Education Act (DSHEA), 230
dietary supplements, 230
    club drugs sold as, 161
    diet aids and, 272–273
    exercise and, 252, 253
    herbal, 273
    labels on, 228, 230
    performance-enhancing, 401

differentiation, embryo, 93–94, 215
digestive system, 180–181, 206
dilation and curettage (D & C), 144
dilation and evacuation (D & E), **145**
disabilities, 10, 140, 246
discretionary calorie allowance, 225
discrimination, 9, 34
diseases. *See also* chronic disease; genetic diseases; illness; infectious diseases; psychological disorders; *specific diseases*
    asymptomatic, **331**
    exercise for prevention/management of, 245–246
    pathogens and, 323–330
disparities, health, 5–11
disposition of body, death/dying and, 420
distress, **28**
Disulfram (Antabuse), 186
diversity, wellness and, 6–11
divorce, separation and, 84, 85
DMT, hallucinogen, 166
DNA (deoxyribonucleic acid), 309, 331
doctor of osteopathic medicine (D. O.), **367**
DOMA (Defense of Marriage Act), 82
dominant gene, 112
dose-response function, **157–158**
double effect, **419**
douche, **134**
drinking. *See* binge drinking; water
DRIs (Dietary Reference Intakes), **217**, 217–218, 237–239
DRIs (dietary reference intakes), 237
driving
    aggressive, 384
    cell phone use during, 385–386
drug abuse, 152–157. *See also* psychoactive drugs
drug(s), defined, **151**. *See also* medications; psychoactive drugs
drug use. *See also* medications; psychoactive drugs
    among Americans, 156
    athletes and, 253
    cardiovascular disease and, 290
    college students and, 154
    ethnicity and, 168
    families/family life, 167
    gender differences in, 155
    legal consequences of, 157
    pregnancy and, 113, 158, 253
    socioeconomic status and, 168
    spirituality and, 156
    stress and, 42
Drug-Induced Rape Prevention and Punishment Act, 161, 399
DSHEA (Dietary Supplement Health and Education Act), 230
dying. *See* death/dying
dysmenorrhea, 94, **95**
dysthymic disorder, 58

E. I. Q. *See* emotional intelligence
E. Q. *See* emotional intelligence
Eastern European Americans, 8, 112
eating. *See* diet(s); nutrition
eating disorders, 276–279, **277**
ebola, 329
EBV (Epstein-Barr virus), 326
EC (emergency contraception), **127**, 128
ECG/EKG (electrocardiogram), **248**, **249**, **294**
eclampsia, **115**
ECT (electroconvulsive therapy), **61**
ectopic pregnancy, **114**
educational attainment
    cardiovascular disease and, 289
    health concerns and, 9–10
    infant mortality rate and, 9, 10
EEG (electroencephalogram), **415**, 415–416

ejaculation, 129
   premature, **98**
ejaculatory duct, **93**
elder abuse, 398
electrical impedance analysis, 265
electrocardiogram (ECG/EKG), **248, 249, 294**
electroconvulsive therapy (ECT), **61**
ELISA (enzyme-linked immunosorbent assay), **334**
embalming, **420**
embolus, 296, **297**
embryo, **108**. *See also* stem cells
   differentiation of, 93–94, 215
   early development of, 109
emergencies
   alcohol, 179
   preparation for, 396
emergency contraception (EC), **127, 128**, 130
emergency medical services (EMS) system, **402**
emotion(s)
   sexual stimulation and, 97
   stress and, 27–28
   strong, 101
   weight management and, 271–272
emotional intelligence (E. Q./E. I. Q.), 101
emotional wellness, 2, 11
emphysema, **193**
employment, alcohol/drug use and, 168
EMS (emergency medical services), **402**
endocrine system, **25**, 32–33
endometrial cancer, 306
endometriosis, 197
endometrium, **95, 129**
endorphins, **25**
endoscopy, **369**
endothelial cells, 288, 293
endurance training, **241**
   frequency of, 251
   intensity of, 250, 251–252
time/duration of, 250
energy
   calories and, 263
   carbohydrates for, 209–212
   drinks, 256
   therapies, 375–377
   weight management and, 263–264, 271, 274
energy use, 350–352
entry inhibitor, **334**
environment, **15**, 17. *See also* air pollution; pollution
   built, 160
   burials/embalming influence on, 421
   carcinogens in, 310
   drug use and, 160
   food crisis and, 347
   global warming, 13, 348–350, **349**
   medicine and, 373
   pregnancy and, 113–114
   seasonal affective disorder, **61**
   stress and, 28
   weight management and, 269
environmental health, 3, 346–361, **347**
   air pollution, 348–352
   Air Quality Index, 348, **349**
   chemical pollution, 355–357
   energy use, 350–352
   hazardous waste, 355–356
   noise pollution, 358–359
   population growth/control, 347–348
   poverty and, 356
   radiation, **356**, 357–358
   sewage and, 353
   solid waste pollution, 353–355
   water quality/pollution, 352–353
Environmental Protection Agency (EPA), 348
environmental tobacco smoke (ETS), **196**, 352

environmental wellness, 3
Environmental Working Group (EWG), 256
enzyme-linked immunosorbent assay (ELISA), **334**
EPA (Environmental Protection Agency), 348
ephedra (ma huang), 253, 273–274
epidemics, 320, 327
epididymitis, **92, 93, 337**
epinephrine, **25**
epithelia, **300**
EPO (Erythropoietin), 253
Epstein-Barr virus (EBV), 326
equipment, exercise, 251
erectile dysfunction, **98**, 100
Erikson, Erik, 66, 67
erogenous zones, **97**
erotic fantasy, **101**
Erythropoietin (EPO), 253
escalation, addictive behavior characteristic, 150
Escherichia coli, 329
essential nutrients, **205, 206**
   antioxidant, **212**, 216–217
   carbohydrates, **208**, 209–212, 219–220, 299
   fats, 207, 209, 218–219
   minerals, **212**, 213, 215
   proteins, 206–207
   water, 216
Essure system, 137
estate, 416, **417**
estrogen, **93**, 290, 303
estrogenic phase, menstrual cycle, **94**
ethnicity
   alcohol abuse and, 177, 187–188
   body image and, 277
   cardiovascular disease and, 286, 291, 292
   contraception and, 138
   diabetes and, 12, 267
   distribution in U.S., 8
   drug use and, 168
   gender and, 79
   genetic diseases and, 112
   health care and, 10
   health disparities among minorities, 5–11
   health insurance and, 379
   heart attack and, 12
   HIV/AIDS and, 11, 332
   income/education and, 10
   suicide and, 7, 79
   wellness and, 7, 9–10
ETS. *See* environmental tobacco smoke
euphoria, **160**
eustress, **28**
euthanasia, 419
evaluation
   complementary/alternative medicine, 377–378
   health information, 16, 368
   mental health professionals, 66
EWG (Environmental Working Group), 256
examinations
   BSE, 304
   exercise and, 248
   testicle self-, 309
excitement phase, sexual response cycle, 97–98
exercise(s), 114, 240–261, **242**
   aging and, 408
   benefits of, 243–247
   body image and, 272
   cancer and, 245
   cardiorespiratory endurance, 240–241, **241**, 243–244, 250, 254
   cardiovascular disease and, 245, 299
   diet and, 255–256
   dietary supplements and, 252, 253
   equipment for, 251
   flexibility, **242**, 248, 252–254
   immune system and, 390
   injuries and, 247, 256–258

injuries from, preventing, 256–258
   isometric, **251**
   isotonic, **251**, 251–252
   muscular strength, **241**, 248, 250–252, 254
   osteoporosis and, 245
   prenatal care, 114
   resistance, **250**
   special health concerns and, 246
   statistics on, 23
   stress management through, 35–36, 390
   water drinking and, 216, 256
   weight management and, 272
exercise program, 247–258
   activity selection for, 248, 249–250
   choosing exercises for, 251
   consistency in, 256
   designing, 247–254
   disabilities and, 246
   flexibility exercises in, 252–254
   frequency of, 250, 251
   instructors/facilities for, 254–255
   intensity and, 393, 397–398
   management/maintenance of, 256–258
   medical clearance for, 392
   personalizing, 259
   physical fitness assessment and, 380–386
   principles of physical training and, 248–249
   progression of, 406
   RICE and, 257–258
   specific skills and, 254
   stretching and, 253–254
   warm-up/cool-down in, 250
exhaustion, GAS stage, 29
expectations, of partner, 73

fallopian tube, **91**
   ectopic pregnancy in, **114**
   gamete intrafallopian transfer (GIFT), **106**
   zygote intrafallopian transfer, **106, 107**
falls, injury from, 388
false negative, test result, **369**
false positive, test result, **369**
FAM (fertility awareness method), **134**, 134–135
families/family life, 84–87. *See also* marriage; parents/parenting
   cycle, 86
   drug use and, 167
   marriage and, 83–84
   step-, 87
   successful, 87
   violence in, 396–398
family history, 13
FAS (fetal alcohol syndrome), **113, 182, 183**
fast-food restaurants, 227
fat(s), 298. *See also* body fat; dietary fat
   trans, 220, 354
   types/sources of, 207, 209
fat-free mass, **242**
fathers, pregnancy tasks for, 109
fatigue, motor vehicle injuries and, 385
fat-soluble vitamins, 214
fatty acids
   omega-3, **208**, 209, 298
   trans, **206**, 207, 315
FBI. *See* Federal Bureau of Investigation
FDA. *See* Food and Drug Administration
FDA (Food and Drug Administration), 228
Federal Bureau of Investigation (FBI), 391, 395
federal legislation. *See* legislation
Federal Trade Commission (FTC), 272–273, 372
feedback, communication skill, 104
fee-for-service plans (indemnity), 378–379
fellatio, **101**
female athlete triad, 268, **269**
female reproductive tract cancer, 305–306
female sexual arousal disorder, 137

females. *See also* women
condoms for, 130, 131
infertility in, **106**, 106–107
sex organs in, 90–91
sexual maturation in, 94–95
sterilization in, 137
FemCap, **132**, 133
fertility, 104–107, **124**, 204–206
fertility awareness method (FAM), **134**, 134–135
fertilization, **104**, 105
in vitro, **106**
fertilized egg, **104**, 105
fetal alcohol spectrum disorder (FASD), 182
fetal alcohol syndrome (FAS), **113**, 182, **183**
fetal development, 108–111
fetal programming, 111
fetus, **91**, **203**
multi-fetal pregnancy reduction, **194**
fiber, 212–213
recommended intake of, 213, 298
sources of, 213
types of, 339–340
fight-or-flight reaction, **25**
financial planning, 409
financial wellness, 3
firearms, 389–390, 393
fires, 388–389
first aid, **402**
fish, 219
flashbacks, LSD-induced, **166**
flexibility, **242**, 248, 252–254
fluid intelligence, **409**
flunitrazepam (Rohypnol), 161
FOCA (Freedom of Choice Act), 142
folic acid, cardiovascular disease and, 292, 298
follicle, **95**
follicle-stimulating hormone (FSH), 94
food(s). *See also* nutrition
additives in, 232
allergies/intolerances to, **232**, 233
antioxidants in, 216–217
chemicals in, 310–311
environment and, 219
genetically modified, 232–233
irradiation, **232**, **367**, 367–368
labels on, 220, 228, 229
organic, **231**, 231–232
personal plan for, 228–233
phytochemicals in, **217**
population and, 226–227
safe handling of, 231
substances in, other, 216–217
trans fat content in common, 220
vegetarian food plan, 225
vitamins in, 213, 214, 216
whole grain, 210–211, 223
food allergy, **232**, 233
Food and Drug Administration (FDA), 95, 137, 175, 228, 252, 372, 373, 377
drug warnings/pregnancy and, 221
Plan B emergency contraceptive approved by, 127
Food and Nutrition Board, 217, 335, 336, 345
food bars, 273
food intolerance, **232**
food irradiation, **232**, **367**, 367–368
food plan, personal, 228–233
food additives and, 232
food labels and, 228, 229
foodborne illnesses and, 228, 231
vegetarian, 225
food safety, pregnancy and, 220
foodborne illnesses, bacteria causing, 228, 231
footwear, exercise, 255
foreplay, **101**
formaldehyde gas, 352

fossil fuels, 348, **349**
fraternal twins, **104**, **105**
fraud, health, 372
free radicals, **216**, **217**
Freedom of Access to Clinics Act, 142
Freedom of Choice Act (FOCA), 142
French Canadian Americans, health concerns of, 8
frequency, endurance training/exercise, 250
fried foods, 310
friendship, 70–71, 120
fruits, 310, 315
FSH (follicle-stimulating hormone), 94
FTC (Federal Trade Commission), 372
fuels
alternative, 351
fossil, 348, **349**
functional fiber, **212**
fungus, **328**

GAD (generalized anxiety disorder), **57**, 57–58
gambling, compulsive, 151–152
gamete intrafallopian transfer (GIFT), **106**
gamma hydroxybutyrate (GHB), 161
gangs, 394
garlic, 376
GAS (general adaptation syndrome), **28**, 38, 39
gastric bypass, 275–276
GDM (gestational diabetes), **115**
gender
alcohol intake and, 177
alcohol use and, 9, 177, 186–187
body image and, 277
cardiovascular disease and, 290
communication and, 75, 77
contraception and, 138
definition of, 7
drug use and, 155
eating disorders and, 276, 277
heart attack and, 9, 290
HIV infection and, 332, 333, 338
injuries and, 385
muscular strength and, 252
oral cancer and, 307
stress and, 9, 29
suicide and, 59–60, 385
tobacco use and, 195, 301, 312, 313
violence and, 392–393
wellness and, 6–8
gender identity, **138**
gender roles, **28**, **29**, 70, 385
gene(s), **11**, **104**, **105**
errors in, 11–12
general adaptation syndrome (GAS), **28**, 38, 39
generalized anxiety disorder (GAD), **57**, 57–58
generic drugs, **365**
genetic diseases, ethnicity and, 112
genetically modified (GM) foods, 232–233
genetically modified organism (GMO), **232**
genetics/heredity, 11–12
body weight and, 268–269
cardiovascular disease and, 290
diversity and, 6
genital herpes, **340**, 340–341
genital warts, **339**
genome, **11**, 11–12, 14
geography, statistics on residential, 10–11
geriatricians, 414, **415**
germ cells, **91**
gerontologists, 414, **415**
gestation period, 206
gestational diabetes (GDM), **115**
GHB (gammahydroxybutyrate), 161
giardiasis, **328**
GIFT (gamete intrafallopian transfer), **106**
glaucoma, **409**

global warming, 13, 348–350, **349**
glucose, **211**, 266–267, 288, 292
glycemic index, **211**, 211–212
glycogen, **211**
GMO. *See* genetically modified organism
goal-setting, behavior change, 22–23
gonads, **91**
gonococcal conjunctivitis, **339**
gonorrhea, **338**, 338–339
Gonzales v. Carhart, 145
government aid, aging and, 414–415
government programs, health insurance, 380
grains, 222, 223. *See also* whole grains
greenhouse effect, 14, 348–350, **349**
greenhouse gases, **349**
grief, 412, 422–425
Guttmacher Institute, 128, 143

HAART (highly active antiretroviral therapy), 335
habits, health, 11, 14–15, 49. *See also* diet(s)
habituation, **150**, **151**
hallucinations, 59, 64, 67, 161, 163
hallucinogens, **165**, 165–166
hangover, alcohol, 178
hantavirus, 329
hardiness, personality, **36**
harm-reduction strategies, 169
Harvard Healthy Eating Pyramid, **217**, 218, 221–225, 270, 273
hate crimes, 394
Hatha yoga, 53, 54
HAV (Hepatitis A virus), 326
hazardous waste, 355–356
HBV (Hepatitis B virus), 326, 341
HCG (human chorionic gonadotropin), 94, 216
HCM (hypertrophic cardiomyopathy), **297**, 297–298
HCV (hepatitis C virus), 326, 341
HDL (high-density lipoprotein), 285, **286**, 287, 299
headaches, 32
health. *See also* environmental health; psychological health; wellness
contraception and, 139
defined, **1**, **2**
disparities, 5–11
education and, 9–10
fats and, 207–209
habits, 11, 14–15, 49
health care. *See also* health insurance
access to, 13–14
choosing primary care physician for, 368–369
complementary/alternative medicine (CAM), **365**, 370–378
conventional medicine, **365**, 366–370
cost of, 378–380
drug use and, 169
end-of-life care, 417–418
ethnicity and, 10
fraud, 372
medical errors in, 371
professional, 364–365
self-care, 362–364
health care proxy, **420**
health information, evaluating, 16, 368
health insurance, 378–380
Health maintenance organizations (HMOs), **379**
health news, evaluating, 368
health savings accounts (HSAs), **379**
health-related fitness, **241**
Healthy People 2010, 5–6
hearing loss, aging and, 410
heart
cardiovascular system and, 181, 283–284, **284**
circulation in, 285
congenital heart defects, **297**

heart attack, **293**, 293–295
  ethnicity and, 12
  gender differences in, 9, 290
heart disease, 292, 293–295. *See also* cardiovascular
    disease
  anger/hostility and, 289
  angina pectoris, 293–294, **294**
  arrhythmias, **294**
  diagnosis/treatment of, 294–295
  exercise and, 246
  less common forms of, 297–298
heavy metal, **353**, 354, 360
height, -weight charts, 264
Heimlich maneuver, **389**
helmets, bicycle, 388
helping others
  alcohol problems, 188
  depression, 61
  drug problem, 170
  dying person, 421
  grieving person, 423
  heart attack victim, 294
hemochromatosis, 112
hemorrhagic stroke, 296, **297**
hepatitis, 326–327, **327**, 340
Hepatitis A virus (HAV), 326
Hepatitis B virus (HBV), 326, 341
hepatitis C virus (HCV), 326, 341
herbal remedies, 62, 273, 376, 377
heredity. *See* genetics/heredity
herpes simplex virus (HSV) types 1/2, 324, 326,
    340–341
herpes viruses, 324, 326, **327**, 340–341
heterosexual, **81**
HEVs (hybrid electric vehicles), 351–352
hierarchy of needs, **64**
high blood pressure, 286–287
high-density lipoprotein (HDL), 285, **286**, 287,
    299
highly active antiretroviral therapy (HAART), 335
hippocampus, 31
histamine, **320**
HIV. *See* human immunodeficiency virus
HIV antibody test, **334**
HIV RNA assay, **334**
HIV/AIDS, 330–336, **331**, 338
  ethnicity and, 11, 332
  global summary, 332
  number people living with, 333
HIV-positive, **334**, 336
HMOs (health maintenance organizations), **379**
home, radiation in, 358
home care, 417–418
home injuries, 388–390, **389**
homeopathy, **373**, 373–374
homeostasis, **26**
homeostatic resilience, 28
homicide, 394
homocysteine, 292
homophobia, 81
homosexual, **81**
honesty, 72
hormonal method, contraception, 122, **123**
hormone(s), **25**, 93–96
  reproductive life cycle and, 93–96
hormone replacement therapy (HRT), 303, 410
hospice, 418, **419**
hospitalist, 371
HPV (human papillomavirus), 327–328, 339–340
HRT (hormone replacement therapy), 303, 410
HSAs (health savings accounts), **379**
HSV (herpes simplex virus) 1/2, 324, 326, 340–
    341
HT (hormone therapy), 131–132, 302–303
human chorionic gonadotropin (HCG), **94**, **106**,
    107

human immunodeficiency virus (HIV) infection,
    330–336, **331**. *See also* acquired immune defi-
    ciency syndrome; HIV/AIDS
  birth control pills and, 124
  contraception methods and, 124
  diagnosis of, 334, 335
  DNA and, 331
  ethnicity and, 11, 332
  gender and, 332, 333, 338
  populations of special concern for, 332–333
  pregnancy and, 331, 332, 335
  prevention of, 336, 337
  sexual contact and, 332–334, 336
  sexual orientation and, 11, 332–333
  symptoms of, 333–334
  transmission of, 331–332
  treatment of, 334–336
human papillomavirus (HPV), 327–328, 339–340
hybrid electric vehicles (HEVs), 351–352
hydrogenation, **206**, 207
hydrostatic weighing, 265
hypertension, 246, **286**. *See also* high blood
    pressure
hypertrophic cardiomyopathy (HCM), **297**,
    297–298
hypertrophy, 288
hypnosis, **374**, 374–375
hypothalamus, **93**
hysterectomy, **139**

"I" statements, 105
identical twins, **104**, **105**
identity
  crisis, **51**
  development of adult, **49**, 49–50
  gender, **138**, 138–139
IDU (injection drug use), 156–157, 332
IED (intermittent explosive disorder), 53, 54
illness, foodborne, 228, 231
immune response, **320**, 321
immune system, **319**, 320–322
  allergies and, 322–323, **323**
  chain of infection, 318–319
  exercise and, 247
  gender differences in, 9
  HIV infection and, 334
  immunization, **322**
  mother's, sexual orientation and, 142
  physical/chemical barriers to infection, 319
  PNI and, 40
  stress and, 31
  supporting, 330
immunity, **320**
immunization, **322**
implants, contraceptive, 126
impotence, 98, 265
in vitro fertilization (IVF), **106**
incest, **401**
income inequality, 9, 10
incontinence, **305**
incubation, **320**, 321
indemnity plans. *See* fee-for-service plans
inequality, income/education, 10
infants/newborns
  ETS and, 196
  herpes viruses in, 340
  infant mortality, 7, 9, 10, **116**, **117**
  infections in, 328, 331, 338
infatuation, **72**
infections, 318–319, **319**
infectious diseases, **4**, 204, 319, 323–345. *See*
    also human immunodeficiency virus (HIV)
    infection
  bacterial, 323–326
  chain of infection, 318–319
  emerging, 328–330

  fungal, **328**
  parasitic worms, **328**
  pathogens associated with, 324
  protozoal, 323, **328**
  rotavirus, 329
  staphylococcus, **323**, 323–324, 325
  streptococcal, 323
  viral, 320, 321, 326–328, **327**
infertility, **106**, 106–107
  treatment for, 106–107
inflammatory response, **320**
influenza, 326, **327**
inhalants, 166–167
injectable contraceptives, 126–127
injection drug use (IDU), 156–157, 332
injuries, intentional. *See* violence
injuries, unintentional, 383–391, **384**
  alcohol-related, 386
  exercise for preventing, 247, 256–258
  exercise-related, 256–258
  gender and, 385
  home, 388–390, **389**
  intentional v. unintentional, 384
  motor vehicle, **384**, 384–387
  prevention of, 390
  work, 390, 390–391
insemination, intrauterine, **106**
insoluble fiber, **212**
insomnia, 37
Institute of Medicine, 335
insulin resistance, 291–292
insurance. *See* health insurance
intact dilation and extraction, **145**
intellectual wellness, 2, 383
intensity, endurance training, 250, 251–252
intentional injuries, **384**. *See also* violence
intercourse. *See* sexual intercourse
intermittent explosive disorder (IED), 53, 54
Internet addiction, 152. *See also* online
    relationships
interpersonal stress, 33
interpersonal wellness, 2, 3, 383
intestate, 416–417, **417**
intimate relationships, 69–89
  capacity for, 48
  challenges in, 72–74
  commitment and, 73, 83, 87
  communication in, 75–78
  conflict/conflict resolution in, 75–78
  dating, 78, 109, 242
  developing, 67, 96–103
  ending, 74
  friendship and, 70–71
  interfaith/intrafaith, 79
  jealousy in, 73
  love/sex/intimacy in, 71–72, 120
  pairing, singlehood and, 78–83
  supportiveness in, 73–74
  unhealthy, 74
intolerances, food allergies and, **232**, 233
intoxication, 149, 156
intracerebral hemorrhage, 296
intrauterine device (IUD), **127**, 127–129, 176, 180
intrauterine insemination, **106**
iron, 112, 113, 124
ischemic stroke, 296
isometric exercises, 251
isotonic exercises, **251**, 251–252
IUD (intrauterine device), **127**, 127–129, 176,
    180
IVF (in vitro fertilization), **106**

jaundice, **327**
jealousy, 73
job-related stress, 33
journaling, 18, 38, 364

Kaposi's sarcoma, 326, **334**
kegel exercises, 114
ketamine, 161
kilocalories, **206**
Koop, C. Everett, 197
Kübler-Ross, Elizabeth, 421

labels
    dietary supplement, 228, 230
    food/dietary supplement, 220, 228, 229, 368
    nutrient claims on, 229
    "organic," 231
    OTC medications, 365
labor
    contractions, **116, 117**
    first stage of, 116–117
    induction, 115, **194,** 223
    pain relief during, 118
    preterm, 115
    second stage of, 117
    third stage of, 118
    transition stage of, **117**
lactation, **119**
lacto-ovo-vegetarians, **225**
lactose intolerance, 112
lacto-vegetarian, **225**
laparoscopy, **137**
Latinos/Latinas, 7, 45
    alcohol use by, 187–188
    cardiovascular disease among, 292
    diabetes in, 267
    drug use/dependence among, 168
    health care for, 10
    health concerns of, 8–9
LBW (low birth weight), **115,** 316
LDL (low-density lipoprotein), **208, 286,** 287, 298,
    299
lead poisoning, 355–356
Lea's Shield, 132–133
legal consequences, drug use/abuse, 157
legislation. *See also* government aid, aging and
    abortion, 141, 142, 145
    anti-tobacco, 197, 198
    double effect, **419**
    drug use, 167
    emergency contraception, 162
    environmental tobacco smoke, 197
    government aid for aging, 414–415
    life-sustaining treatment, 418–419
    nutrition-related, 207
legumes, **206,** 267
leisure, injuries, **390**
leukemia, **300**
leukoplakia, 313
Levonorgestral IUD (Mirena), 127–128
life expectancy, 5, 265, **413,** 413–415
    gender differences in, 9, 413
life purpose, 67
lifestyle
    choice, **4**
    college students and, 13
    culture and, 10–11
    death causes and, 4, 5
    weight management and, 269, 270–272, 273
    wellness, 14–20
life-support systems, **415**
lightening, **108**
lipoproteins, 208, 286, 287, 298, 299
listening, communication skill, 90
liver disease. *See* hepatitis
living will, **419**
locus of control, **16,** 16–17
loneliness, 53
loss of control
    addictive behavior, 130
    nicotine and, 189

love
    commitment and, 73, 83, 87
    intimacy/sex and, 71–72, 120
    pleasure/pain of, 72
    transformation of, 72
low birth weight (LBW), **115,** 316
low-back pain, 247
low-density lipoprotein (LDL), **208, 286,** 287, 298,
    299
loyalty, friendship and, 70
LSD (lysergic acid diethylamide), 252, 258
lung cancer, 301–302, 309, 310–311
    ETS cause of, 315
    smoking and, 193
lymphatic system, **300**
lymphoma, **300,** 301
lysergic acid diethylamide (LSD), 161

ma huang (ephedra), 253, 273–274
magnetic resonance imaging (MRI), **294**
mainstream smoke, **315**
maintenance, behavior change, 18, 25–26
malaria, **328**
male condoms, **129,** 129–131
males
    alcohol abuse by, 288
    condoms for, **129,** 129–131
    sex organs of, 91–92
    sterilization of, 136–137, **137**
malignant tumors, **300**
mammogram, **303**
managed-care plans, **379**
management, exercise program, 406–409
mania, **61,** 61–62
manipulative/body-based methods, CAM and,
    375
manual vacuum aspiration (MVA), **145**
marijuana, 56
    cannabis products, 164–165
    dependence on, 165
    medical, 56, 165
    pregnancy and, 165
marriage, 83–84. *See also* families/family life; inti-
    mate relationships
    benefits of, 83
    cohabitation and, **78,** 78–81
    issues in, 83
    median age of, 81
    role of commitment in, 83
    same-sex, 82
    sterilization contraception and, 138
Maslow, Abraham, 47–48
masturbation, **100,** 100–101
mature understanding of death, **417**
maximal oxygen consumption (VO_{2max}), **250**
MDMA (methylenedioxymethamphetamine), 161
meat, 310
media
    global warming in, 351
    health information in, 368
    tobacco use as emulating, 190
    violence in, 392
Medicaid, **380**
medical doctor, **367**
medical errors, 371
medical marijuana, 56, 165
Medicare, **380**
medications. *See also* drug(s), defined; drug use
    abortifacients, 128
    antibiotics, **324,** 325, 326, 329
    antidepressant, 63
    antiviral, 328, 334
    drug dependence and, 169
    errors in, 371
    generic, **365**
    medical abortion, 195

over-the-counter, 161, 166, **363,** 363–364
    self-medication and, 363–364
    sleep, 48, 145
meditation, **40,** 156
Mediterranean diet, 221–222
melanoma, 306, **307**
men
    communication advice for, 77
    contraception involvement by, 140
    heart attack in, 290
    hypertension in, 290
    injuries among, 385
    sexual assault and, 399
    stress and, 29
    suicide in, 59–60
menarche, **94, 95**
meningitis, 323
menopause, 410–411
menses, **94, 95**
menstrual cycle, **94, 95**
    amenorrhea/absence of, **269**
menstrual problems. *See* dysmenorrhea; premen-
    strual dysphoric disorder; premenstrual
    syndrome
mental health. *See* psychological health
menthol, cigarettes, 191–192
mercury, 356
metabolic syndrome, 291–292
metabolism, **176**
    alcohol, 176, 178
metastasis, **300**
methamphetamine, 161, 163
methicillin-resistant staphylococcus aureus
    (MRSA), 325
methotrexate, 146
methylenedioxymethamphetamine (MDMA), 161
methylphenidate (Ritalin), 159, 164
MFPR (multi-fetal pregnancy reduction), **145**
micronutrients, vitamins/organic, **212,** 213–216
migraines, 42
milk, 224
mind-body interventions, 374–375
mindfulness, 40
minerals, **212,** 213, 215
    toxic effect of megadoses of, 215
minority, America's aging, 413–414
Mirena (Levonorgestral IUD), 127–128
miscarriage, 114–115, **140**
misoprostol, 195
mitral valve prolapse (MVP), **298**
moments of relaxation, 49
mood disorders, **58,** 58–62, **59**
    depression, 58–62, **59**
    mania/bipolar, **61,** 61–62
motivation
    behavior change, 15–17, 25
    drug use, 155
    quitting smoking, 198–199, 202
    tobacco use, 189–191
motor vehicle crashes, BAC and, 180
motor vehicle injuries, **384,** 384–387
motorcycles/mopeds, 387
mourning, 423
MRI (magnetic resonance imaging), **294**
MRSA (methicillin-resistant staphylococcus
    aureus), 325
MSA (Master Settlement Agreement), 197
mucus method, fertility awareness methods, 135
multi-fetal pregnancy reduction (MFPR), **145**
murmur, 298, **299**
muscular endurance, **241**
muscular strength, **241,** 248, 250–252, 254
music, relaxation technique, 42
mutuality, friendship and, 70
MVA (manual vacuum aspiration), **145**
MVP (mitral valve prolapse), **298**

mycoplasmas, **323**
MyPyramid, **217**, 218, 221–225, 270, 273
myths
   cancer, 311
   contraception, 155

The National Center for Complementary and Alternative Medicine (NCCAM), 371, 377
National Cholesterol Education Program (NCEP), 287, 298, 299
National Institute for Occupational Safety and Health (NIOSH), 58
National Institute of Mental Health (NIMH), 58
National Institutes of Health (NIH), 262, 266, 371, 372
National Weight Control Registry, 274
Native Americans. *See* American Indians
Native Hawaiians, 10, 168, 186. *See also* ethnicity
natural method, contraception, **123**
NCCAM (National Center for Complementary and Alternative Medicine), 371, 377
NCEP (National Cholesterol Education Program), 287, 298, 299
nervous system, 25, 81
neurotransmitters, **157**
nicotine, **189**
   addiction to, 189
   clove cigarettes/bidis, 195–196
NIH (National Institutes of Health), 262, 266, 371, 372
nitrogen dioxide (NO_2), 348
NO_2 (nitrogen dioxide), 348
noise pollution, 358–359
non-rapid eye movement (non-REM) sleep, **37**
nonreactive resiliency, 28
nonverbal communication, 103
norepinephrine, 25
normality, compared with psychological health, **49**
Northern Europeans, 7, 56, 112
nuclear power, 357–358, **358**
nutrition, 56, 205–239, **330**
   antioxidants, **212**, 216–217
   calories and, 218
   carbohydrates, **208**, 209–212, 219–220, 299
   DASH diet, 218, 286, 299
   diet planning for, 217–227
   Dietary Reference Intakes, **217**, 217–218, 237–239
   essential nutrients and, **205, 206**
   fast-food restaurant eating strategy for, 227
   food allergy/intolerance, **232**, 233
   Healthy Eating Pyramid, **217**, 218, 221–225, 270, 273
   labeling of foods/dietary supplements, 220, 363, 368
   minerals, **212**, 213, 215
   personal food plan for, 225
   prenatal, 113
   stress management through, 36

OA (osteoarthritis), 373, 410
obesity, 262, 263, **265**, 275. *See also* body fat; weight management
   cancer and, 311
   cardiovascular disease and, 287–288
   deaths from, 5, 419
   definition of, **265**, 266
   diabetes and, 265–266
   exercise and, 246, 391, **417**
   life expectancy and, 265
   type 2 diabetes and, 246, 266
   waist circumference and, 417, 422, 423
obsession, **58, 59**
obsessive-compulsive disorder (OCD), **58, 59**
Occupational Safety and Health Administration (OSHA), 358–359

occupational wellness, 3
OCD (obsessive-compulsive disorder), **58, 59**
OCs (oral contraceptives), **123**, 123–125
oils, 221–222
older adults, suicide in, 49–60, 413
omega-3 fatty acids, **208**, 209, 298
one drink, **176**
online pornography, 103
online relationships, 80
openness, 100
opioids, **160**
opportunistic infection, **331**, 335
optimism, 52–53
optometrist, **367**
oral cancer, 307, 309
oral contraceptives (OCs), **123**, 123–125
oral sex, 101, 102, 139, 331, 336, 337, 339, 341
oral-genital stimulation, 101
organ donors, 420
organic foods, **231**, 231–232. *See also* micronutrients
organizations, websites and
   alcohol use, 201–204
   cardiovascular disease, 316–317
   childbirth-related, 120
   communication/intimacy, 89
   contraception-related, 128, 148
   drug use, 173
   environmental health, 360–361
   health care, 381
   injuries/violence, 404
   leading health, physical activity recommendations by, 385
   nutrition-related, 235
   physical fitness-related, 260
   preconception care/pregnancy-related, 231
   STDs-related, 344–345
   stress-related, 45
   tobacco use, 201–204
   weight management-related, 281
   wellness-related, 22–23
orgasm, **97**
orgasmic dysfunction, **98**
OSHA (Occupational Safety and Health Administration), 358–359
osteoarthritis (OA), 373, 410
osteoporosis, 213, **215**, 245, 246, 389, **411**
OTC (over-the-counter) medications, 161, 166, **363**, 363–364, 365
ovarian cancer, 306
ovary, **91**
overgeneralizing, 7
overload, **249**
over-the-counter contraceptives, 130
over-the-counter (OTC) medications, 161, 166, **363**, 363–364, 365
ovulation, **94, 95**
ovum, **91**
ozone layer, **350**

pacemaker, 294, 298
Pacific Islander Americans, 168, 186. *See also* ethnicity
   health concerns of, 11
PAD (peripheral arterial disease), 292, 293
pain relief, during labor, 118
pairing, singlehood and, 78–83
palliative care, 418, **419**
pandemics, **327**
panic disorder, **56, 57**
Pap test, **124, 305**
paraphilia, 145
parasites, 326, 328, 342
parasitic worms, **328**
parasomnia, 103
parasympathetic division, **25**

parents/parenting, 142
   becoming, 84–85
   family life cycle in, 117
   single, 86–87
   styles of, 85–86
The Partial Birth Abortion Ban Act, 142
partial vegetarians, **225**
particulate matter (PM), 348, 357
partners
   choosing, 78
   civil unions/ same-sex marriage and, 112
   contraception communication with, 139
   expectations of, 73
   HIV-positive, revealing by, 336
   informing, STDs and, 336, 343
   physician-patient, 369
   same-sex, 81
   separation/divorce and, 84
PAS (physician-assisted suicide), **419**
passion, 98–99
passive euthanasia, **419**
pathogens, 323–330
PCBs (polychlorinated biphenyls), **353**
PCP, hallucinogen, 166
peer counseling, 44, 64, 169
pelvic inflammatory disease (PID), 124, 128–129, 136, 157, 338, 339
penis, **91**
PEP (postexposure prophylaxis), 335
percent body fat, **263**
peripheral arterial disease (PAD), 292, 293
permanent contraception, **136**, 136–139, **137**
permissiveness, parental, 86
persistent vegetative state, 418, **419**
personal contract, behavior change, 20
personal flotation device, **390**
personal safety, 383–405
   campus violence and, 401
   food, 371
   food handling, 231
personality
   stress and, **26**, 27–28
   type A, B, and C, 27
personalized plans
   behavior change, 18–20
   exercise program, 259
   food plan, 228–233
   stress management, 56–57
pesticides, **356**
pharmaceuticals, 366
pharmacological properties, drugs, **157**
pharmacopoeia, **374**
phobia
   simple, **74**
   social, **74**
   specific, **74**
physical activity, 218, **242**. *See also* exercise
   cardiovascular disease and, 287
   classifying levels of, 249
   weight management and, 269, 271, 273
physical dependence, **153**
physical education, 241
physical fitness, **240**, 240–243, **241**, 260. *See also* exercise; exercise program
   aging and, 407–408
   assessment of, 380–386
   body composition in, **242**
   cardiorespiratory endurance and, 240–241, **241**, 243–244, 250, 254
   definition of, 380–382
   flexibility and, **242**, 248, 252–254
   muscular strength/endurance in, **241**, 248, 250–252, 254
   physical activity for, 218, 385–386
   skill-related, **382**
physical wellness, 2

physician-assisted suicide (PAS), **419**
physician-patient partnership, 369
physicians, 367–368, 377–378
    when to see, 363
phytochemicals, **217**
PID (pelvic inflammatory disease), 124, 128–129, 338, 339
pinworms, 328
pipe smoking, 195
pituitary gland, **93**
PKC enzyme, 40
placebo, **62**
    effect, **158**, 374
placenta, **108**
placenta previa, **115**
placental abruption, **115**
Plan B, contraception, 127, 128, 130
plant stanols/sterols, 298
plant sterols. *See* plant stanols/sterols
plaques, **193**, **293**
platelets, **284**, 285
PM (particulate matter), 348, 357
PMDD (premenstrual dysphoric disorder), **95**
PMS (premenstrual syndrome), **95**
Pneumocystis pneumonia, **334**
pneumonia, **323**
PNI (psychoneuroimmunology), **30**
podiatrist, **367**
Point-of-service (POS) plans, **379**
Poison Control Center, 389
poisoning, 389
    alcohol, 178
    lead, 355–356
    mercury, 356
pollution. *See also* air pollution
    air, 348–352
    chemical, 355–357
    industrial, 311
polychlorinated biphenyls (PCBs), **353**
polypeptide supplements, 253
polyps, **303**
population growth, 347–348
pornography, **103**
portion sizes, 228, 229, 271
POS (Point-of-service) plans, **379**
positive attitude, 49, **49**, 51. *See also* self-concept
positive growth resiliency, **28**
postexposure prophylaxis (PEP), 335
postpartum depression, **119**
postpartum period, **118**, 118–119, **119**
post-traumatic stress disorder (PTSD), 40, 45, **58**, **59**, 76–77, 424
potassium, **286**, 351
poverty, 188, 243, 356
PPOs (preferred provider organizations), **379**
precontemplation, 17
preeclampsia, **115**
preferred provider organizations (PPOs), **379**
pregnancy
    alcohol use during, 113, 182, 281–282
    caffeine during, 114, 220
    changes in woman's body during, 107–108
    childbirth classes, 114
    cocaine use during, 162
    complications of, 114–116
    drug use during, 113, 158, 253
    early stages of, 107–108
    ectopic, **114**
    environmental hazards during, 113–114
    fathers' tasks during, 109
    HIV infection and, 331, 332, 335
    loss of, 114–116
    marijuana use during, 165
    nutrition during, 219
    prenatal care, 113–114
    smoking during, 113–114, 196–197, 201, 204

    STDs and, 114
    tests, 107
    unplanned, 139
premature birth, **115**
premature ejaculation, **98**
premenstrual dysphoric disorder (PMDD), **95**
premenstrual syndrome (PMS), **95**
premenstrual tension, **95**
prenatal care, 113–114
preparation, behavior change, 17
prepuce, **91**
presbyopia, 410, **411**
prescription drugs. *See also* medications
    spending on, annual, 370
    weight-loss, 275
preterm labor, 115
primary care physician, choosing, 368–369
prions, **328**
private sector, anti-tobacco action in, 319
problem solving, 50–51
procrastinating, behavior change, 25
professional care, 364–365
professional help, for psychological disorders, 64–66
progestational phase, menstrual cycle, **94**
progesterone, **95**
progestins, **93**
progressive overload, exercise principle, 249
progressive relaxation, **52**
proof value, **176**
prostaglandin cream, 137
prostate cancer, 303–305
prostate gland, **93**
prostate-specific antigen (PSA), **304**
prostitution, **104**
protease inhibitor, **334**
proteins, **206**, 206–207
    AMDRs for carbohydrate/fat and, 208
    complete/incomplete, 206–207
    dietary supplement, 253
    recommended intake of, 207
protozoa, 323, **328**
PSA (prostate-specific antigen), **304**
psychiatrists, number practicing, 64
psychoactive drugs, **149**, 149–174, **151**. *See also* nicotine
    addictive behavior and, **151**
    alcohol use with, 179
    behavior change strategy and, 266
    club drugs, 161, 252
    commonly used, 159
    contents in, unknown, 156
    cost of, economic, 167
    date rape drugs, 161
    dependence potential of, 154, 155–156
    depressants, **160**, 160–162
    dose-response function in, 157–158
    drug abuse and, 152–157
    drug testing and, 167, 169
    effects on body of, 157–158
    future issues for, 167–171
    hallucinogens, **165**, 165–166
    health care and, 169
    inhalants, 166–167
    legalization of, 167
    methamphetamines, 161, 163
    motivation for using, 155
    opioids, **160**
    performance-enhancing, 401
    pharmacological properties of, **157**
    religion/spirituality motivation for using, 156
    representative, 158–167
    risks of, 155–157
    stimulants, **162**, 162–164, 253
    substance dependence and, 152–157, **153**
    tolerance and, **153**

    user factors/response, 158
    user/nonuser profiles, 153–155
psychodynamic model, 87
psychological disorders, 31, 54–64
    agoraphobia, **74**
    anxiety disorders, 55–58, 60
    choosing mental health professional, 89
    generalized anxiety disorder (GAD), **57**, 57–58
    mood disorders, **58**, 58–62, **59**
    panic disorder, **74**
    professional help for, 64–66
    schizophrenia, **62**, 62–64
    self-help for, 64
    summary of, 89–90
psychological health, 47–68, **64**, 247
    anger and, 54
    communication and, 53
    defense mechanisms and, 51–52, 53
    defining, 64–66
    growing up and, 49–50
    intimacy and, 65, 67
    loneliness and, 72
    normality v., 49
    optimism and, 52–53
    self-actualization and, 64–65
    self-esteem in, 48, 49, 50–51
    values and, 67
psychological normality, **65**
psychology, 288–290
    stress and, 40
psychoneuroimmunology (PNI), **30**
psychotherapy, 57, 79
PTSD (post-traumatic stress disorder), 40, 45, **58**, **59**, 76–77, 424
puberty, **94**, **95**
pubic lice, **342**
public health systems, 5
Puerto Rican Americans, 10
pulmonary circulation, 283, **284**
pulmonary disease, chronic obstructive, 193
pulmonary edema, **297**
pulmonary heart disease, 193, 297
purging, **277**

Qigong, 376, **377**
QMS (quadruple marker screen), **111**
quadruple marker screen (QMS), **111**
Quinlan, Karen Ann, 418
quitting, smoking, 198–199, 202
quitting, tobacco use, 198–199, 202

rabies, 324
racial discrimination, 9, 44
radiation, 311–312, **356**, 357–358. *See also* ultraviolet (UV) radiation
radiation sickness, **358**
radon, **358**
randomized controlled trials (RTCs), 367
rape. *See* sexual assault
rapid eye movement (REM), **37**
RDAs. *See* Dietary Reference Intakes
realism, 48
    self-talk, 52
recessive gene, 112
reciprocity, friendship and, 70
recommended intake
    carbohydrate, 210, 212
    fat, 208–209, 210
    fiber, 213, 298
    protein, 207, 210
    sodium/potassium, 220–221, 298
    water, 216
rectal cancer. *See* colon/rectal cancer
recycling, 354
refined carbohydrates, whole grains v., 210–211
Reiki, 376, **377**

reinforcement
addictive behavior characteristic, 150
behavioral model, **85**
relapse, behavior change, 18
relationships. *See also* intimate relationships
aging and, 409
competitiveness in, 73
depression and, 80
online, 80
relaxation
moments of, **49**
music for, 42
progressive, **52**
response, **52**, 53
techniques for, 39–42
religion, 51
intimate relationships and, 79
REM (rapid eye movement), **37**
remission, **303**
repetitive strain injuries (RSIs), **390**, 390–391
reproductive life cycle, 93–96
reservoir, **318**, **319**
residential geography, statistics on, 10–11
resiliency, 36
resistance, **28**
exercises, **250**
resources. *See* organizations, websites and
respect, 97
respiratory system, 257, 300, 307, 308, 311–312
response, behavioral model, **85**
restaurants, fast-food, 227
resting metabolic rate (RMR), **269**
retarded ejaculation, **98**
retirement, 409–410
reverse transcriptase inhibitors, **334**
reversibility, exercise principle, **249**
reversible contraception, 123–136
Rh factor, **113**
RHD (rheumatic heart disease), 298
rheumatic fever, **299**
rheumatic heart disease (RHD), 298
RICE (rest/ice/compression/elevation) principle,
257–258
risk factors, **1**, **2**. *See also* substance dependence;
specific diseases
Ritalin (methylphenidate), 159, 164
RMR (resting metabolic rate), **269**
Roe v. Wade, 141
Rohypnol (flunitrazepam), 161
role models, 17, 49
rotavirus, 329
RSIs (repetitive strain injuries), **390**, 390–391
RTCs (randomized controlled trials), 367

SAD (seasonal affective disorder), **61**
safer sex, 104, 147
safety. *See* personal safety
safety belts, 386
salmon, omega-3 fatty acids in, 208
Salmonella, 228
salt, sodium/potassium and, 220–221
same-sex marriage, civil unions and, 82
same-sex partnerships, 81
SAMHSA (Substance Abuse and Mental Health Services Administration), 154, 167
sanitary landfill, **353**
sarcoma, **300**, 326, 334
sarcopenia, 380
SARS (severe acute respiratory syndrome), 329–
330
saturated fats, 298, 315
scabies, 342
Schiavo, Terri, 418
schizophrenia, **62**, 62–64
school violence, 394
scrotum, **91**

SDM (Standard Days Method), 134–135
seasonal affective disorder (SAD), **61**
secondary reinforcers, **302**, **303**
sedation, **160**
sedative-hypnotics, **160**. *See also* depressants, CNS
selective estrogen-receptor modulators (SERMs),
303
selective serotonin reuptake inhibitors (SSRIs), 130
self-actualization, 47–49, **48**, **49**
self-care, 362–364
self-concept, **49**, 68, 69–70
self-disclosure, 103
self-efficacy, **15**
self-esteem, 48, **49**, 50–51, 69–70, 271–272
self-help, 64
self-medication, 363–364
self-talk, 17, **51**, 52
self-treatment, 363–364
seminal vesicles, **93**
sense of humor, 51
separation, divorce and, 84, 85
SERMs (selective estrogen-receptor modulators),
303
severe acute respiratory syndrome (SARS), 329–
330
sewage, 353
sex. *See also* sexual behavior; sexual intercourse
addiction to love and, 152
biological, 93
chromosomes, **93**
cybersex, 103–104, **104**
defined, **8**
HIV infection and, 332–334, 336
love/intimacy and, 71–72, 120
safer, 104
sober, 104
wellness and, **6–7**, 6–8
sexsomnia (sleep sex disorder), 103
sexual anatomy, 90–92
sexual assault (rape), 162, 163, **398**, 398–401
child sexual abuse, 400
date rape, **398**, 398–399
dealing with, 399–400
sexual behavior, 100–104
agreed-on, 104
atypical/problematic, 102–103
celibacy, **100**
communication about, 104, 105
decision making about, 101, 143
foreplay, **101**
oral sex, 101, 102, 139, 331, 336, 337, 339, 341
privacy and, 104
prostitution and, **104**
responsible, 104
touching in, 101
sexual coercion, **103**
sexual functioning, 96–100. *See also* sexuality
masturbation and, **100**, 100–101
products for enhancing, 99
sexual dysfunctions, **98**, 98–100
sexual stimulation and, 97
sexual harassment, 400–401, **401**
sexual intercourse
anal sex and, 100
HIV infection from, 332–334
sexual maturation
female, 94–95
male, 95–96
sexual orientation, 11, **81**, 100
HIV infection, 332–333
same-sex partnerships and, **81**
sexual problems, 102–103, 127, 135–137
sexual response cycle, 97
sexual stimulation, 97
sexuality, **91**, 96
aging and, 96

commercial, 103–104
communication about, 104, 105
sexually transmitted diseases (STDs), 104, 114,
123, 124, 319, 330–345. *See also* acquired immune deficiency syndrome; human immunodeficiency virus
bacterial vaginosis, **342**
chlamydia, 337–338
condoms and, 129, 343
contraception and, 122, 124, 129, 131, 136, 139
education about, 342
gender differences and, 9
gonorrhea, **338**, 338–339
Hepatitis B virus, 326, 341
HIV/AIDS, 330–336, **331**
human papillomavirus, 327–328, 339–340
major, 330–342
pregnancy and, 114
prevention of, 337, 343
syphilis, **340**, 341–342
women and, 338
sexually transmitted infections (STIs), 330
shock therapy. *See* electroconvulsive therapy
shyness, 57
sickle-cell disease, 8, 112
sidestream smoke, **191**
SIDS, **116**, **117**
simple phobia, **56**, **57**
single parents, 86–87
singlehood
pairing and, 78–83
statistics on, 81
skill-related fitness, **242**
skin cancer, 306–307
skin patch, contraceptive, 125
skinfold measurements, 265
sleep
deprivation, 37
problems, 48, 50, 103
sex during, 103
stress and, 36–37
sleep apnea, 37
sleep sex disorder (*sexsomnia*), 103
sleeping pills, 48
smog, 348
smokeless tobacco. *See* spit tobacco
smoking, 188
chronic bronchitis from, **193**
chronic obstructive pulmonary disease from, 193
cigar/pipe, 195
cumulative effects from, 194
effects on nonsmokers, 196–197
emphysema from, **193**
immediate effects of, 192
long-term effects of, 192–194
lung cancer from, 193
during pregnancy, 113–114, 201, 204
quitting, 19, 198–199, 202
snacks, 271
SO_2. *See* sulfur dioxide
sober sex, 104
social anxiety, behavior change for, 67
social phobia, **56**, **57**
social security, 414, **415**
social stress, 33
social stressors, 33
social support, 33, 34–35
socioeconomic status
cardiovascular disease and, 289
contraceptive use and, 138
drug use and, 168, 261
health insurance and, 379
sodas, 270
sodium, 220–221, 286, 298
solid waste, 353–355. *See also* hazardous waste
soluble fibers (viscous), 212

somatic nervous system, **26**
special health concerns, 358–359, 391
specificity, exercise principle, 248–249
speeding, 384
sperm, **91**
  count, 93
spermicide, 133–134
spermicides, 130
sphygmomanometer, 286
spiritual wellness, 2, 3, 35, 38, 87, 156
spirituality, drug use motivation of, 156
spit tobacco (smokeless), 194–195
sponge, contraceptive, 130, **132**, 133
spontaneous abortion (miscarriage), 114–115, **140**
squamous cell carcinoma, **307**
stability, self-concept and, 68
stages of change, 17–18
stalking, **396**, 397
Standard Days Method (SDM), 134–135
staphylococcus, **323**, 323–324, 325
state dependence, **162**, **163**
statistics. *See also* costs
  abortion, 125, 143, 145, 146
  alcohol use, 184, 186, 283, 285
  annual mean temperature, 350
  cancer, 301, 302, 306, 307, 311
  cell phone use while driving, 385–386
  death causes, 4, 5, 79, 280, 292, 311, 313
  drug use, 156, 162, 166, 167, 169
  energy use, 350
  health care costs, 378
  HIV/AIDS, 332, 333, 336
  income, median, 409
  infectious diseases, 319, 323, 347
  injuries, 384, 385–386, 388
  marital status, 78, 79, 81, 84, 85
  obesity, 262, 263, 275, 382
  on older Americans, 414
  pollution, 348
  population, 347
  significance of, 368
  on smoking, 21, 188, 193, 194, 199
  STDs, 331, 338, 341
  suicide rate, 59, 78
  twins, 106
  violence, 393, 394–395, 397
  whole grain consumption among Americans, 210
statutory rape, **398**
STDs. *See* sexually transmitted diseases
stem cells, 407
stepfamilies, 87
stereotyping, 7
sterilization, **136**, 136–139, **137**
  female, 137, 176
  male, 136–137, **137**
steroids. *See* anabolic steroids
stillbirth, 115
stimulants, CNS, 84, **162**, 162–164, 253
  amphetamines, 162–163
  caffeine, 114, 164
  cocaine, 162
stimulus, behavioral model, **85**
STIs (sexually transmitted infections), 330
strength training exercises, 248, 250–252, 254
  isometric exercises, **251**
stress, 24–46, **25**, 409. *See also* stressors
  academic, 32
  alarm stage of, 28
  allostatic load, 29–30, **30**
  behavior change and, 25
  campus violence and, 45
  cardiovascular disease and, 30–31, 289
  college-related, 32–33, 41–42
  common sources of, 31–34
  conditions linked to, specific, 39–41
  counterproductive coping strategies, 55–56, 57

  defined, 32–37
  emotional response to, 27–28
  environment and, 28
  ethnicity and, 15
  experience as a whole of, 36–37
  gender differences in, 9, 29, 38
  genital herpes and, 341
  hormones, **25**, 37
  immune system and, 31
  interpersonal, 41
  job-related, 33
  journal, 57
  meditation and, **52**, 53
  past experiences and, 36
  perceptions of, 38
  personality and, **26**, 27–28
  physical responses to, 24–27
  PKC enzyme and, 40
  post-traumatic stress disorder, 40, 45, **76**, 76–77
  psychological problems related to, 40
  sense of humor and, 51
  social, 33
  symptoms of, 42
  test anxiety, 27, 44
  weight management and, 272
  wellness and, 28–31
  women and, 37, 38
stress management, 34–42, 273
  cognitive techniques for, 38–39
  counterproductive coping strategies, 42
  deep breathing, 40–41
  exercise for, 35–36
  meditation for, **40**
  nutrition for, 36
  overview of strategies for, 37
  personalized plan for, 56–57
  problem solving for, 50–51
  relaxation techniques for, 39–42
  sleep and, 36–37
  social support, 34–35
  support groups for, 57
  time management and, 37–38
  visualization, 40
  writing and, 38
stress response, **25**
stressors, 24–28, **25**, 33–34, 42–43
stretching, 253–254
stroke, 9, 193, **294**, 295–297
subarachnoid hemorrhage, 296
subcutaneous fat, **263**
substance abuse, **153**
Substance Abuse and Mental Health Services Administration (SAMHSA), 154, 167
substance dependence, **153**. *See also* codependency
  alcohol abuse and, 183–188
  marijuana, 165
  prevention of, 170–171
  psychoactive drugs, 152–157
  risk factors for, 155–156
  state dependence, **162**, **163**
  treatment for, 169–170
success rehearsal, for test anxiety, 59
suction curettage, 144, **145**
sudden cardiac death (cardiac arrest), **294**
sudden infant death syndrome (SIDS), **116**, **117**
suffocation, 389
sugar, 219, 232
suicide, 7, 49, 60, 79
  gender and, 59–60, 385
  myths about, 82
  among older adults, 59–60
  physician-assisted, **419**
  rate, 59
  warning signs of, 59–61
sulfur dioxide (SO_2), 348
sunscreen, 308

supplements. *See* dietary supplements; herbal remedies
support groups, 43
  peer counseling and, 64, 169
  quitting smoking, 198
  stress management and, 57
supportiveness, 73–74
surgery, 370
  coronary bypass, **294**, 295
  gastric bypass, 275–276
  weight loss, 275–276
surgical method, contraception, **123**
surrogate, **420**
sympathetic division, **32**
synesthesia, **166**
syphilis, **340**, 341–342
systematic desensitization, for test anxiety, 59
systemic circulation, 283, **284**
systemic infection, **319**
systole, **284**

Tai chi, 41
tanning salons, 308
target behaviors, **15**, 19
target heart rate range, **250**, 251
tasks of mourning, 423
tax, cigarette, 198
Tay-Sachs disease, 8, 112
TB (tuberculosis), **324**, 324–325
TCM (traditional Chinese medicine), 372–373, **373**
technology, solid waste from discarded, 354
teenagers
  contraceptive use by, 138, 139
  dietary challenges with, 226
  divorce and, 84
  statistics on, 4
  STDs and, 338
  tobacco use by, 189–190
temperature method, contraception, 135
temperature, trends in average, 349–350
tension headaches, 32
tension-release breathing, 54
teratogens, **113**
terrorism, 330, 395–396
test anxiety, 27, 44
testator, 416, **417**
testes, **125**
testicular cancer, 309
testis, **91**
testosterone, **93**
thalassemia, 112
THC, 164
therapeutic touch, 376, **377**
Thornburgh v. American College of Obstetricians and Gynecologists, 142
thrombus, 296, **297**
TIA (transient ischemic attack), **297**
tickborne infections, 325
time management, 37–38, 73
time pressures, 33
time-action function, drug use effect, **158**
time/duration, endurance training, 250
tips for today
  cancer prevention, 314
  cardiovascular disease, 314
  contraception, 146
  death/dying, 425
  diet, 233
  environment, 359
  exercise, 258
  health care, 380
  injuries/violence, 402
  intimate relationships, 88
  pregnancy, 119
  psychoactive drugs, 171
  psychological health, 65

STDs, 343
stress management, 57
tobacco use, 199
weight management, 279
wellness, 21
tobacco/tobacco use, 42, **176**, 188–199
additives in, 191
advertising of, 301, 305, 307
cardiovascular disease and, 192–193, 285, 299
children, 189–190
cost to society of, 197
deaths from, 4, 5, 300, 309–310
environmental tobacco smoke, **196**, 352
gender differences in, 9, 195, 301, 312, 313
individual action against, 198
legislation on, 197, 198
mainstream smoke, **315**
motivation for, 189–191
MSA on, 197
organizations related to, 326–327
other forms of, 194–196
quitting, 198–199, 202
sidestream smoke, **191**
smokeless, 301
social/psychological factors in, 189
teenagers and, 189–190
user profile by ethnicity/age/education, 188
Tolerable Upper Intake Level (UL), 218
tolerance
nicotine, 189
substance dependence and, **153**
withdrawal and, 189
tolerance/withdrawal, 189
total fiber, **212**
touching, 101
foreplay and, **101**
therapeutic touch, 376, **377**
toxic shock syndrome (TSS), **132**, 323
toxin, **319**
traditional Chinese medicine (TCM), 372–373, **373**
tranquilizers, **160**
trans fats, 220
trans fatty acids, **206**, 207
transient ischemic attack (TIA), **297**
transition, labor stage, **117**
treatment
centers, 169
withholding/withdrawing, 418–419
trichomoniasis, **342**
triglycerides, 288
trimesters, pregnancy, 108–110. *See also* fetal development
TSS (toxic shock syndrome), **132**, 323
tubal sterilization, **137**
tuberculosis (TB), **324**
tumors, **299**, 299–300
twins, 104, 105, 106
Type 1 diabetes, 266
Type 2 diabetes, 245–246, 266

U. S. Department of Agriculture (USDA), 360, 365
U. S. Supreme Court, 418
UL (Tolerable Upper Intake Level), 218
ultrasonography, 110–111, **111**, **303**
ultraviolet (UV) radiation, 306, **307**
umbilical cord, **108**
Uniform Donor Card, **420**
unintentional injuries, 383–391, **384**
United Nations, 347
urethra, **91**
urethritis, **337**
USDA (U. S. Department of Agriculture), 218, 221–225, 231
USDA Center for Nutrition Policy, 352
user factors, physical effects of drug use, 158
uterine cancer, 306

uterus, **91**
UV (ultraviolet) radiation, 306, **307**

vaccines, **322**, 343
VAE (voluntary active euthanasia), 419
vagina, **91**
vaginal contraceptive ring, 125–126
vaginal spermicides, 130, 133–134
values, 50, 51, 68
vas deferens, **93**
vasectomy, 136–137, **137**
vasocongestion, **97**
vegans, **225**
vegetables, 222, 223–224, 310, 315
cruciferous, **217**
vegetarians, 225
vehicles, hybrid/electric, 351–352
veins, **284**
venae cava, 283, **284**
ventricles, **284**
viable fetus, **186**
violence, 391–402, 404
alcohol-related, 179, 277, 393
assault, 393–395
campus, 391–392, 401
against children, 397–398
date rape, **398**, 398–399
elder abuse, 398
factors contributing to, 391–393
family/intimate, 396–398
gang-related, 394
gender differences in, 392–393
homicide, 394
interpersonal v. collective, 395
school, 394
sexual assault, 398–401
terrorism, 395–396
what to do about, 395, 401
workplace, 394
viral hepatitis, 326–327
viruses, 320, 321, 326–328, **327**. *See also* human papillomavirus
visceral fat, **263**
viscous fibers (soluble), **212**
vision, aging and, 410
visualization, 17, **40**
vitamin B-6, 214
vitamin B-12, 214, 292
vitamins, **212**, 213–216
VO$_{2max}$ (maximal oxygen consumption), **250**
voluntary active euthanasia (VAE), 419
vulva, **90, 91, 125**

warts, genital, **339**
water, 352–353
contamination/treatment of, 352–353
exercise and, 216, 256
recommended intake for, 216
water-soluble vitamins, 214
websites. *See* organizations, websites and
weight management, 218, 262–282
acceptance/change and, 276
aging and, 408
basic concepts, 262–268
body composition and, **242**, 262–263, 264–265
body fat excess and, 265–266, 268–270
body image and, 268, **269**, 272, 276
body mass index and, 264–265, **265**
calories and, 270–271
diet and, 218, 274, 280
diet sodas and, 270
diet/eating habits and, 269, 270–271
eating disorders and, 276–279, **277**
emotions and, 271–272
energy balance in, 263–264, 271, 274
genetic factors in, 268–269

lifestyle factors in, 269, 270–272, 273
obesity definition and, **265**, 266
personal weight guidelines, 268
physical activity and, 269, 271, 273
physiological factors in, 269
psychosocial factors in, 270
stress and, 272
weight problem approaches, 272–276
weight-loss programs for, 272, 274–275
wellness, 1–23. *See also* psychological health
body fat distribution and, 266–267
body fat excess and, 265–266
continuum, 2
dimensions of, 1–3
diversity and, 6–11
emotional, 2, 11
environmental, 3
ethnicity and, 7, 9–10
exercise for total, 243, 247
factors influencing, 11–14
financial, 3
gender and, 6–8
Healthy People 2010 goals for, 5–6
intellectual, 2
interpersonal, 2, 3
for life, 21
lifestyle management and, 14–20
occupational, 3
physical, **2**
physical activity for, 242–243
self-efficacy in, **15**
sex/gender and, 6–8
spiritual, 2, 3, 35, 38, 87, 156
stress and, 28–31
West Nile virus, 329
Western blot, **334**
Western medicine. *See* conventional medicine
WHO (World Health Organization), 193, 212, 318, 395
whole grains, 210–211, **211**, 223
widows, 413
wills, 416–417, **417**
wine, 176
withdrawal, **153**
withdrawal method, contraception, **134**, 134–135
withdrawal, tolerance and, 189
WOAR (Women Organized Against Rape), 399
women. *See also* females; pregnancy; sexual assault
alcohol abuse by, 288
cardiovascular disease and, 290
communication advice for, 77
contraception use among American, 138
date-rape prevention for, 399
HIV/AIDS in, 332, 333, 338
osteoporosis and, **411**
sexual assault guidelines for, 399–400
STDs and, 338
stress and, 29
violence to, 396
widowed, 413
Women Organized Against Rape (WOAR), 399
work addiction, 152
work injuries, **390**, 390–391
workplace
drug use/testing in, 167, 169
radiation in, 358
violence in, 394
World Health Organization (WHO), 193, 212, 318, 395
writing, 18, 38, 364

yoga, 41

zygote intrafallopian transfer (ZIFT), **106, 107**